Textbook of
EAR, NOSE AND THROAT DISEASES

Textbook of
EAR, NOSE AND THROAT DISEASES

Twelfth Edition

Editors

Mohammad Maqbool MBBS DLO MS FICS
Ex-Professor and Head
Department of Otorhinolaryngology
Government Medical College
Srinagar, Jammu and Kashmir, India

Suhail Maqbool MBBS MS
Assistant Consultant
Department of Otorhinolaryngology
King Fahad Medical City
Riyadh, Kingdom of Saudi Arabia

Foreword

Suresh C Sharma

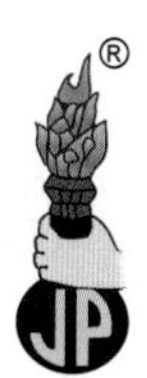

JAYPEE BROTHERS MEDICAL PUBLISHERS (P) LTD

New Delhi • London • Philadelphia • Panama

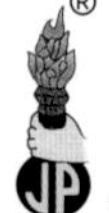

Jaypee Brothers Medical Publishers (P) Ltd.

Headquarters
Jaypee Brothers Medical Publishers (P) Ltd.
4838/24, Ansari Road, Daryaganj
New Delhi 110 002, India
Phone: +91-11-43574357
Fax: +91-11-43574314
Email: jaypee@jaypeebrothers.com

Overseas Offices
J.P. Medical Ltd.
83, Victoria Street, London
SW1H 0HW (UK)
Phone: +44-2031708910
Fax: +02-03-0086180
Email: info@jpmedpub.com

Jaypee-Highlights Medical Publishers Inc.
City of Knowledge, Bld. 237, Clayton
Panama City, Panama
Phone: + 507-301-0496
Fax: + 507-301-0499
Email: cservice@jphmedical.com

Jaypee Medical Inc.
The Bourse
111, South Independence Mall East
Suite 835, Philadelphia, PA 19106, USA
Phone: + 267-519-9789
Email: joe.rusko@jaypeebrothers.com

Jaypee Brothers Medical Publishers (P) Ltd.
17/1-B, Babar Road, Block-B, Shaymali
Mohammadpur, Dhaka-1207
Bangladesh
Mobile: +08801912003485
Email: jaypeedhaka@gmail.com

Jaypee Brothers Medical Publishers (P) Ltd.
Shorakhute, Kathmandu
Nepal
Phone: +00977-9841528578
Email: jaypee.nepal@gmail.com

Website: www.jaypeebrothers.com
Website: www.jaypeedigital.com

Textbook of Ear, Nose and Throat Diseases

First Edition: 1982 *Second Edition:* 1984 *Third Edition:* 1986 *Fourth Edition:* 1988
Fifth Edition: 1991 *Sixth Edition:* 1993 *Seventh Edition:* 1996 *Eighth Edition:* 1998
Ninth Edition: 2000 *Tenth Edition:* 2003 *Eleventh Edition:* 2007

Twelfth Edition: 2013

ISBN: 978-93-5090-495-4

Printed at Replika Press Pvt. Ltd.

Dedicated to

All medical undergraduate students
who may wish
to pursue ear, nose and throat (ENT)
surgery as a specialty

Contributors

Abdullah S AlAmro MD FRCPC
Consultant
Radiation Oncologist
CEO
King Fahad Medical City
Riyadh, Kingdom of Saudi Arabia

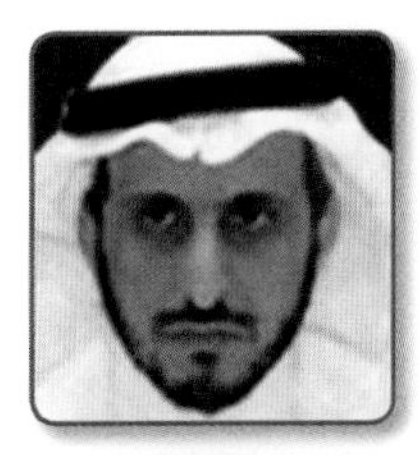

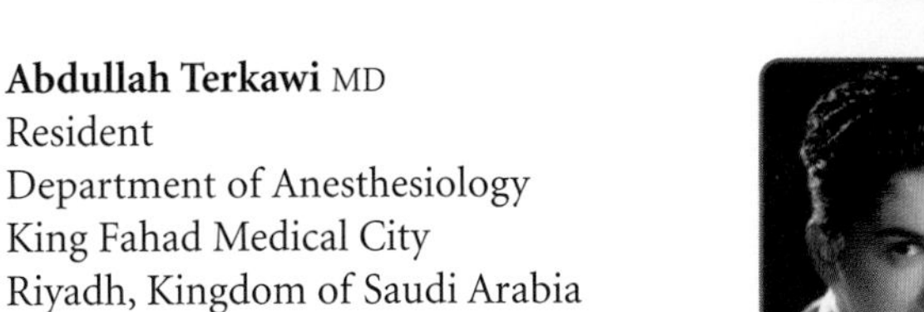

Abdullah Terkawi MD
Resident
Department of Anesthesiology
King Fahad Medical City
Riyadh, Kingdom of Saudi Arabia

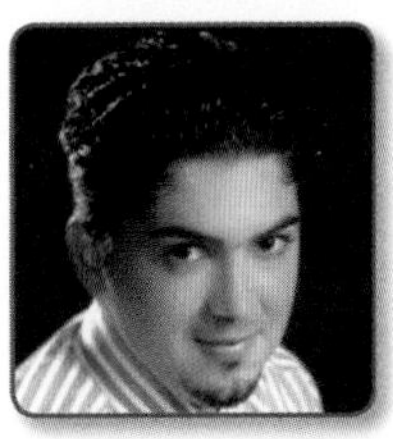

Bilal A Raja MS
Consultant ENT Surgeon
Jammu and Kashmir Health Services
Jammu and Kashmir, India

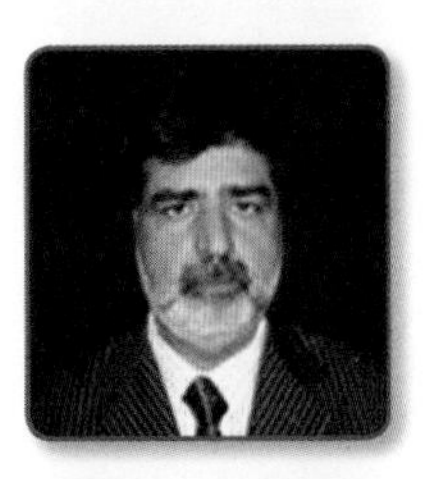

Ibreez Ajaz (Medical Student)
Mymensingh Medical College
Bangladesh

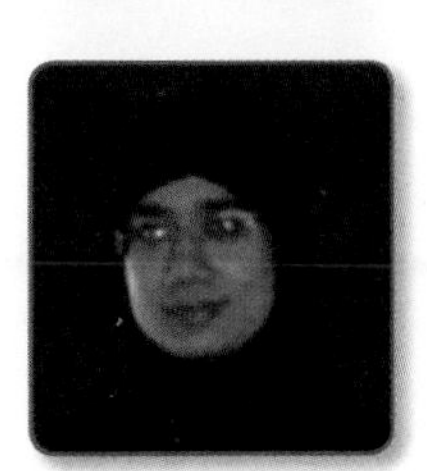

Imtiaz Majid Qazi MS FICS
Consultant Otorhinolaryngology Surgeon
Zain and Al-Sabah Hospitals
Safat, Kuwait

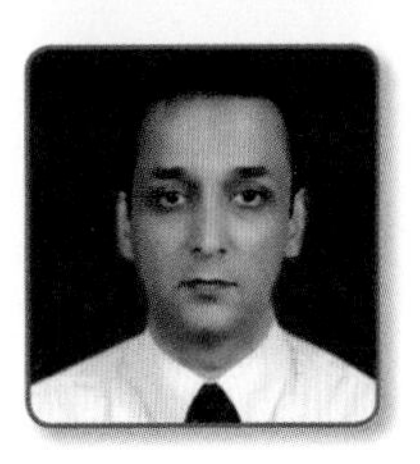

Khalid H Al-Qahtani MD FRCSC
Consultant, Head and Neck Surgeon
Chief of Staff
King Abdulaziz University Hospital
Riyadh, Kingdom of Saudi Arabia

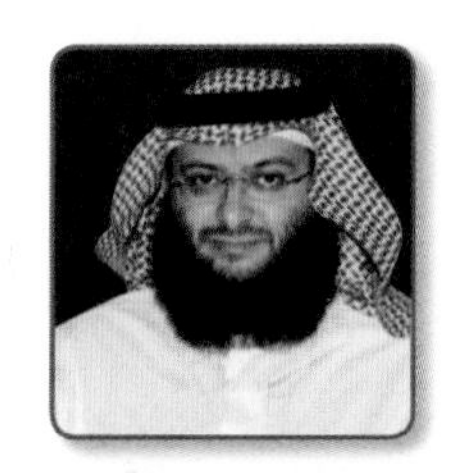

Mohammad Maqbool
MBBS DLO MS FICS
Ex-Professor and Head
Department of Otorhinolaryngology
Government Medical College
Srinagar, Jammu and Kashmir, India

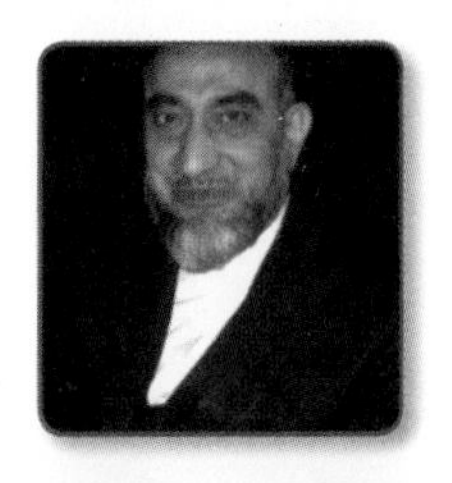

Rafiq Ahmad Pampori MS
Consultant and Head
Department of Otorhinolaryngology
Principal
Government Medical College
Srinagar, Jammu and Kashmir, India

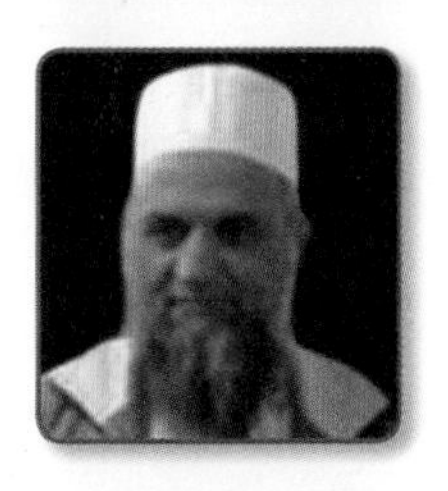

Saleh F AlDhahri MD FRCSC
Chief
Otorhinolaryngology/
Head and Neck Surgery
King Abdulaziz University Hospital
King Saud University
Riyadh, Kingdom of Saudi Arabia

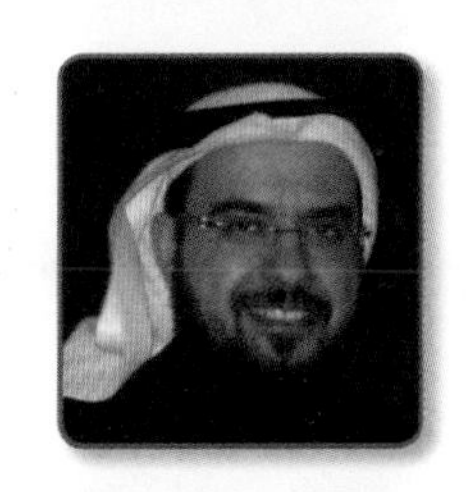

Suhail Maqbool MBBS MS
Assistant Consultant
Department of Otorhinolaryngology
King Fahad Medical City
Riyadh, Kingdom of Saudi Arabia

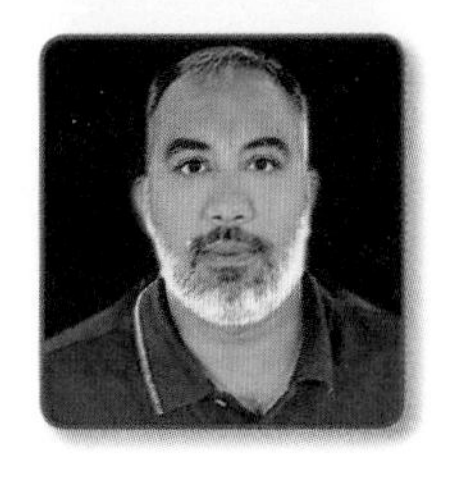

Foreword

Dear Reader,

As an ENT practitioner, who has spent over 30 years in the practice and teaching of this wonderful specialty, I am glad to write the foreword for the twelfth edition of the *Textbook of Ear, Nose and Throat Diseases.*

What makes it easy (and a touch difficult!) to write the foreword is my strong personal relationship with the editors. I have known Professor Mohammad Maqbool for over 30 years, especially for his academic excellence and desire to improve the standard of ENT knowledge among medical graduates and general practitioners. Dr Suhail Maqbool, who was my student, has made me proud by producing the book of high quality.

I find this compact yet comprehensive review a complete source of accurate information for medical students. The book is presented in an easy-to-read manner with the figures and pictures of the high quality of variety of clinical situations. I am sure that the book will not only benefit the undergraduate students but also prove to be a handy-quick review for the general practitioners. The editors have indeed done a commendable job by writing the textbook of an uncompromising standard.

My hope and belief is that the book will continue to contribute to the knowledge of the students and the wider medical community.

Suresh C Sharma
Professor and Head
Department of Otorhinolaryngology
Head and Neck Surgery
All India Institute of Medical Sciences
New Delhi, India

Preface to the Twelfth Edition

This edition has taken a longer span to appear than the previous editions of this book, but among other reasons for the delay, serious attempt has been made to thoroughly revise the book and update relevant important information. Naturally, this has taken time.

Constant effort has been made to present the information in a very simple manner to benefit the originally intended readers, the medical undergraduate students. General practitioners will find the book handy too. A few new chapters on management of neck masses, chemotherapy in head/neck tumors, otologic concerns in a syndromic child, and histopathology of common ENT diseases have been written. Additionally, Multiple Choice Questions (MCQs) have been added after every section. New pictures and figures have been included.

We are thankful to our esteemed colleagues, who have contributed to various chapters, new and old. We must particularly thank Shri Jitendar P Vij (Group Chairman), Mr Ankit Vij (Managing Director), Mr Tarun Duneja (Director-Publishing) and other staff of M/s Jaypee Brothers Medical Publishers (P) Ltd, New Delhi, India, for their help and cooperation. A special thanks to Ibreez Ajaz (medical student) for her most helpful contribution in initial proofreading and online research.

We hope, this humble effort proves valuable for the students and meets their expectations.

Mohammad Maqbool
Suhail Maqbool

Preface to the First Edition

Though there are quite a few books on otorhinolaryngology now available in the country, omission of some important topics or common conditions is noticed in most of these books. As such, a student or a clinician feels handicapped and has to waste a lot of time in looking from book to book for a particular topic or information. A humble effort has been made to prepare a comprehensive *Textbook of Ear, Nose and Throat Diseases* which would provide all the necessary details and conception to the reader. I hope and pray that all the readers of the textbook, undergraduate and postgraduate students, academicians, and general practitioners will be benefitted.

I owe personal thanks to my departmental colleagues particularly to Dr Ab Majid, Dr Ghulam Jeelani and Dr Rafiq Ahmad for their constant interest and contribution to the text.

I must particularly thank Shri Jitendar P Vij of M/s Jaypee Brothers Medical Publishers (P) Ltd, New Delhi, India, for his help and cooperation. I would feel grateful to any suggestion and healthy criticism from readers.

Mohammad Maqbool

Contents

Section 1: EAR

Section 2: NOSE

Section 3: THROAT

Introduction

Preliminary Considerations in Examination

HISTORY TAKING

Before proceeding to the examination of a patient, a detailed and proper history taking is a must. The relevant points to be noted may vary from one organ to another, hence are described at the beginning of each section.

The examination room should be reasonably large and noise free.

Most of the ear, nose and throat areas lend themselves to direct visualization and palpation but a beam of light is needed for proper visualization of the inside of the cavities.

Hands should be free for any manipulation. This is achieved, if a beam of light is reflected by a head mirror or head light. Usually the head mirror is used. The head light serves the same purpose in the operation theater.

HEAD MIRROR

It consists of a concave mirror on a head-band with a double box joint. The head mirror should be light as it is worn for long periods of time and may cause headache. The purpose of the double box joint is to enable the mirror to be as close to the examiner's eye as possible. The center of the mirror has a hole about 2 cm in diameter.

The focal length of the head mirror is generally 8 to 9 inches (25 cm). It is the distance at which the light reflected by the mirror is sharply focussed and looks brightest. It is also the distance where most people can see and read clearly.

The head mirror is worn in such a way that the mirror is placed just in front of the right eye (in right handed persons). The examiner looks through the hole in the mirror and thus binocular vision is retained.

LIGHT SOURCE

The light is provided from an ordinary lamp fixed in a metallic container with a big convex lens and fitted on a movable arm which slides on a rod with a firm base (Bull's eye lamp) or a revolving light source provided with ENT treatment unit (**Fig. 1**). This light source is kept behind and at the level of the patient's left ear. Light from this source is reflected by the head mirror worn by the examiner.

POSITION OF THE PATIENT

The patient should remain comfortably seated. Young children usually do not permit the examination in this position and need assistance. The assistant sits in front of the examiner and holds the child in his/her lap (**Fig. 2**). The legs of the child are held inbetween the thighs of the assistant. One hand of the assistant holds the child's hands across his chest while the other hand stabilizes the child's head.

POSITION OF THE EXAMINER

The examiner sits in front of the patient on a stool or revolving chair (**Fig. 3**). The legs of the examiner should be on the right side of the patient's legs.

EXAMINATION EQUIPMENT

The following are the instruments routinely used for ENT examination (**Fig. 4**).

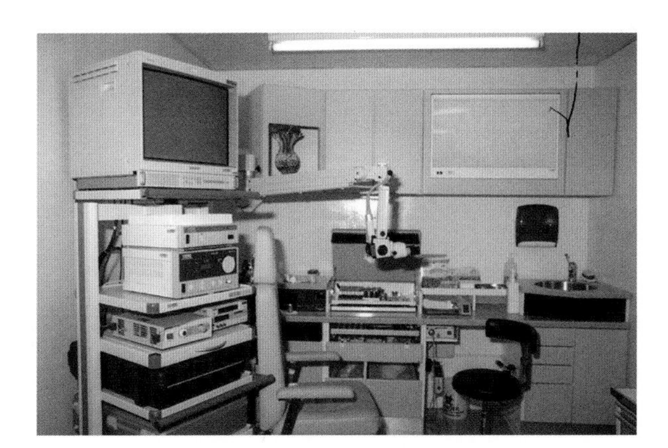

Fig. 1: ENT treatment unit

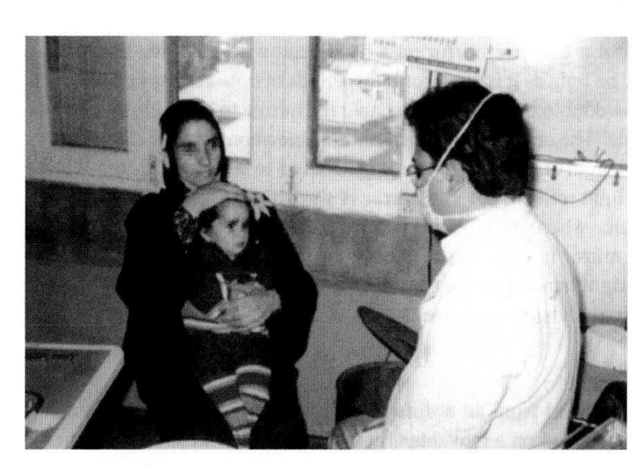

Fig. 2: Mother holding child for examination

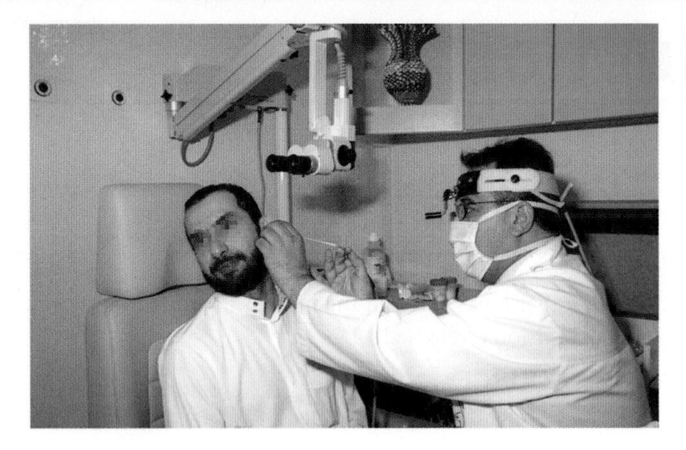

Fig. 3: Position of the patient for ENT examination

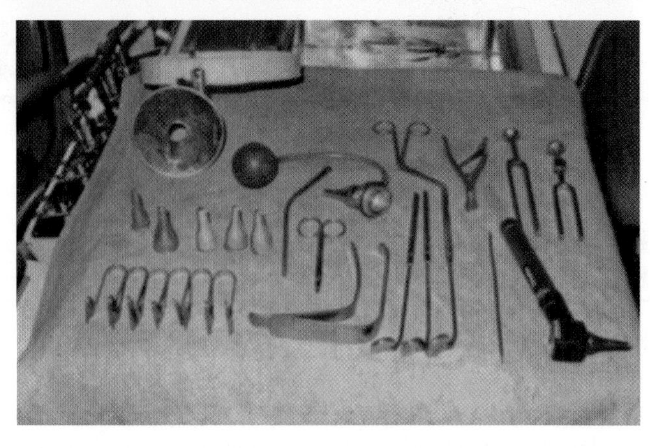

Fig. 4: Common instruments used in ENT outdoor examination

1. Tongue depressor
2. Nasal specula
3. Ear specula
4. Holm's sprayer
5. Laryngeal mirrors
6. Postnasal mirrors
7. Seigel's speculum
8. Eustachian catheter
9. Ear forceps
10. Nasal forceps
11. Tuning forks
12. Probes
13. Ear syringe
14. Auroscope.

Besides, a sterilizer, Cheatle's forceps, spirit lamp and few small labeled bottles containing the commonly used solutions, paints and ointments are also needed.

SUCTION APPARATUS

A suction apparatus with suction tubes and catheters of various sizes is very helpful for cleaning the discharges to allow proper examination. It is also used for removing wax from the ears of the patients who have wax along with CSOM, where water should not be syringed in.

Section 1

EAR

Section Outline

- Development of the Ear
- Anatomy of the Ear
- Physiology of the Ear
- History Taking with Symptomatology of Ear Diseases
- Examination of the Ear
- Congenital Diseases of the External and Middle Ear
- Diseases of the External Ear
- Diseases of the Eustachian Tube
- Acute Suppurative Otitis Media and Acute Mastoiditis
- Chronic Suppurative Otitis Media
- Complications of Chronic Suppurative Otitis Media
- Nonsuppurative Otitis Media and Otitic Barotrauma
- Adhesive Otitis Media
- Mastoid and Middle Ear Surgery
- Otosclerosis
- Tumors of the Ear
- Otological Aspects of Facial Paralysis
- Ménière's Disease and Other Common Disorders of the Inner Ear
- Ototoxicity
- Tinnitus
- Deafness
- Hearing Aids and Cochlear Implant
- Principles of Audiometry
- MCQs on Ear

Chapter 1

Development of the Ear

The knowledge of the development of the ear is important for the diagnosis and therapy of the various diseases of the ear. It is also necessary to know the various anatomical variations that the surgeon may encounter on the table.

The two functional parts of the auditory mechanism have different origins. The sound conducting mechanism takes its origin from the branchial apparatus of the embryo, while the sound perceiving neurosensory apparatus of the inner ear develops from the ectodermal otocyst.

Development of the External and Middle Ear

The structures of the outer and middle ear develop from the branchial apparatus (**Figs 1.1 and 1.2**). During the 6th week of intrauterine life, six tubercles appear on the first and second branchial arches around the first branchial groove. These tubercles fuse together to form the future pinna.

The first branchial groove deepens to become the primitive external auditory meatus, while the corresponding evagination from the pharynx, the first pharyngeal pouch, grows outwards. By the end of the second fetal month, a solid core of epithelial cells grows inwards from the primitive funnel-shaped meatus towards the epithelium of the pharyngeal pouch. By the 7th month of embryonic life, the cells of the solid core of epithelium split in its deepest portion to form the outer surface of the tympanic membrane and then extend outwards to join the lumen of the primitive meatus. Thus, congenital atresia of the meatus may occur with a normally formed tympanic membrane and ossicles, or with their malformation depending upon the age at which development gets arrested.

The first pharyngeal pouch becomes the eustachian tube, middle ear cavity and inner lining of the tympanic membrane. The cartilages of the first and second branchial arches proceed to form the ossicles.

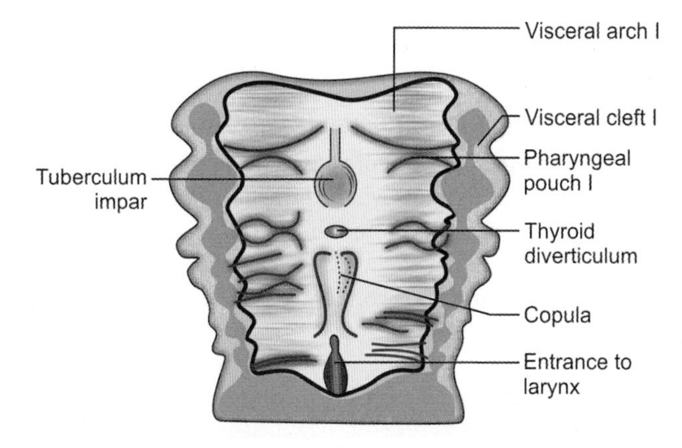

Fig. 1.1: Visceral arches, clefts and pharyngeal pouches

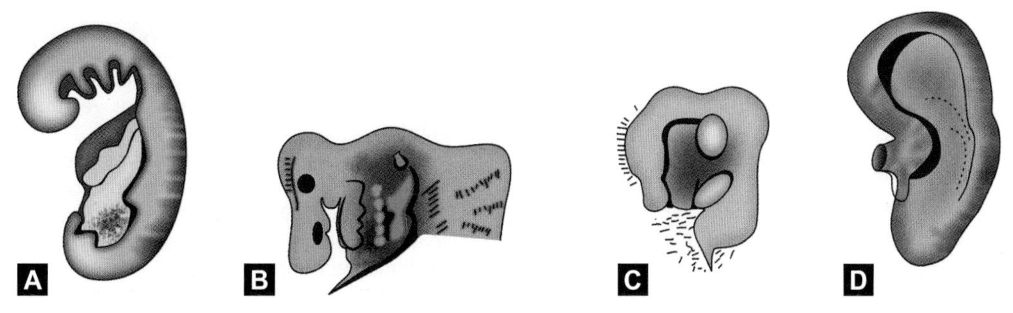

Figs 1.2A to D: Development of the pinna: (A) Primordial elevations on the first and second arches; (B and C) Progress of embryonic fusion of the hillocks; (D) Fully developed configuration of the auricle

The malleus and incus basically develop from the Meckel's cartilage of the first branchial arch. From the second branchial arch develop the stapes, lenticular process of the incus and the handle of malleus.

The foot plate of the stapes is formed by the fusion of the primitive ring-shaped cartilage of the stapes with the wall of the cartilaginous otic capsule. The ossicles are fully formed at birth.

As the ossicles differentiate and ossify, the mesenchymal connective tissue becomes looser and allows the space to form the middle ear cavity. The air cells of the temporal bone develop as out-pouchings from the tympanum, antrum and eustachian tube. The extent and pattern of pneumatization vary greatly between individuals. Failure of pneumatization or its arrest is believed to be the result of middle ear infection during infancy. The mastoid process is absent at birth and begins to develop during the second year of life by the downward extension of the squamous and petrous portions of the temporal bone. This is of importance in infants where the facial nerve is likely to be injured during mastoidectomy through the postaural route. In order to avoid injury to the facial nerve, the usual postaural incision is made more horizontally.

Points of Clinical Importance

- Hearing impairment due to congenital malformation usually affects either only the sound conducting system or only the sensorineural apparatus because of their entirely different embryonic origin, but occasionally both can be affected
- The particular malformation present in each case depends upon the time in embryonic life, at which the normal development was arrested, as well as upon the portion of the branchial apparatus affected
- Failure of fusion of the auricle tubercles leads to the development of an epithelial-lined pit called preauricular sinus
- Failure of canalization of the solid core of epithelial cells of the primitive canal leads to atresia of the meatus
- At birth, only the cartilaginous part of the external auditory canal is present and the bony part starts developing from the tympanic ring which is incompletely formed at that time.

The best indication of the degree of middle ear malformation in cases of congenital atresia is the condition of the auricle. As the auricle is well-formed by the 3rd month of fetal life, a microtia indicates arrest of development of the branchial system earlier in embryonic life with the possibility of absent tympanic membrane and ossicles.

Development of the Inner Ear

At about the 3rd week of intrauterine life a plate-like thickening of the ectoderm called otic placode develops on either side of the head near the hindbrain. The otic placode invaginates in a few days to form the otic pit. By the 4th week of embryonic life, the mouth of the pit gets narrowed and fused to form the otocyst that differentiates as follows (**Fig. 1.3**):

i. At four and a half weeks the oval-shaped otocyst elongates and divides into two portions—endolymphatic duct and sac portion, and the utriculosaccular portion.
ii. By the seventh week arch-like out-pouchings of the utricle form the semicircular canals. Between the seventh and eighth weeks, a localized thickening of the epithelium occurs in the saccule, utricle and semicircular canals to form the sensory end organs.

Evagination of the saccule forms the cochlea, which elongates and begins to coil by the 11th week. A constriction between the utricle and saccule occurs and forms the utricular and saccular ducts, which join to form the endolymphatic duct.

The mesenchyme surrounding the otocyst begins to condense at the sixth week and becomes the precartilage at the seventh week of embryonic life. By the 8th week, the precartilage surrounding the otic labyrinth changes to an outer zone of true cartilage to form the otic capsule. The inner zone loosens to form the perilymphatic space.

The perilymphatic space has three prolongations into surrounding osseous otic capsule, viz. the perilymphatic duct, the fossula ante fenestram, and the fossula postfenestram.

Development of the Bony Labyrinth

In the otic capsule, the cartilage attains maximum growth and maturity before ossification begins. The endochondral bone initially formed from the cartilage is never removed and is replaced by periosteal haversian system as occurs in all other bones of the body, but remains as primitive, relatively avascular and poor in its osteogenic response. The first ossification center appears around the cochlea in the 16th week. By the twenty-third week, the ossification is complete.

Points of Clinical Importance

- The labyrinth is the first special organ which gets differentiated when the other organs have not yet budded out in the embryo
- The vestibular apparatus gets developed before the cochlea and is less prone to disease than the cochlea
- The labyrinth is fully formed by the fourth month of intrauterine life and maximum anomalies of the labyrinth occur during the first trimester of pregnancy.

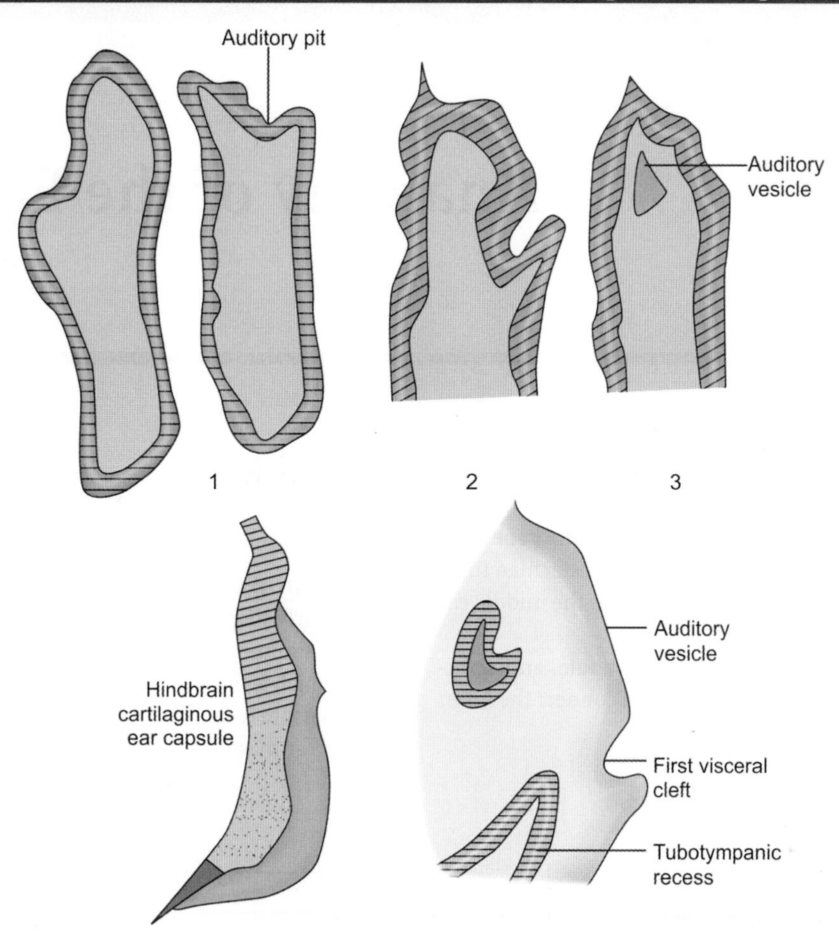

Fig. 1.3: Development of the inner ear

Chapter 2

Anatomy of the Ear

Anatomically the ear is divided into three parts (**Fig. 2.1**):

i. *External ear*: The external ear consists of the pinna, the external auditory canal and the tympanic membrane
ii. *Middle ear*: The middle ear cavity with the eustachian tube, and the mastoid cellular system is termed as the middle ear cleft.
iii. *Inner ear*: It comprises the cochlea, vestibule, and semicircular canals. Vestibulocochlear nerves connect the inner ear with the brain.

External Ear

PINNA

This consists of auricular cartilage covered by skin. The cartilage is irregularly shaped and is continuous with the cartilage of the external auditory meatus, except between the root of helix and tragus which is filled by fibrous tissue. This cartilage-free gap is called incisura terminalis and is utilized in making an end-aural incision for mastoid surgery (**Fig. 2.2**).

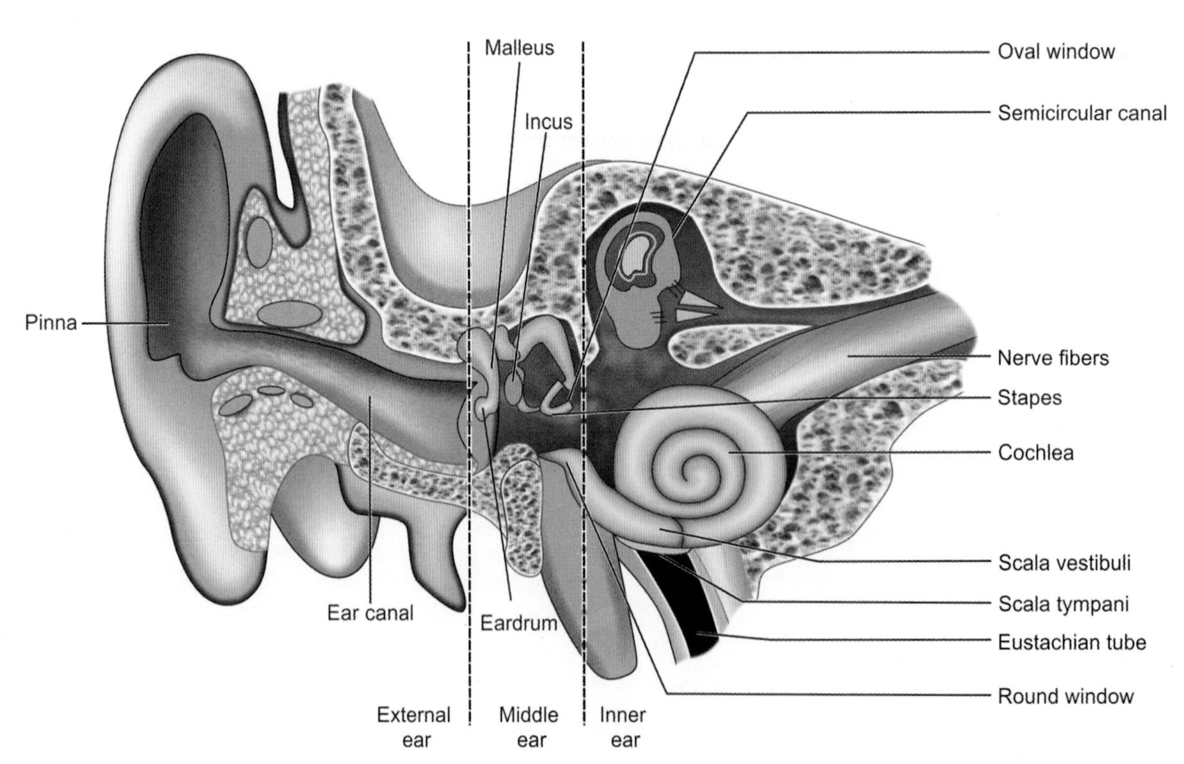

Fig. 2.1: Section of the external, middle and inner ear

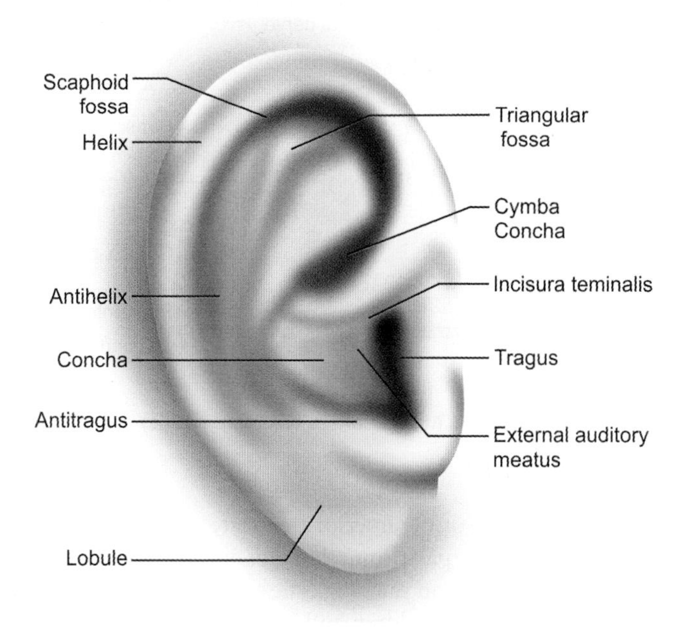

Fig. 2.2: Parts of the pinna

Blood Supply

The anterior surface of the pinna is supplied by the branches of the superficial temporal artery while its posterior surface is supplied by the posterior auricular artery, a branch of the external carotid.

Nerve Supply

The upper two-thirds of the anterior surface of the pinna is supplied by the auriculotemporal nerve (branch of the mandibular division of the V nerve) and the lower one-third by the greater auricular nerve(C_2-C_3). On the posterior surface of the pinna, the lower two-thirds is supplied by greater auricular nerve and upper one-third by the lesser occipital nerve(C_2).

EXTERNAL AUDITORY CANAL

This tortuous canal is 24 mm in length from the outer opening to the tympanic membrane. It has the cartilaginous and bony portions. The lateral-third is cartilaginous and the medial two-thirds is bony. The cartilaginous meatus is directed inwards, upwards, and backwards while the bony meatus is directed inwards, downwards and forwards producing an "S" shaped curvature of the canal. The skin of the cartilaginous meatus has hair follicles, and sebaceous and ceruminous glands.

The dehiscences in the cartilage of the anterior wall of the external auditory canal (*fissures of Santorini*) are important as infection can travel from the external auditory canal to the parotid gland and vice versa.

The bony meatus is formed by the tympanic and squamous portions of the temporal bone. Prominent bony spines may appear in the canal at the squamotympanic and tympanomastoid sutures. The skin of the bony meatus is thin, firmly adherent to the periosteum contains no hair follicles or glands and shows epithelial migratory activity. The anterior half of the canal is supplied by the auriculotemporal nerve while the posterior half by the tenth nerve through the *Alderman's or Arnold's nerve.* Sensory supply to part of the concha is by the facial nerve through the nervus intermedius, thus providing the anatomical basis for herpetic eruption in this part of the concha in the Ramsay Hunt syndrome. The posterior portion of the canal wall may also receive supply from the facial nerve (nerve of Wrisberg or nervus intermedius).

TYMPANIC MEMBRANE

This is a grayish-white membrane, set obliquely in the canal and separates the external ear from the middle ear. The membrane is convex towards the middle ear. The tympanic membrane consists of two parts, the pars tensa, below the anterior and posterior malleolar folds and the pars flaccida (Shrapnell's membrane), above the malleolar folds (**Fig. 2.3**).

The handle of the malleus is attached to the tympanic membrane. The point where the tip of the handle ends is the point of maximum concavity and is called umbo. In the upper part of the membrane, the short process of malleus is seen. The anterior and posterior malleolar folds run anteriorly and posteriorly from the short process of the malleus. The cone of light extends anteroinferiorly from the umbo (**Fig. 2.4**).

The pars tensa has three layers. The outer layer of squamous epithelium is continuous with the skin of the external auditory canal. The middle layer of fibrous tissue consists of radial and circular fibers and the inner layer is formed by the mucosa of the middle ear.

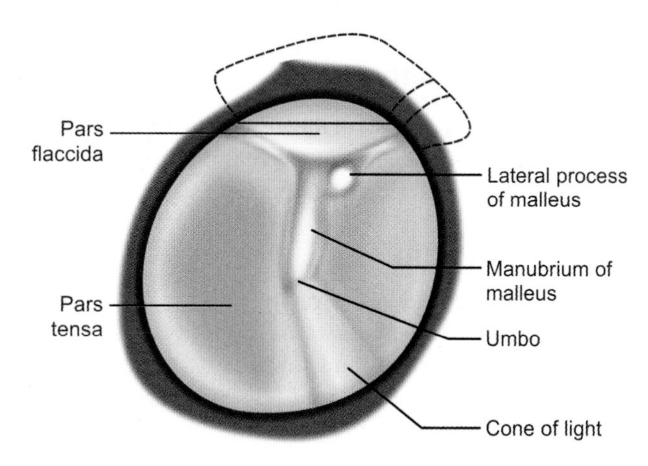

Fig. 2.3: Anatomy of the right ear tympanic membrane

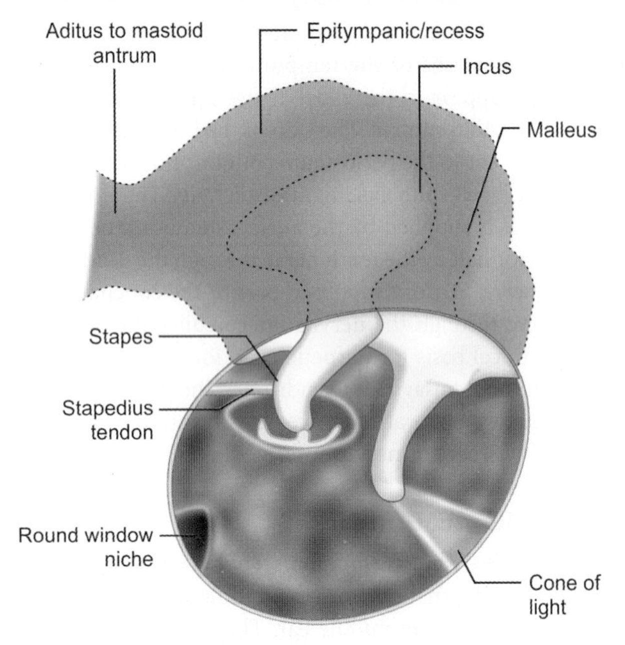

Fig. 2.4: Right tympanic membrane and relationship of ossicles

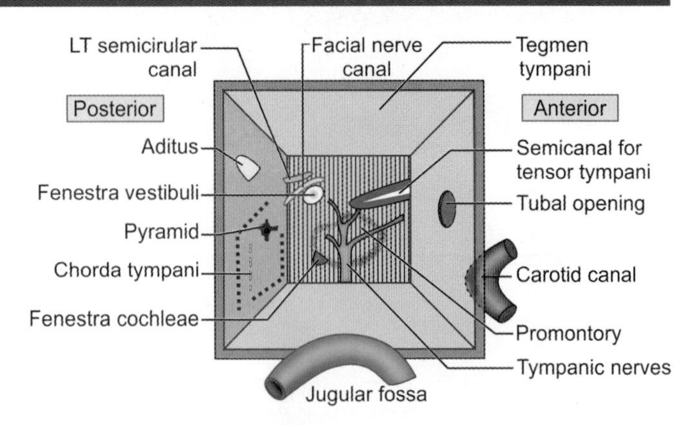

Fig. 2.5: Middle ear cavity (diagrammatic)

The pars flaccida has only an outer epithelial and inner mucosal layer. It is devoid of the middle fibrous layer. The major portion of the tympanic membrane is formed by the pars tensa. Pars tensa is thickened at the periphery to form the fibrocartilaginous annulus, which fits in the grooved tympanic sulcus of the bone. This groove is deficient above in the form of a notch, called the notch of Rivinus. From the ends of this notch, the anterior and posterior malleolar folds extend down and attach to the lateral process of the malleus.

The nerve supply of the membrane is derived internally from the tympanic plexus and externally by the auriculotemporal nerve in its anterior half and by the auricular branch of vagus (Alderman's nerve) in its posterior half.

Middle Ear Cleft

The middle ear cleft consists of the eustachian tube, the middle ear cavity, the aditus ad antrum, the mastoid antrum and the air cells of the mastoid (**Fig. 2.5**).

EUSTACHIAN TUBE

This connects the middle ear cavity with the nasopharynx. It is directed upwards, backwards and outwards from its nasopharyngeal opening and towards its upper opening in the anterior walls of the middle ear. Its upper-third towards the middle ear is bony while the rest of the tube is a fibrocartilaginous passage. The nasopharyngeal end of the tube which is on the lateral wall of the nasopharynx, just behind the posterior end of the inferior turbinate normally remains closed. The tensor palati muscle helps in opening the tubal end on swallowing and yawning. The eustachian tube is short, straight and wide in children and is thought to predispose to middle ear infection.The nerve supply of the eustachian tube is derived from tympanic plexus and the sphenopalatine ganglion.

MIDDLE EAR CAVITY

The middle ear cavity lies between the tympanic membrane laterally and the medial wall of the middle ear formed by the promontory, which separates it from the inner ear.

Medial Wall

The medial wall of the middle ear is marked by a rounded bulge produced by the basal turn of the cochlea called the promontory. Processus cochleariformis is a projection anteriorly and denotes the start of the horizontal portion of the facial nerve. The oval window lies above and behind the promontory and is closed by the foot plate of stapes. The round window lies below and behind the promontory, faces posteriorly and is closed by the secondary tympanic membrane (**Fig. 2.6**).

Just above the oval window and promontory is the horizontal portion of the facial nerve lying in its bony (fallopian) canal. In about 10 percent individuals, the canal may be dehiscent thus exposing the nerve to injury or infection. The horizontal semicircular canal projects into the medial wall of the tympanic cavity, above the facial nerve.

The posterior part of the medial wall of the tympanic cavity is divided into three depressions by two bony ridges called the ponticulus and the subiculum. The upper-most groove above the ponticulus is the oval window region, the lower-most groove below the subiculum is the round window region, and the middle one between the two ridges is the tympanic recess.

The chordal ridge is a ridge of bone which runs laterally from the pyramidal process to the chorda tympani aperture.

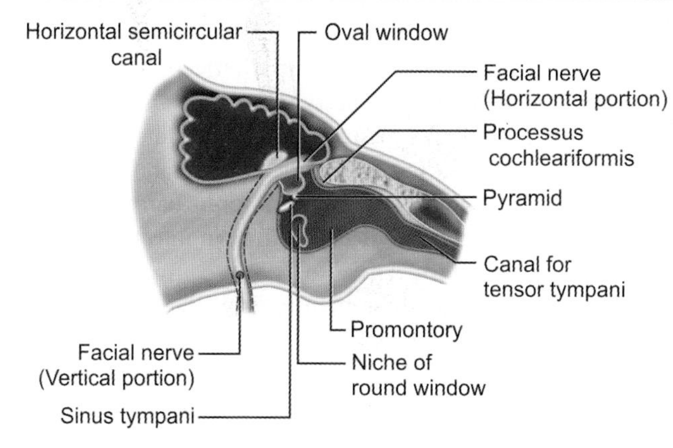

Fig. 2.6: Medial wall of the tympanic cavity

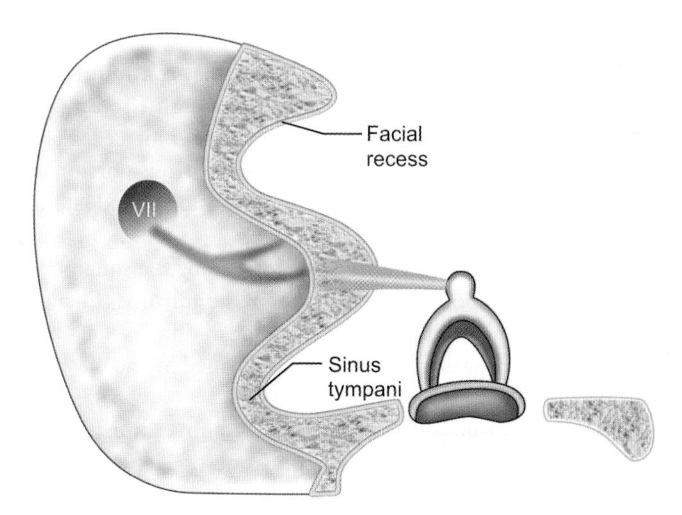

Fig. 2.7: Section through the posterior wall of middle ear at the level of the oval window

Facial recess: This recess is bounded laterally by the deep aspect of the posterosuperior part of the tympanic annulus, superiorly by the short process of incus and medially by the facial nerve which separates this recess from the sinus tympani (**Fig. 2.7**). This recess may serve as a route to the middle ear for anterior cholesteatoma. This recess is explored during the posterior tympanotomy procedure and the surgically created limits of the recess are (1) The facial nerve medially (2) The chorda tympani laterally and (3) Fossa incudis superiorly.

Sinus tympani: Sinus tympani and the facial recess (suprapyramidal recess) lie deep to the posterior tympanic sulcus and immediately posterior to the oval and round windows. The sinus tympani starts above at the oval window niche, occupies a groove deep to the descending portion of the facial nerve and to the pyramid and passes behind the round window niche to the hypotympanum. This area is commonly infiltrated with cholesteatoma associated with retraction of the posterior segment of the tympanic membrane. As shown in the **Figure 2.7**, the facial recess is superficial to the sinus tympani and is separated from it by the descending portion of the facial nerve and processus pyramidalis. In intact canal wall tympanoplasty, sinus tympani is not clearly seen so that there is a danger that the cholesteatoma may be left *in situ* with this technique.

Anterior Wall

This wall of the middle ear cavity has three openings. The eustachian tube opening is seen in the lower part of the anterior wall. A thin plate of bone separates the eustachian tube and the middle ear from the internal carotid artery. The canal for tensor tympani muscle is above the opening of the eustachian tube. Two more openings are present, the upper one being the canal of Huguier that transmits the chorda tympani from the middle ear, and the lower opening is called the glaserian fissure, which transmits the tympanic artery and the anterior ligament of the malleus.

Posterior Wall

The posterior wall in its upper portion shows an opening called the aditus ad antrum, which leads from the attic to the mastoid antrum. Below the aditus is a conical projection called pyramidal process, which transmits the stapedial tendon to its insertion into the neck of stapes. At the pyramidal process the vertical portion of the facial nerve passes deep to the posterior canal wall. Lateral to the pyramid is the opening for the chorda tympani.

Floor

It is formed by a thin plate of bone which separates it from the dome of the jugular bulb. This floor may be deficient sometimes and thus the jugular bulb may project into the tympanic cavity.

Roof

It is formed by the tegmen tympani which is formed partly of the petrous part of the temporal bone and partly by the squamous portion of the temporal bone. This wall separates the middle ear cavity from the middle cranial fossa. The petrosquamous suture may persist and form a pathway for the spread of infection.

Lateral Wall

The lateral wall is formed by the tympanic membrane and partly by bone above and below and accordingly the cavity of the middle ear is divided into three parts:

i. *Mesotympanum:* It is the portion of the middle ear cavity which lies medial to the tympanic membrane.
ii. *Epitympanum (attic):* It is the portion of the cavity which lies above the level of the horizontal portion of the facial

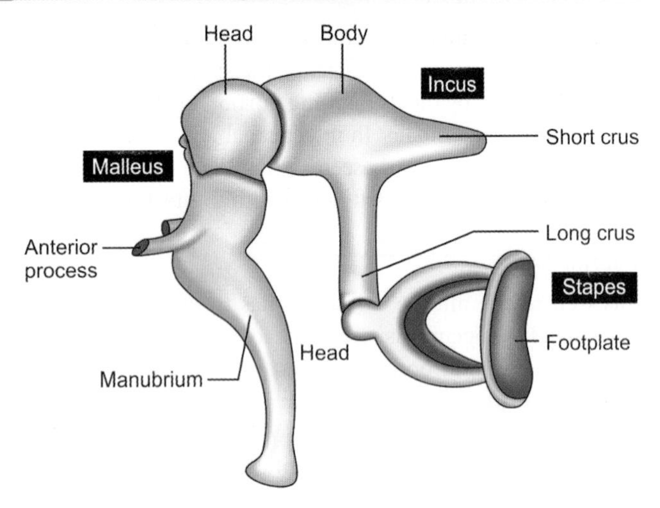

Fig. 2.8: Bony ossicles

nerve, medial to the horizontal part of the squama (outer attic wall).

iii. *Hypotympanum:* It is the part of the cavity which lies below the tympanic sulcus.

Contents of the Middle Ear Cavity

The middle ear cavity contains air, three bony ossicles (**Fig. 2.8**), intratympanic muscles, the tympanic plexus, chorda tympani nerve and the arteries and veins.

The three ossicles are the malleus, incus and the stapes.

The malleus is a hammer shaped bone with a head, handle, neck, anterior and lateral processes. The handle is attached to the tympanic membrane whereas the head which lies in the attic articulates with the body of the incus.

The incus is anvil shaped and has a body, a short process and a long process. The body articulates with the head of malleus and the long process with the head of stapes via the lenticular process.

The stapes is stirr-up shaped and has a head, neck, anterior crura, posterior crura and a footplate.This footplate is firmly attached to the oval window by the annular ligament.

The two intratympanic muscles are the tensor tympani and stapedius. The former arises from the canal above the eustachian tube and its tendon turns round the processus cochleariformis to be inserted into the neck of malleus. The muscle is supplied by a twig from the mandibular division of the fifth cranial nerve. Tensor tympani draws the tympanic membrane medially making it tense.

Stapedius muscle arises within the pyramid and is inserted into the neck of stapes. It is supplied by the facial nerve. Stapedius makes the ossicular chain taut, dampening loud sounds thus protecting the inner ear.

The *tympanic plexus* is formed by the ramifications of the tympanic nerve (*Jacobson's nerve*) which is a branch of the glossopharyngeal nerve. It is joined by the caroticotympanic nerves which arise from the sympathetic plexus around the internal carotid artery. The tympanic plexus lies on the promontory. In addition to supplying the middle ear cleft it also sends a root to the lesser superficial petrosal nerve which is parasympathetic and is secretomotor to the parotid gland.

The mucosa of the middle ear is thrown into folds by the intratympanic structure. These folds and compartments are surgically important as these help to limit the spread of the disease and transmit blood vessels to the ossicles.

Prussak's space is a small space between the Shrapnell's membrane laterally and the neck of malleus medially. It is bounded below by the short process of the malleus and above by the fibers of the lateral malleolar fold.

MASTOID ANTRUM

It is an air chamber in the temporal bone that communicates anteriorly with the tympanic cavity through the aditus. Posteriorly, it communicates with the mastoid air cells. The medial wall of the antrum is formed by the petrous portion of the temporal bone and in this wall lie the posterior and lateral semicircular canals (**Fig. 2.9**).

The lateral wall of the antrum is formed by the squamous portion of the temporal bone. The roof of the antrum is formed by tegmen antri which separates it from the middle cranial fossa and the posterior wall and the floor are formed by the mastoid portion of the temporal bone.

Surgical anatomy: The antrum lies above and behind the projection of a bone called the spine of Henle, on the posterosuperior angle of canal wall. The cribriform area of the bone above and behind this spine is the site for the antrum which lies about 13 mm deep from the surface in adults and only 3 mm deep in infants.

The surface anatomy of the antrum is marked by a triangular area called the Macewen's triangle which is bounded

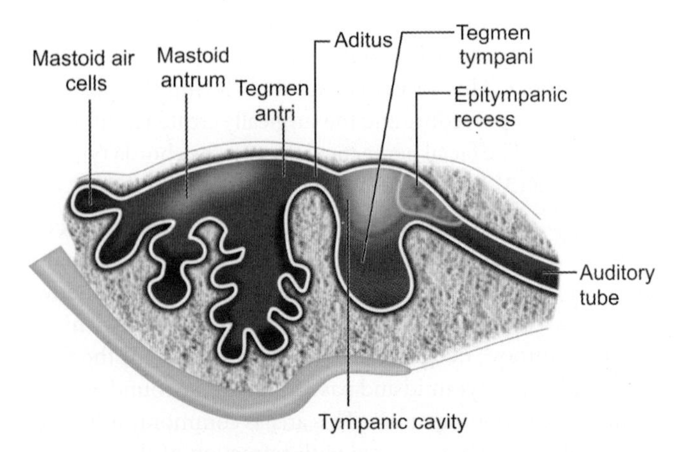

Fig. 2.9: Middle ear cleft

above by the posterior root of zygoma and anteriorly by the posterosuperior canal wall. Behind, the triangle is completed by a line which is tangential to the posterior canal wall below and cuts the posterior root of the zygoma above.

The petrosquamous suture may persist in adult life (Korner's septum) and form a false bottom of the antrum which may mislead the surgeon and lead to incomplete removal of the disease.

Mastoid Process

The mastoid process is not present at birth and starts developing at the end of the first year and reaches its adult size at puberty. It develops posterior to the tympanic portion of the temporal bone. In infancy the mastoid process being absent, the facial nerve emerges lateral to the tympanic portion from the stylomastoid foramen and is likely to get injured by the usual postaural incision.

Mastoid Air Cells

During development of the mastoid process, the bone is normally filled with marrow. Only the mastoid antrum and a few periantral cells are present at birth. With development, the mastoid process becomes cellular in a majority of cases (80%) where air cells are large and the intervening septae are thin, which is regarded as normal. In some cases, the mastoid remains diploic (*acellular*) wherein others the cellularity is completely absent (*sclerotic*). Here are various theories to explain the deficient pneumatization. (1) *Wittmaack theory* which states that infantile otitis media interferes with the resorption of the diploic cells (2) Tumarkins theory which states that failure of pneumatization occurs because of failure of middle ear aeration due to eustachian tube dysfunction and(3) Diamant and Dahlberg suggest that dense bone is congenital and is a normal anatomic variant.

Air cell groups of the mastoid: From the antrum, the cellular system extends into the adjacent bone and is grouped as follows **(Fig. 2.10)**:

1. Periantral cells
2. *Tip cells:*
   a. *Superficial:* The superficial cells lie superficial to the posterior belly of the digastric muscle.
   b. *Deep tip cells:* These lie deep to the attachment of the posterior belly of digastric. The superficial and deep tip cells are separated by the digastric ridge, the facial nerve lies anterior to this ridge.
3. *Perisinus cells:* These are present around the sigmoid sinus.
4. *Perilabyrinthine cells:*
   a. Around the labyrinth within the petrosa.
   b. Supralabyrinthine, above the arch of the superior semicircular canal.
   c. Infralabyrinthine, below the labyrinth.
   d. Retrolabyrinthine, behind the labyrinth.

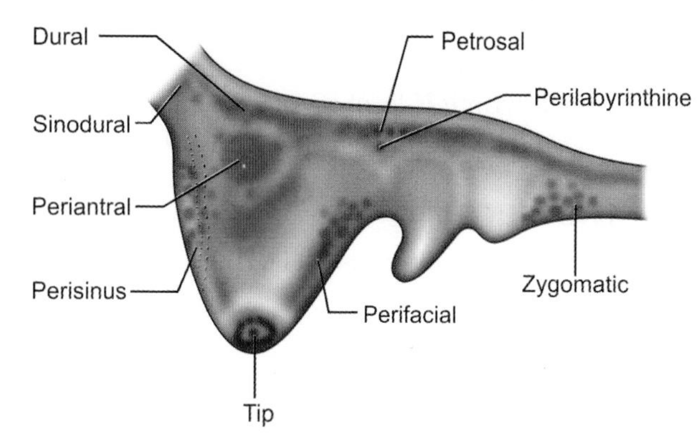

Fig. 2.10: Different groups of mastoid air cells

5. *Retrofacial cells:* These are present behind the vertical portion of the facial nerve.
6. *Petrosal cells:* Air cells may invade the body and apex of the petrous bone and may be present under the trigeminal ganglion, around the internal carotid artery or around the eustachian tube (peritubal cells).
7. Hypotympanic cells tracts.
8. *Zygomatic cells:* These extend forwards into the zygoma.

Antrum threshold angle It is a triangular area of bone and is formed above by the horizontal semicircular canal and fossa incudis, medially by the descending part of the facial nerve and laterally by the chorda tympani.

Sinodural angle: It is the angle between the tegmen antri and the sigmoid sinus.

Solid angle: This lies medial to the antrum formed by a solid bone in the angle formed by the three semicircular canals.

Trautmann's triangle: The triangle lies behind the antrum, bounded by the sigmoid sinus posteriorly, the bony laby¬rinth anteriorly and the superior petrosal sinus superiorly. Infection can travel through this to the posterior cranial fossa.

Cranial nerves in relation to the middle ear cleft: Apart from the 7th cranial nerve which is related to the middle ear cleft there are other nerves like 9th, 10th and 11th cranial nerves which emerge from the jugular foramen just medial to the jugular bulb and may be involved in glomus tumors. Ganglion of the 5th cranial nerve lies in a shallow depression on the anterior surface of the petrous apex. The 6th cranial nerve runs along the posterior surface of the petrous apex in the posterior cranial fossa, enroute to Dorello's canal which is formed by the petroclinoid ligament of the sphenoid bone.

Inner Ear

The inner ear is a structure of winding passage, the labyrinth, situated in the temporal bone. It is an important organ of hearing and balance. It has two parts:

i. Bony labyrinth
ii. Membranous labyrinth.

The bony labyrinth is lined by endosteum. Between the membranous and bony labyrinth lies the perilymph.

BONY LABYRINTH

The bony labyrinth has three parts (**Fig. 2.11**):

i. Vestibule
ii. Cochlea
iii. Semicircular canals.

Vestibule

It is the central part of the labyrinth. On its lateral surface is the opening of the oval window which is closed by the footplate of the stapes. On the posterior portion of the medial wall of the vestibule is an opening for the aqueduct of the vestibule.

Semicircular Canals

These are three in number. The superior canal lying transverse to the long axis of the petrous part, forms the arcuate eminence on the anterior surface of the petrosa. The posterior semicircular canal lies in a plane parallel to the posterior surface of the petrosa. The lateral canal lies in an angle between the superior and posterior canals making a bulge on the medial wall of the attic and aditus ad antrum. Each semicircular canal has an ampulated end which opens independently into the vestibule and a nonampulated end. The nonampulated end of the superior and posterior semicircular canals unite to form a common channel—crus commune. The three canals open by five openings into the vestibule, posteriorly.

Bony Cochlea

The bony cochlea lies in front of the vestibule and is like a snail shell. It has two and three-fourth turns, coiling around a central bony axis called the modiolus. The basilar membrane of the membranous cochlea is attached to the osseous spiral lamina (In the attached margin of this spiral lamina is the spiral canal of the modiolus) and the outer surface of the membranous cochlea is attached to the inner wall of the bony cochlea thus dividing the bony cochlea into three compartments, the upper scala vestibuli, the lower scala tympani and the membranous cochlea or the scala media.

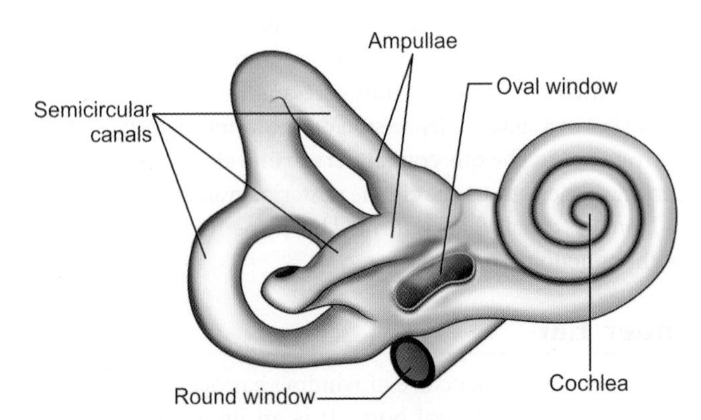

Fig. 2.11: The bony labyrinth

MEMBRANOUS LABYRINTH

The membranous labyrinth is filled with endolymph and comprises of the following (**Fig. 2.12**):

i. The saccule and utricle
ii. The membranous semicircular ducts within the corresponding bony canals
iii. The ductus cochlearis in the bony cochlea.

SACCULE AND UTRICLE

The utricle lies in the upper part of the vestibule while the saccule lies below and in front of the utricle. The ducts from the saccule and utricle join to form the endolymphatic duct which occupies the bony aqueduct of the vestibule. The saccule is also connected by a small duct called ductus reuniens with the duct of the cochlea.

Membranous Semicircular Ducts

These open into the utricle by five openings. One end of each duct near the utricle is dilated and is called the ampulla which houses the vestibular receptor organ. The vestibular receptor organ is a specialized neuroepithelium called crista. The sensory cells have cilia, which project into a gelatinous substance probably secreted by the supporting cells. The gelatinous substance is dome-shaped in the ampullae and is called the cupula. In the utricle and saccule, the specialized epithelium

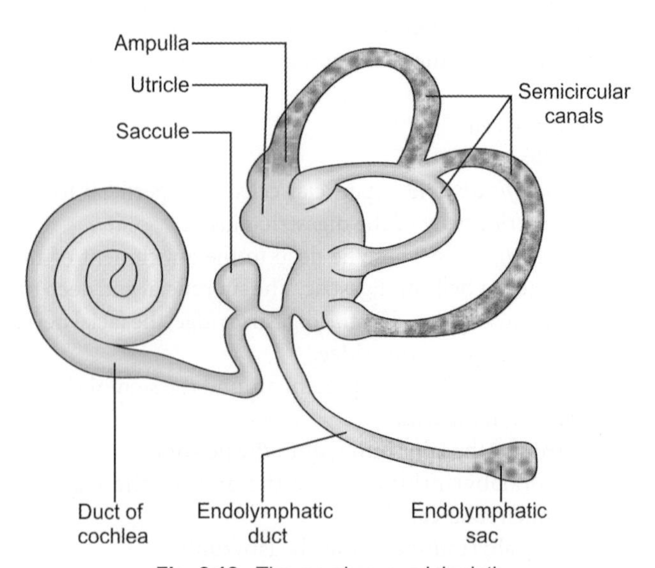

Fig. 2.12: The membranous labyrinth

is called, macula, which lies in a horizontal plane in the utricle and vertical plane in the saccule. The gelatinous substance lying above the neuroepithelium is flat in the saccule and utricle and contains a number of crystals embedded in it, known as statoconia (otoliths).

Ductus Cochlearis (Scala Media)

The membranous duct lies in the bony canal of cochlea. It is roughly triangular, with a base formed by the basilar membrane. The basilar membrane stretches from the osseous spiral lamina to the spiral ligament, which is a thickened endosteum on the outer wall of the bony canal. Continuous with the spiral ligament are the cells richly supplied by blood vessels and capillaries on the outer bony wall called stria vascularis. The other side of the triangle is formed by another membrane called the Reissner's membrane which stretches from the osseous spiral lamina to the outer bony wall.

The scala media or ductus cochlearis ends as a blind tube, dividing the bony cochlear canal into two passages, the upper chamber called scala vestibuli and lower passage known as scala tympani. The two passages communicate with each other at the apex of the modiolus through a narrow opening called the helicotrema. The scala vestibuli communicates with the middle ear through the oval window that is closed by the footplate of stapes. The scala tympani communicates with the middle ear through the round window which is closed by the *secondary tympanic membrane* (**Fig. 2.13**).

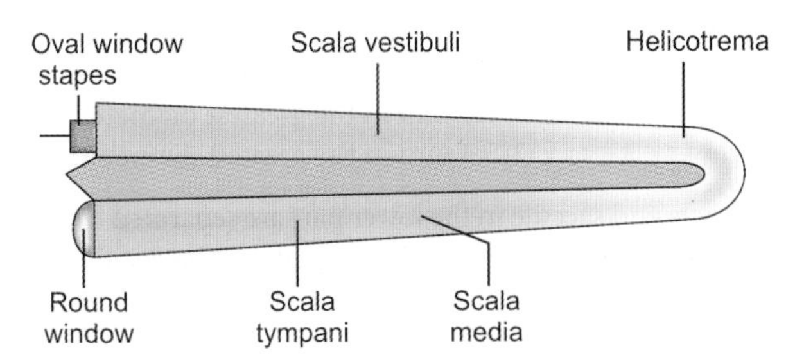

Fig. 2.13: Longitudinal section of cochlea

Organ of Corti

It is the sense organ of hearing and lies on the basilar membrane. It has three components namely hair cells, supporting cells and the gelatinous membrane called the tectorial membrane. There are two types of hair cells, the outer and inner hair cells. The hair cells are supported by pillars of Corti that enclose a space called the *tunnel of Corti.* This tunnel contains a fluid called cortilymph that resembles perilymph in composition. The nerve fibers around the hair cells pass through the osseous spiral lamina into a long bony canal of modiolus (Rosenthal's canal) which contains the spiral ganglion (**Figs 2.14A and B**). The inner hair cells are arranged in one row and are flask-shaped. They develop earlier than outer hair cells and are more resistant to damage by noise or ototoxic drugs and are supplied mainly by afferent nerve fibers from spiral ganglion. The outer hair cells are arranged in three or more layers and are cylindrical in shape. They develop later than inner hair cells and are easily damaged by noise or ototoxic drugs. The nerve supply is mainly efferent from olivocochlear bundle. Each cochlear sends innervation to the both sides of brain.

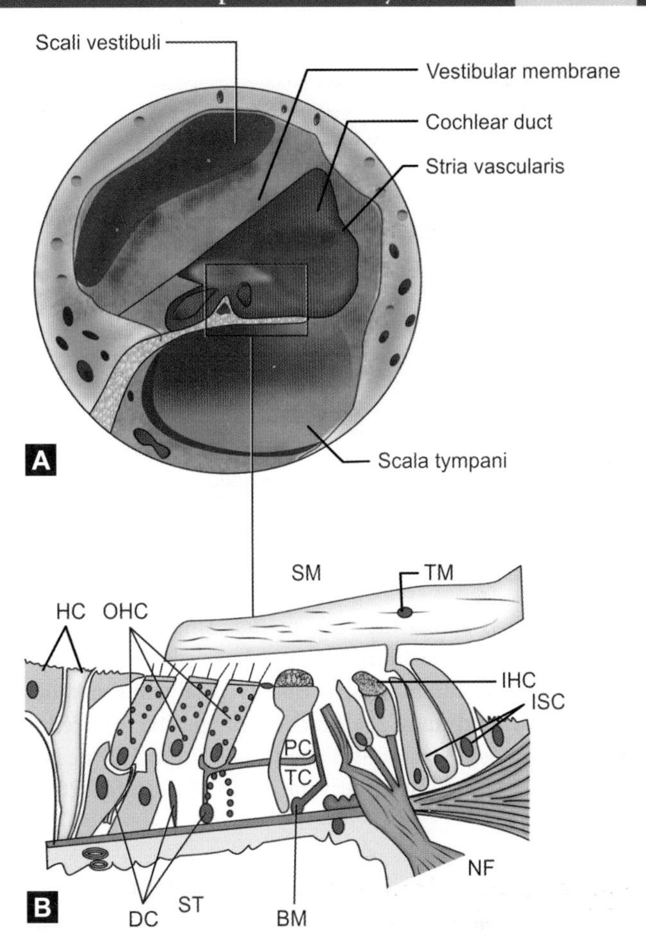

Figs 2.14A and B: (A) Inner ear structures (B) Organ of Corti. SM = Scala media, TM = Tectorial membrane, OHC = Outer hair cells, IHC = Inner hair cells, DC = Deiter's cells, BM = Basilar membrane, PC = Pillars of Corti, TC = Tunnel of Corti, ISC = Inner supporting cells, ST = Scala tympani, NF = Nerve fibers, HC = Hensen's cells

Blood supply of the internal ear: The arterial supply of the internal ear is derived from the internal auditory artery.

This artery usually arises from the anterior cerebellar artery which is a branch of the basilar artery. The internal auditory artery passes down the internal auditory canal and divides to supply the vestibule and cochlea (**Fig. 2.15**).

The organ of Corti has no direct blood supply and depends for its metabolic activities upon diffusion of oxygen from the

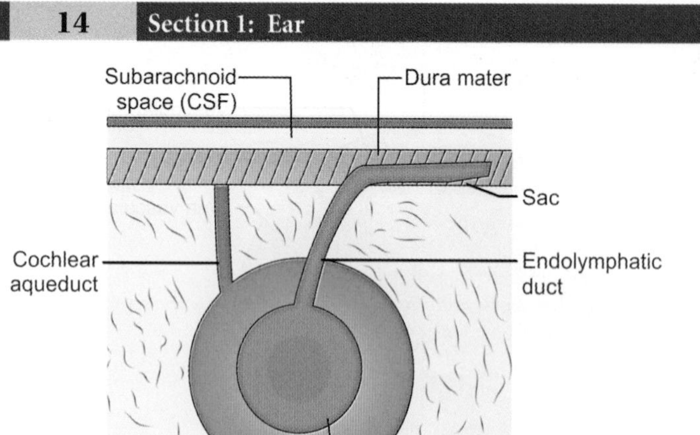

Fig. 2.15: Blood supply of labyrinth

stria vascularis across the scala media. This arrangement is necessary for the acoustic insulation of hair cells from inevitable noise arising in blood vessels. Energy producing metabolic processes depend upon the function of specific intracellular enzymes. Oxygen tension is highest (44-78 mm Hg) near the stria vascularis and lowest near the organ of Corti (16-20 mm Hg).

Average Physical Data of the Ear

EXTERNAL AUDITORY MEATUS

Length	2.3-2.9 cm
Size of lumen at entrance	0.9 cm vertically 0.65 cm horizontally
Diameter	0.7 cm
Area of external opening	0.3-0.5 cm^2
Volume	1.04 cm^3
Resonance frequency	3000-4000 Hz

TYMPANIC MEMBRANE

Diameter along the manubrium	8.5-10 mm
Diameter perpendicular to manubrium	8-9 mm
Height of cone (inward displacement of umbo)	2 mm
Area	85 mm^2
Effective area	55 mm^2
Thickness of whole membrane	0.1 mm
Weight	14 mg

MIDDLE EAR CAVITY

Total volume	2.0 cm^3
Volume of ossicles	0.5-0.8 cm^3
Height	15 mm
Anteroposterior dimension	13 mm
Transverse diameter	6 mm upper part 2 mm center 4 mm lower part

Malleus

Weight	23 mg
Total length	7.6-9.1 mm
Length from the end of manubrium to the end of lateral process	5.8 mm

Incus

Weight	25-30 mg
Length along long process	7.0 mm
Length along short process	5.0 mm

Stapes

Weight	2.86 mg
Height	3.26 mm
Length of footplate	2.64-3.36 mm
Width of footplate	1.41 mm
Area of footplate	1.65-3.76 mm^2

Oval Window

Dimension	1.2 × 3 mm

Round Window

Dimension	2.25 × 1.0-1.25 mm
Area	2 mm^2

Tensor Tympani Muscle

Length	23-26 mm
Area	5.5 mm^2
Stapedius Muscle	
Length	6.3 mm
Area	4.9 mm

Inner Ear

MEASUREMENTS OF INNER EAR

Vestibule	6-7 mm in length 5 mm maximum diameter 3 mm minimum diameter
Saccule	1-1.6 mm in the greatest diameter
Utricle	2-5.3 mm in the greatest diameter

Utricle and saccule in the lower part are separated by 1 mm distance, in the upper part they are in contact. The distance from the anterior part of the oval window to the saccule is 0.75 mm, 1 mm or 1.6 mm depending upon the level, whether high or low.

The anterior part of the oval window to internal auditory meatus	1.75 mm
Upper part of window to utricle	0.5 mm
Posterior and more inferior part of window to utricle	1-1.6 mm
Anterior part of stapedial base of proximal extremity of cochlear duct	0.3 mm

Footplate diameter 2.5-3 mm, width 2 mm, thickness of footplate varies with calcification or bone formation, it may be only 00.425 mm, i.e. usually about 0.4 mm.

(Surgical significance: The surgeon should not move the stapes more than 0.1 mm.)

Cochlea

Number of turns	2-1/6–2-7/9
Volume (including vestibule proper)	98.1 mm^3

Scala Vestibuli

Volume (including vestibule proper)	54 mm^3

Scala Tympani

Volume	37.4 mm^3

Cochlear Duct

Volume	6.7 mm^3
Length	35 mm
Shortest fluid estimated as pathway	20 mm

Helicotrema

Area	0.08-0.2 mm^2

Basilar Membrane

Length	13.52 mm

Width varies on the average 6.25 mm fold from the basal end to a position near the apex, from a minimum of 0.08 mm to a maximum of 4.498.

Number of transverse fibers 24,000.

Organ of Corti

Cross-sectional area varies about 4.6-fold from a minimum of 0.0053 mm^2 to a maximum of 0.0223 mm^2.

Number of inner hair cells	3,300
Number of outer hair cells	12,000

Spiral Ligament

Area 0.543 mm^2 at the basal end and 0.042 mm^2 at the apex.

Ganglion Cells

Total number	25,614
Mastoid air cell volume: Approximately	1.5 cm^3

A comparative composition of inner ear fluids is given in **Tables 2.1** and **2.2** above gives the origin and absorption of inner ear fluids.

Table 2.1: Comparative composition of inner ear fluid

	Subjective/measure	Blood	CSF	Perilymph	Endolymph
1.	Sodium in mEq/liter	141	141	135-150	13-16
2.	Potassium mEq/liter	5	2.5	7-8	140-160
3.	Chloride mEq/liter	101	126	135	120-130
4.	Magnesium mg/100 ml	2	2	2	–
5.	Protein total	7000	10-25	70-100	20-30
6.	CO_2	27	18	10	20
7.	Phosphorus mg/100 ml	2	1	1-3	0.8-1.3
8.	pH	7.35	7.35	7.2	7.5

Table 2.2: Origin and absorption of inner ear fluids

Origin			Absorption
Perilymph			
	i.	From CSF	Through aqueduct of cochlea in subarachnoid space
	ii.	Direct blood filtrate from the vessels of spiral ligament.	
Endolymph			
	i.	Secreted by stria vascularis or by the adjacent tissues of outer sulcus.	Saccus endolymphaticus
	ii.	Derived from perilymph across Reissner's membrane.	Stria vascularis

Chapter 3

Physiology of the Ear

The pinna which plays a role of sound collection in some lower animals does not seem to play this function in human beings. The external auditory canal acts as a channel for the conduction of sounds from the auricle to the tympanic membrane and adds resonance to it, amplifying it by 10-12 decibels.

Physiology of Hearing

Sound is conducted from the external auditory canal through the tympanic membrane and ossicles to the cochlea which is the sensory organ of hearing. The impulses pass from the inner ear through the nerves to central connections and the auditory cortex in the brain, where the message is perceived.

The hearing mechanism thus involves two components:

i. The sound conducting mechanism (transmission)
ii. The perceptive neural mechanism (transduction)

The sound conducting system extends from the external auditory canal to the cochlear fluids.

PHYSIOLOGY OF THE CONDUCTIVE MECHANISM

The functions of the ear include hearing and maintenance of balance.

The tympanic membrane and ossicles not only conduct the sound but also increase its pressure before it is transmitted to the cochlea. This increase in sound pressure provided by the tympanic membrane and ossicles is necessary to overcome the impedance (resistance) to the sound transmission, and is called impedance matching function of the middle ear.

IMPEDANCE MATCHING OF MIDDLE EAR

Transmission of sound from the middle ear containing air to the cochlea containing fluid would have been difficult as this means sound transmission from air to fluid. Because of the difference in the acoustic properties of the two media, most of the sound would be reflected back (impeded) and this would mean a loss of about 99.9 percent of acoustic energy. Nature has, thus, provided with middle ear impedance matching system which overcomes this resistance by increasing the sound pressure. The function is affected by the following:

i. The large effective surface area of the tympanic membrane (55 mm^2) compared to the small surface area of the footplate of stapes (3.2 mm^2) provides a magnification of about 17 times. This is called hydraulic ratio.
ii. The greater length of the handle of malleus compared to the long process of incus (1.3:1) called ossicular chain lever ratio also provides some gain in the transmission.

The result of the two gains, the hydraulic ratio and the ossicular lever ratio ($17 \times 1.3 = 22$) is known as the transformer ratio.

This is how the middle ear functions as the sound pressure transformation mechanism and helps in impedance matching of the sound.

The tympanic membrane, while preferentially feeding the oval window with sound waves, also gives a protection to the round window. It shields the round window from the direct impact of the sound waves and thus allows it to function as a release point necessary for fluid displacement of the inner ear.

The reconstruction of the middle ear transformer mechanism and round window protection form the principles of tympanoplasty.

BONE CONDUCTION OF SOUNDS

Besides air conduction, the sounds are also transmitted through bone, which may be due to vibration of the skull by the subject's own sound waves, the free-field sound energy or by application of the vibrating body directly to the skull.

The stimulation of the sense organs by the bone conducted sounds occurs as a result of compressional mechanism of the skull or by the inertia (lagging behind) of the ossicles and mandible as the skull vibrates. The lagging behind of the mandible produces vibration of the cartilaginous meatus which is then transmitted to the ear.

FUNCTIONS OF THE MIDDLE EAR MUSCLES

The basic function of the intratympanic muscles, the stapedius and tensor tympani, is to protect the inner ear from damage due to high intensity sounds. Loud sounds reflexly stimulate the muscles, which cause stiffness of the ossicular chain and thus less of sound is passed into the inner ear. As these muscles have a latent period of contraction of 10 msec, these do not provide protection from sudden explosive sounds. A sound intensity of 70–90 dB above the hearing threshold is required to elicit the stapedial reflex.

Besides this reflex function the intratympanic muscles help in supporting the ossicular chain.

FUNCTIONS OF EUSTACHIAN TUBE

Eustachian tube helps in aeration of the middle ear. Normally, an aerated middle ear cavity is essential for proper functioning of the tympanic membrane and ossicles and provides a hypotympanic air bubble for the movement of the round window membrane.

The eustachian tube helps in equalization of pressure in the middle ear. As the atmospheric pressure decreases, as during ascent in an aeroplane, the air in the middle ear cavity gets absorbed and a negative pressure develops inside the middle ear cavity. This can be equalized by frequent swallowing movements which open the eustachian tubes. Failure to open the tubes results in their closure (locking) and produces serous otitis media.

A similar situation occurs during the decompression phase in pressurized chambers.

FUNCTIONS OF THE MASTOID CELLULAR SYSTEM

The function of cellularity of the mastoid is not very clear. However, it may serve the following functions:

1. It may be an air reservoir for the middle ear cavity.
2. It may be insulating chambers protecting the labyrinth from temperature variations.
3. It may provide resonance to sound.

SENSORINEURAL MECHANISM OF HEARING

Once the sound waves are transmitted, the footplate of stapes causes movement of the cochlear fluids. It produces a wave which causes displacement of the basilar membrane. The organ of Corti gets stimulated and results in generation of cochlear microphonics.

The nerve impulses (action potentials) are carried to the central connection **(Figs 3.1 and 3.2)**.

PITCH DISCRIMINATION IN THE COCHLEA

There are different theories of hearing which try to explain pitch discrimination in the cochlea:

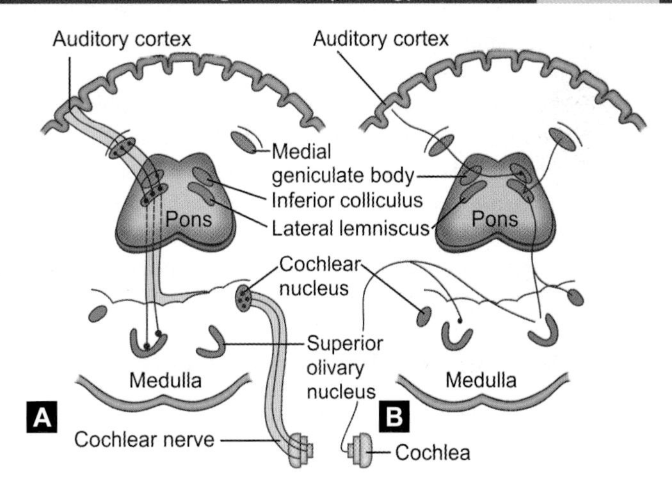

Figs 3.1A and B: The auditory nervous pathway: (A) Afferent fibers; (B) Efferent fibers

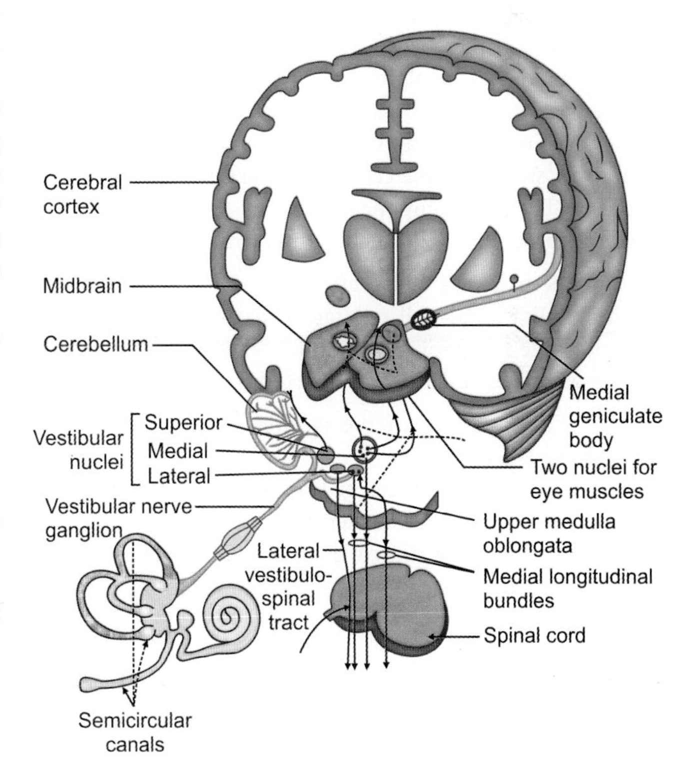

Fig. 3.2: Vestibular pathways to brain

1. *Place theory (Helmholtz' theory):* According to this theory, the perception of pitch depends on movements of the point of maximum displacement of the basilar membrane. Thus each pitch would cause vibration of its own place on the basilar membrane.
2. *Telephonic theory:* Rutherford's telephonic theory assumes that pitch discrimination depends upon the rate of firing of the action potentials in the individual nerve fibers, the

frequency analysis is then done by the central nervous system.

3. *Volley theory (Wever's theory):* This theory is a combination of place and telephonic principles and assumes that the place principle is applicable to higher frequencies which cause maximum displacement of the basilar membrane near the base. The low tones displace the whole of the basilar membrane and are represented in the auditory nerve by nerve fiber responses.

Physiology of the Vestibular System

The vestibular system plays a role in maintaining equilibrium in addition to visual and proprioceptive mechanisms.

Semicircular canals: The canals are sensitive to changes of angular velocity. The movements of endolymph stimulate the vestibular end organ, crista ampullaris. During angular acceleration or deceleration, the endolymph due to its inertia lags behind and thereby exerts pressure within the ampulla. As soon as, the constant velocity of rotation is attained and inertia overcomes, the initial stimulation ceases. Once angular acceleration or deceleration ceases, the endolymph being still in motion, stimulates the crista ampullaris but in the reverse direction. The slow component of the nystagmus is always in the direction of the flow of endolymph (Ewald's law).

Utricle: The hair cells of the utricular macula are stimulated by the gravitational pull on statoconial membrane, which is responsible for static labyrinthine reflexes resulting from centrifugal forces and also responsible for linear acceleration.

Saccule: The functions of the saccule are not very clearly understood at present.

There is a constant discharge from the vestibular labyrinth conducted through the 8th nerve to the central vestibular connections which keep the cortex informed about the changes in position and posture of head and thus help in maintaining the equilibrium.

ELECTRICAL POTENTIALS IN THE COCHLEA

Two main types of potentials have been identified:

i. The steady or resting state potentials
ii. Superimposed AC voltage fluctuations due to acoustic stimulation.

The most striking finding is a positive potential of some 80 mV in the scala media called the endolymphatic potential (EP).

Insertion of the electrode into a hair cell reveals a negative potential of about 80 mV so that there is an overall potential difference of 160 mV between the scala media and the interior of the hair cells, a striking high voltage difference to be found across a cell membrane. A small positive potential of about 5 mV is also noted in the scala vestibuli.

It has been found that the microphonic potentials are a composite of several electrical activities. These are as follows:

1. *Auditory nerve action potential (AP):* This consists of an aggregate of the action potentials of the individual nerve fibers. These potentials are similar to those of other nerves, e.g. a spike discharge preceded by a latent period and followed by a refractory period.
2. *Cochlear microphonics (CM):* This is the main component and confers upon the cochlear potentials. It has two elements—CM 1, which is oxygen dependent and is abolished by oxygen lack or by death of the individual and CM 2, about 10 percent of the whole, which can still be elicited for several hours after total oxygen deprivation or death. The origin of CM is conclusively shown to be the physical stimulation of the hair cells.
3. *Summation potential (SP):* This also results from acoustic stimulation and consists of a change in EP which may be in the positive or the negative sense (SP^+ and SP^-). Unlike CM, it does not follow the actual instantaneous values of the sound stimulus, but is proportional to the RMS (root mean square) acoustic pressure.

Summation potential becomes the most conspicuous at higher sound levels, beyond the point at which distortion begins in CM. It is thought to originate in the hair cell reticular lamina area like CM but is probably the product of a different mode of differential vibration between the organ of Corti and the tectorial membrane.

Cochlear hydrodynamics means that the cochlear fluids vibrate instantaneously from window to window. These movements are those of a fluid column vibrating back and forth without significant compression and rarefaction of its constituent molecules. This means that a sound wave as such does not travel through the cochlear fluids.

EFFERENT COCHLEAR SYSTEM

Within the auditory nerve, there are about 500 centrifugal fibers coursing from the brainstem to the hair cells. Anatomical studies show that they originate in the superior olivary nucleus. About one-fifth of them are of homolateral origin and the remainder from the opposite side. Ramussen has defined several separate bundles of these fibers which converge upon and merge with the auditory nerve.

Masking

The masking of a tone by a louder sound of approximately similar frequancy is called ipsilateral direct masking. This mechanism is an independent of the central nervous system.

Remote masking: It is the term used to describe changes in the threshold of a tone caused by a masking sound in a different frequency range.

To get the same degree of masking, a higher intensity of masking sound is required than necessary for direct masking.

Transcranial masking: It is due to acoustical leakage of a masking sound around the head to the opposite ear.

Central masking: It results from the intermingling of the central connection of the two ears.

Distortion in the Ear

There are several forms of sound distortion to which the ear, in common with other acoustic devices, is subjected. These are as follows:

Frequency distortion: The preferential transmission of certain frequencies as compared to others occurs when the secondary system into which the sound is transmitted from the primary system cannot reproduce all frequencies with the same relative amplitude as does the primary system. In this sense, the relative loss of high frequency components in low pass filters is an example of frequency distortion.

Phase distortion: Changes in the phase relationships of the constituent frequencies of a complex sound constitute phase distortion.

Amplitude distortion: It refers to the inability of a given system to reproduce the incident waveform properly. Both simple and complex wave motions can be affected by amplitude distortion.

Chapter 4

History Taking with Symptomatology of Ear Diseases

Deafness

Deafness or hearing impairment is an important otological symptom. It may be unilateral or bilateral. The various points to be noted are the following:

1. *Onset:* Whether the onset was gradual or sudden. Sudden deafness may occur after head injuries, blast injuries, viral infections and vascular causes, etc.
2. *Duration:* Deafness which is present since birth may be due to genetic causes, due to prenatal intake of drugs like thalidomide or if the mother suffered from rubella during pregnancy. Prolonged labor and otitis media, measles, mumps and meningitis during infancy are also important causes of deafness. Deafness of recent origin in adults may be due to traumatic, inflammatory, neoplastic, vascular and metabolic causes.
3. *Nature of deafness:* A deaf patient may hear better in noisy surroundings (paracusis willisii, characteristic of otosclerosis). In cochlear lesions, patients do not hear at conversational intensity but get irritated by loud sound (recruitment). Fluctuant deafness occurs in secretory otitis media and Ménière's disease.
4. *History of drug intake:* Drugs like salicylates, aminoglycosides, quinine and cytotoxic drugs are known to be ototoxic.
5. *Occupation:* People working in noisy surroundings are more prone to hearing impairment (acoustic trauma).
6. *Family history:* Otosclerosis has a familial predisposition.

Hard of hearing: A person is said to be hard of hearing, if he or she has a hearing loss which can be helped by medical and/ or by surgical treatment, or has learned speaking naturally as a partially hearing child or adult. Rehabilitation measures like providing amplification (hearing aid), and speech and auditory trainings can help in restoring verbal communication. Provided the treatment is started early in life, such a person can be educated with normal hearing children and in later life will have the same employment opportunities as normal hearing people.

Deaf: A person is said to be deaf if he or she has a severe hearing loss with little or no residual hearing. Such a person's hearing is nonfunctional for ordinary purposes of life. When measured with an audiometer the hearing loss for speech is 82 dB or worse (normal hearing is from 0 to 25 dB). A deaf person should be educated and trained in a deaf school.

TINNITUS

Tinnitus is first important symptom of salicylate poisoning. Tinnitus associated with periodic episodes of deafness and vertigo constitutes Ménière's syndrome. Wax in the external auditory canal, aero-otitis media, infections of the ear, acoustic trauma and otosclerosis may be associated with tinnitus. Pulsatile tinnitus is seen in glomus jugulare and AV shunts. Fluctuant deafness, fullness in ears and tinnitus are found in secretory otitis media.

VERTIGO

Meticulous history is an important diagnostic tool as far as vertigo is concerned. The first thing to ascertain is whether the vertigo is really vertigo (a sense of rotation) or a syncopal attack in which the patient gets a blackout, falls momentarily and quickly regains consciousness, or just giddiness.

Vertigo with a discharging ear indicates labyrinthitis. Vertigo of central origin is associated with other neurological features. Positional vertigo is seen in critical postures only. Upper respiratory catarrh followed by vertigo may indicate viral labyrinthitis or vestibular neuronitis.

Patients taking ototoxic drugs may also get vertigo. Unilateral hearing loss with vertigo is characteristic of acoustic neuroma.

EAR DISCHARGE (OTORRHEA)

Discharge from the ear is a common manifestation of ear disease. The discharge is commonly due to middle ear pathology but may also be due to the infections of the external auditory canal. The discharge may be serous, mucoid, mucopurulent, purulent, blood stained, or watery. It may be scanty or profuse.

Serous discharge is found in allergic otitis externa. Mucopurulent discharge is commonly due to benign chronic suppurative otitis media and the extension of the disease process to mastoid air cells. A purulent discharge usually signifies an underlying bone eroding process in the middle ear like cholesteatoma. The discharge in this condition is usually scanty and foul-smelling. This type of discharge may occur in otitis externa also. Blood-stained discharge is a feature of malignancy, glomus jugular and granulations. Watery discharge in the ear may be CSF due to trauma or because of diffuse otitis externa.

EARACHE (OTALGIA)

Pain in the ear may occur due to lesions in the ear itself or due to the conditions in the surrounding areas (referred otalgia) (**Fig. 4.1**).

Painful lesions of the ear include the following:

1. *External ear*
   a. Furunculosis
   b. Impacted wax or foreign body
   c. Perichondritis
   d. Diffuse otitis externa
   e. Otomycosis
   f. Myringitis bullosa
   g. Ramsay-Hunt's syndrome
   h. Traumatic lesions within the external auditory canal.
2. *Middle ear*
   a. Acute suppurative otitis media
   b. Acute mastoiditis
   c. Aero-otitis
   d. Dull aching pain may be due to secretory otitis media or as a complication of chronic ear disease
   e. Malignant lesions in the ear may be associated with earache.

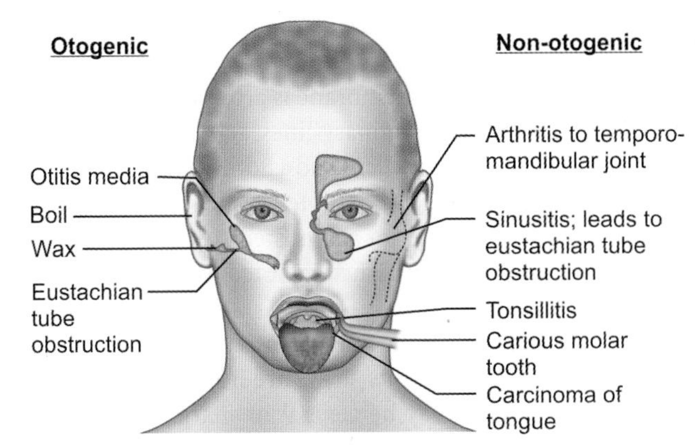

Fig. 4.1: Causes of earache

Referred Otalgia

The ear itself being normal, otalgia may be a symptom of lesions affecting various anatomical sites in the head and neck. The external ear is supplied by 5th and 10th cranial nerves. These nerves also supply various structures of the head and neck. Similarly, the 9th cranial nerve besides supplying the middle ear is also sensory to portions of the oropharynx and base of the tongue. The pain may also be referred to the ear through C2 and C3 supplying the auricle and skin of the postaural region. The important causes of referred otalgia are as follows:

1. *Via the auriculotemporal nerve* (branch of 5th cranial nerve):
   a. *Dental causes:* Impacted wisdom tooth, caries, gingivitis, tooth abscess, etc.
   b. *Lingual causes:* Ulcerative and malignant lesions of anterior two-thirds of the tongue.
   c. *Temporomandibular joint lesions:* Arthritis, trauma and malfunction.
   d. *Lesions of the floor of mouth:* Ulcerative and malignant lesions.
2. *Via the greater auricular nerve and facial nerve:* Cervical spine lesions, neck lesions (inflammatory, traumatic, neoplastic, etc.), herpes.
3. *Via the glossopharyngeal nerve*
   a. *Tonsillar lesions:* Inflammation, abscess, malignancy, foreign body, etc.
   b. *Tongue (posterior one-third) lesions:* Carcinoma, foreign body, etc.
   c. *Nasopharyngeal lesions:* Carcinoma, adenoid hypertrophy.
4. *Via the vagus nerve*
   a. *Pharyngeal lesions:* Carcinoma, foreign body, abscess.
   b. *Laryngeal lesions:* Carcinoma, inflammation, etc.

TULLIO PHENOMENON

This term is applied to a condition where the subject gets attacks of dizziness or/vertigo by loud sounds. The vertigo is due to stimulation of the ampullary cristae by the sound waves. The phenomenon may occur in patients having labyrinthine fistulae, and in those who have undergone fenestration operation.

HYPERACUSIS (PHONOPHOBIA)

This term is applied to a condition when the subject complains of increased sensitivity to sounds.

The sounds appear as uncomfortably loud to the patient. This phenomenon occurs in cases suffering from stapedius muscle paralysis as after suprastapedial facial nerve paralysis and in cases of congenital syphilis (Hennebert's sign).

Chapter

5

Examination of the Ear

Methods of Examination of the Ear

The auricle, external auditory canal and the postaural region are thoroughly inspected for the shape and size of the auricle, color changes in the skin, swelling, ulcer or a previous operative scar.

The lesions of the pinna may be congenital, traumatic, inflammatory or neoplastic. The infection to auricle or external canal may spread from scalp and the skin lesions may be eczematous. The auricle stands out prominently and the postauricular groove gets obliterated in furunculosis. The auricle is displaced downwards and outwards in mastoiditis with subperiosteal abscess.

The movements of the auricle and tragus are tender in otitis externa (furunculosis)—Tragus sign.

The mastoid region is examined for edema, abscess or postaural fistula as occurs in mastoiditis. Mastoid tenderness is elicited at the tip and at the cymba concha for the antrum which indicates an underlying infection. Edema at the site of exit of the mastoid emmissory vein (Griesinger's sign) occurs in lateral sinus thrombosis.

OTOSCOPY

The inside of the external auditory canal is examined conveniently using a head mirror, light source and an ear speculum. The examination may also be done by using a battery or electric otoscope. This gives some magnification and is useful in examining children and infants, and for bedside examination of patients, but any manipulation with an instrument while using the otoscope is impossible.

For a proper view of the inside of the canal, the pinna is gently pulled backwards and upwards in adults and downwards and outwards in infants to straighten the canal. A proper sized speculum is used to inspect the canal. Swelling due to a furuncle may be visible in the cartilaginous canal. Wax or debris may be filling the canal which is removed for deeper examination. Sagging of the posterosuperior canal wall occurs in mastoiditis.

The nature of ear discharge is noted and the discharge is cleaned by a cotton tipped applicator.

The ear canal is examined for edema, redness or granulations. A polypoidal mass may be seen in the canal due to chronic suppurative otitis media, glomus jugulare and malignancy. A deeper look into the canal shows the tympanic membrane or its remnants.

The tympanic membrane appears as a grayish white, translucent membrane set obliquely inside the canal. The important landmarks on the membrane are as follows:

1. The short process of the malleus appears as a small projection in the upper anterior part of the pars tensa. This landmark is least obliterated in disease.
2. The anterior and posterior malleolar folds radiate forwards and backwards from this projection separating the pars flaccida above from the pars tensa below.
3. The short process is followed down to note the handle of the malleus which is directed downwards and backwards, ending at the umbo.
4. From the umbo a cone of light is seen radiating anteroinferiorly.
5. Sometimes the long process of the incus may be seen through the posterior part of the pars tensa, below the posterior malleolar fold.

The pars tensa of the membrane is arbitrarily divided into four quadrants by two imaginary lines. A vertical line passes down along the handle of malleus and a horizontal line intersects it at the umbo, dividing the pars tensa into anterosuperior, anteroinferior, posteroinferior and posterosuperior quadrants. Abnormalities of the membrane are noted with respect to the quadrant involved.

1. *Integrity:* The membrane may be intact or perforated. The site of perforation and its shape are noted. A perforation of the pars tensa may be central or marginal. A central perforation may be small or large, but the intact rim of membrane is seen around the margins of the perforation. A perforation is called marginal if no rim or annulus is seen around or on side of the margin of the perforation.

A marginal perforation is an indication of an unsafe disease. A perforation in the pars flaccida or attic perforation indicates an underlying cholesteatoma.

2. *Color changes in the tympanic membrane:* The tympanic membrane normally appears as a grayish white membrane. A congested membrane with prominent blood vessels is seen in the early stage of acute otitis media while a dull lustreless membrane is seen in secretory otitis media. A blue discoloration of the membrane occurs in hemotympanum and the flamingo pink reflex is seen in otosclerosis (Schwartze's sign).
3. *Position of the membrane:* Normally the position of the membrane is maintained by the pressure of air column on its either side. A bulging congested drum is seen in exudative stage of acute otitis media. A retracted membrane may occur in aero-otitis, serous otitis media, and adhesive otitis media. The retracted membrane appears dull, lustreless, with absent or distorted cone of light and has a reduced mobility. The handle of the malleus appears more horizontal and the short process more prominent.
4. *Mobility of the membrane:* The mobility of the membrane is tested by the Valsalva's method and by siegalization. The hypermobile areas of the membrane indicate scarring of the membrane. Restricted mobility is due to adhesive otitis media or fluid in the middle ear cavity.

EXAMINATION WITH SIEGEL'S SPECULUM

This speculum consists of a 10 diopter lens and a side tube connected with a rubber bulb. An air tight system is produced in the canal and pressure is increased in the bulb. The speculum is helpful for the following reasons.

1. It gives a magnified view of the membrane.
2. It is helpful to assess the mobility of the membrane.
3. The speculum is used to elicit the fistula sign.
4. By varying the pressure, discharge through the perforation can be sucked out as well as medication can be put into the middle ear.

EXAMINATION UNDER MICROSCOPE

For better and detailed examination of the middle ear cleft, examination under a microscope is of great help to the otologist (**Fig. 5.1**). It is done as an OPD procedure.

Examination of Ear with an Operating Microscope

In modern otological clinics a microscope is essential to inspect all quadrants of the drum adequately. Pus and debris may be aspirated and disease in the attic, margin or center of the tympanic membrane confirmed (**Fig. 5.2**).

Evaluation of Ear Disease

FISTULA TEST

Erosion of the bony part of the vestibule (usually the lateral semicircular canal) by trauma or by an ear disease exposes the membranous labyrinth to the external pressure changes. If the labyrinth is functioning, its stimulation will lead to a subjective feeling of vertigo and vomiting and may be associated with nystagmus. The presence of the erosion (fistula) can be demonstrated by the following ways:

1. Alternately compressing and releasing the tragus against the external meatus. This alters the pressure in the canal and stimulates the labyrinth.
2. By moving the polyp or granulations in the ear by a cotton tipped applicator.
3. By increasing and decreasing the pressure in the canal with a Siegel's speculum.

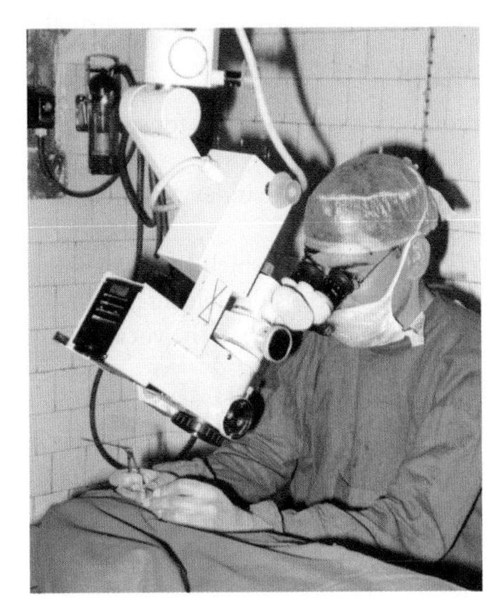

Fig. 5.1: Examination under the microscope

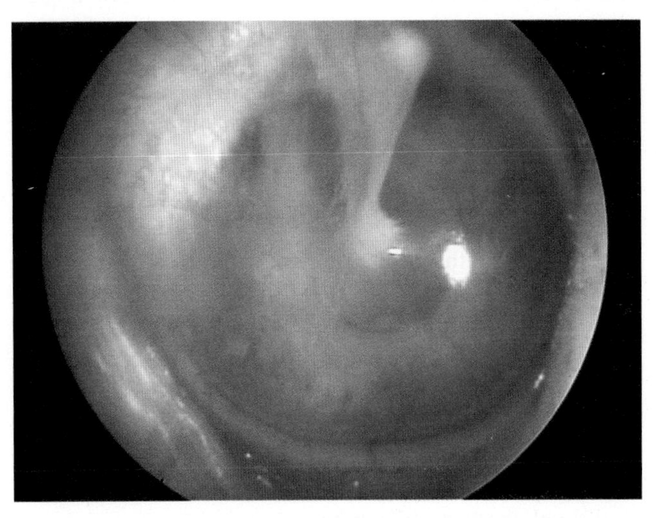

Fig. 5.2: Otoscopic view of normal tympanic membrane

The subjective feeling of giddiness, nausea or vomiting with or without nystagmus indicates a *positive fistula sign* which indicates that there is a fistula in the labyrinth, and that the labyrinth is still functioning.

The fistula sign may be false-negative or false-positive.

False-negative fistula sign: This means that there is a fistula in the labyrinth but the fistula test is negative. This occurs in a dead labyrinth.

False-positive fistula sign: This means that there is no fistula in the labyrinth but the fistula test is positive. This occurs in congenital syphilis due to the deformed hypermobile footplate and is called Hennebert's sign. It may also occur after stapedectomy.

EUSTACHIAN TUBE PATENCY

The patency of the eustachian tube can be demonstrated by various tests. However, a patent eustachian tube is not necessarily an index of normal function of the tube.

The nasopharynx is examined by a posterior rhinoscopy or by a nasopharyngoscope.

Valsalva's Test

The patient is asked to close the mouth and pinch the nostrils and then to blow out, thus increasing the pressure in the nasopharynx. This opens up the eustachian tube and allows air to pass into the middle ear cavity. The outward movement of the tympanic membrane is seen through the ear speculum. The test is useful to know the mobility of the membrane as well as the patency of the eustachian tube. This test may normally be negative.

Politzerization

The tip of the nozzle of the Politzer's rubber bag is placed in one nostril and the other nostril closed over it by fingers. The patient is given some water to swallow. At the movement of swallowing, the air in the bag is compressed. The air thus enters the eustachian tube as it opens up on swallowing. The outward movement of the tympanic membrane indicates a patent eustachian tube.

Eustachian Catheterization

An eustachian catheter of a proper size is passed through the nose into nasopharynx. The tip of the catheter is turned into the eustachian orifice and air is blown down the catheter into the eustachian tube. The movement of the tympanic membrane is observed through the canal or the passage of the air through the tube is heard by an auscultation tube, one end of which is placed in the patient's ear and the other end in the examiner's ear. The sound heard by the examiner indicates the passage of air through the eustachian tube.

Method

The nasal cavity is anesthetized by the local use of 4 percent lignocaine spray, the eustachian catheter is passed along the floor of the nasal cavity without touching it, the tip of catheter pointing downwards till the catheter reaches the posterior wall of nasopharynx. The catheter is brought forwards gently till the tip hooks against the posterior edge of the soft palate. Now the tip of catheter is rotated by 90° outwards which approximates it with the pharyngeal end of the eustachian tube. The ring on the proximal end of the catheter indicates the direction of the tip of the catheter. A Politzer's bag nozzle is attached to the proximal end of catheter and is squeezed to allow the air to be blown into the eustachian tube through the catheter. If the tip of the catheter is rotated through 180° towards the other side of the nasopharynx the patency of the eustachian tube of the other side can be assessed. After the process is over, the catheter is brought back to the position as it was passed into the nasal cavity and withdrawn gradually from the nasal cavity without touching its sides and floor.

Functional Examination of Ear

The tests of hearing are intended to measure the ability to hear sounds (quantitative) and to test and compare the efficiency of the conductive and perceptive parts of the auditory apparatus (qualitative).

Qualitative testing is done by tuning forks and pure tone audiometer and quantitative by speech (live or recorded) and pure tone audiometer.

All tests should be carried out in a quiet room. In quiet places, normal distance at which speech of conversational level can be heard is about 20 feet, whereas the whispered voice (using residual air) should be understood at 12 feet. But most rooms do not allow more than a 12 feet range, so it is customary to consider 12 feet for both speech and whisper as the normal standard.

VOCAL INDEX

It is the relation between hearing loss for speech and whispered voice.

In conductive deafness the index is small and there is little difference between the two.

In perceptive deafness in which loss is mainly confined to high tones, there may be considerable discrepancy between the hearing for speech and whisper, so the vocal index is high.

THRESHOLD FOR SPEECH

In a person with normal hearing this threshold is zero but in a person with moderate degree of hearing loss it may be 40-45 dB.

SPEECH AUDIOMETER

A trained speaker speaks into a microphone certain words which are transmitted to the listener through a pair of head phones. Adjustments are made on the attenuator, which is so adjusted that when the dial is at zero at least 50 percent of the test material is heard.

PURE TONE AUDIOMETER

It is used to determine the threshold of hearing for pure tones within a selected band of frequencies. The tones are electrically produced and can be varied both in frequency and intensity. The range of frequencies available may be fixed at octave or half octave intervals between 64 and 8,192 cycles/sec (if Helmoltz scale is used) or there may be continued sweep between 0 and 10,000 cycles/sec.

Intensity can be varied, usually in 5 dB steps from 0 to 100 dB and the intensity dial is so calibrated that at zero for each selected frequency a person with normal hearing can just hear the test tone.

As sound at a level of 60 dB or more can be heard in the untested ear, it is advisable to use a masking apparatus. Masking is essential when there is considerable difference in the hearing acuity between the two ears, and when testing by bone conduction to get correct results.

The value of the pure tone audiometer test depends upon the following:

i. Accuracy of the audiometer.
ii. The way in which the test is carried out.
iii. Intelligence of the patient.

Each ear should be tested separately for all frequencies (usually 7) with masking of untested ear when necessary. For bone conduction, masking of the untested ear is essential. Only four tones are tested (256-2,048 cycles/sec).

The various hearing tests are described below.

VOICE TESTS

Speech tests though less accurate are simple and easily understandable to the patient. The conversational and whispered voice tests are conducted in reasonably quiet surroundings. The material for speech tests may be spondee words or numbers. Spondee words are bisyllabic words having an equal stress on both syllables like arm-chair, toothbrush, mousetrap, cough-drop, etc. Whispered voice is used at the end of normal expiration and is thus easily standardized than conversational voice.

Method: Each ear is tested separately. The other ear being masked by the finger on tragus or rubbing the nontest ear with a piece of paper. The distance at which the patient can hear the conversational and whisper voice in a reasonably quiet surrounding are noted. The distance is reduced for whisper voice in high frequency loss than for conversational voice. In conductive deafness there is little difference in distance at which each can be heard.

TUNING FORK TESTS

Tuning forks provide a simple, easy and reliable method of testing the hearing. A set of 256, 512, 1024, double vibration forks is commonly used. The following tests are commonly in use:

i. Rinne's test
ii. Weber's test
iii. Absolute bone conduction test.

Rinne's Test

The fork is struck gently on the elbow, knee cap, hypothenar eminence or a rubber pad and held in such a way so that the prongs vibrate against the ear in line with the external canal at a distance of about 1 inch (**Fig. 5.3**). The air conduction of the sound is compared with bone conduction. To test the bone conduction, the foot piece of the fork is placed on the mastoid. The patient is asked to indicate which of the two is louder or where he hears for the longer time.

Interpretation

1. Normally air conduction is better than bone conduction, which is called Rinne's positive. In patients with sensorineural deafness, both air and bone conduction of sound are diminished but air conduction is still better than bone conduction. This is called Reduced Rinne's positive.
2. Rinne's negative means that bone conduction of the sound is better than air conduction and signifies conductive deafness.
3. Sometimes air conduction of sound equals bone conduction and indicates mild conductive deafness.
4. At times, the test may be false-negative. A patient with severe unilateral sensorineural loss may indicate that he hears the bone conducted sound in the affected ear (test ear) with poor or no response to the air conduction, therefore, indicating negative Rinne's test. But in reality, this is false as he is hearing this bone conducted sound

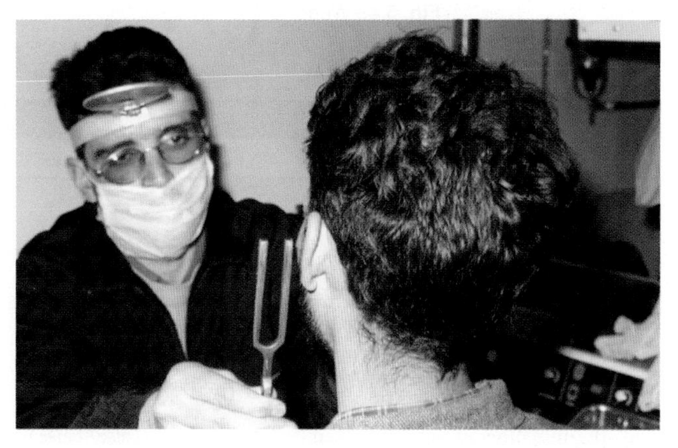

Fig. 5.3: Rinne's test

across the skull through the normal ear. In these cases, the test is repeated by masking the normal ear while testing the affected ear. Barany's noise box can be used for masking the ear.

The results of the Rinne's test are given in **Table 5.1**.

Weber's Test

A vibrating tuning fork is held either on the vertex, root of nose or on the upper incisor teeth (**Fig. 5.4**). The patient may hear the sound equally on both the sides, in the center of the head, or the sound may be lateralized to one side.

Interpretation

1. When the sound is heard in the center of the head or equally on both sides it is called Weber's centralized and is found in normal persons or may occur in patients having bilateral, symmetrical conductive hearing loss.
2. If the sound is heard louder on one side than the other, then it is called Weber's lateralized to that particular side. Weber's test gets lateralized to the deaf ear in conductive deafness and towards the normal ear in sensorineural deafness.

Absolute Bone Conduction (ABC) Test

This compares the absolute bone conduction of the patient with that of the examiner. The hearing of the examiner is considered to be normal. The vibrating fork is held on the mastoid of the patient, closing the external meatus firmly with the tragus, the patient is asked to signal when he no longer hears the sound (**Fig. 5.5**). The fork is then transferred by the examiner to his own mastoid closing the external meatus. The absolute bone conduction of the patient is thus compared with that of the examiner.

Interpretation

1. If the examiner still hears the vibration of the fork, when the patient has stopped hearing it, then the absolute bone conduction of the patient is said to be reduced. This is found in perceptive deafness.
2. If the examiner also does not hear the sound of the fork when the patient has stopped hearing it, then absolute bone conduction is regarded as normal.
3. The test is absolute and thus it cannot get prolonged.

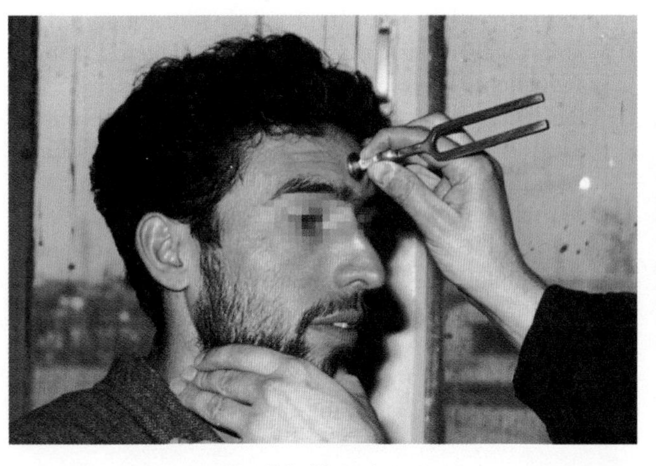

Fig. 5.4: Weber's test

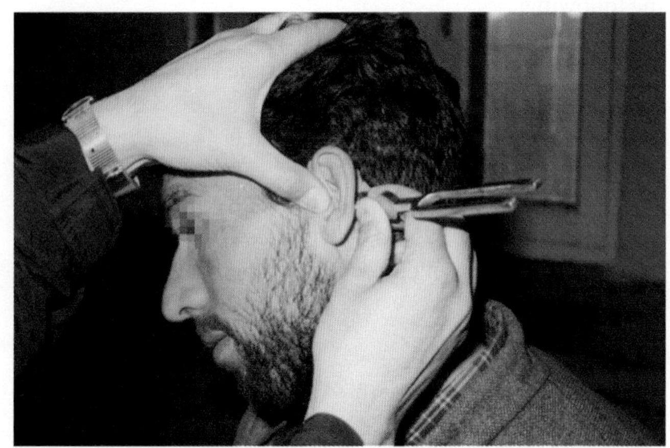

Fig. 5.5: Absolute bone conduction test

Table 5.1: Results of Rinne's test

Tuning for results	Nomenclature	Interpretation
1. AC > BC	R+	Normal
2. AC > BC (both reduced)	R+ (reduced)	Perceptive deafness
3. AC = BC	R=	Slight conductive deafness
4. AC only, No BC	R+ infinitely	Severe perceptive deafness
5. BC > AC	R–	Conductive deafness
6. BC only, other ear masked	R– infinitely	Very severe conductive deafness
7. BC only, other ear left Unmasked	R–(False) False negative Rinne	Very severe or total perceptive deafness

Schwaback's Test

The test is performed to determine the state of bone conduction in presence of air conduction. This test is conducted like the absolute bone conduction test but without occluding the external auditory canal.

Radiological Examination of the Ear

Plain X-rays of the temporal bone help in determining the extent of middle ear and mastoid disease, the condition of the ossicles and the extent of pneumatization. The following views are of common use (**Figs 5.6A to D**):

Towne's view: The patient's head lies in contact with the film and the direction of the beam is 25-35° fronto-occipital (**Figs 5.7 and 5.8**).

It demonstrates both the mastoids on same film providing a contrast with the normal side. The following points are noted:

i. Degree of pneumatization or sclerosis.
ii. Mastoid antrum and air cells.
iii. Semicircular canals (superior and lateral) may appear in the film.
iv. Internal auditory meatus.
v. Ossicles like malleus and incus.

Haziness or destruction of bony partitions, cavity formation or erosion should be noted and compared with the other side.

Lateral oblique view: The patient's head is placed in a lateral position. The ray is directed 30-35° caudally. Each side is taken separately. It is useful in providing information regarding the following:

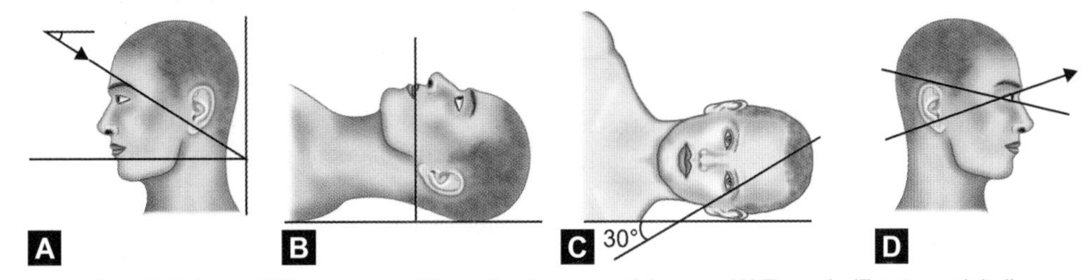

Figs 5.6A to D: Different view of X-ray for diseases of the ear: (A) Towne's (Fronto-occipital); (B) Submento-vertical view; (C) Stockholm-B view (Lateral-oblique); (D) Stenvers view (Oblique-posterior anterior)

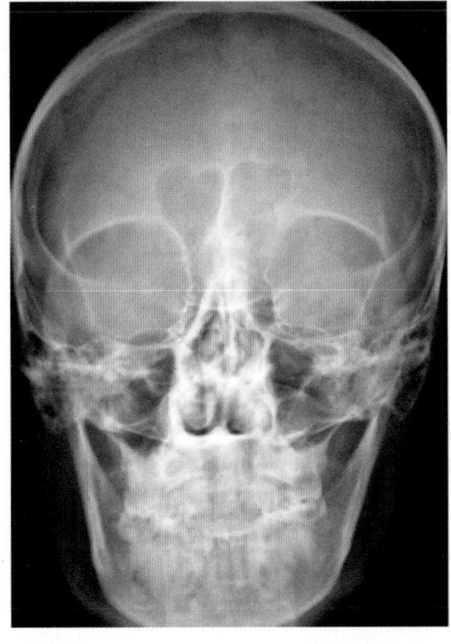

Fig. 5.7: Towne's view

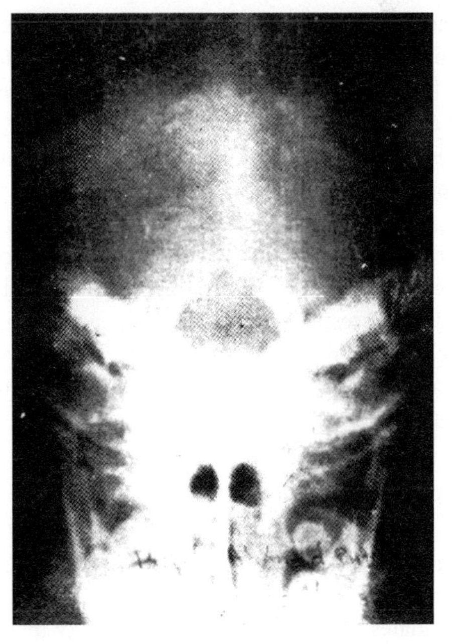

Fig. 5.8: X-ray of the skull, Towne's view showing sclerotic mastoids with bilateral cavities (cholesteatoma)

i. Relationship of the sinus plate to the air cells and thus helps in determination of the posterior extent of the pneumatization.
ii. Superiorly the dural plate, the floor of the middle fossa is visible.
iii. Aditus, attic and antrum are demonstrated.

The external auditory canal and tympanic cavity are obscured by the bony labyrinth.

Stenver's projection: This is an oblique view of the skull, taken separately for each side at an angle of 12.5°. The view is taken mainly to demonstrate following structures:

i. The upper border of petrous bone
ii. The internal auditory meatus
iii. The superior semicircular canal
iv. Ossicles like malleus and incus.

Transorbital view of the petrous apex: This view demonstrates both petrosa on the same film and is commonly taken to visualize the internal auditory meati. A difference of 1 mm or more is significant.

Owen's projection: This is an oblique view which demonstrates the attic, aditus, and antrum. The ossicles are shown clearly within the external auditory canal.

X-ray base of the skull: The submentovertical view may be required to study the mastoids, auditory canals, petrousapex, bony eustachian tube and carotid canal.

CT SCAN

Computerized axial tomography (CAT) is the most accurate noninvasive neurodiagnostic test available. This test was invented by Hounsfield who received the Nobel prize for physics in 1979. The scanner has a diagnostic accuracy of 98 percent and the great advantage is that it is noninvasive and the radiation involved is only one-third of the dose for a single lateral skull radiograph.

The CAT scanner is capable of producing pictures in a wider range of densities than the conventional X-ray procedures. It clearly pin-points pathology like tumors, intracranial bleeding, infarcts, cysts, abscesses, hydrocephalus, aneurysms and various eye and ear, nose, throat (ENT) lesions. Vascular structures can also be seen following the injection of an iodized contrast material in the patient.

Advantages of CT Scanning

1. It provides a speedy and accurate diagnosis.
2. Pin-pointing of the pathological spots facilitates in accurate surgery.
3. It eliminates the need for painful and risky investigations and exploratory surgery.

Contrast Radiography

Radiographic examination after instillation of a radio-opaque dye may be done for eustachian salpingography and to demonstrate the lesions of the internal auditory meatus.

The dye may be put either through the nasopharyngeal orifice of the tube to demonstrate the block in the tube or alternatively, it may be injected into the middle ear through a tympanic membrane perforation if it is present, or a fine needle is used to put the dye into the middle ear.

Dye injected into the middle ear determines the patency of the tube as well as helps in assessing eustachian tube function by tympanic cavity clearance study.

In 8th nerve tumors the internal auditory meatus study is done by injecting the contrast material through a cisternal puncture.

Nuclear Magnetic Resonance

Nuclear magnetic resonance (NMR) or magnetic resonance imaging (MRI) is now used in advanced centers as a noninvasive scanning procedure and is superior to CT scan in some ways. It is based on the magnetic processes of the atomic nuclei. The nuclei are aligned in a strong magnetic field and a radiofrequency pulse applied. After this pulse is removed, the nuclei return to their original orientation emitting a radiofrequency signal. The image is created by specially encoding the emitted radiofrequency signal.

ADVANTAGES OF MRI

1. It is a noninvasive procedure and is safe even when used repeatedly and even in pregnancy.
2. The sagittal, coronal and even oblique sections can be taken to find the exact extent and location of the tumor.
3. Fractures are better visualized.
4. Tumors are better differentiated from muscles and blood vessels than by CT scanning.
5. Arteries and veins can be differentiated.

DISADVANTAGES OF MRI

1. The cost is very high and thus a limitation.
2. Small calcifications may be missed.
3. There is lack of bone details.
4. Patients with any metallic foreign body, e.g. pacemakers, metallic prosthesis, aneurysm clips cannot be imaged and these may have to be removed, as they may sometimes act as sharp, lethal missiles.

Examination of the Vestibular Apparatus

While examining the vestibular system a detailed neurological check-up including that of the cranial nerves is done for proper assessment of the lesion.

CRANIAL NERVES

The 5th cranial nerve is tested by eliciting the corneal reflex. The cornea is touched with a cotton wisp and normal brisk closure of the eyes occurs. This reflex may be diminished or absent in cerebellopontine angle tumors.

The 7th cranial nerve is frequently involved by the cholesteatoma, malignancy of ear or acoustic neuroma and is tested to determine the site of lesion.

NYSTAGMUS

Nystagmus is the rhythmic oscillatory movement of the eyes and has two components, slow and quick.

Nystagmus can be of the following types:

1. Central, with other signs of intracranial disease.
2. Ocular, with signs of ocular disease.
3. Vestibular, with vertigo and some loss of hearing.

It can also be classified as follows:

First degree nystagmus: Present only when patient looks in the direction of the quick component.

Second degree nystagmus: Also present when the patient looks straight in front.

Third degree nystagmus: If still present when the patient looks in the direction of the slow component.

Under anesthesia, the quick component is eliminated and only the slow or vestibular movement takes place and results in conjugate deviation.

In labyrinthine nystagmus there is a slow component of vestibular origin and a quick component which is of cerebral origin. Each labyrinth tries to deviate the eyes slowly to the opposite side due to its tonic activity and thus normally the effect is neutralized so that the eyes remain in midline. When one utricle is stimulated due to disease or caloric stimulation, the eyes get deviated slowly to the opposite side. When the cerebral cortex becomes aware of this deviation, it brings in effect the correcting reflex, thus bringing the eyes quickly back to the original position. The reverse occurs when the labyrinth is hypoactive or dead, i.e. the quick component to the opposite side and slow component to the affected side.

The vestibular nystagmus is fine, always horizontal and does not last for more than six weeks.

Central nystagmus (due to involvement of the central connections) may be horizontal, vertical or rotatory, is coarse and lasts for a longer time.

How to look for nystagmus: The patient is placed in good light and the examiner faces the patient. The patient's head is kept steady and he is asked to follow the direction of the finger tip of the examiner, which is moved across the field of vision in various directions. The jerking of eyes appears at the extreme range of vision in normal individuals and should not be mistaken for labyrinthine nystagmus.

If the labyrinth is irritated on one side, spontaneous nystagmus occurs towards that side and when the labyrinth is destroyed, the nystagmus occurs towards the opposite side.

The function of the vestibular system may be evaluated by stimulating the labyrinth and noting the change in its response. Induced nystagmus may be produced by the following tests:

i. Caloric test
ii. Rotation test
iii. Optokinetic test.

The Caloric Test

In this test the labyrinth is stimulated by the changes in temperature. This is done by irrigating the external auditory canal with hot and cold water.

Commonly the lateral semicircular canal is tested. The patient lies supine on the table. The head end of the table is inclined 30° forwards. This is done because the anterior end of the horizontal semicircular canal is about 30° higher than its posterior end. In this position, the horizontal canal thus assumes a vertical plane for easy stimulation.

Cold caloric test: About 5 cc of ice cold water is injected into the external auditory canal. This cools down the surrounding bone and the temperature variation is transmitted to the labyrinth. Convection currents are set-up in the endolymph and thus the labyrinth is stimulated. Nystagmus occurs and its duration nystagmus is compared on both sides. Normally the nystagmus persists for about two minutes. This is a simple test but is less informative.

Bithermal caloric test (differential caloric test) or Fitzgerald and Hallpike test: This test is done by irrigating the external auditory canal with water having a temperature 7° above body temperature (44°C) and 7° below body temperature (30°C). The canal is irrigated by the water at these temperatures for 40 seconds.

The onset and duration of the nystagmus with each stimulation is graphically recorded (calorigram—**Figs 5.9A to D**). An interval of about 5 minutes should be allowed between the tests. Cold stimulation produces nystagmus towards the opposite side and hot stimulation produces nystagmus towards the same side. The duration of nystagmus is measured on both sides. If nystagmus persists for less than the average time, it is called canal paresis (hypoactive). Sometimes caloric responses are enhanced in one particular direction (directional preponderance). This is due to the loss of tonus elements and commonly occurs towards the normal ear.

Nystagmus may be observed unaided or with the help of Frenzel's glasses worn by the patient to prevent optic fixation and provide magnification of the eye movements. Thus low intensity nystagmus, which may not be visible to the naked eye, becomes obvious.

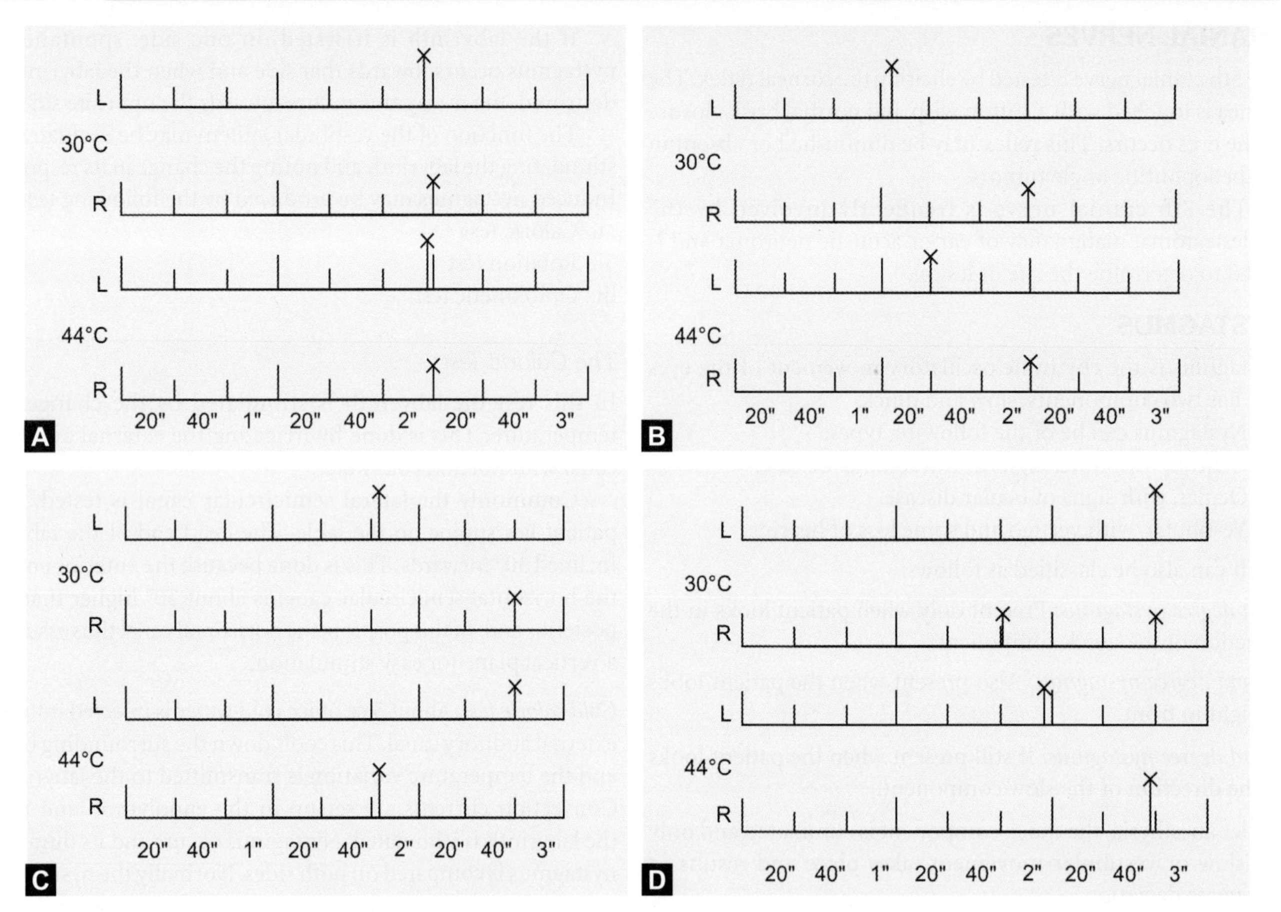

Figs 5.9A to D: Calorigram: (A) Normal; (B) Left canal paresis; (C) Left directional preponderance; (D) Right directional preponderance

Caloric test with Dundas-Grant apparatus: In patients with perforation of the tympanic membrane water cannot be injected into the external canal. In such patients the Dundas-Grant metallic coil is used. Ethyl chloride is sprayed over the coil and air is passed by pressing the attached rubber bulb. As the air passes through the coil, it gets cooled and enters the ear, thus producing cold caloric responses in the ear.

Rotation Test

The patient is placed on a revolving Barany's chair which is rotated at the rate of ten revolutions per second. The chair is then suddenly stopped and the postrotational nystagmus noted. Both labyrinths are stimulated at the same time, hence, the test is not of much significance.

Optokinetic Test

A white rotating drum with black vertical lines is used. The drum rotates on a horizontal plane. The patient is seated at a distance of 3 feet from the drum. The drum rotates to one side and then to the other. The patient follows the vertical lines on the drum to either side. The drum is stopped and eyes are examined for nystagmus. A normal person has nystagmus of both sides. In central vestibular lesions, the nystagmus of one side is suppressed.

ELECTRONYSTAGMOGRAPHY

It is an extremely useful method for recording the eye movements. The apparatus is shown in **Figure 5.10**. The corneoretinal potential method utilizes the electric potential between the cornea and retina. An electric field exists between the cornea (electrically-positive) and the retina (electrically-negative). Electronystagmography (ENG) detects movements of these electric fields and records them onto a continuous tracing. The electrodes are placed lateral to each eye and on the forehead between the eyes. The main advantage of ENG is that some patients reveal nystagmus which is not readily visible on naked eye examination. ENG recordings also allow for quantification and the provision of a permanent record of the nystagmus (**Fig. 5.11**). Characteristic tracings are seen in peripheral and central vestibular disorders, congenital nystagmus and cerebellar disorders. This technique allows the recording of nystagmus with the eyes closed or open. It provides a base line

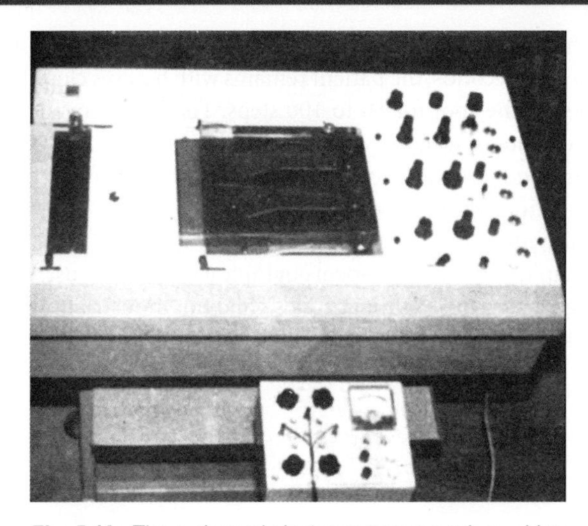

Fig. 5.10: Three-channel electronystagmograph machine

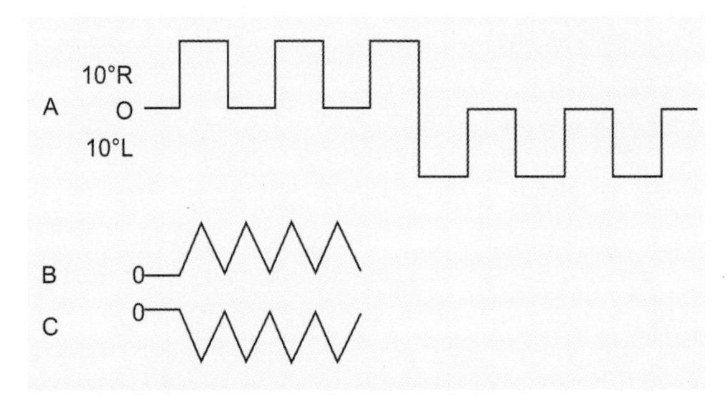

Fig. 5.11: Typical electronystagmographic records: (A) Calibration record; (B) Nystagmus towards right; (C) Nystagmus towards left

record and subsequent changes are compared with this tracing. It also allows the evaluation of other parameters of nystagmus in terms of duration, intensity, velocity and latency of onset.

The special advantage of electronystagmography in determining the qualitative and quantitative changes of nystagmus is made use of in the following tests as well:

1. *Rotation tests:* Rotation activity is grossly diminished by ototoxic drugs like streptomycin, neomycin, etc. when frequency and amplitude of nystagmus are both affected, while gross asymmetry of the reaction is seen in vestibular neuronitis. Normal frequency but reduced amplitude on the rotation testing is seen in Ménière's disease.
2. *Optokinetic tests:* Marked asymmetry of nystagmus on optokinetic tests usually suggests a central lesion of the vestibulo-optic system.
3. *Eye tracking tests:* In this test eye movements in response to a visual pendular simulus are recorded which normally produces a sinusoidal curve. A nonsinusoidal curve is always due to central lesions while sinusoidal with superimposed nystagmic movements can occur in peripheral lesions.

Positional Test

Positional nystagmus can be induced by placing the patient's head in different positions. The procedure is explained to the patient.

Nystagmus is looked for after asking the patient to lie down and sit up with the head turned 90° to the right, to the left and backwards. The patient is taken backwards for about 10 seconds, if the nystagmus appears, the position is maintained for 30 seconds. Observation is made concerning the latent period, direction, duration and fatiguability. Fine, horizontal, fatiguable nystagmus occurs in vestibular lesions and benign positional vertigo. Rotatory or horizontorotatory nystagmus which is nonfatiguable is seen in central lesions.

Romberg's test

This test is conducted by asking the patient to stand upright with the heels together. The patient may be asked to close the eyes. The patient falls towards the direction of the slow component of peripheral labyrinthine nystagmus. In case of the central lesion the patient swings or fall towards the direction of the quick component.

Past Pointing

The patient has a sensation of objects turning away from him which, he voluntarily attempts to compensate by touching a fixed object. This effect is due to presence of vertigo.

Cupulometry

It is a rotation test to assess the vestibular function by utilizing minimal stimuli. It was devised by Jongkees and coworkers in 1952. A special turning chair is used in which the patient sits with his feet free of the floor and his head immediately above the axis of his rotation in the upright position, inclined 30° forwards to bring the two lateral semicircular canals in the horizontal plane.

Subthreshold acceleration is given to the turning chair and maintained till every reaction has ceased. It is then suddenly stopped. This is repeated at different velocities. The duration of after-sensation and after-nystagmus are recorded on a logarithm scale. The record is called cupulogram.

The test is based on the fact that the cupulae of the semicircular canals respond to the angular acceleration, i.e. the increasing speed of rotation. Angular acceleration which when maintained for 20 sec is sufficient to evoke a just recordable nystagmus is known as threshold. Normal threshold for nystagmus without optic fixation is 0.15°/sec^2 and with optic fixation, it is 1°/sec^2.

Craniocorpography

Craniocorpography provides a rapid graphical recording of the combined results of the Romberg and the Unterberger tests for the pathological discrimination of the spinal vestibular system. The basis of craniocorpography is the Unterberger test, established as the most sensitive method for accurate clinical studies of the spinal vestibular system. Unterberger gave special consideration to the rotation of the human body in the slow phase of the nystagmus after a caloric stimulation.

In the craniocorpograph test, which does not last more than sixty seconds, the patient remains with his eyes closed and walks on the spot for 80 to 100 steps. The craniocorpograph test considers walking deviation and lateral balance of the patient and provides more explicit information allowing better discrimination between central and vestibular peripheric perturbations or a combination of both.

Rapidity of the craniocorpograph test makes it useful for group screening, examination of children, industrial medical checkups, legal medicine, driving test, etc.

Chapter

6

Congenital Diseases of the External and Middle Ear

Anomalies of the Pinna

The pinna arises from a series of six tubercles which develop on the first and second branchial arch around the primitive meatus at about the 6th week of intrauterine life. The development is complete by the 4th month of fetal life.

The arrest of development may result in various deformities.

ANOTIA

This refers to the absence of the pinna.

MICROTIA

This is the term for an abnormally small and deformed pinna (**Fig. 6.1**), while macrotia indicates an abnormally large pinna. The cases of absent pinna can be given a prosthesis or treated by plastic reconstruction using moulded rib cartilage.

ACCESSORY AURICLES

These present as small elevations of skin often containing the cartilage, just in front of the tragus or the helix (**Fig. 6.2**). They need surgical removal if the patient desires.

PREAURICULAR SINUS

These are blind tracks lined by squamous epithelium occurring in the region of the auricle, usually near the tragus and root of the helix. These arise because of incomplete fusion of the tubercles during development (**Fig. 6.3**).

COLLAURAL FISTULAE

These have an upper opening in the floor of the external auditory meatus and the lower opening behind the angle of jaw at the anterior border of sternomastoid.

These skin tracks usually get infected and, therefore, are treated by dissection of the tract and excision. The tract may lie deep to facial nerve.

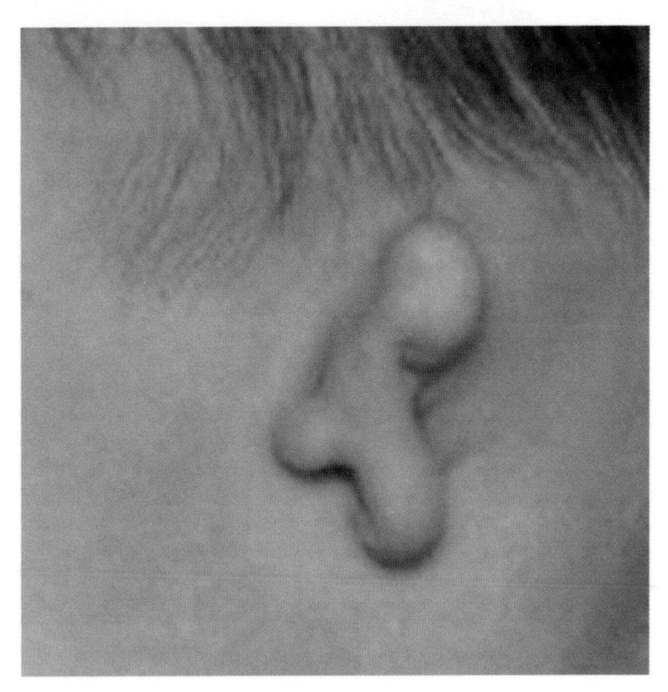

Fig. 6.1: Microtia

DERMOID CYSTS

These may occasionally occur in relation to the pinna.

Malformations of the pinna are commonly associated with a deformed canal. Many minor variations in the shape of the pinna may occur.

DARWIN'S TUBERCLE

It is small elevation on the posterosuperior part of the helix. This is an inherited condition and is homologus to the tip of the ear in mammals.

WILLDERMUTH'S EAR

The antihelix is more prominent than helix. The lobule may be absent or adherent to the side of the head.

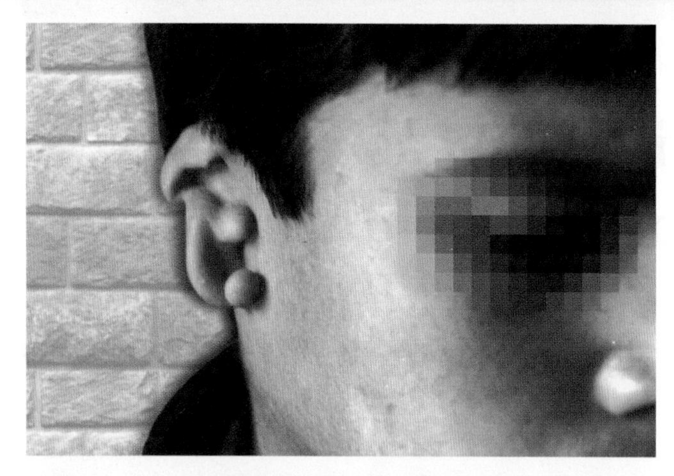

Fig. 6.2: Accessory auricles

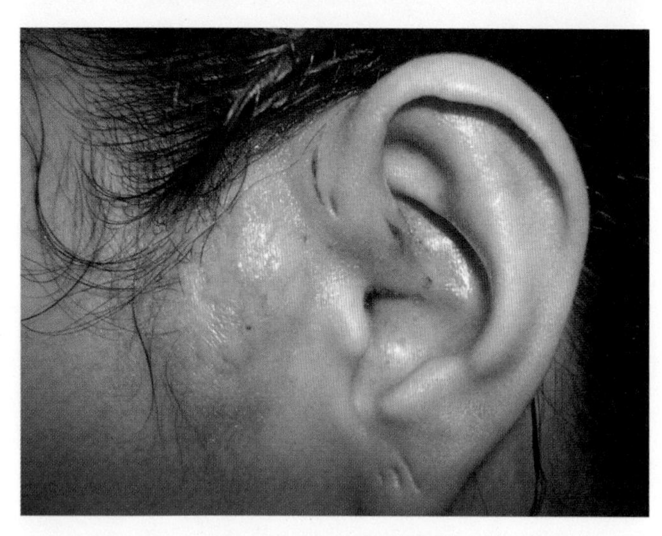

Fig. 6.3: Preauricular sinus

BAT EAR

This deformity consists of an abnormal protrusion of the pinna with absence of the antihelix. Major degree of the deformity require surgery, the aim is to create an antihelix and thus reduce the prominence of the auricle.

Lop ear is a more severe variant of bat ear.

Anomalies of the External Auditory Canal

The congenital abnormalities of the external auditory canal may present as follows:

i. Complete atresia
ii. Shallow depression
iii. Changes in the curvature of the canal.

These conditions are usually associated with abnormalities of the middle ear. The malformed external canal is usually filled with dense bone, sometimes cartilage and dense fibrous tissue may also be present.

Anomalies of the Middle Ear

The congenital conditions of the middle ear may present as follows:

OSSICULAR DEFORMITIES

Malleus is the most frequently malformed ossicle. It may be fused with the incus or be adherent to the walls of the epitympanum. A similar deformity may involve the incus. The stapes may show the congenital fixation of its foot-plate.

ABNORMAL COURSE OF THE FACIAL NERVE

Congenital dehiscence of the bony canal of the facial nerve may occur and the nerve may take an abnormal course thereby exposing it to trauma during surgery.

MANDIBULOFACIAL DYSOSTOSIS

Congenital atresia in association with other malformations occurs in *mandibulofacial dysostosis* (Treacher-Collins syndrome). The severity of the deformity may vary. The deformation usually involves the structures of the first and second branchial arches. Its usual features include the following:

1. Hypoplasia of the middle third of the face including the malar prominence.
2. Hypoplasia of the mandible.
3. Congenital atresia of the ear with microtia.
4. Ocular deformities like antimongoloid shape of the palpelpebral fissures, notching of the lower eyelids and atrophic lid margins.

TREATMENT OF CONGENITAL ATRESIA OF THE CANAL AND MIDDLE EAR DEFORMITIES

It is very important to know of the deformities beyond the atresia so that the results of surgery can be predicted to some extent. When conventional radiography is of little help, more details are provided by tomography.

Surgical exploration is the treatment of choice. Cases having bilateral congenital atresia should be operated early, usually around 18 months to 2 years. This period corresponds to the timing for acquisition of speech. The cases suffering from unilateral disease develop normal speech, therefore, in such cases surgery can be delayed.

The aim of surgery is to reconstruct the hearing mechanism and to create an external meatus.

Chapter 7

Diseases of the External Ear

The diseases affecting the auricle may be congenital, inflammatory, traumatic or neoplastic.

Perichondritis

It is the inflammation of the perichondrium of the auricular cartilage.

ETIOLOGY

It may be due to infection following trauma of the pinna itself or to the cartilaginous meatus due to spread of infection from a furuncle, or may follow an operative procedure on the ear. Sometimes the infection may follow an insect bite.

CLINICAL FEATURES

The patient complains of burning pain in the ear.

The pinna is red hot, swollen and markedly tender. Since the perichondrium carries the blood supply to the auricular cartilage, it may get necrosed and may crumble producing a deformed pinna (**Fig. 7.1**).

TREATMENT

Systemic antibiotics are given in heavy doses in addition to the analgesics and anti-inflammatory drugs. Magnesium sulphate paste may be applied. If the condition does not respond to conservative treatment and proceeds to abscess formation, then multiple incisions are given to drain the pus and pressure bandage is applied.

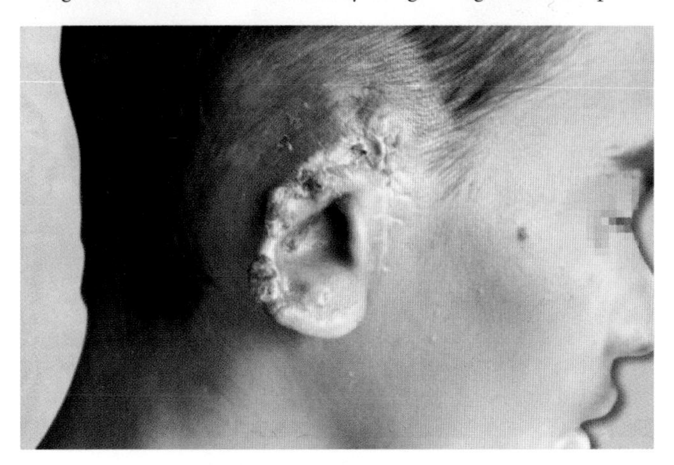

Fig. 7.1: Perichondritis (right pinna)

Hematoma of the Auricle

Trauma to the auricle is common in boxers. This results in formation of a tense fluctuant swelling under the auricular skin. A little collection of blood may not require any treatment except pressure bandage but a big hematoma requires aspiration or incision drainage with pressure dressing to prevent its recurrence. Antibiotics are given to prevent secondary infection. Recurrent injury, particularly, in boxers and wrestlers produces a deformity of the pinna called cauliflower ear or boxer's ear (**Fig. 7.2**).

Frostbite of the Pinna

The pinna being exposed to variations in temperature and the blood vessels being superficial (deep only to the skin), extremes

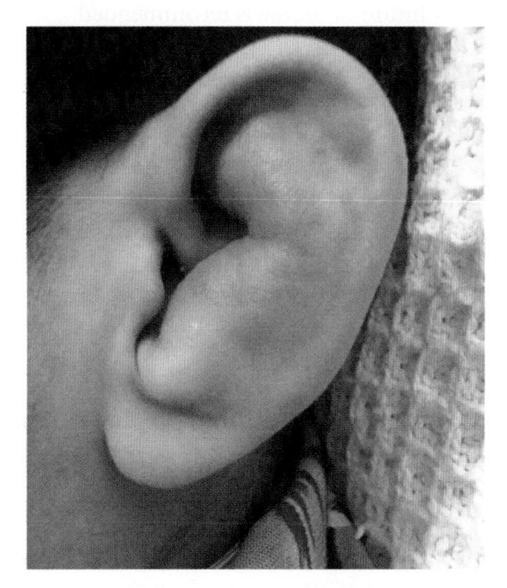

Fig. 7.2: Auricular hematoma

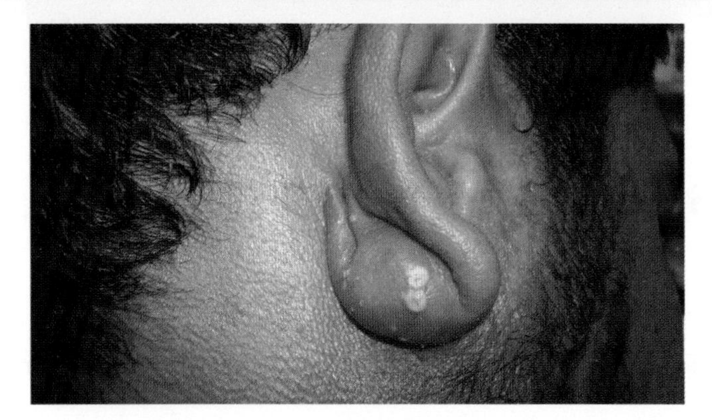

Fig. 7.3: Infected sebaceous cyst of lobule of pinna

of cold affect it readily. Frostbite occurs particularly in the upper and outer portions of the pinna.

TREATMENT

Treatment involves slow thawing. Vasodilator drugs like nicotinic acid and nylidrine are also prescribed (**Fig. 7.3**).

As a preventive measure, exposure to cold should be avoided.

Pseudocyst Pinna

A soft cystic swelling may develop on pinna due to collection of fluid under the skin. There is no definite cyst wall. The exact etiology is not known but possibly this extravasation of fluid is due to trauma of which the patient may be unaware.

TREATMENT

Aspiration or incision drainage under aseptic precuations is done followed by pressure bandage. In case of recurrence, removal of the necrosed cartilage and painting of the wound with a weak solution of iodine is recommended.

Otitis Externa

It is the inflammation of the skin lining the external auditory canal.

Otitis externa may be acute or chronic, and localized (furunculosis) or diffuse. It is also classified as infection and reactive otitis externa.

FURUNCULOSIS

Etiology

It is the staphylococcal infection of the root of the hair follicle and sebaceous gland, occurring in the cartilaginous meatus. The bony meatus is not involved as it does not contain any hair follicles or sebaceous glands.

The infection usually follows trauma to the canal caused by pricking or abrasion at attempts to clean the ear.

Clinical Features

The patients complain of severe pain in the ear. Since there is absence of subcutaneous tissue, the inflammatory exudate produces great pressure on the nerve endings. There may be pain on opening the jaws.

The furuncle produces a red, swollen area in the canal, and may partially obliterate its lumen. The movements of the tragus or any part of the pinna are very painful. Sometimes, the infection can cause cellulitis in the postaural region, obliterating the postaural groove. The auricle stands out forwards and outwards. The infection may lead to perichondritis and postaural lymphadenitis. Usually, there is no deafness and X-ray of the mastoid in doubtful cases shows clarity of air cell system in contrast to mastoiditis.

Treatment

In the early stages, furunculosis is treated by analgesics and hot fomentation. Packing of the canal with gauze soaked in 10 percent icthyol in glycerine is helpful. It reduces the edema and supports the canal wall thus helping to reduce the pain. Most of the cases of furunculosis are helped by the above treatment. Antibiotics are given for severe cases. Penicillinase resistant antibiotics like cloxacillin are preferable. When the abscess is pointing, it needs drainage.

CHRONIC DIFFUSE OTITIS EXTERNA

It is a chronic infection of the ear canal. Acute exacerbations of this condition may occur. The skin of the pinna may also get involved (**Fig. 7.4**).

Etiology

The inflammation of the canal skin may be a part of seborrheic dermatitis or a generalized skin disorder such as eczema. The

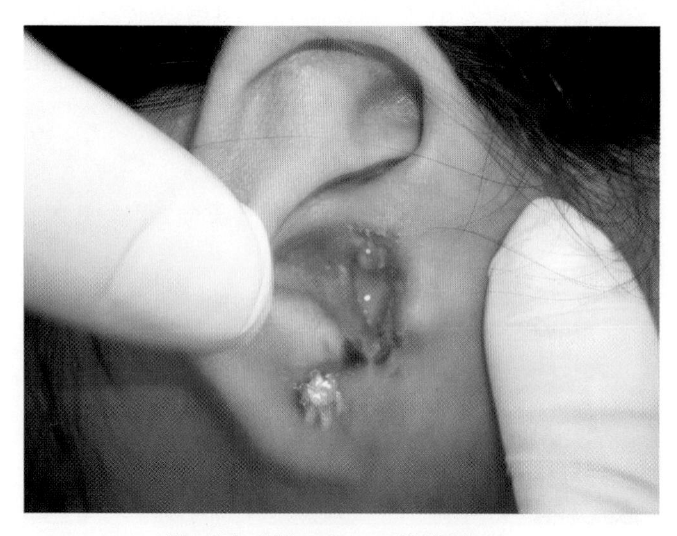

Fig. 7.4: Otitis externa with discharge

discharge of chronic otitis media may irritate the skin of the canal and produce its inflammation. Organisms commonly found are of the gram-negative group such as *Proteus* and *Pseudomonas aeruginosa.*

Clinical Features

The common symptoms of this disease are itching, pain, discharge and excessive desquamation. Sometimes impairment of hearing may also be a complaint.

The canal appears narrowed, and the skin is red, swollen and dry. The epithelial debris may be seen filling the canal. The discharge is scanty, thick and foul smelling.

The tympanic membrane should be examined by gently passing the speculum into the canal. Scalp and other areas of the skin are examined for skin lesions.

Treatment

Local treatment is necessary and very helpful. The debris and discharge are cleaned. A piece of ribbon gauze soaked in any antibiotic-hydrocortisone preparation is put in the canal and frequently changed. Antibiotic-hydrocortisone drops are used for a few weeks. Systemic antibiotics may be prescribed for a few days initially. Water is avoided in the ear. The canal wall should not be traumatized. Attention is given to the underlying or associated skin disease.

Otomycosis

ETIOLOGY

It is a fungal infection of the ear. The common fungi involved are *Aspergillus niger*, *Aspergillus fumigatus* and *Candida albicans*. The disease is more frequent during the rainy season as the increase in humidity leads to the rapid growth of the fungus. The condition may follow from swimming in infected water.

CLINICAL FEATURES

Itching and irritation in the ear are common. The patient may complain of discomfort in the ear which may amount to actual pain. Sometimes a scanty discharge is also present.

The canal wall is hyperemic and the fungal debris is seen in the canal with some discharge.

Aspergillus niger produces black colonies and *Candida albicans* presents as white granules resembling wet blotting paper. When the debris is removed, then tympanic membrane looks normal.

TREATMENT

The fungal debris is cleaned. Local applications of nystatin in glycerine drops or other local fungicidal preparations like clotrimazole are helpful. Two percent salicylic acid in alcohol drops is keratolytic and may be prescribed after removal of the fungal debris.

Malignant Otitis External

ETIOLOGY

This is a fulminating, severe form of otitis externa, particularly seen in elderly people and diabetic patients. The causative organism is usually *Pseudomonas aeruginosa.*

CLINICAL FEATURES

The production behaves like a malignant process and causes destruction of the tissues of the canal, preauricular and postauricular tissue, and may cause facial nerve paralysis.

TREATMENT

Heavy doses of antibiotics like gentamicin or carbenicillin, local cleaning and debridement of necrotic tissues and control of the underlying diabetes are recommended.

Keratosis Obturans (Canal Wall Cholesteatoma)

ETIOLOGY

The condition is due to abnormal desquamation of the epithelium in the deep external auditory canal.

CLINICAL FEATURES

The desquamated epithelium assumes properties similar to cholesteatoma and causes bony erosion of the canal wall with destruction of surrounding tissues.

- The condition may be associated with chronic bronchitis or bronchiectasis.
- The patients may present with deafness or pain.

TREATMENT

Periodical removal of this mass of desquamated epithelium is done preferably under general anesthesia.

Foreign Bodies in the External Auditory Canal

Foreign bodies in the ear are common in children who may put beads, peanuts, beans, pieces of lead pencil (inanimate), etc. into the ear. Grains of maize and paddy are commonly found both in children and adults particularly during the harvest season. Live insects like bedbugs, mosquitoes and cockroaches (animate) may enter the ear. Flies may lay eggs in patient with CSOM which hatch out to form maggots.

CLINICAL FEATURES

The patient may present with pain in the ear and deafness. Injury may occur to the canal wall or the tympanic membrane by the foreign body itself or by improper attempts at its removal.

TREATMENT

1. A living foreign body may be killed by instilling some oily drops into the ear. This suffocates and kills the insect which can be then removal by forceps or syringe.
2. Metallic foreign bodies, glass beads and small-sized foodgrains may be removed by syringing.

If the foreign body is in the outer part of the canal, an ear hook may be useful for its removal by expert with the patient in the proper position.

The foreign bodies lying deep in the meatus in children and in patients who are apprehensive are removed under general anesthesia. Impacted foreign bodies may need a postaural approach for removal.

Impacted Wax in the External Canal

Wax is a mixture of secretions of the ceruminous and sebaceous glands of the external auditory canal. It also contains shedded epithelium and dust particles.

CLINICAL FEATURES

The wax may get accumulated and impacted in the canal wall producing symptoms of deafness, discomfort, itching and pain. The pain occurs because of pressure on the nerve endings. Tinnitus and vertigo may occur.

The external canal shows a dark brown plug of wax filling the canal and obscuring the view of the tympanic membrane.

TREATMENT

The wax may be removed with a curette or by syringing. Hard wax may be softened by using oily substances, sodium bicarbonate in glycerine drops or by a number of other wax solvents instilled for a few days before syringing. Removal with curette (Jobson-Horne probe). The curette should be used gently without traumatizing the ear canal. The tip of the curette should be kept in view to avoid blind digging in the canal or damaging the tympanic membrane.

Syringing: Syringing of the ear may be necessary to remove the wax or a foreign body. It should not be done if there is perforation of the tympanic membrane or a history of ear discharge.

The patient is seated in a proper position with the head stabilized and suitably drapped to prevent water spilling on his clothes. The water for irrigation (usually tap water) is brought to the body temperature. A proper sized syringe is filled with this water and the jet of water from the nozzle is directed along the posterosuperior canal wall. The fluid and the debris are collected in the kidney-shaped tray held below the ear. A few syringefuls of fluid may be needed for proper removal of the wax. If the wax or foreign body is directly hit by the stream of water, it moves deeper and may get impacted. Excessive force used while syringing may damage the canal wall or the tympanic membrane. If the water used is not at body temperature, it produces caloric stimulation with symptoms of giddiness and vomiting. The canal should be mopped dry after syringing.

Bullous Myringitis

ETIOLOGY

Myringitis bullosa is a viral infection characterized by formation of vesicles on the tympanic membrane and on the adjacent skin of the deep meatus.

CLINICAL FEATURES

The main symptom is severe pain the ear. Otoscopy reveals a congested tympanic membrane with vesicles on its surface, commonly in the upper part. The membrane is mobile.

TREATMENT

Treatment is symptomatic by analgesics. In some cases, a picture of encephalitis may develop a complication. No attempt should be made to puncture the vesicles.

Traumatic Perforations of the Tympanic Membrane

ETIOLOGY

Perforation of the tympanic membrane may occur due to foreign bodies usually pointed objects, and improper curetting or syringing. The damage may also occur due to direct violence like a slap or in blast injuries. The membrane may get damaged in head injury.

CLINICAL FEATURES

The patient complains of pain the ear, deafness and sometimes blood-stained discharge.

Examination reveals the perforation with ragged edges and the membrane may show areas of ecchymosis.

TREATMENT

If the patient is seen shortly after injury, the external canal is packed with a sterile cotton plug. Systemic antibiotics and decongestant drops in the nose are used to prevent infection of the middle ear through the eustachian tube.

No topical drops are used in the ear. The perforation usually heals by itself. Sometimes cautery, patching or myringoplasty may be needed.

Chapter 8

Diseases of the Eustachian Tube

Acute Salpingitis (Acute Tubal Catarrh)

It usually follows acute rhinitis and leads to acute otitis media if not treated well in time. The epithelial lining of the tube becomes congested and edematous resulting in tubal blockage without involving the middle ear.

CLINICAL FEATURES

The patient complains of blockage of the ear. On swallowing, the feeling of blockage is temporarily relieved. There may be occasional earache.

Symptoms continue as long as the nasal catarrh persists and clear up when the cold settles down.

TREATMENT

Rest in a ventilated room, nasal decongestants and antihistaminics are all which are needed. Treatment of acute rhinitis and improvement in the general health hastens the recovery.

Chronic Salpingitis

It presents with chronic tubal obstruction without any active disease in the tympanic cavity.

The predisposing factors include adenoiditis, chronic infection in the nose and sinuses, and nasal allergy.

CLINICAL FEATURES

The presenting symptom is intermittent deafness with discomfort. Otoscopy shows a retracted tympanic membrane that does not move on Valsalva's maneuver. The tuning form test and audiogram show mild to moderate conductive deafness.

TREATMENT

Any infection or allergy is to be controlled. Nasal decongestants and antihistaminics should be prescribed.

Politzerisation or eustachian catheterisation is done after the infection has been controlled.

Myringotomy with grommet insertion may be needed for middle ear aeration.

Adenoidectomy in children is done to prevent recurrence.

Chapter

9

Acute Suppurative Otitis Media and Acute Mastoiditis

Acute Suppurative Otitis Media

Acute suppurative otitis media is a pyogenic bacterial infection of the middle ear. It is a common disorder occurring at all ages and particularly in children.

ETIOLOGY

The predisposing factors include the following:

i. Nasopharyngeal or nasal packs
ii. Adenoids
iii. High deviated nasal septum
iv. Nasal polypi
v. Rhinitis and sinusitis
vi. Tumors of the nose and nasopharynx
vii. *Anatomical factor:* Short, straight and wide Eustachian tube in young children.
viii. Carelessness on the part of mother in keeping the baby in a flat position while feeding, thus allowing milk to regurgitate into the nasopharynx and to the middle ear cavity through the eustachian tube.

Eustachian tube is the most common route by which infection travels from the nose and nasopharynx to the middle ear. The attack usually follows a common cold or influenza. The viral infection damages the mucosal barrier and bacteria invade as secondary organisms. The most common organisms include *Haemophilus influenzae*, *Pneumococcus* (particularly in infants, diabetics, and in the aged), *Moraxella catarrhalis*, *beta haemolytic Streptococci*, *Staphylococcus aureus*, nonhemolytic *Streptococcus*, etc.

The other path through which infection may reach the middle ear is a traumatic perforation in the tympanic membrane.

Sometimes infection of the middle ear may follow an imperfectly sterile operative procedure on the middle ear.

PATHOLOGY AND CLINICAL PRESENTATION

Various stages which occur during this disease process are the following:

Stage of tympanic congestion: The mucoperiosteum of middle ear reacts to the invading organism by hyperemia. During this stage, the patient complains of pain and sensation of fullness in the ear. The tympanic membrane looks congested. There occurs no significant hearing loss at this stage. **Figures 9.1 and 9.2** show normal and inflamed tympanic membranes respectively.

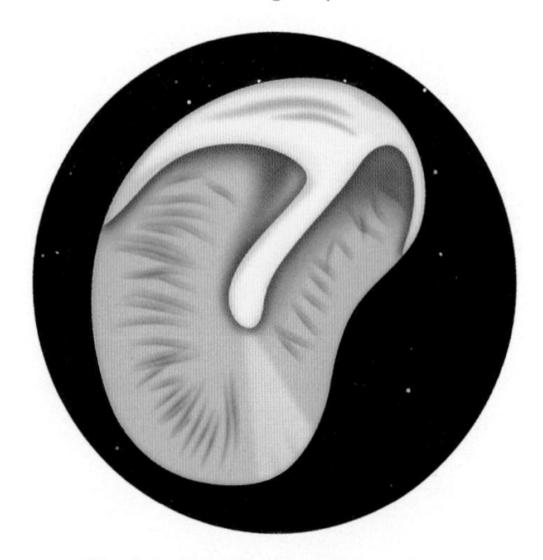

Fig. 9.1: Normal tympanic membrane

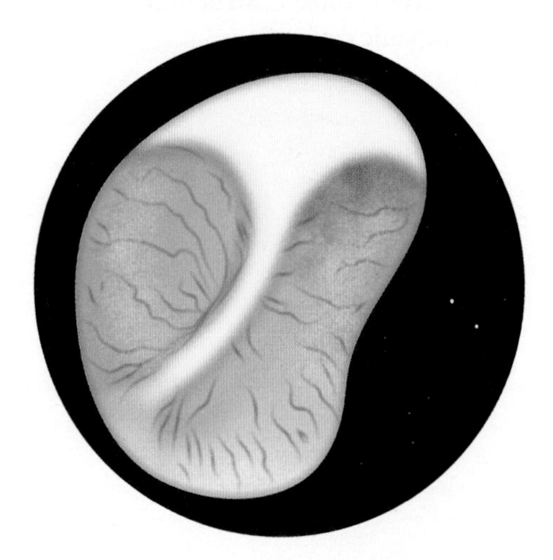

Fig. 9.2: Acute otitis media

Stage of exudation: As the inflammatory process progresses, an exudate collects in the tympanic cavity. The patient complains of marked pain in the ear with deafness. The tympanic membrane shows bulging and looks more congested. Constitutional symptoms like fever and malaise occur.

Stage of suppuration: The pent up inflammatory exudate causes pressure necrosis and perforation of the tympanic membrane. The perforation is central. The intensity of pain diminishes but hearing loss persists. The mucosa of the middle ear if seen through the perforation is much congested and thickened. The discharge is serosanguinous at the onset and mucopurulent later on. **Figures 9.3A to D** show various types of tympanic membrane perforations.

Radiological examination of the mastoid at this stage shows clouding of the air cells but the bony partitions between the air cells remain intact.

Stage of convalescence or recovery: The disease starts subsiding and the recovery process begins. However, in case where proper treatment is not instituted and also depending upon the severity of infection and individual resistance, the disease process may involve the mastoid air cells.

Stage of acute mastoiditis: Continued infection in absence of the proper therapy causes hyperemia and thickening of the mucoperiosteum, thus impeding the drainage of secretions and promoting stasis. Hyperemic decalcification of the wals of the mastoid air cells causes the smaller air cells to coalesce into large cavities and this leads to bony erosion.

SYMPTOMS

The pain in the ear which had diminished in intensity following the stage of superuration intensifies with increase

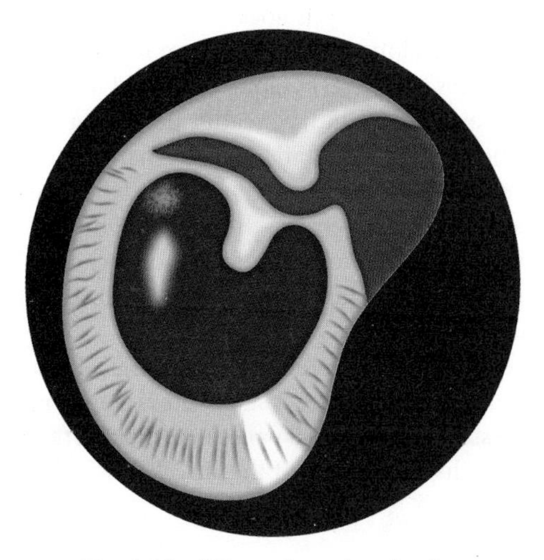

Fig. 9.3A: Kidney-shaped perforation

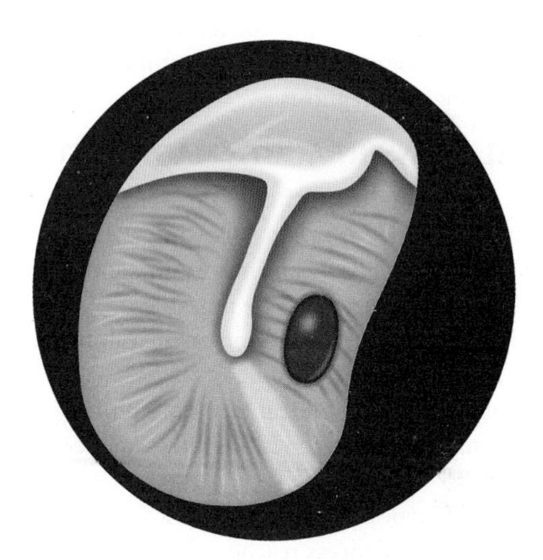

Fig. 9.3B: Small central perforation

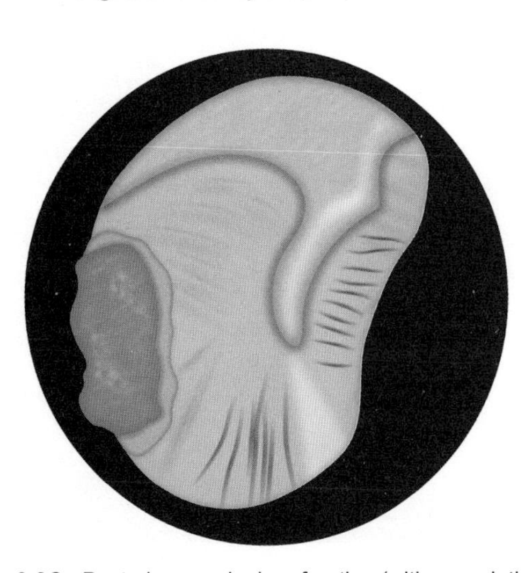

Fig. 9.3C: Posterior marginal perforation (with granulations)

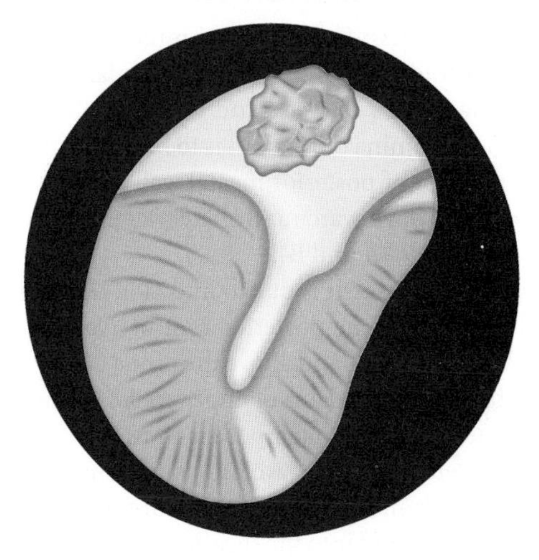

Fig. 9.3D: Attic perforation (with cholesteatoma)

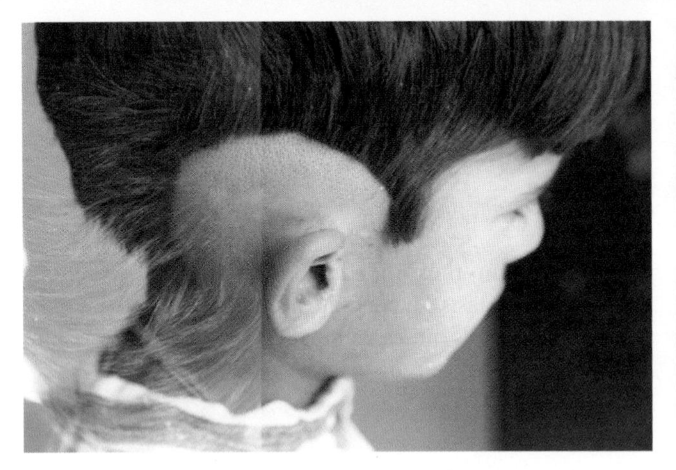

Fig. 9.4A: Mastoid abscess right ear

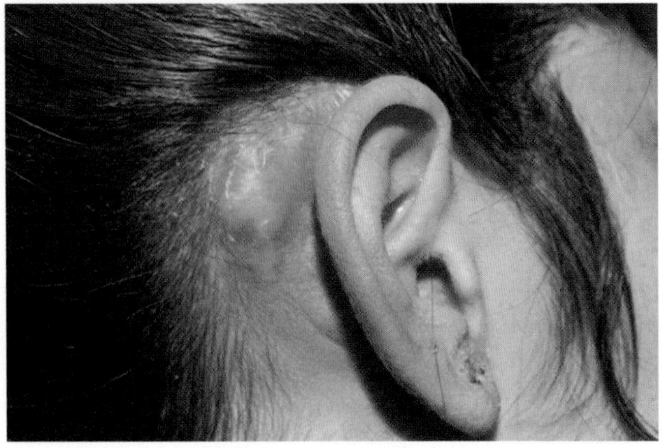

Fig. 9.4B: Postaural abscess

in deafness and profuse discharge continues to drain from the ear. Constitutional symptoms like fever and bodyache recur. Diagnosis is radiological with X-ray mastoids or CT temporal bone confirming the diagnosis.

CLINICAL SIGNS IN ACUTE MASTOIDITIS

Ear discharge, usually profuse, purulent or creamy, for more than two weeks duration following an attack of acute suppurative otitis media is an important sign of coalescent mastoiditis. The discharge may be pulsatile.

Sagging of the posterosuperior canal wall occurs due to periostitis adjacent to the antrum.

The mucosa of the middle ear through a central perforation of the tympanic membrane, if visible, shows marked congestion and thickening.

Mastoid tenderness is another significant sign that occurs as the inflammatory process reaches the cortex.

ABSCESSES IN RELATION TO MASTOIDITIS

i. *Postaural abscess:* This is most common form presenting over mastoid. In young children and infants pus collects over Macewen's triangle and can pass along vascular channel of lamina cribrosa. It is to be differentiated from furunculosis of posterior meatal wall as it pushes pinna forwards to downwards and obliterates the retroauricular sulcus (**Figs 9.4A and B**).

ii. *Zygomatic abscess:* It is due to infection of zygomatic air cells situated at the posterior root of zygoma. Swelling appears in front of and above the pinna (**Fig. 9.5**). There may be associated edema of upper eyelid. Pus here colelcts superficial or deep to temporalis muscle.

iii. *Bezold's abscess:* Here, swelling is present in the upper part of neck and it forms because of pus going through the tip of mastoid into the sheath of sternocleidomastoid muscle or via the digastric muscle to the chin.

iv. *Citelli's abscess:* The abscess is found in the digastric triangle of neck, as pus goes throught the inner table of mastoid tip along posterior belly of digastric muscle.

v. *Meatal abscess:* Here, swelling is formed in the deep part of the external auditory meatus, pus going through the wall between antrum and bony external auditory meatus.

vi. *Retromastoid abscess:* It is formed behind the mastoid along mastoid emissary vein, on the occipitotemporal suture.

Constitutional symptoms like fever, bodyache, malaise and loss of appetite are the other accompanying features of the acute mastoid infection.

Deafness is usually conductive. Radiological examination of the mastoid in the coalescent stage shows clouding of the air cells with destruction of all cell partitions, thus there occurs loss of clarity and distinctiveness of the air cells.

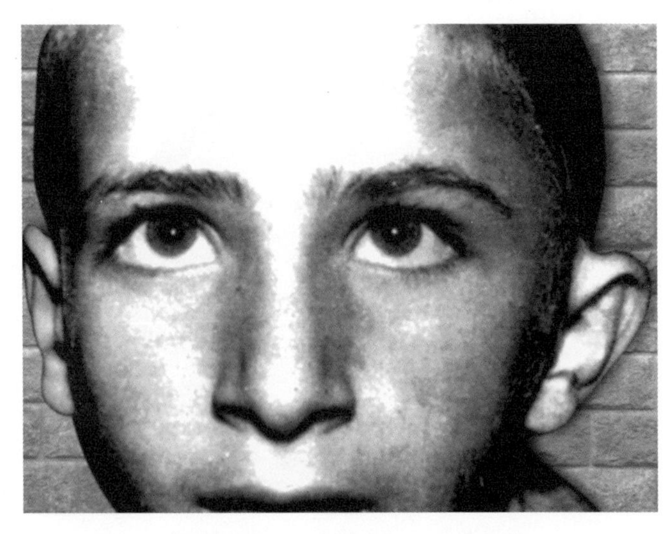

Fig. 9.5: Zygomatic abscess left side

The coalescent stage if not treated may lead to the complications.

TREATMENT

Acute suppurative otitis media: In the initial stages of the disease, nasal decongestants, antihistaminics, analgesics and antibiotics like amoxicillin, ampiclox or cephalosporins are given for about 1 to 2 weeks time to cure the disease. Attention should be given to any nasal or nasopharyngeal pathology.

During the stage of exudation when the pain is severe and the drum appears bulging, *myringotomy* is advisable besides the conservative line of treatment as described above. Myringotomy provides drainage to the pent-up secretions and relieves the pain without the tissue necrosis of the tympanic membrane. Besides the systemic antibiotics (preferably following a culture sensitivity test of the ear discharge), the external canal should be cleaned of the discharge by suction or dry mopping and local antibiotic drops instilled.

Mastoid surgery is reserved for those who start to develop a subperiosteal abscess, any other complications or show no response after 48 hours of intravenous antibiotic therapy.

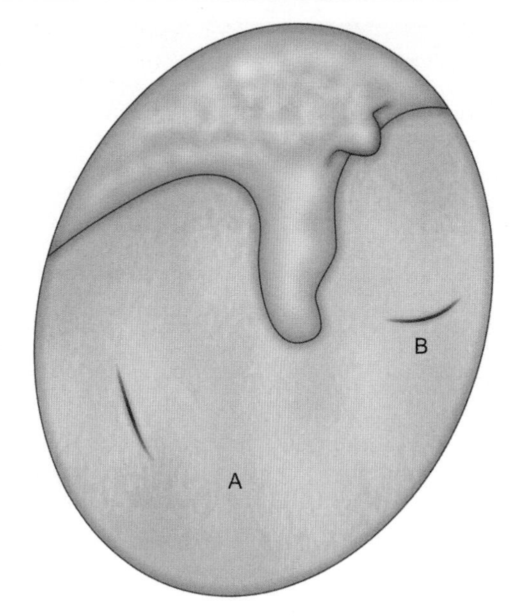

Fig. 9.6: Myringotomy incision: (A) Posteroinferior quadrant. (B) Anterosuperior quadrant

Myringotomy

INDICATIONS

The common indications of this procedure are the following:

1. Cute suppurative otitis media, particularly during exudative stage when the drum is bulging or the patient has severe pain.
2. In cases where deafness persists even after apparent control of acute suppurative otitis media.
3. In secretory otitis media, for aeration of the middle ear (grommet insertion) and removal of secretions.
4. In adhesive otitis media—for aeration.
5. Aero-otitis media.
6. In Ménière's disease, myringotomy sometimes gives dramatic relief though the exact mechanism is not known.

PROCEDURE

It should be performed under the operating microscope under general anesthesia. There are two types of incisions—posterior myringotomy and anterior myringotomy incisions (**Fig. 9.6**).

Posterior myringotomy: A J-shaped incision is made in posteroinferior quadrant of the tympanic membrane as this is most accessible area, is relatively less vascular and there are less chances of damage to the ossicular chain. In cute otitis media small 3-4 mm incision is generally all that is required.

Anterior myringotomy: This is done for the insertion of grommets and for facilitating aspiration of serous effusion by providing a second opening in secretory otitis media (**Fig. 9.7**).

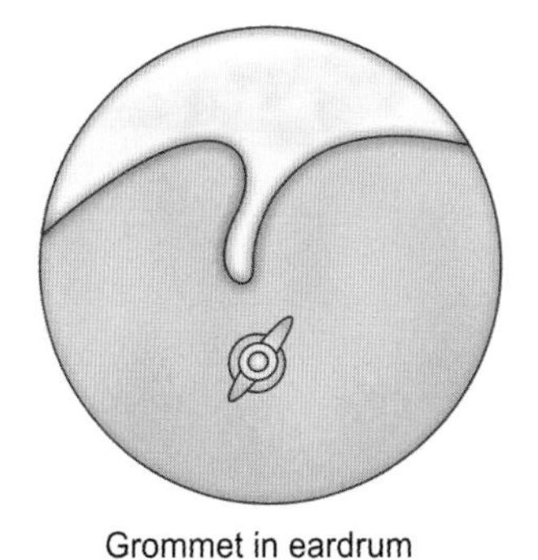

Grommet in eardrum

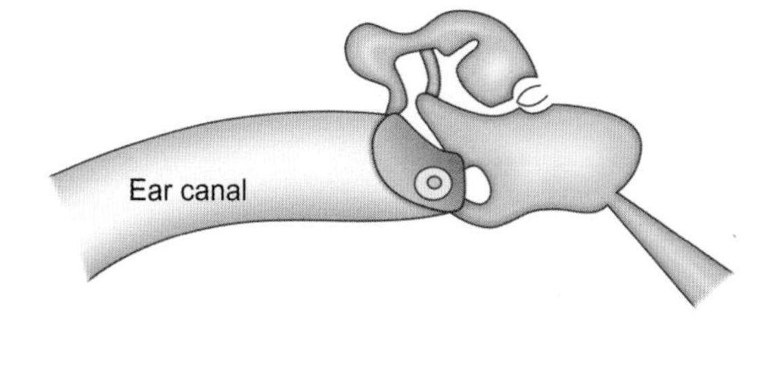

Grommet tube seen in cross section

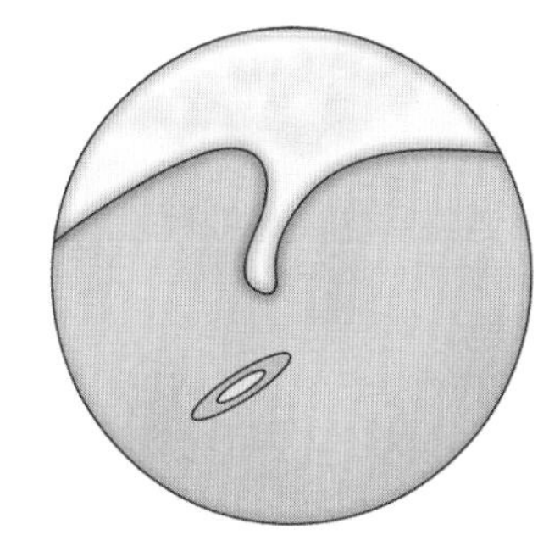

Insertion of grommet

Fig. 9.7: Grommet tube seen in cross-section

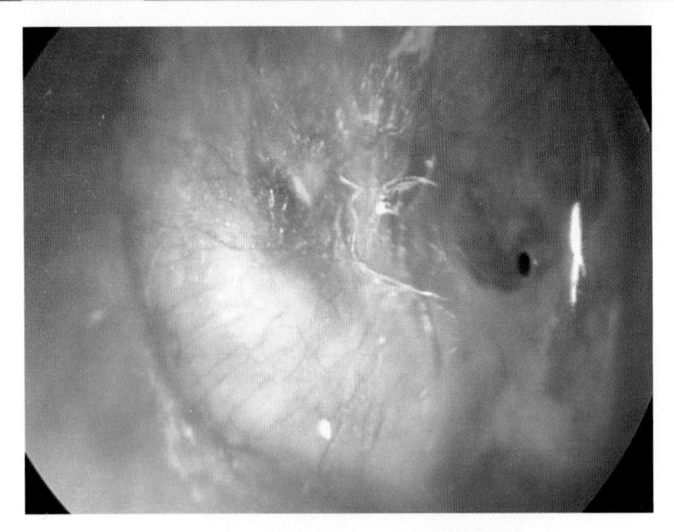

Fig. 9.8: Pin hole perforation of tympanic membrane

POSTOPERATIVE CARE

In cases of purulent discharge drainage is encouraged by daily mopping. Medication with antibiotics, and nasal decongestants are prescribed (**Fig. 9.8**).

If a grommet has been introduced, the patient is warned against getting water into the ears (**Fig. 9.9**). The grommet usually gets extruded after 6 to 8 months.

COMPLICATIONS

These include incudostapedial joint dislocation, injury to the chorda tympani nerve, and injury to the jugular bulb which may be projecting into the middle ear due to a dehiscence in its floor.

GRADENIGO'S SYNDROME

This symptom complex occurs when the process of acute mastoiditis involves the cell tracts leading to petrous apx and causing petrositis. The presenting features include otorrhea, trigeminal neuralgia (headache, retro-orbital pain) and sixth nerve palsy. This is probably due to edema involving the sixth nerve in the *Dorello's caal.*

TREATMENT

This includes mastoid exploration and exenteration of the cell tracts leading to petrous apex.

MASKED MASTOIDITIS

Those cases of acute mastoiditis which do not present with the typical symptoms and signs are grouped under the term *masked or latent mastoiditis.* This is usually the result of inadequate treatment with antibiotics, which slow the process but do not completely check the disease. The acute symptoms subside but the patient is not completely well. There is a dull aching pain with some amount of deafness and low grade fever. On examination, the tympanic membrane shows an inflammatory thickening and congestion of the tympanic mucosa is evident. Some amount of postaural periosteal thickening with mastoid tenderness is present. Radiological examination reveals the coalescent process of the mastoid.

Treatment

Treatment is cortical mastoidectomy.

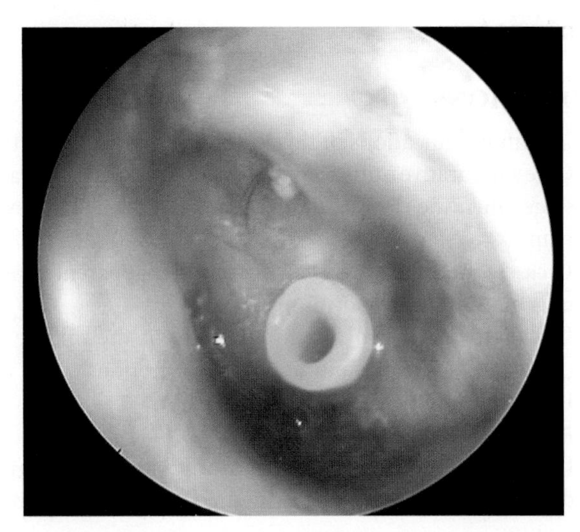

Fig. 9.9: Grommet in posteroinferior quadrant

Chapter 10

Chronic Suppurative Otitis Media

Chronic suppurative otitis media (CSOM) is a chronic inflammatory process involving the middle ear cleft producing irreversible pathological changes. It is of two types: The tubotympanic type and the atticoantral type.

Tubotympanic Type (Safe Type)

This is a benign type of CSOM confined only to the middle ear cleft.

PATHOLOGY

1. *Persistent mucosal disease:* Infection reaches the middle ear either through the eustachian tube or through a perforated tympanic membrane. Repeated infection of middle ear leads to hyperplasia of its mucosa. These hyperplastic mucosal proliferations trap the infection which is responsible for its chronicity. In some cases especially in sclerotic mastoids, mucosal proliferation leads to polyp formation (**Figs 10.1A and B**).
2. *Cholesterol granuloma:* The middle ear gets ventilated through the eustachian tube. When there is mucosal hypertrophy, it may block the posterior portion of the tympanum, thus creating vacuum which leads to extravasation of blood into the middle ear. This provokes a foreign body reaction resulting in the formation of cholesterol granuloma. The tympanic membrane appears blue in this condition.

Blue-drum is progressive middle ear deafness accompanied by blue-gray discoloration of the drum head and cloudiness of the mastoid cells on X-ray, caused by the accumulation of a dark brown slimy fluid or "sludge" in the middle ear and mastoid process. There is also an extremely vascular granulation tissue containing numerous cholesterol crystals, blood pigments, and giant cells. It occurs in cellular mastoids. Forster described such cases in children first in 1947.

The blood cholesterol level is raised to over 300 mg/100 ml. The condition usually arises in the posterosuperior part of the middle ear filling the attic. Swab culture is usually found to be sterile.

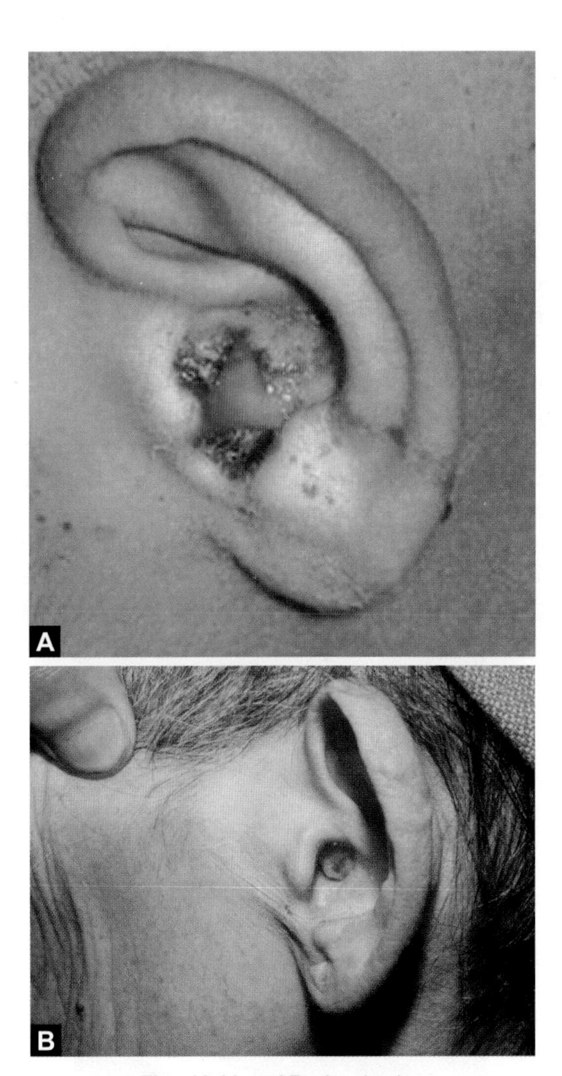

Figs 10.1A and B: Aural polyp

Tubotympanic type of CSOM may further be subdivided into two types:

1. *Tubal type:* In this variety, the infection ascends through the eustachian tube and the underlying cause of infection lies either in the nose, sinuses or the nasopharynx. This type is

usually seen in children from the low socioeconomic strata and often involves both ears.

2. *Tympanic type:* In this variety, the infection reaches the middle ear through a defect in the tympanic membrane, usually a large central perforation (persistent perforation syndrome). This is usually seen in adults and often involves one ear only. There is usually profuse discharge which responds to antibiotics and recurs with the introduction of water into the ear.

The author has removed one *Ascaris lumbricoides* from the middle ear cavity of a girl of 8 year age, coming out of the perforation of the tympanic membrane due to CSOM. The Ascaris had crawled up from upper respiratory tract (**Fig. 10.2**).

CLINICAL FEATURES

1. *Tubal type:* There is profuse bilateral mucopurulent discharge with a running nose.

   On examination, the external auditory canal is seen full of mucopurulent discharge and there is usually an anterior perforation of the tympanic membrane. On nasal examination, a deviated nasal septum, features of sinusitis or adenoids may be seen.

   Pure tone audiometry reveals mild-to-moderate hearing loss.
2. *Tympanic type:* It is usually seen in adults who complain of deafness and repeated infection of the ear. On examination, discharge is seen in the external auditory canal. A large central defect is visible in the tympanic membrane. Granulations and polypi may be seen in the middle ear. These patients complain of improved hearing when the external auditory canal is full of pus, which deteriorates when the pus is mopped off. This is because pus seals the defect of the tympanic membrane so that the transmission of sound waves is better in the presence of pus.

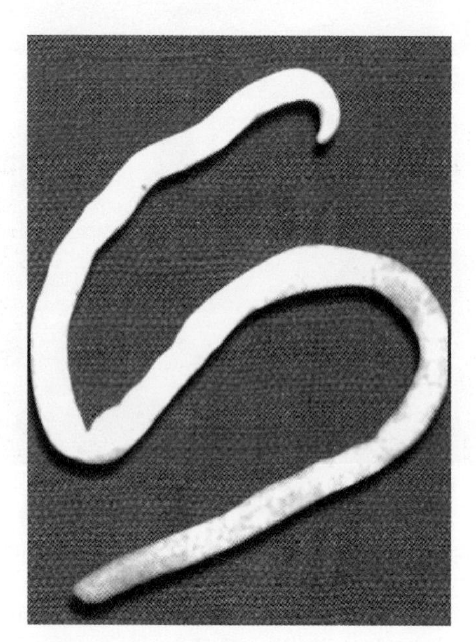

Fig. 10.2: *Ascaris lumbricoides* removed from the middle ear cavity of a girl

Patch test: A cigarette paper or a piece of gelfoam is placed on the tympanic membrane perforation and the patient asked if he hears better. If the hearing improves it means that the patient will be benefited by myringoplasty alone.

INVESTIGATIONS

1. Tuning fork tests and pure tone audiometry is done for hearing assessment.
2. Culture sensitivity test of the discharge helps in selection of proper antibiotics.
3. X-ray of the mastoids and paranasal sinuses may be needed in some cases.
4. Examination of the ear under microscope.

TREATMENT OF TUBOTYMPANIC DISEASE

The aim of the treatment is to control the infection, treat the underlying cause, keep the ear dry and finally reconstruct the hearing mechanism.

1. *Treatment of underlying cause:* Proper attention should be paid to any abnormality of the nose, paranasal sinuses and nasopharynx, and if found, it should be adequately treated.
2. *Aural toilet:* Daily aural toilet is an essential step for keeping the ear dry. This may be done by dry mopping, i.e. cleaning the ear with a sterile cotton tipped probe. Aural toilet is better performed under the microscope and the ear examined in detail for any pathology that may otherwise be missed by the naked eye.
3. *Culture sensitivity:* Culture sensitivity of the discharge is done to select proper antibiotics. Both systemic as well as local antibiotics are used. Local antibiotics are used as ear drops and include neomycin, gentamicin, quinolones and chloramphenicol with or without hydrocortisone.

SURGICAL MANAGEMENT (TUBOTYMPANIC TYPE)

The aim of surgery is to provide a safe, dry and a hearing ear.

1. *Adenoidectomy, septoplasty and antrum* washes may be required in some cases, where the predisposing factors are in the nose and paranasal air sinuses.
2. *Aural polypectomy:* Aural polypectomy should be done under general anesthesia using the microscope. The aural polyp should be removed with utmost care as it may be attached to the oval or round window or the facial nerve.
3. *Myringoplasty:* When the ear has become dry, the tympanic membrane defect should be sealed off so as to prevent further infection of the middle ear as well as to improve the hearing.

MYRINGOPLASTY

Pre-requisites for Myringoplasty

1. The ear should be dry for at least six weeks before myringoplasty is done.
2. The eustachian tube should be patent.
3. There should be no focus of infection in the nose, paranasal sinuses and nasopharynx.
4. There should be an adequate cochlear reserve.

Advantages of Myringoplasty

1. To prevent further infection of ear.
2. To improve the hearing or to prevent further deterioration in hearing.
3. To prevent complications.
4. To prevent tympanosclerosis (drying effect of air has been implicated as an etiological factor for tympanosclerosis).

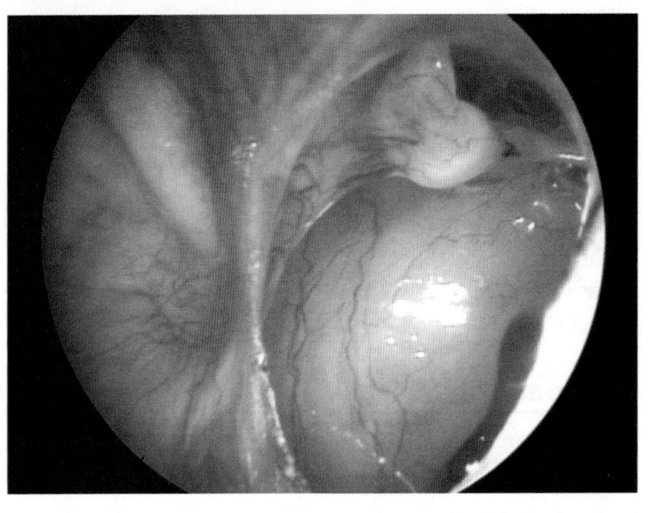

Fig. 10.3: Posterior TM perforation incudostapedial joint is visualized

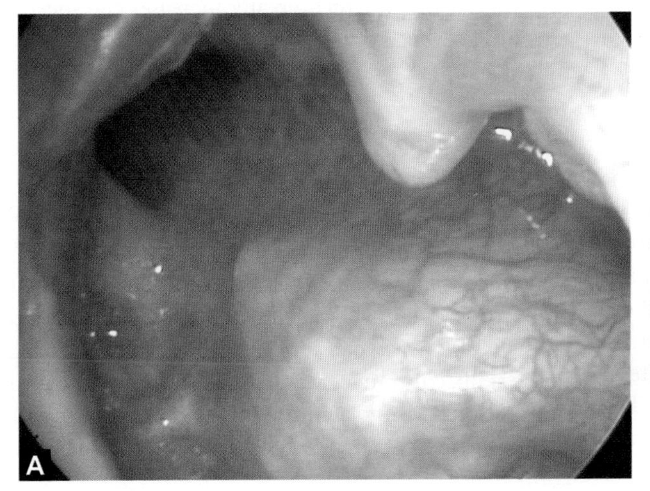

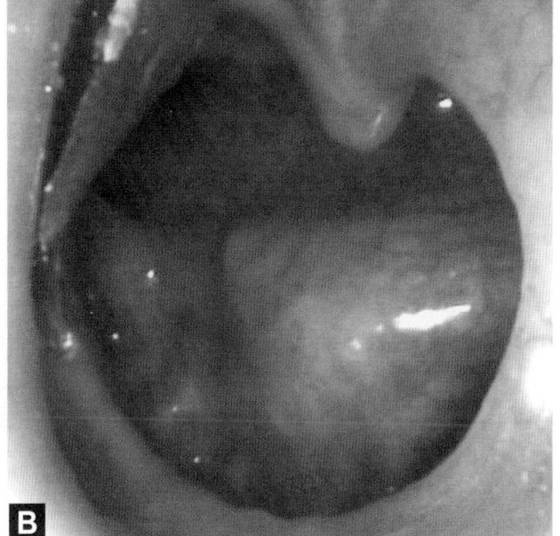

Figs 10.4A and B: Subtotal TM perforation

5. To enable proper fitting of the hearing aid.
6. To enable recruitment in certain professions.

Graft Material

The temporalis fascia is the most commonly used material for myringoplasty. To obtain this, an incision is made in the postaural groove just above the pinna. The incision goes right through skin and superficial fascia exposing the underlying temporalis fascia. It becomes easy to dissect the fascia if normal saline is injected under it, which separates it from the muscle. The fascia is then allowed to dry up before use. Temporalis fascia has also been successfully used as a homograft by preserving a large piece of fascia in 70 percent alcohol or in 0.02% aqueous cinlit preservative and using it in a number of cases.

Tragal perichondrium and homograft tympanic membrane are also used by some.

Procedure (Figs 10.3 and 10.4)

Onlay technique: The bed for the graft is prepared by elevating the canal skin adjacent to the annulus and the outer squamous epithelial layer of the drum remnant. The graft is applied and kept in position by gel foam soaked in antibiotic solution.

Inlay (underlay) technique: This is suitable for a large posterior perforation especially when the anterior remnant is thin and atrophic. The rim of the perforation is removed and adjacent mucosa is sacrificed. The tympanic membrane remnant along with the annulus is lifted anteriorly. The middle ear is packed with gel foam soaked in antibiotic solution. Then the graft is placed under the tympanic membrane remnants, posteriorly it lies over the canal wall.

Postoperative Care

Antibiotics and nasal decongestants are prescribed.

If the underlay technique has been used the patient is instructed to do the Valsalva maneuver from the second day to facilitate contact between the graft and the bed. The gauze pack is removed on the 10th day, and gel foam is removed after 3 weeks.

Atticoantral Disease (Unsafe Type)

The atticoantral disease involves the attic, antrum and the posterior tympanum. An important feature of this variety is that it is a bone-eroding disease, therefore, exposes the adjacent structures with resultant complications and hence it is termed dangerous or unsafe variety of chronic suppurative otitis media (**Fig. 10.5**). The main pathological feature is the formation of "cholesteatoma" and the inflammatory granulation tissue which cause erosion of the bone.

CHOLESTEATOMA

This term is a misnomer for neither is it a tumor nor does it necessarily contains cholesterol crystals. Cholesteatoma is a sac of keratinized desquamated epithelium in the middle ear cleft, resting on a fibrous tissue layer called the matrix. The constant desquamation of the keratinized epithelium causes accumulation of epithelial debris in the middle ear cavity which becomes secondarily infected. In simpler terms, cholesteatoma is squamous epithelium in an abnormal site in the middle ear which possesses bone-eroding properties. The bone erosion is due to two things: (a) Pressure effects produced by bone remodeling, (b) Enzymatic activity at the margins of the cholesteatoma which greatly increases the speed of bone erosion. The levels of these osteoclastic enzymes increase in the presence of bacterial infection (**Fig. 10.6**).

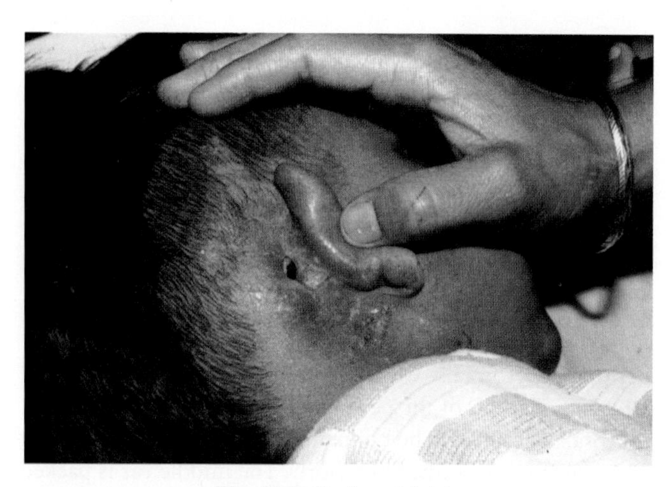

Fig. 10.5: Postaural fistula

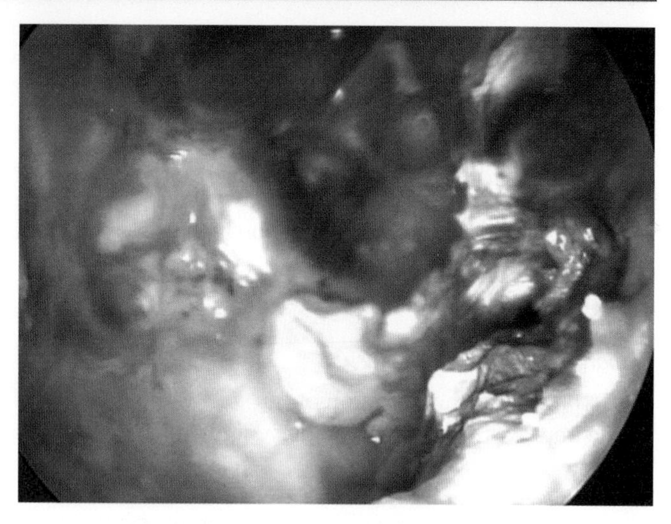

Fig. 10.6: Attic retraction with cholesteatoma

Classification

Cholesteatoma is classified as congenital or acquired.

The acquired variety is further divided into primary acquired cholesteatoma, and secondary acquired cholesteatoma.

Congenital cholesteatoma: Cholesteatoma is thought to be of embryonic origin. It is believed that during development, epithelial cell nests get trapped in the parietal bone or elsewhere in the skull, continue to desquamate and enlarge causing bony destruction. It is most commonly found in the middle ear or within the temporal bone particularly the petrous apex. CT is confirmatory.

Primary acquired cholesteatoma: In this variety, the cholesteatoma occurs in the attic or in the posterior part of the tympanic cavity, where there has not been any predisposing chronic otitis media.

Secondary acquired cholesteatoma: In this variety, the cholesteatoma develops in the ears which have suffered from the active chronic disease with defects in the tympanic membrane.

Etiology of Primary Acquired Cholesteatoma

The exact cause for the development of cholesteatoma is not yet known. The following theories have been put forward:

1. *Metaplasia:* Because of repeated infections, squamous metaplasia of the low cuboidal epithelium of the middle ear occurs, which subsequently leads to development of cholesteatoma. This theory did not find much favor.
2. *Immigration theory:* It is believed that cholesteatoma is derived from the immigration of squamous epithelium

from the deep meatal wall and tympanic membrane, though the precise mechanism is not known. Some authors believe that it is the special growth potential of the squamous epithelium of the membrane and deep meatal wall along with the presence of embryonal connective tissue in a relatively acellular mastoid, which leads to the formation of cholesteatoma. They believe that recurrent acute middle ear infection in childhood acts as a stimulus for the process of cholesteatoma formation.

3. *Invagination theory:* Tumarkin suggests that as a result of inadequate ventilation in the attic because of infantile otitis, there occurs a collapse and invagination of the pars flaccida and thus a dimple formation results. Gradually, the squamous epithelium goes on collecting in this pocket and the sac enlarges forming a cholesteatoma.

Clinical Features

The main complaint in an uncomplicated ear is of discharge and deafness. The discharge is purulent, foul smelling and scanty in amount, occasionally blood stained. The deafness is of slow onset, progressive, and may be associated with tinnitus. However, the development of earache, vertigo, vomiting and headache signify the onset of complications. The tympanic membrane reveals an attic perforation, or a posterosuperior marginal perforation and granulations which are reddish in color, unlike the pale polypoidal mucosa of tubotympanic variety. The fistula sign may be positive. The demonstration of epithelial lumps or cholesteatoma flakes is diagnostic.

Investigations of Atticoantral Disease

1. *Hearing assessment:* This usually reveals conductive deafness unless the inner ear has also been involved.
2. *Bacteriology:* The culture usually reveals a mixed group of organisms like *Proteus* spp., *Pseudomonas aeruginosa, Pseudomonas pyocynaeous, E. coli* and anaerobic bacteria. These are only secondary invaders in the disease.
3. *Radiology:* X-ray of the mastoids, usually Towne's, Schuler's and Law's lateral views and CT scan of the temporal bone are taken to study the extension of the disease. The mastoids are usually sclerotic, hypocellular or acellular. There may be seen an area of bone destruction, i.e. cavity formation which has sclerosed margins.

Treatment of Atticoantral Disease

The aim of treatment in cholesteatoma is to make the ear safe by eradicating the disease and to prevent its recurrence. Also of importance is the reconstructive surgery of the damaged ossicles and the membrane (tympanoplasty).

Depending upon the extent and location of the disease and degree of deafness, various surgical procedures are undertaken like atticotomy, modified radical mastoidectomy, radical mastoidectomy, mastoidectomy with tympanoplasty or combined approach tympanoplasty (CAT).

Tuberculous Otitis Media

It is not an uncommon disease, particularly in India. It occurs almost always secondary to pulmonary tuberculosis.

ROUTES OF INFECTION

1. Tubercular bacilli usually reach the middle ear through the eustachian tube. The coughed out sputum from the infected lungs reaches the tube and the bacilli travel to the middle ear.
2. Drinking unpasteurized milk of infected cows can cause the infection.
3. Tubercular otitis media may also be blood borne.

CLINICAL FEATURES

The diagnosis is made by following characteristics:

1. Slow onset of disease
2. Painless condition
3. The discharge is thin, scanty and odorless
4. The tympanic membrane is pale yellow to rosy-pink in color.
5. The posterior part of membrane is bulging and the anterior part shows dilated blood vessels.
6. Perforations in the membrane are usually multiple and may be associated with pale granulations.
7. Hearing loss is disproportionate to other symptoms. Confirmation is done by stained smear, culture of the discharge or by biopsy of the granulations.

Treatment is by the usual antitubercular therapy. Advanced cases may require surgical intervention after the active disease is under control.

Chapter

11

Complications of Chronic Suppurative Otitis Media

The infections of the middle ear cleft are always threatening by way of the possibility of their extension to the adjacent intracranial tissues. Various complications can arise because of direct spread of infection through the preformed pathways or by the bone eroding disease like cholesteatoma or by osteothrombophelibitis through intact bone.

The common complications that can occur are given in **Table 11.1** and shown in **Figure 11.1**.

Labyrinthitis

Pyogenic inflammation of the labyrinth may result from acute otitis media, following operations on the stapes or through preformed pathways like fracture lines.

In chronic suppurative otitis media (CSOM), cholesteatoma may cause erosion of the semicircular canals, usually of the lateral semicircular canal or the stapes footplate and promontory, thus exposing the labyrinth to the infective process.

Similarly removal of polypi or granulations arising from the promontory may result in labyrinthitis.

Labyrinthitis may be circumscribed (paralabyrinthitis) or diffuse.

In the circumscribed variety the bony capsule is eroded and membranous labyrinth is exposed (fistula formation). Labyrinthitis is localized to the area of the fistula only. The patient complains of attacks of dizziness with nausea and vomiting in addition to the ear discharge.

In diffuse labyrinthitis, depending upon the severity of the infection the attack may be mild, when the inflammatory exudate is serofibrinous with only a few round cells. This type is called diffuse serous labyrinthitis. If the inflammatory process continues the exudate becomes purulent, then the condition is known as diffuse purulent labyrinthitis. The patient suffers from severe attacks of vertigo. The infective process from the labyrinth may cause intracranial complications.

The vestibular symptoms like dizziness, vomiting and loss of balance are the more important presenting symptoms. The patient lies on the sound ear and looks towards the diseased ear. The hearing is not markedly affected in serous labyrinthitis. In purulent labyrinthitis the vestibular symptoms are more severe in nature with intense giddiness, frequent vomiting and marked deafness. Spontaneous nystagmus is present towards the healthy side. The patient lies in bed curled up on the side of his healthy ear. Vomiting may persist for a few days.

The recovery usually starts after two weeks and is complete within 4 to 6 weeks of the attack as by this time the central mechanism compensates for the loss of one labyrinth.

Table 11.1: Complications of CSOM

	Meningeal	Nonmeningeal
1.	Extradural abscess	Mastoiditis
2.	Perisinus abscess	Petrositis
3.	Venous sinus	Facial nerve paralysis thrombosis
4.	Otitic hydrocephalus	Brain abscess
5.	Meningitis	Labyrinthitis
6.	Subdural abscess	Retropharyngeal abscess

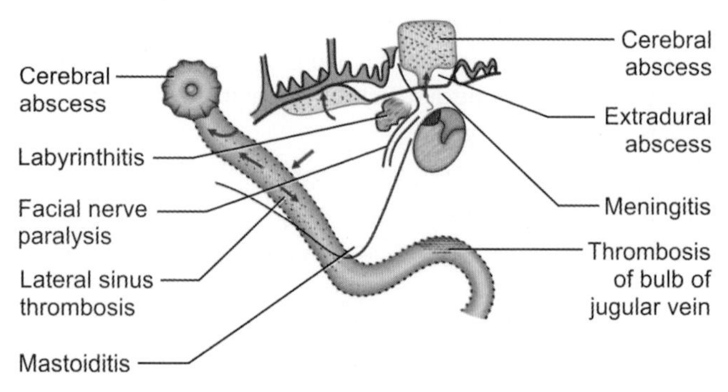

Fig. 11.1: Complications of chronic suppurative otitis media

TREATMENT

Labyrinthitis arising from an attack of acute otitis media is treated by an intensive course of antibiotics besides other general measures like bed rest and prescribing vestibular sedatives.

Labyrinthitis which is due to chronic ear disease is an absolute indication for surgery, which means mastoid exploration and removing the disease process. Antibiotics only control the infection and prevent its further spread. Before undertaking surgery, the hearing level and the condition of the other ear must be known for if the affected ear is functionally better, then an attempt should be made to preserve the labyrinth at operation.

In more extensive cases, where the whole labyrinth is involved and destroyed with loss of function, labyrinthectomy should be performed so that no pockets of the infection persist.

Otogenic Intracranial Infection

Infection spreads from the middle ear cleft to the intracranial structures usually directly. It may travel upwards into the middle cranial fossa or backwards into the posterior fossa. The infection passes through the planes of the dura mater, venous sinuses, subdural space and pia-arachnoid to the brain tissue.

Coalescent bony erosion in acute otitis media or the cholesteatoma in chronic otitis media exposes the adjacent structures to the infective process. When the infection reaches the dura or the sinus wall, these tissues respond by the formation of granulations and there may occur extradural and perisinus abscess.

If the dura fails in limiting the infection, it gets necrosed and subdural abscess may occur from where the meninges get involved.

Invasion of brain tissue: Thrombophlebitis of the blood vessels or the venous sinuses occurs as the result of infection and it is thought to be the cause of invasion of the brain tissue. The infection may also travel to the brain tissue through the perivascular space. Focal necrosis and liquefaction may follow, with abscess formation in the brain. The abscess cavity gets encapsulated, expands and presents as a space-occupying lesion.

CLINICAL FEATURES OF THE INTRACRANIAL INFECTION

In an ear disease, threatening intracranial spread, the patient may complain of headache, vomiting, and nausea. The site and severity of the headache is variable. Changes occur in the temperature and pulse rate. Changes in the level of consciousness may occur, drowsiness progressing to coma occurs in an uncontrolled disease. Giddiness may be a feature, indicative of labyrinthine or cerebellar involvement. In an established intracranial disease, epileptic fits may occur. Neck rigidity results from irritation of the basal meninges. Nystagmus is common in cerebellar abscess. Aphasia is an evidence of the involvement of the dominant hemisphere.

Extradural Abscess

Extradural abscess is the most common otogenic intracranial complication. It consists of collection of pus between the bone and the dura mater. It may develop in the middle or the posterior cranial fossa.

CLINICAL FEATURES

Headache in acute or chronic otitis media may be the only suggestive feature. The patient has a feeling of being unwell. He complains of malaise and may have low grade fever. Most cases are diagnosed at the time of ear surgery. Treatment consists of opening the abscess and evacuating its contents by the removal of the bone till the healthy dura is exposed.

Sinus Thrombophlebitis

Lateral sinus thrombosis occurs due to direct extension of the disease from the mastoid and is often preceded by the perisinus abscess. Thrombosis generally follows a chronic ear disease and *Streptococcus haemolyticus* is a common causative organism, although other gram-negative organisms like *E. coli*, *Pseudomonas pyocyaneus*, etc. have been isolated. Thrombosis of the sinus is a response to the infection and an attempt to limit the disease process. As the infection spreads, thrombosis may extend to the adjacent continuing sinuses. A cerebellar abscess may develop and septicemia usually follows.

CLINICAL FEATURES

The patient with an ear disease presents with rigors. The temperature shows sudden rise and fall. There occurs severe shivering and profuse sweating. The fever is of the remittent type (*picketfence curve*). Between the attacks the patient seems well. There may occur thrombosis of the mastoid emissary vein, with resultant edema over the mastoid process (*Greisinger's sign*). In advanced stages, changes of the intracranial hemodynamic system may occur and the patient may present with a cerebellar abscess.

Lillie-Crowe test or sign: This helps to decide which lateral sinus is diseased. When one lateral sinus is occluded by thrombosis, digital compression of the opposite jugular vein produces dilatation of the retinal veins on the normal side as seen on fundoscopy.

Tobey-Ayer test: In unilateral sinus thrombosis pressure on the jugular vein of the normal side produces a quick rise of CSF pressure equivalent to that of bilateral jugular pressure in a normal subject while compression of the vein on the affected side produces little change in the pressure of cerebrospinal fluid.

MANAGEMENT

The blood examination shows leukocytosis and blood culture during the attack helps in isolation of the organism.

Most patients should receive heavy doses of antibiotics like injectable combinations of two or more antibiotics like ampicillin, chloramphenicol, a cephalosporin and an aminoglycoside. In chronic ear disease, the mastoid must be explored, sinus plate exposed and the perisinus abscess drained. The sinus is exposed till healthy dura is seen and the state of the sinus is assessed. A healthy sinus is blue in color and easily compressible. In thrombosis the sinus is discolored and feels cord-like. When an intrasinus abscess is suspected, it should be drained by incising the sinus and bleeding, if any, is controlled by packing. In some cases, to limit the spread of thrombosis the internal jugular vein may need ligation. The role of anticoagulants is controversial, however, such therapy has a role if thombosis is progressive.

Otitic Hydrocephalus

This complication of the ear disease results because of sinus thrombosis which has upset the intracranial hemodynamics. If the occluding thrombus involves both the sinuses, a marked rise of intracranial venous pressure occurs. The thrombosis may spread to other sinuses also. This affects the absorption of CSF by the arachnoid granulations that produces a rise in the CSF pressure which lead to otitic hydrocephalus.

CLINICAL FEATURES

The patient presents with headache, vomiting and blurred vision.

Papilledema is a striking finding. Other localizing signs of raised intracranial pressure like 6th nerve palsy may occur. Lumbar puncture shows CSF under marked pressure (over 300 cm of water) but it does not show any biochemical change and is sterile.

TREATMENT

Active medical and surgical treatment is given for sinus thrombosis. The lumbar puncture is done to reduce the cerebrospinal fluid pressure.

Otogenic Brain Abscesses

Brain abscess is usually a complication of chronic ear disease. The majority of brain abscesses are associated with other intracranial lesions.

Extension of infection to the middle fossa produces temporal lobe abscess while cerebeller abscess occurs because of spread of infection to the posterior fossa. Further there may occur metastatic abscesses in the brain because of thrombophlebitis or embolic phenomenon. The abscesses form within the white matter and expand by further destruction towards the ventricles. Subsequently cerebral edema, encephalitis, focal necrosis and liquefaction occurs. The microglial and mesodermal tissues of the blood vessels try to limit the spread by the formation of a capsule of fibrous tissue around the abscess. The capsule may even undergo hyaline degeneration and calcification.

Finally, an abscess may rupture into the ventricle or subarachnoid space. An expanding abscess and the associated edema cause a rise in intracranial pressure with tentorial herniation and impaction of cerebellar tissue.

The commonly found organism in the brain abscesses are *Staphylococcus aureus*, *Staphylococcus albus*, *Streptococcus pyogenes*, gram-negative organisms like *E. coli*, *B. proteus*, *Pseudomonas pyocyaneus* and anaerobic bacteria.

CLINICAL FEATURES

The initial invasion of brain tissue is obscured by other intracranial complications like meningitis or sinus thrombosis. The signs and symptoms are those of increased intracranial tension and focal symptoms depending upon the part of the brain involved.

The initial presenting features are headache and vomiting followed by drowsiness and the changes in pulse and temperature. As the disease progresses, drowsiness proceeds to stupor and coma.

Focal Signs

Visual field: In temporal lobe abscess, perimetry may demonstrate homonymous hemianopia.

Aphasia: Abscess of the dominant temporal lobe interferes with speech. Nominal aphasia, i.e. inability to name the common objects is frequent.

As the abscess spreads involvement of the motor tracts occurs and manifests as paralysis of the limbs. Ocular paralysis may be the presenting feature of temporal lobe abscess.

Signs of Cerebellar Abscess

1. Nystagmus which is usually horizontorotatory, slow, coarse with the quick component towards the diseased side.
2. Muscle incoordination occurs, which is detected by dysdiadochokinesia and the finger nose test.
3. Asynergia on walking, the patient staggers to the side of the lesion.
4. Romberg's sign is positive, i.e. the patient when asked to stand with heels together and eyes closed, falls towards the side of the lesion.
5. Muscular atonia and pendular tendon jerks are other features of cerebellar abscess.

MANAGEMENT OF OTOGENIC BRAIN ABSCESS

Once the brain abscess is suspected, the opinion of the neurosurgeon should be obtained and the patient investigated.

1. Funduscopy gives a clue about papilloedema.
2. Provided there is no marked rise in intracranial pressure, lumbar puncture may be done.
3. Plain X-ray of the skull may show a displaced pineal body or gas within the abscess cavity. The other important localizing investigations include angiography, ventriculography, electroencephalography, tomography and scanning.

Treatment

Heavy doses of antibiotics are given to localize the abscess.

Once the abscess has been diagnosed and localized it is tapped through an appropriate burr hole. Frequent aspirations may be needed to obliterate the abscess cavity. Treatment of the ear disease is important as, unless the primary focus of infection is removed, tapping of the brain abscess only will not help. Treatment of the ear disease usually means exploration of the mastoid and removing the cholesteatomatous debris. In those centers where proper neurosurgical facilities are not available, the otologist usually while performing the mastoidectomy in such cases, puts an aspirating needle into the temporal lobe or in the posterior fossa and may hit on the abscess cavity and successfully tap the abscess.

Chapter 12

Nonsuppurative Otitis Media and Otitic Barotrauma

Nonsuppurative Otitis Media

The disease is characterised by accumulation of a nonpurulent effusion in the middle ear cleft. Controversy has arisen concerning the nature and etiology of the effusion and because of this various names have been given to this condition, viz. secretory otitis media, serous otitis media, otitis media with effusion and glue ear, etc. The term secretory otitis media has now passed into common usage. The usual age group involved is 5 to 10 years.

ETIOLOGY

Various theories have been put forward to explain the effusion in the middle ear.

1. *Vacuum theory:* This theory maintains that negative pressure in the middle ear is the pathogenic factor. As a result of this negative pressure which results because of blockage of eustachian tubes due to any cause, fluid comes out of the mucosal vessels into the middle ear.
2. *Allergy:* Secretory otitis media is considered by some authors as a manifestation of upper respiratory tract allergy. Proponents of this theory believe that because of anatomic continuity and on embryological basis, mucosa of nose, paranasal sinuses and nasopharynx responds in a like manner to allergic stimulus, with resultant edema and effusion in the middle ear.
3. There is now a general agreement about secretory otitis media being a low-grade inflammatory condition. There is still speculation as to the exact causative agent, whether bacterial or viral, and the predisposing factors. Eustachian tube dysfunction has been implicated as a predisposing cause and may be due to the following causes:
   i. Hypertrophied nasopharyngeal tonsils (adenoids) and nasopharyngeal carcinoma.
   ii. Mucosal diseases of the nose and paranasal sinuses (sinusitis).
   iii. Cleft palate, septal deviation, polyps in the nose.
   iv. Inadequate treatment of acute otitis media.
   v. Hypogammaglobulinemia.
   vi. Radiotherapy of the head and neck region.
   vii. Passive smoking.

CLINICAL FEATURES

1. The cardinal symptom is deafness, often noted by parents and teachers. Deafness is usually worse with an attack of common cold.
2. Earache, usually mild is complained by the patient and sometimes a woolly feeling or a feeling of fluid in the ear may be experienced.
3. Tinnitus may be present.

Signs: The tympanic membrane is usually dull, lustreless, retracted with restricted mobility and the landmarks may be prominent.

The fluid level may be visible (hairline) and sometimes air bubbles are seen inside the tympanic cavity. Chronic cases may show chalk patches suggestive of tympanosclerosis.

INVESTIGATIONS

Tuning fork tests and audiometry impedance and pure tone reveal conductive deafness, reduced compliance and flat curve.

X-ray of the postnasal space usually reveals hypertrophied adenoid tissue and X-ray examination of the paranasal sinuses may reveal other predisposing factors like polyposis, mucosal hypertrophy or fluid level.

Allergic tests to determine the allergen and further desensitization may be required.

Treatment of this condition is not satisfactory. It can be classified as medical or surgical.

MEDICAL TREATMENT

This consists of nasal decongestants (local or systemic), antihistamines or steroids for allergy, and mucolytic agents like bromhexine, chymotrypsin and urea. Some studies have indicated that these measures help clear effusion in about 15 percent of children within a month of this treatment.

To improve the drainage of effusion from the middle ear, procedures like Valsalva's maneuver, politzerization or eustachian catheterization may prove helpful.

SURGICAL TREATMENT

1. Myringotomy and suction of glue with the insertion of grommet for the aeration of the middle ear is helpful in majority of the cases. Sometimes double myringotomy is needed when secretions in the middle ear are very thick.
2. Treatment of the underlying predisposing factor by antral lavage, polypectomy, adenotonsillectomy, septoplasty or functional endoscopic sinus surgery (FESS) may be needed.

Acute Otitic Barotrauma

This is a noninfective inflammatory lesion.

CAUSAL FACTORS

It is caused by the establishment of a pressure differential between the air filled middle ear cleft and the atmospheric environment of the patient.

A patient with a perforated drum cannot develop otitic barotrauma unless the middle ear is loculated. There should be a major change in atmospheric pressure to cause this condition, as occurs usually in aviation and deep sea diving, on an intact tympanic membrane and inefficiently functioning eustachian tube.

The eustachian tube has two parts, the medial collapsible part and lateral rigid patent part, so air can be blown through it easily but it cannot be sucked out. Thus the pressure difference does not occur during ascent in an aircraft when the middle ear pressure tends to be higher than the atmospheric pressure, but it occurs during descent when the middle ear pressure becomes progressively lower than the atmospheric pressure and, therefore, air tries to suck in through the eustachian tube. This is not possible unless the eustachian tube is actively opened by muscular action. So, symptoms develop during descent both in an aircraft and in deep sea diving.

PATHOLOGY

Patients with complete physical obstruction of the eustachian tube suffer from atmospheric pressure changes. They first feel severe pain on ascent in an aircraft and the pain is relieved either by rupture of the drum or by descent.

Pressure equalization: Potentially patent or completely obstructed eustachian tubes fail to maintain adequate pressure equalization during rapid changes of atmospheric pressure.

During ascent the relative pressure in the middle ear rises. The tympanic membrane bulges outwards, increasing the capacity of the middle ear cavity, thus limiting slightly the pressure increase. Finally, the elasticity of the eustachian tube is overcome and air is discharged through the tube and pressure is equalized. This is a passive procedure and requires no active measures to be taken by the subject, though equalization takes place much earlier if the subject swallows. If he does not swallow or move his pharynx he will be conscious of an increasing feeling of fullness in his ears and an increasing depression of auditory acuity, until he feels a cracking at the back of his nose, when the discomfort in his ear disappears and his hearing returns to normal.

The two ears may not react synchronously so that the patient may feel alternating discomfort and deafness in the two ears. This is not normally painful but in a person who has suffered recently from barotrauma the drum becomes very sensitive to stretching and pain is very easily induced.

During descent in an aircraft (unlike ascent) pressure equalization in the middle ear does not take place passively and with the rise in atmospheric pressure, an unequal loading of the two surfaces of tympanic membrane develops which results in impaired hearing. The tympanic membrane becomes indrawn, and a feeling of discomfort becomes noticeable. The patient then swallows, the eustachian tube opens and symptoms are relieved by a rush of air into the middle ear. The sequence then begins again.

If swallowing does not help, the patient attempts the Valsalva's maneuver and if this too is not successful, the continued descent increases the symptoms until pain becomes intense and deafness severe.

Pressure changes: Atmospheric pressure does not increase in direct proportion to the decrease in altitude. Pain and physical changes in the middle ear are partly due to the atmospheric pressure displacing the tympanic membrane inwards but mainly due to the negative pressure leaving the walls of the blood vessels in the mucosa unsupported.

Chapter 13

Adhesive Otitis Media

Adhesive otitis media is a condition marked by adhesions that developed as a result of previous inflammation in the middle ear cavity (**Fig. 13.1**).

Etiology

Most otologists believe adhesive otitis media is a complication of inadequately treated acute otitis media. The condition may follow chronic suppurative otitis media or secretory otitis media.

Pathology

Pathological changes occur both in the middle ear mucosa and the tympanic membrane. Adhesions develop by way of organization of the inflammatory exudate and connective tissue proliferation from the inflamed mucosa. The mobility of the ossicles and the membrane is diminished and ankylosis of the ossicles may occur.

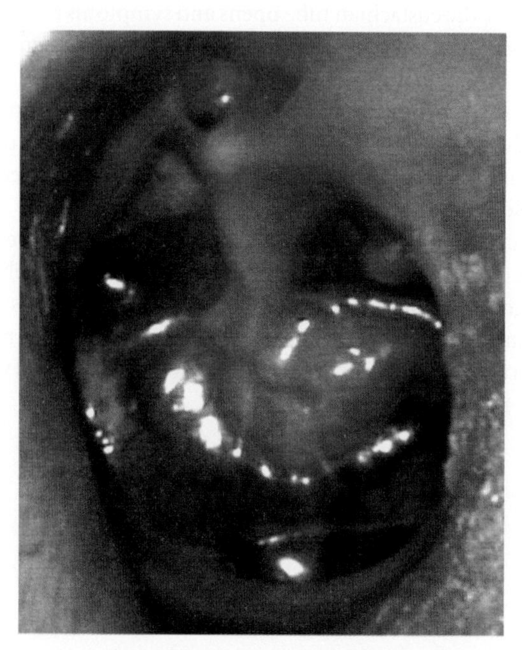

Fig. 13.1: Adhesive otitis media

Clinical Features

Symptoms: The main symptom is deafness though tinnitus may be present.

Signs: The tympanic membrane shows retraction and chalk patches. Mobility of the membrane is impaired and scarring may be present. Tuning fork tests and audiometry show conductive deafness.

Treatment

Some cases of adhesive otitis media with adequate hearing require no treatment.

Patients with marked deafness may either be prescribed a hearing aid or advised surgery. However, the results of surgery are not always successful because of further adhesion formation.

The surgical procedures undertaken are the following:

1. Grommet insertion
2. Exploratory tympanotomy wherein adhesions are broken, ossicles and membrane freed and silastic sheets are placed in the middle ear cavity to avoid further adhesions.

Tympanosclerosis

It was first described by Von Troltsch in 1869. Tympanosclerosis means deposition of plaques of collagen with calcareous deposits in the submucosa of the middle ear cavity. When confined to the tympanic membrane, it is called a chalk patch or myringosclerosis. Small plaques may not hamper the functioning of the middle ear but larger deposits on the oval window hamper hearing. Tympanosclerosis is usually an end result of otitis media when healing takes place and excessive collagen gets deposited. The exact etiological factor remains unknown though the drying effect of air to which the middle ear is exposed after perforation and severe acute otitis media may be the causative factors. Studies have demonstrated the presence of tympanosclerosis in 40 percent of children with ventilation tubes. Tympanosclerosis may be difficult to differentiate from otosclerosis when the tympanic membrane is normal and only the ossicles are involved. There is no family history but a past history of otitis media is usually present. Tympanotomy may be needed to differentiate the two conditions.

TREATMENT

Small plaques may not need any treatment. Chalk patches can be removed before placing the graft in myringoplasty. If the ossicles are involved, removal of the tympanosclerotic deposits does not help as there occurs scarring and adhesions. Silastic sheets may be put in to prevent adhesion formation.

In fixation of the foot plate of stapes, stapedectomy may be helpful but in more severe cases fenestration is the method of choice for restoration of hearing.

Chapter

14

Mastoid and Middle Ear Surgery

Incisions for Exposure of Middle Ear Cleft

Postaural incision (William Wilde): This incision for exposure of mastoid process follows the curve of the postaural fold, beginning above at the upper attachment of the auricle, downwards to the tip of mastoid.

As the mastoid process in infants is not fully developed, the usual postaural incision might injure the facial nerve and thus incision in this age group should be almost horizontal.

The incision has the following advantages. It provides a wide open field, therefore, facilitates a thorough exenteration of the mastoid cells and provides an access for unexpected extension of disease process and also allows to deal with complications.

Endaural incision (Kessel-Lempert): The incision is made in the cartilage free gap, filled with fibrous tissue (incisura terminalis). It is extended upwards parallel to the helix.

The lower part of the incision is made at the junction of the cartilaginous with the bony meatus and it is curved from the 3 o'clock position in the canal through the 12 o'clock position to reach the floor of the canal at the 6 o'clock position. The incision is deepened through the periosteum which is separated upwards and backwards exposing the bony cortex of the mastoid.

This incision gives a direct access to the external osseous meatus, tympanic membrane and tympanic cavity with the result that the cavity is better constructed with regard to the meatus and postoperative care of the cavity can be better performed.

Permeatal incision (Rosen): This incision is started from the 12 o'clock position, 2 mm away from the annulus, is swept posteriorly so that it is 6 mm away from the annulus at the center and meets the annulus again the 6 o'clock position inferiorly.

Surgical Procedures for the Discharging Ear

The commonly performed operations on the middle ear and mastoid are given below (**Fig. 14.1**). Instruments used for mastoid surgery are shown in **Figure 14.2**.

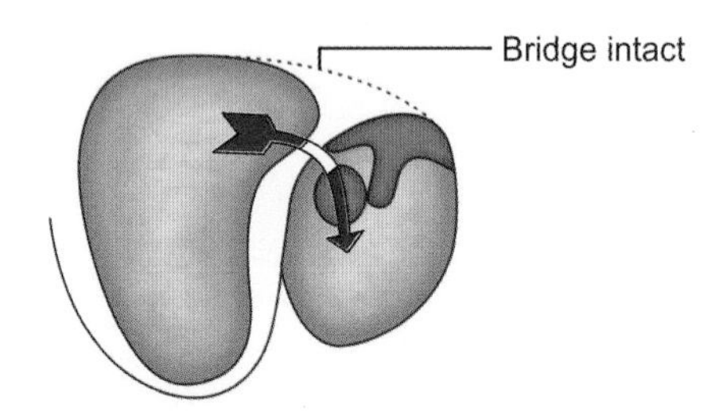

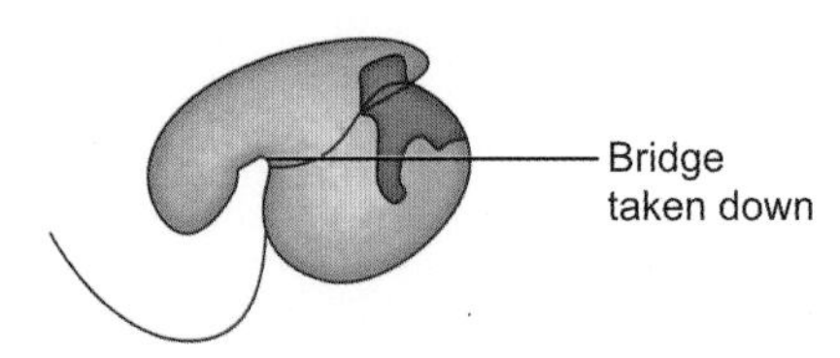

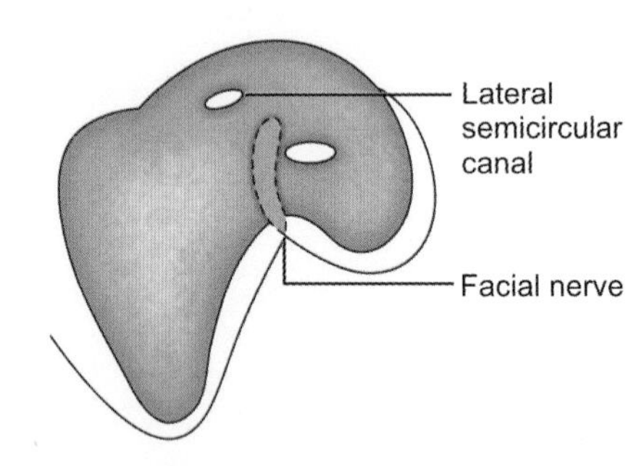

Fig. 14.1: Types of mastoidectomy

CORTICAL MASTOIDECTOMY (SIMPLE OR CONSERVATIVE MASTOIDECTOMY, SCHWARTZE OPERATION)

This operation was described by Schwartze in 1873. It involves the removal of all accessible mastoid air cells without disturbing the middle ear. The osseous superior and posterior meatal walls are kept intact. The cells are followed from the antrum, inferiorly

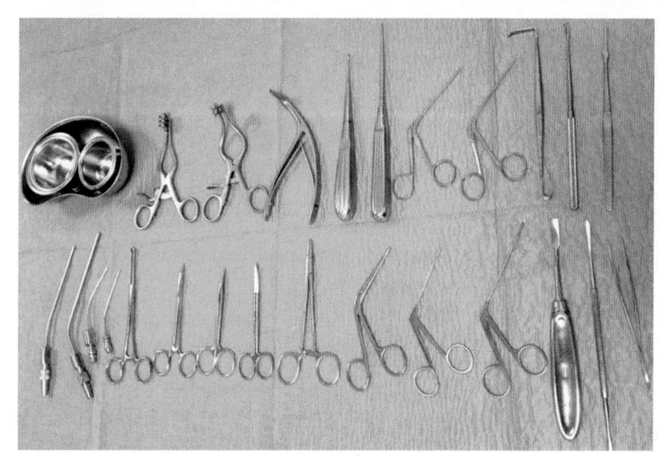

Fig. 14.2: Instruments used for mastoid surgery

to the mastoid tip, posteriorly to the sinus plate, superiorly to the tegmen plate, and anteriorly to the limit of pneumatization in the posterior root of the zygoma.

Indications

1. Acute mastoiditis refractory to medical treatment
2. Masked mastoiditis
3. Subperiosteal abscess
4. Bezold's abscess
5. Labyrinthectomy
6. Preliminary to exposure of saccus endolymphaticus for Menier's disease.

Steps of Operation

The hair is shaved for about 5 cm round the ear. A curved incision is made 1.25 cm behind the pinna. The upper end of the incision extends anteriorly above the auricle to the level just above the external auditory canal while the lower end extends to the mastoid tip. The incision is deepened right to the bone and after cauterizing the bleeding points a self-retaining mastoid retractor is applied. The mastoid cortex is exposed and Mecewen's triangle is identified. Removal of the bone is started in this area either using an electric drill or a hammer and gouge. The mastoid antrum is identified by seeing the aditus in its anterior wall and the lateral semicircular canal in its medial wall. The mastoid cells are then traced and removed. The wound is closed with interrupted silk sutures after putting a corrugated drain at the lower end of the wound. A pressure dressing is applied. The external auditory canal is packed with a ribbon gauze.

Postoperative Care

Antibiotics are given postoperatively.

The drain is removed after 24 to 48 hours and the stitches are removed after one week.

Complications

1. Facial nerve paralysis
2. Dislocation of the incus
3. Injury to the lateral sinus or dura
4. Hematoma.

RADICAL MASTOIDECTOMY

The procedure involves removal of the disease from the mastoid antrum and tympanum converting both of them into a single, smooth walled cavity accessible freely through the external auditory canal. During this procedure the malleus, incus, chorda tympani and remnants of the tympanic membrane are also removed.

Indications

1. Unsafe type of chronic suppurative otitis media (CSOM)
2. Cholesteatoma
3. Complicated CSOM
4. Malignant disease of the middle ear.

Operative Steps

The mastoid antrum is entered as in cortical mastoidectomy. The partition wall between the external meatus and the antrum is progressively lowered to the level of the tympanomastoid suture. The facial bridge is removed together with the anterior and posterior buttresses. This is followed by the removal of the tympanic membrane, malleus, incus and all mucoperiosteal lining. Meatoplasty is done to create a flap which lines the cavity and widens the meatus. The cavity is packed with ribbon gauze impregnated with bismuth iodoform paraffin paste (BIPP) or an antibiotic ointment. The pack helps to keep the meatal flap in position, prevents canal stenosis and controls bleeding. The wound is closed with interrupted silk sutures and a pressure bandage applied.

Complications

1. Facial palsy
2. Injury to the sigmoid sinus causing severe bleeding from the sinus
3. Injury to dura mater
4. Meningitis and other intracranial complications
5. Suppurative labyrinthitis by displacement of the stapes
6. Severe conductive deafness
7. Unhealed cavity and persistent ear discharge
8. Mucous cyst.

Postoperative Care

Antibiotics are administered. The pack and stitches are removed on the 6th day. Packing should thereafter be replaced at weekly intervals until epithelialization is complete.

MODIFIED RADICAL MASTOIDECTOMY

This is a procedure performed to eradicate the mastoid disease in which the epitympanum, mastoid antrum and external canal are converted into a common cavity and made accessible to the outside through the meatus. This differs from the radical operation in that the tympanic membrane remnants and the healthy ossicular remnants are retained to preserve hearing. The procedure is similar to radical mastoidectomy in that the superior and posterior osseous meatal walls are removed, meatal flap constructed and the cavity is exteriorized.

Atticoantrostomy (*Bondy's mastoidectomy*) is a type of modified radical mastoidectomy which is indicated for cases of primary acquired cholesteatoma with perforation in the pars flaccida and intact pars tensa with the disease limited to the attic and antrum.

Atticotomy (epitympanotomy): This is a procedure used when cholesteatoma is limited to the epitympanic or attic region. The cavity is widely exposed and subsequently cleaned.

Mastoidectomy with tympanoplasty: This operation involves the eradication of disease in the middle ear and mastoid and to reconstruct the hearing mechanism. It is indicated in those cases where the disease is widespread throughout the mastoid and middle ear. It is then necessary to completely eradicate the disease in the mastoid which can only be done by the removal of the posterior canal wall. The principles of radical mastoidectomy apply and the goal is to achieve eradication of disease and exteriorization of the mastoid cavity with reconstruction of the sound conducting mechanism. It may be done as a one-stage procedure or as a two-stage procedure.

MASTOID OBLITERATION OPERATION

The aim of the operation is to eradicate the disease when present and to obliterate the mastoid cavity to lessen the problems of permanent cavity in the mastoid. Various materials like fat, blood clots, temporalis muscle and cortical bone have been used for this purpose.

Tympanoplasty

This is an operative procedure of reconstruction of the sound conducting mechanism of the middle ear. This is based on the following principles:

1. Restoration of sound pressure transformer mechanism of the middle ear.
2. Sound protection of the round window.

   Various types of tympanoplasty techniques are aimed to achieve these physiological principles.

PREREQUISITIES OF TYMPANOPLASTY

1. There should be adequate air-bone gap with good cochlear reserve.

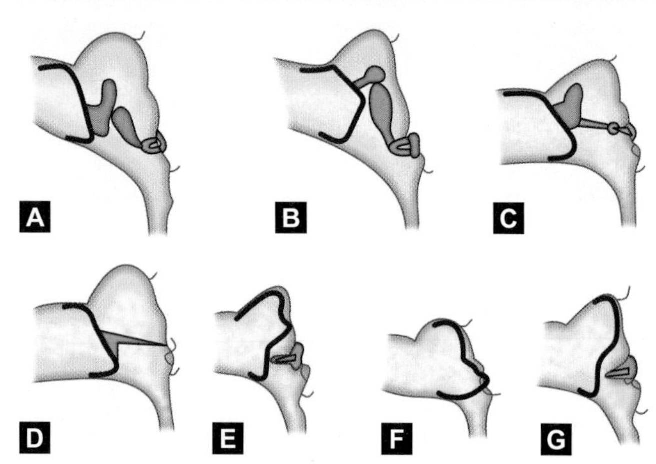

Figs 14.3A to G: Various types of tympanoplasty: (A) Type I, (B) Type II 'a', (C) Type II 'b', (D) Type II 'c', (E) Type III, (F) Type IV, and (G) Type V

2. The middle ear and mastoid should be free of disease to ensure success of the reconstructive procedure.
3. The eustachian tube should ideally be functioning to allow proper aeration of the middle ear cleft, which is necessary for optimal functioning of the ossicular chain and tympanic membrane.

TYPES OF TYMPANOPLASTY

Based on the physiological principles, there are five types of tympanoplastic procedures(Wullstein's tympanoplasty technique) (**Figs 14.3A to G**).

Myringoplasty: This means repair of the tympanic membrane perforation only.

- Type I — Includes myringoplasty but also involves exploration of the middle ear to rule out any other pathology. Ossicular chain is intact and mobile.
- Type II — Malleus handle is absent, reconstruction of the tympanic membrane is done over the malleus remnant and the long process of incus.
- Type III — The malleus and incus are missing. The reconstruction is done by placing the tympanic membrane graft over the head of a mobile stapes (*Columella type* as in birds).
- Type IV — There is loss of middle ear components. A shallow cavity is constructed by placing the graft over the round window to create a hypotympanic air bubble. The mobile footplate of stapes is exposed to sound waves.
- Type V — There is loss of middle ear components and the footplate of stapes is fixed. Fenestration of the lateral semicircular canal is done for sound waves to enter the ear. The round window is shielded by the graft. This type of reconstruction is very rarely done these days.

CONTRAINDICATIONS OF TYMPANOPLASTY

1. In presence of residual disease like cholesteatoma.
2. In ear disease with intracranial complications.
3. Malignant disease of ear.
4. High-risk patients like diabetics, who are prone to fulminating infections.

Prosthesis in use for reconstruction of the ossicles include cartilage struts strengthened with stainless steel wires, cortical bone pieces, homograft ossicles and synthetic material like total ossicular replacement prosthesis (TORP) and partial ossicular replacement prosthesis (PORP).

COMBINED APPROACH TYMPANOPLASTY

This operative procedure was developed and promoted, as an alternative to wide access techniques in the management of chronic suppurative otitis media.

A combined approach implies a combined access, transmeatal and transmastoid on either side of an *intact* posterosuperior bony canal wall.

Soft tissue approach is by the postaural incision. Periosteal tissues are separately incised and elevated. Bone over the mastoid cortex and the root of zygoma is exposed.

Meatal skin is elevated from the posterosuperior aspect of the meatus and then in continuity with the surface epithelium of any tympanic membrane remnant.

Cortical mastoid operation is performed and the incus and head of malleus are exposed in the attic. Posterior tympanotomy is done to view the hypotympanum. This consists of opening the facial recess from its mastoid aspect.

The posterior canal wall is thinned down and the disease is removed in continuity. The main aim of combined approach tympanoplasty (CAT) is eradication of disease, avoidance of open mastoid cavity, and reconstruction of the sound transformer mechanism.

Advantages

1. It avoids the mastoid cavity, therefore, its problems.
2. The canal wall is preserved, therefore, better reconstruction of tympanum is possible.

Disadvantages

1. Residual and recurrent cholesteatoma are possibilities.
2. It is a difficult and time consuming procedure.

Contraindications

The following are the contraindications to CAT:

1. Extensive disease in the middle ear and mastoid.
2. Intracranial complications.
3. Malignant disease of the ear.

Chapter 15

Otosclerosis

Otosclerosis is primarily a disease of the bony labyrinth which produces effects upon the middle and inner ear functioning. The primary change is the formation of new spongy bone and the chief secondary effect is ankylosis of the footplate of stapes.

The term "otosclerosis" is a misnomer which has resulted from the mistaken idea that ankylosis of the stapes occurs due to chronic sclerosis of the tympanic mucosa. The disease actually involves formation of new spongy bone so a better term used by otologists is "otospongiosis" which refers to the active phase of the disease characterised by the presence of vascular spaces containing highly cellular fibrous tissue. The term 'otosclerosis' refers to the final stage consisting of highly mineralized bone, which is more cellular and thicker than the normal bone. Both stages may be seen together in a single focus.

Etiology

The exact cause of the disease is not known and various theories have been put forward to explain its etiology.

1. *Heredity:* There is a family history in about 70 percent of the cases and evidence goes in favor of an autosomal dominant inheritance.
2. *Racial distribution:* The disease is common in Indians and in Whites while it is rare in Negroes, Chinese and Japanese.
3. *Age of onset:* The disease process usually begins between 15 to 35 years in approximately 90 percent of the cases.
4. *Sex:* Otosclerosis is more common in females.
5. *Sites of predilection:* Fossula ante-fenestram is the most common site for otosclerosis. It is a 2 to 3 mm area in front of the oval window up to the processus cochleariformis where remnants of the embryonic cartilage persist which may later on lead to new bone formation in susceptible cases. The other common sites are fossula postfenestram, round window, footplate of stapes, and the infracochlear region below the internal auditory meatus.

   New bone formation occurs to fill up these clefts and this bony growth may fix up the stapes producing the typical clinical picture. In 70 to 80 percent of both temporal bones are affected with a striking similarity of location and extent of the lesions in the two ears.
6. *Aggravating factors:* Pregnancy and puerperium may initiate or increase the deafness in otosclerosis.

Pathology of Otosclerosis

Gross pathology: The otosclerotic focus can be distinguished from the labyrinthine capsule by its whiter chalky color or that the overlying mucoperiosteum appears thickened and vascular, contrasting with the bluish appearing avascular normal footplate.

There are four macroscopical types:

Type I — Early focus, at least half of the footplate remains thin.

Type II — Fairly advanced lesion involving whole of the footplate which can be still fractured and removed.

Type III — Advanced lesion involving footplate, which is thickened, but the footplate can still be differentiated from the oval window niche.

Type IV — Obliterative type of focus. The bone is continuous with otic capsule.

Histopathology of otosclerosis: Histopathology reveals that the normal endochondral bone of the bony labyrinth is replaced by new bone, which is spongy, more cellular and more vascular. The osteocytes are more numerous and the amount of basophillic cementum in the ground substance is increased.

Types of Otosclerosis

1. *Histological otosclerosis:* This type of otosclerosis does not produce any symptoms during life but is revealed only at postmortem.
2. *Clinical otosclerosis:* This is of the following types:
   a. *Stapedial otosclerosis:* The otosclerotic focus may produce ankylosis of the stapes causing conductive deafness.
   b. *Cochlear otosclerosis:* The otosclerotic process encroaches upon the membranous labyrinth producing sensori-neural deafness.

c. *Mixed:* Otosclerosis causes both fixation of the stapes and involvement of the labyrinth so that there is mixed hearing loss.

Clinical Features

Deafness is a common and outstanding symptom. It is usually bilateral in 80 percent of cases and tends to be symmetrical in progress and degree. The onset of deafness is insidious and the progress is usually slow.

Paracusis willisiana: A feature of deafness in a majority of these cases is the presence of paracusis willisi, i.e. the ability to hear speech better in noisy surroundings, like in public transport, machine shops, engine rooms, etc. In these places a normal person raises his voice above the noise level and above the threshold of the otosclerotic patient and thus the patient has no difficulty in hearing. Tinnitus is a usual complaint and may be unilateral or bilateral.

Vertigo may be an occasional symptom.

Physical Findings

Otoscopy reveals the tympanic membrane as intact and mobile. In 2 percent of cases, a flemingo-pink tinge may be seen through the tympanic membrane known as *Schwartze sign,* which is indicative of a highly vascular active otosclerotic focus.

Tuning fork tests reveal conductive deafness.

Gelle's test: Place a vibrating tuning fork on mastoid process, then increase pressure in external auditory canal by Seigle's speculum and ask patient if there is any change in intensity of sound after increasing the pressure in EAC. In normal subjects, there will be decrease in perceived sound whereas in otosclerosis there will be no change as the footplate of stapes is already fixed.

Tympanometry may reveal a A's type of curve. Pure tone audiometry usually shows bilaterally symmetrical air bone gap and in few cases may show a dip in the bone conduction curve (Carhart's notch).

Carhart's notch: This is a pure tone audiometric finding and is characteristic of otosclerosis. There is a dip in the bone conduction curve which corresponds to 5 db loss at 1000 Hz, 10 db loss at 1500 Hz and 15 db loss at 2000 Hz and then back to 5 db loss at 4000 Hz. This is probably due to the loss of the insertial component of the footplate of the stapes, which is fixed in otosclerosis.

Differential Diagnosis of Otosclerosis

The following diseases with an intact tympanic membrane producing conductive deafness are commonly confused with otosclerosis. The characteristic features of these conditions are considered below:

1. *Secretory otitis media*
   i. The disease is common in young children.
   ii. Earache may be the presenting feature.
   iii. The tympanic membrane is dull, may be retracted and shows restricted mobility.
   iv. A fluid level may be visible.
   v. Impedance audiometry shows reduced compliance and negative pressure.
2. *Adhesive otitis media*
   i. A history of previous middle ear disease is usually available.
   ii. Conductive deafness is usually unilateral.
   iii. The tympanic membrane shows areas of scarring and chalk patches and is retracted with restricted mobility.
3. *Ossicular chain disruption*
   i. The history is suggestive of head injury or previous ear surgery.
   ii. It is usually a unilateral condition.
   iii. Impedance audiometry shows increased compliance.
   iv. Stapedial reflex is absent.
   v. Tympanotomy is diagnostic.
4. *Congenital ossicular fixation*
   i. Deafness is present since birth, is nonprogressive, and usually unilateral.
   ii. Associated congenital abnormalities are present.
   iii. Tympanotomy gives the final diagnosis.
5. *Vander Hoeve's syndrome*
   Blue sclerae with osteogenesis imperfecta constitute this syndrome. There are usually pathological fractures in long bones. When the temporal bone is involved, it may simulate otosclerosis. The Schwartze sign is absent and acoustic reflex cannot be elicited.
6. *Paget's disease*
   This is a disease of bones in which osteolytic and osteoblastic processes cause softening of the bones, fractures and deformities. When the temporal bone is involved it can lead to deafness like in otosclerosis. The stapedial reflex is always present, and the Schwartze sign may also be present. Radiological examination shows osteolytic lesions of the bones with mottled appearance.
7. *Tympanosclerosis*
   Chalk patches will be seen on the tympanic membrane, a conductive hearing loss is seen, there is a previous history of middle ear disease and tympanometry will show reduced mobility.
8. *Persistent stapedial artery*
   This is a rare condition in which the large artery covers the footplate and immobilizes the stapes, resulting in conductive deafness. Tympanotomy is diagnostic.

Treatment

Majority of the patients with deafness due to stapedial otosclerosis can be assisted either by medical or surgical methods.

Medical treatment: The prescription of a hearing aid can help patients overcome the difficulty in hearing. The function of the hearing aid is to amplify the sound waves and this overcomes the resistance to sound transmission. Hearing aid is advised when surgery is contraindicated or refused by the patient. In the early stages of the disease sodium fluoride 20 mg thrice a day for 6 months to 1 to 2 years has been used with varying results. Sodium fluoride reduces osteoclastic bone resorption and increases osteoblastic bone formation.

Surgical treatment: Rapid advances of surgery for otosclerosis have taken place in recent years. The surgery is aimed to allow normal transmission of sound and has taken three main directions.

1. *Bypassing the stapes:* This involves making an opening in the lateral semicircular canal (fenestration operation). This produced an open mastoid cavity and the patient suffered from residual hearing loss, so the procedure did not gain favor.
2. *Mobilization of the stapes:* The ankylosed stapes was mobilized at the operation. However, the hearing improvement only proved partial and reankylosis of the stapes occurred frequently.
3. *Stapedectomy (Shea's technique):* This is the treatment of choice nowadays. The stapes is removed and replaced by a prosthesis like teflon piston, wire, gelfoam, stainless steel piston and similar other prosthesis.

Stapedectomy

OPERATIVE PROCEDURE

It is usually done under local anesthesia but may be done under general anesthesia. Permeatal incision is made from the 6 o'clock to 12 o'clock position, 6 mm lateral to the tympanic annulus at the center. The tympanomeatal flap is elevated, the chorda tympani nerve is identified and preserved and any bony overhang of the posterior canal wall removed. The ossicles are palpated with a probe and stapedial fixation is confirmed. The stapedius tendon is cut, incudostapedial joint disarticulated, crura broken and a hole made in the footplate of stapes by a fine straight pick which should not go too medially as the utricle lies only 1 mm medial to the footplate of stapes. The stapes should not be moved more than 0.1 mm. A teflon or stainless steel piston is hooked around the long process of incus and fitted in the hole made in the footplate of stapes. The tympanomeatal flap is put back and the external auditory canal packed with gelfoam (**Figs 15.1A to D**).

COMPLICATIONS

1. Injury to the chorda tympani and facial nerve
2. Tear in the tympanic membrane
3. Hemotympanum
4. Perilymph fistula
5. Sensorineural hearing loss
6. Labyrinthitis
7. Acute otitis media
8. Necrosis of the long process of incus and slipping of the prosthesis
9. Postoperative granuloma
10. Subluxation of the footplate.

CONTRAINDICATIONS FOR STAPEDECTOMY

1. Otitis media
2. Young children
3. Poor cochlear function
4. Cochlear otosclerosis
5. Only functioning ear
6. Second ear (i.e. stapedectomy done on one side should not be done on the other ear)
7. Perforation of the tympanic membrane (Stapedectomy should be done only as a second stage operation after myringoplasty)
8. Otosclerosis causing mild conductive deafness
9. Extensive tympanosclerosis
10. Malignant otosclerosis
11. Pregnancy.

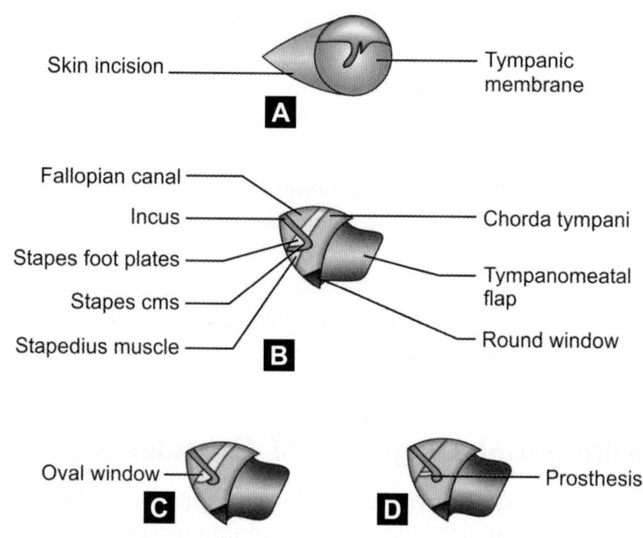

Figs 15.1A to D: Surgical steps of stapedectomy: (A) Incision in the ear canal, (B) Middle ear structures exposed on tympanotomy, (C) View, following removal of stapes, and (D) Placement of prosthesis from incus to oval windows

Table 15.1: Differences in deafness caused by adhesive otitis media and stapedial otosclerosis

Deafness	Adhesive otitis media	Stapedial otosclerosis
Type Onset	Conductive Common before 15 years	Conductive Uncommon before 15 years
Family history	Nil	70% positive
Sex incidence	Equal	Females 2:1 males
History of otitis media	50% positive	Nil
Paracusis willisi	Absent	Usually present
Tympanic membrane	Abnormal always	Usually normal
Eustachian tube	Blocked usually	Uncommonly blocked

Differences in deafness caused by adhesive otitis media and stapedial otosclerosis are given in **Table 15.1**.

PROGNOSIS

In 90 percent of the cases, the results are good, in 8 percent no change occurs and in 2 percent results are poor. Hence, only one ear should be operated upon at one time because chances of sensorineural loss, however small, are still present. Successful results have been reported with laser stapedectomy using argon and KTP lasers.

Advantages include a bloodless fenestra and reduced risk of subluxation of the footplate but the disadvantages are a high cost and vestibular symptoms due to an increase in the perilymph temperature.

Cochlear Otosclerosis

It is defined as the presence of an otosclerotic lesion in the capsule of the cochlea, clinically characterised by sensorineural type of deafness. It may be associated with stapedial fixation when it is known as combined or mixed otosclerosis. The diagnosis of pure cochlear otosclerosis without the involvement of stapes can be suspected in any patient who has developed bilateral progressive sensorineural deafness in early adult life.

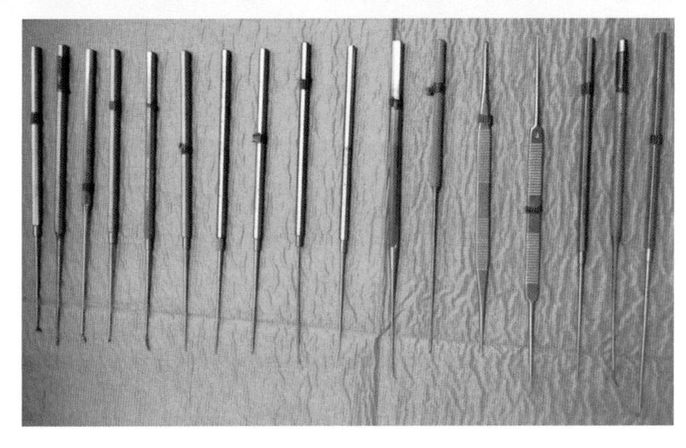

Fig. 15.2: Instruments for micro ear surgery

TREATMENT (FIG. 15.2)

Surgery has no place in the treatment of pure cochlear otosclerosis. Oral therapy with sodium fluoride in moderately large doses is given with a hope that it causes recalcification and inactivation of the otosclerotic focus.

Other indications for fluoride treatment are the following:

1. Malignant otosclerosis
2. When surgery is contraindicated
3. After stapedectomy.

Malignant Otosclerosis

It is cochlear type of otosclerosis which starts in early life and progresses rapidly producing severe sensorineural hearing loss. The Schwartze sign is strongly positive. Stapedectomy is contraindicated. Fluoride therapy and prescription of a hearing aid are the treatment for this condition.

Chapter 16

Tumors of the Ear

Tumors of the External Ear

BENIGN TUMORS OF THE AURICLE

The tumors of the external ear are uncommon. Benign lesions which may affect the external ear include hemangiomas, papillomas, chondromas and fibromas.

MALIGNANT TUMORS OF THE AURICLE

Squamous cell carcinoma and basal cell carcinoma are the two types of malignancies which usually involve the auricle.

Squamous Cell Carcinoma

It usually presents as a small superficial ulcer having rolled up margins which progresses causing destruction of the cartilage (**Figs 16.1 and 16.2**). The regional lymph nodes usually get involved. Biopsy confirms the diagnosis.

Complete surgical excision of the lesion is done with care being taken to achieve tumor free margins. Tumor free margins are ensured intraoperatively by sending biopsies from all the edges of the defect created postremoval of the lesion and getting a histopathological confirmation before a repair of the defect is attempted. The local defect is usually corrected by skin grafts. Large lesions may require total excision of the pinna.

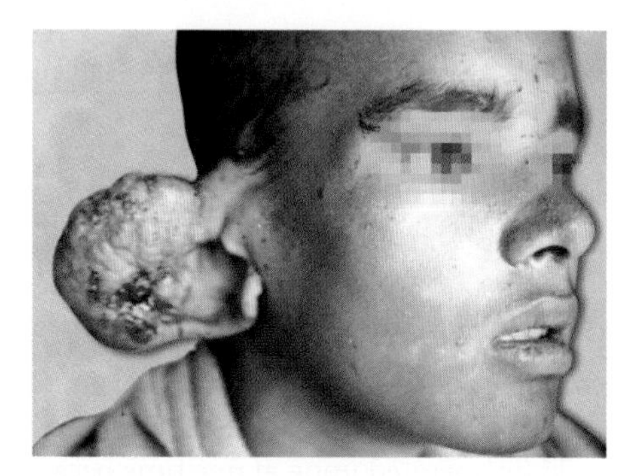

Fig. 16.1: Squamous cell carcinoma (right pinna)

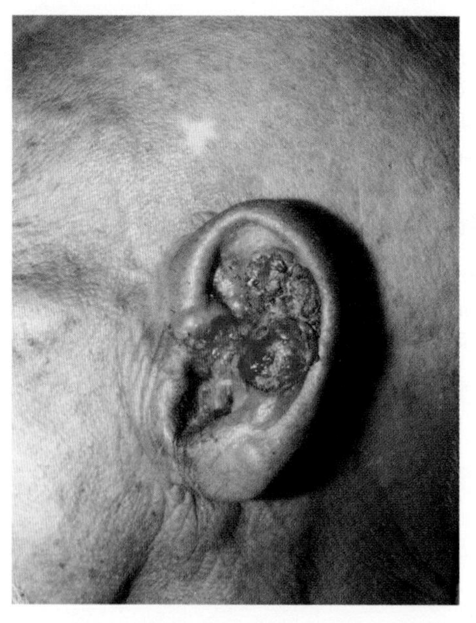

Fig. 16.2: Malignancy of left external auditory canal and pinna

Basal Cell Carcinoma (Rodent Ulcer)

This type usually presents initially as a raised pigmented plaque with a tendency to form crusts. Common sites involved are the border of helix, meatal entrance and the tragus. Surgical excision is the treatment of choice. Advanced cases require wide excision and postoperative radiotherapy.

BENIGN TUMORS OF THE EXTERNAL AUDITORY MEATUS

The common benign lesions are exostoses, osteoma and adenoma. Sometimes angioma, papilloma, fibroma and chondroma may also occur.

Exostoses

Exostoses present as hemispherical smooth bony outgrowths from the canal wall. These are usually multiple and the condition is usually bilateral. The exact cause is not known but it was thought that repeated swimming in cold water could be an etiological factor. Exostoses usually do not produce any symptoms unless these outgrowths obliterate the lumen of the canal.

When exostoses are small and symptomless, no treatment is needed but when these outgrowths become large in size, they are removed using a drill and cutting burr.

Osteoma

Osteoma is a smooth, solitary, rounded, pedunculated tumor from the outer part of the bony meatus, usually from the region of tympanosquamous or the tympanomastoid suture. Treatment is removal by cutting through the pedicle.

Adenoma

Benign tumors may arise from both the types of glandular tissues in the external canal. So, the adenoma could be of following types:

i. Sebaceous adenoma
ii. Ceruminoma.

Sebaceous adenoma: The tumor arises from sebaceous glands and is usually seen as smooth, skin-covered swelling in the outer part of the meatus. Treatment is surgical excision.

Ceruminoma (Hidradenoma): This tumor arises from the ceruminous glands of the meatal skin. The lesion presents as a firm, skin-covered mass which may be sessile or pedunculated.

Treatment is wide local excision because chances of its recurrence and turning malignant are marked.

MALIGNANT TUMORS OF THE EXTERNAL AUDITORY MEATUS

Carcinoma

The external auditory meatus is not a common site for carcinomas. The disease is usually seen in cases having long-standing suppurative disease. The most common histologic types of EAC cancer are squamous cell, basal cell, and glandular tumors including adenoid cystic, mucoepidermoid and adenocarcinoma. Other rare lesions include sarcomas, melanoma, sebaceous cell carcinoma and metastatic lesions. By far, the most common of these is squamous cell carcinoma which accounts for approximately 90 percent of all cases. The patient presents with blood-stained discharge and pain in the ear and on examination, an ulcer or a bleeding mass is seen in the canal. Diagnosis is dependent upon biopsy, and biopsy of any canal lesion which is unresponsive to routine therapy is essential. Other suggested diagnostic studies include temporal bone CT scans, and angiography if there appears to be involvement of the great vessels. The adjacent auricular lymph nodes may be involved. Surgery for external canal cancer varies from a minimal "sleeve excision" of the external canal to lateral temporal bone resection to subtotal and total temporal bone resection.

Adenocarcinoma

The tumor may primarily arise from the glands of the external auditory canal and its differentiation from squamous cell carcinoma is difficult on clinical grounds.

Biopsy is confirmatory and surgery followed by radiotherapy is the treatment of choice. Depending upon the extent of involvement, surgery may be limited to radical mastoidectomy or even subtotal resection of the temporal bone may be needed to remove the disease.

Tumors of the Middle Ear

GLOMUS TUMORS

Nonchromaffin paraganglionic tissue is present in the dome of the jugular bulb or along the course of Jacobson's and Arnold's nerve or sometimes in the mucosa of the middle ear. A tumor arising from this tissue is known as glomus tumor, *chemodectoma* or nonchromaffin paraganglioma (**Fig. 16.3**). These tumors are histologically benign but locally behave like malignant tumors (**Fig. 16.4**). According to their location, they are named as glomus jugulare, arising from the jugular bulb, glomus vagale, arising from the vagus and glomus tympanum, arising from the promontory.

Histology

The histopathological features include a highly vascular tissue with sheets of eosinophilic epitheloid cells and nerve fibrils.

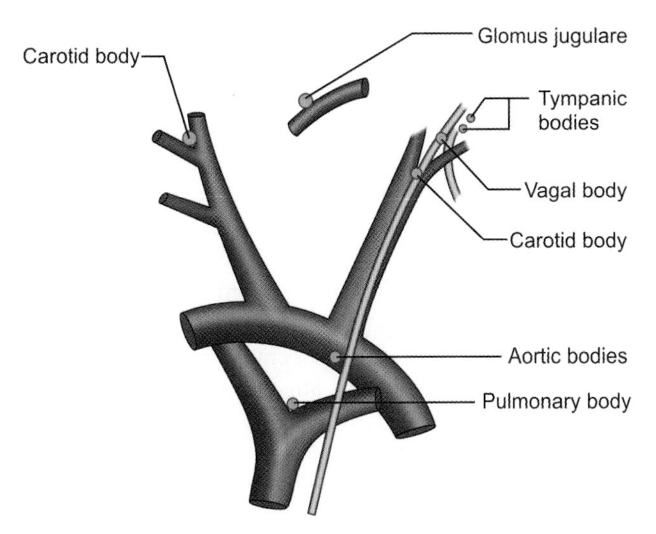

Fig. 16.3: Sites where chemodectoma can occur

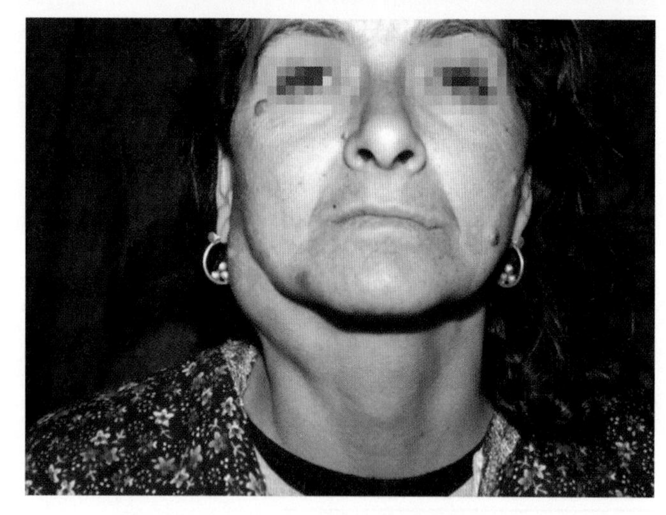

Fig. 16.4: Chemodectoma: Carotid body tumor

Clinical Features

The tumor commonly occurs in elderly females. Depending upon the origin and spread of the tumor, symptoms may be aural, neurological, or combination of the two groups:

1. *Aural symptoms:* The tumor presents in the ear with tinnitus, usually pulsatile, deafness, and blood-stained discharge.
2. *Neurological symptoms:* The tumor which primarily arises from the jugular bulb subsequently involves the adjacent cranial nerves in the jugular foramen and produces symptoms of their involvement. The 7th and 8th cranial nerve involvement produces asymmetry of the face, dizziness and perceptive deafness.

   Pain is not the usual feature unless infection is present.

Signs

Otoscopically, a reddish blue mass may be seen behind the tympanic membrane—a rising sun appearance.

Browne's sign: Increasing the pressure in the external auditory canal by the Siegel's speculum makes the tumor mass more prominent and red, with increased pulsations. As the pressure is increased above systolic pressure, blanching occurs and pulsations disappear to reappear again on release of the pressure.

Once the tumor perforates the drum-head, it presents as a bleeding vascular polypoidal mass in the canal. A bruit may be heard over the ear. Evidence of cranial nerve paralysis may be present and mostly the 7th, 8th, 9th, 10th and 11th cranial nerves are involved.

Classification of Glomus Jugular Tumor Oldring and Fisch's (1979)

Classification of the glomus jugular tumor is as follows:

Type A: Tumor confined to the middle ear
Type B: Tumor confined to the middle ear and mastoid without destruction of infralabyrinthine part of the temporal bone
Type C: Tumor in middle ear and mastoid with destruction of infralabyrinthine part of the temporal bone and destruction of the petrous apex
Type D: Tumor extending intracranially.

Staging of Glomus Jugular Tumor

Stage I: Tumor limited to hypotympanum.
Stage II: Tumor involves tympanomastoid cavities.
Stage III: Spreads to intracranial structures.

Investigations

1. A baseline audiogram is obtained. Hearing tests may show conductive or sensorineural loss
2. X-ray examination of the mastoids is of little value though it may show areas of bone destruction and enlargement of jugular foramen
3. CT scan of temporal bone with contrast is valuable. Erosion of jugular plate is diagnostic (Phelps's sign)
4. MRI/MRA will usually show a 'salt and pepper' lesion on T2-weighed images, although very small lesions may be missed.
5. Bilateral four-vessel angiography is helpful in diagnosing the extent of the tumor, and assess the collateral circulation.
6. Biopsy from the tumor mass is confirmatory but should be done very carefully as the tumor is very vascular and bleeds profusely. The clinical features, CT and Angio scans are usually sufficient to diagnose this tumor and biopsy is rarely if ever indicated to confirm this diagnosis.

Histopathology: It reveals nests of nonchromaffin staining cells clustered among vascular channels lined by epithelioid cells.

Treatment

Small tumors are excised. Larger lesions may be treated by radiotherapy followed by surgery. Careful angioembolization of selected identified feeding vessels is done to reduce intraoperative bleeding and ensure complete removal of these lesions. Sometimes radiotherapy is given postoperatively for recurrent/residual tumors or for those patients who are not fit otherwise for surgery.

MALIGNANT TUMORS OF MIDDLE EAR CLEFT

Mesenchymal Tumors

Embryonal rhabdomyosarcoma: Rhabdomyosarcoma is a malignant tumor of striated muscle origin. It is derived from primitive mesenchyme that has retained its capacity for skeletal muscle differentiation. Rhabdomyosarcoma of the head and neck is primarily a disease of the first decade of life, and it is the most common soft tissue sarcoma in childhood. Approximately 90 percent of all cases of rhabdomyosarcoma are diagnosed in individuals younger than 25 years, and within this group, 60 to 70 percent are younger than 10 years. Embryonal rhabdomyosarcoma is the most common subtype observed in children, accounting for approximately 60 percent of all cases in this age group. The tumors can occur at any site, but they are most commonly observed in the genitourinary region or the head and neck region. Treatment of rhabdomyosarcoma is a multimodality effort. Initial efforts are aimed at surgical resection of the tumor, always followed by chemotherapy and typically ending with a standard course of radiation. The principles of surgical and radiation therapy are based on the site of involvement and the extent of disease, whereas the chemotherapeutic options depend on risk factors.

Eosinophilic granuloma: Eosinophilic granuloma is a granulomatous disease of unknown etiology which may affect the temporal bone chiefly in children and young adults. Osteolytic lesions occur and involvement of the temporal bone may present as a polypoid mass in the posterior canal wall followed by pain and infection. It is often confused with chronic otomastoiditis. X-rays show unifocal or multifocal osteolytic lesions and histology shows proliferation of histiocytes. Conservative surgery with steroids and radiotherapy has proved useful in such patients.

Epithelial Tumors

The disease commonly affects elderly males and squamous cell carcinoma is the common variety of malignancy involving this region.

The patient usually gives a history of long-standing ear discharge. With the onset of malignancy, the discharge becomes blood stained and may be profuse. Hearing loss becomes progressive and more marked and facial nerve paralysis may occur. Pain in the ear is an important symptom.

Examination reveals the friable bleeding mass in the external meatus and biopsy confirms the disease.

X-ray of the temporal bone shows bone destruction and the extent of involvement.

A combination of radical surgical excision followed by radiotherapy is the treatment of choice.

Tumors of the Inner Ear

ACOUSTIC NEUROMA (FIG. 16.5)

Auditory or 8th nerve tumors are common intracranial tumors and account for 80 percent of all tumors of the cerebellopontine angle and 8 percent of the brain tumors.

Acoustic neuroma is a benign tumor and may be associated with multiple neurofibromatosis (von Recklinghausen's disease) in which case it may be bilateral.

Origin

These tumors arise from the distal neurilemmal portion of the 8th nerve, usually from the vestibular division, hence also called neurilemomma. The tumor represents neoplasia of the Schwann cells and is correctly called vestibular schwannoma.

Spread

In most cases, the tumor arises in the distal neurilemmal portion of the vestibular division of the 8th nerve inside the internal acoustic meatus. It grows out of the meatus into the cerebellopontine angle. The adjacent nerve roots in the cerebellopontine angle get stretched. Extratemporal spread in the posterior fossa leads to increased intracranial pressure.

Histopathology

The tumor consists of interlacing bundles of spindle-shaped cells. A typical feature of these tumors is that spindle-shaped nuclei of adjacent cells get aligned in columns parallel to one another (palisading of the nuclei) forming ribbon-like fasciculated structures called *Verocay bodies (Antoni type A)*. Sometimes, there is an evidence of degeneration and nuclei are seen scattered in connective tissue fibrils (*Antoni type B*).

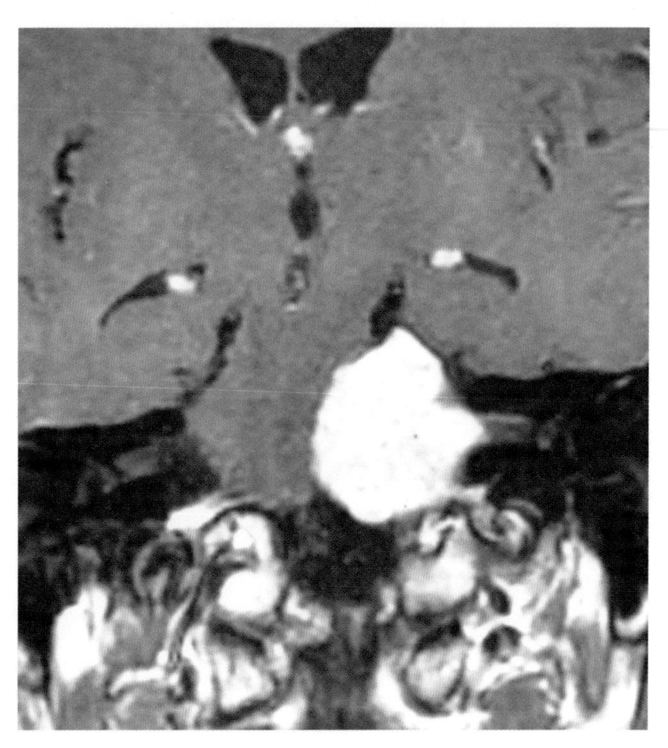

Fig. 16.5: Axial MRI showing acoustic neuroma

Clinical Features

The tumor is common in the 4th to 6th decades of life and is commoner in females than males with a ratio of 3:2. Although the tumor most commonly arises from the vestibular nerve, the earliest symptoms are usually auditory. The slow-growing progressive changes of the vestibular nerve produce little disturbance due to central adaptation. The earliest symptom is most often progressive, unilateral perceptive deafness frequently associated with tinnitus. The patient has difficulty in understanding speech. Sometimes, vertigo is the presenting symptom. The other presenting features may be due to involvement of adjacent structures like cranial nerves, and in late cases symptoms of increased intracranial pressure may occur. The trigeminal nerve is the first to be affected causing diminished corneal reflex, pain and tingling and numbness along the nerves distribution. Facial paralysis and diplopia herald raised intracranial pressure. Once the tumor involves the cerebellum, cerebellar symptoms appear. Blindness and coma precede death.

Neurological Evaluation

1. Ophthalmic examination is done for nystagmus, signs of papilloedema and corneal reflex.
2. *Sensory nerve examination*
   a. *Corneal reflex* reflects on the integrity of the trigeminal nerve. Loss of this reflex may be an early sign of the disease.
   b. *Facial nerve examination:* The posterior aspect of the external auditory canal should be examined for the presence of decreased sensation (Teal's sign).

As the tumor grows larger, there may be evidence of involvement of the cerebellum, adjacent brainstem and other cranial nerves.

Investigations

1. Pure tone audiometry reveals unilateral sensorineural deafness.
2. Discrimination of speech is markedly reduced as detected by *speech audiometry*.
3. *Loudness recruitment* is usually absent.
4. *Tone decay* is markedly present (> 30 db above threshold).
5. *Vestibular evaluation* reveals a hypoactive labyrinth in most patients. Caloric tests show canal paresis.
6. *Radiological investigation:* To demonstrate the erosion or widening of the internal auditory meatus. CT (Air meatography) of the internal auditory meatus is very useful. A difference of even 1 mm in diameter of internal auditory meatus on the two sides is significant of this pathology. Late cases may show marked erosion of the internal auditory meatus.
7. *Other investigations* like tomography, angiography, posterior cranial fossa myelography and CSF protein analysis are helpful procedures in the diagnosis of acoustic neuroma.
8. *MRI* is now considered to be a standard investigation for the diagnosis of vestibular schwannoma. It can pick-up lesions as small as 2 mm with a positive predictive value of more than 90 percent.
9. *Auditory brainstem response:* Interaural latency difference of wave V of more than 0.3 ms and wave I to wave V inter peak difference of more than 4 ms is highly suggestive of the disease.

Treatment

Total removal of the tumor is the treatment of choice. Various approaches have been suggested depending on the size of the tumor.

The translabyrinthine route and the middle cranial fossa approach are carried out for the tumor limited to the meatus. The added advantage of these approaches is that the facial nerve is preserved. The suboccipital approach is adopted for the large tumors.

Chapter 17

Otological Aspects of Facial Paralysis

Facial Paralysis

The course of facial nerve is shown in **Figure 17.1. Figure 17.2** shows a case of facial paralysis.

Otological Aspects of Facial Paralysis

ANATOMY AND COURSE OF FACIAL NERVE

Facial nerve is a mixed nerve having a motor and sensory root. It supplies muscles of facial expression and carries secretomotor fibers to lacrimal, submandibular and sublingual salivary glands and taste sensation from anterior two-third of tongue. It also supplies sensory twigs to concha and retroauricular regions.

There are three divisions of facial nerve.

1. Intracranial—from pons to internal acoustic meatus.
2. Intratemporal—from internal acoustic meatus to stylomastoid foramen.
3. Extratemporal—from stylomastoid foramen to its peripheral branches.

It is the intratemporal part of facial nerve which is of primary concern to an ENT surgeon.

A number of conditions in the middle ear can involve the nerve, some of these include: CSOM (Cholesteatomas), ASOM (Acute Suppurative Otitis media), tumors of middle ear, fracture of temporal bone; more often in transverse fractures, Bell's palsy, herpes zoster oticus (Ramsay Hunt syndrome); and last but not the least following ear surgery.

The sheath that surrounds facial nerve through its course in the fallopian canal consists of periostium, epineurium and perineurium. Surgical decompression of facial nerve

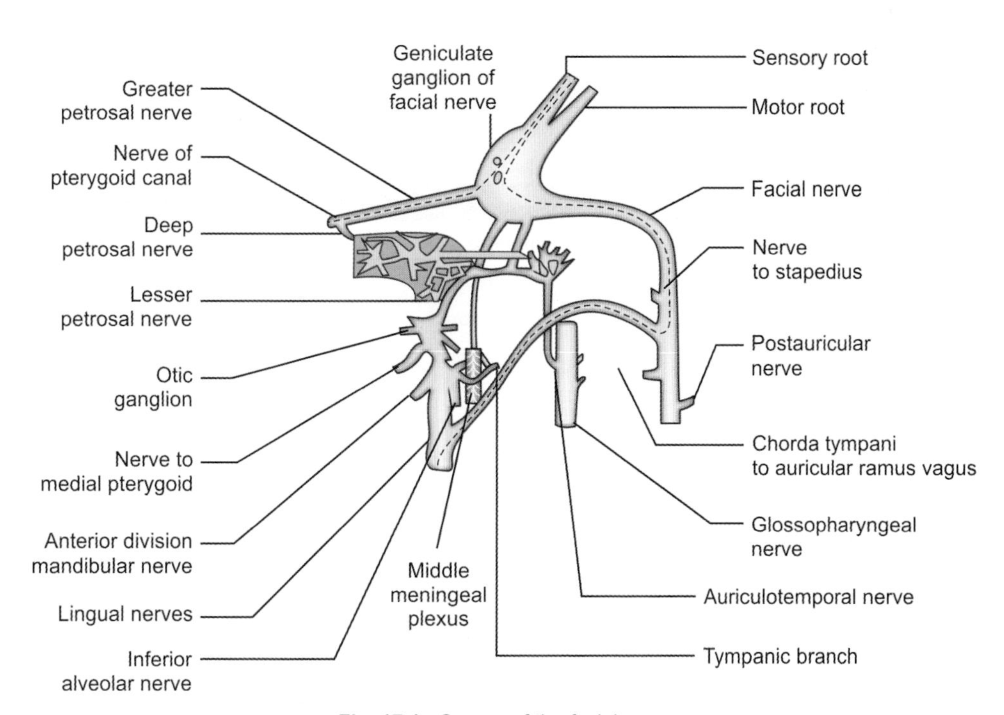

Fig. 17.1: Course of the facial nerve

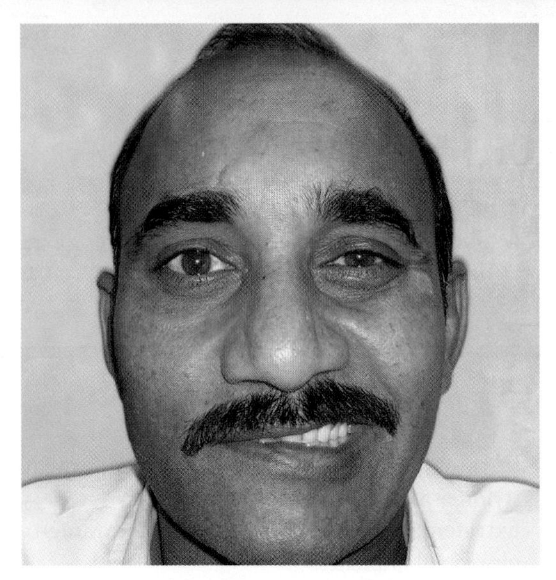

Fig. 17.2: Right sided facial paralysis

involves opening of perineurium. Although this procedure is controversial in cases of Bell's palsy and herpes zoster oticus but it has a definitive role in primary facial tumors and in cases of trauma where the nerve is disrupted and it is necessary to find the proximal and distal ends for repair.

PATHOLOGY OF FACIAL NERVE INJURY

Sunderland (1978) has described five possible degrees of injury facial nerve can undergo.

1st degree	Compression
2nd degree	Interruption of axoplasm and myelin
3rd degree	Disruption of endoneurium
4th degree	Disruption of endoneurium and perineurium
5th degree	Transsection of the nerve.

This classification is more comprehensive than the previous classification of neuropraxia, axonotmesis and neurotmesis prescribed by Seddon (1943).

Pathological processes causing facial paralysis in patients with Bell's palsy or herpes zoster usually do not progress beyond first or second degree which accouts for recovery in most of the cases.

Etiology

The etiology of facial paralysis is shown in **Table 17.1**.

FACIAL NERVE PARALYSIS DUE TO OTITIS MEDIA

1. *ASOM:* In about 6 percent of the population, the facial canal shows a bony dehiscence, with the result that any acute infective process like acute suppurative otitis media can lead to edema of the facial nerve and hence its paralysis. The treatment is of the infective process, and facial palsy recovery occurs with the control of the infection.
2. *Herpes zoster of the facial nerve (Ramsay Hunt's syndrome):* Herpetic infection of the geniculate ganglion is often associated with facial palsy accompanying auditory and vestibular symptoms. The vesicular eruptions usually occur on the concha, antihelix, antitragus and external auditory canal. The treatment in such cases is symptomatic. Steroids sometimes help.
3. *CSOM:* In cases of chronic suppurative otitis media (atticoantral variety), the cholesteatoma causes bone erosion and hence exposes the facial nerve to the disease process, with resultant paralysis. In such cases, mastoid exploration is done and the cholesteatoma removed. The recovery depends upon the extent of damage, the nerve has suffered from the disease.

Table 17.1: Etiology of facial nerve paralysis

Intracranial	Intratemporal	Extratemporal
1. Meningitis	1. Acute suppurative otitis media	1. Parotid malignancy
2. Tumors particularly in cerebellopontine angle	2. Cholesteatoma a. Accidental b. Surgical	2. Trauma
3. Posterior inferior cerebellar artery thrombosis	3. Trauma: a. Accidental b. Surgical	
4. Poliomyelitis	4. Bell's palsy	
5. Disseminated sclerosis	5. Acoustic neuroma	
6. Trauma	6. Neuroma of facial nerve	
	7. Glomus jugular	
	8. Malignancy of middle ear cleft	
	9. Ramsay Hunt syndrome	

FACIAL PARALYSIS DUE TO SURGERY ON THE MIDDLE EAR AND MASTOID

The facial nerve can get damaged during surgical procedures on the middle ear cleft. The nerve courses on the medial wall of the middle ear anteriorly from the processus cochleariformis, above the promontory and the oval window to the pyramidal process where it takes a bend, to start its vertical portion and comes out of the temporal bone through the stylomastoid foramen.

Facial paralysis due to surgical trauma can occur in the following situations:

1. In infants, because of lack of development of the mastoid process, the standard postaural incision damages the nerve, so the incision is placed more horizontally to avoid the nerve.
2. During mastoidectomy, one should identify the plane of the lateral semicircular canal, and avoid working at any level more medial than this to avoid nerve damage.
3. The compact bone of the digastric ridge gives the plane of the stylomastoid foramen. This should be kept in mind while working on the mastoid tip, otherwise the nerve gets damaged.
4. The gouge and drill work should be parallel and in the line of the facial nerve. Bony work across the line of the canal damages the nerve.
5. During radical mastoidectomy, while removing the outer attic wall or the bony bridge, the nerve may be cut and hence the surgeon should be careful at this stage.
6. Curettage of the middle ear is not advisable as it can damage the nerve.
7. While lowering the facial ridge, the bone should be cut along the line of the nerve and one should not go deep to the tympanomastoid suture line.
8. The nerve may get damaged during stapedectomy during currettage of the bony overhang of the posterior canal wall or at the time of work on the footplate.

Management of Postoperative Facial Paralysis

In case the facial paralysis is noted immediately after the operation, the damage to the nerve is more severe. Immediate exploration is done and if a bone piece is found piercing the nerve, it is removed or the hematoma drained. If the nerve is cut, its ends are brought together and sutured or a graft may be needed to bring the edges together. The graft is taken from the greater auricular or crural nerve of the leg.

If the paralysis develops later on, it signifies a lesser damage, probably that the nerve is exposed and paralysis is because of edema or due to pressure of the tight pack. In such cases, pack removal and steroids help to reduce the edema and the paralysis recovers.

Bell's Palsy

Bell described this idiopathic infranuclear lesion of the facial nerve. There is complete or partial paralysis of the muscles of facial expression of the whole of one side of the face, of sudden onset and there is no evidence of any symptom or sign of disease of the ear or central nervous system. It is thought to be an autoimmune disease. Probably, the paralysis is caused by the ischemia of the arterioles within the fallopian canal.

CLINICAL FEATURES

The paralysis is usually of sudden onset with a history of exposure to cold, sometimes associated with earache. In a vast majority of cases, the paralysis is incomplete and recovery occurs over a period of one to six months. In a smaller group of cases, the paralysis remains a permanent feature.

INVESTIGATIONS (FIG. 17.3)

Many topographical and electrodiagnostic tests have been described to know the exact site of lesion and the severity of the damage that the nerve has suffered. To know the level of lesion of the facial nerve, the various tests used are the following:

1. *Schirmer's test:* Blotting paper strips (3 cm × 5 cm) are placed under both the lower eyelids, and after sometime wetting of the blotting paper on the two sides is compared. If the facial nerve lesion is above the geniculate ganglion, lacrimation on the affected side will be less as the greater superficial petrosal nerve is involved.

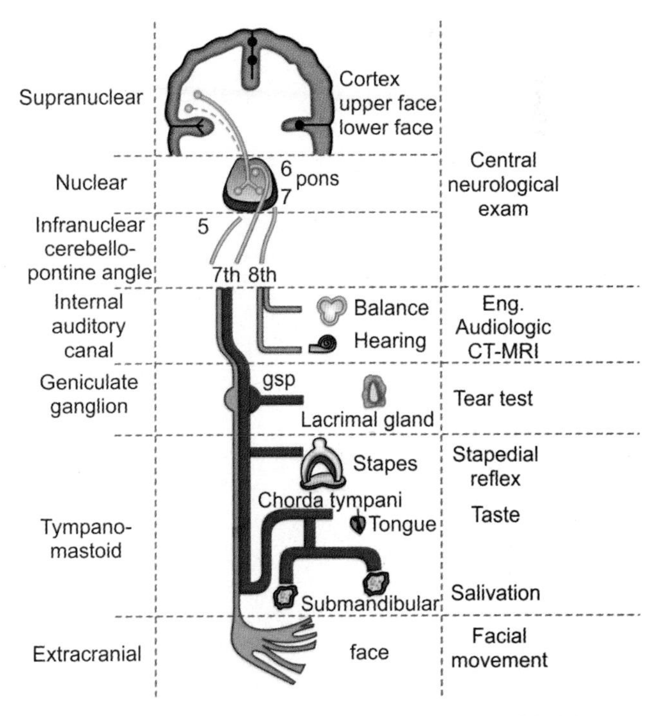

Fig. 17.3: Topographical and electrodiagnostic tests of facial nerve

2. *Acoustic reflex:* If the lesion is above the nerve to stapedius, this reflex is absent and the patient will complain of discomfort and pain on hearing loud sound (*phonophobia*).
3. *Electrogustometry:* An electrode is placed on the tongue and a current of 3 to 10 mA is given. Normally, a metallic taste is perceived. If the lesion is above the level of the chorda tympani nerve, the taste sensation of the affected side is absent.

TREATMENT

Various drugs, like vasodilators (nicotinic acid, nylidrine) vitamins (B_1, B_{12} and B_6) have been tried without much efficiency.

It has now been seen that prednisolone 80 mg/day and tapered off for 9 days is most effective.

Injections of ACTH gel have given better results than cortisone. Usually 60 IU are given intramuscularly daily for about a week.

Surgical treatment: Stellate ganglion block has proved useful in some cases. The role of facial nerve decompression in Bell's palsy is controversial. It is not a definite treatment for the disease but only tries to lay a ground work for the recovery by relieving the pressure on the nerve.

Hemifacial Spasm

It is a rare condition characterized by violent hemifacial muscular contractions without actual paralysis, seen in older patients. In severe cases the condition becomes intolerable and resistant to all sorts of treatment except facial nerve resection to cause complete facial paralysis.

Important Points

In facial nerve palsy one should ask the history of:

a. Trauma especially head injuries and penetrating injuries
b. Previous mastoid and middle ear surgery
c. Ear discharge and/or ear pain
d. Slow progressive paralysis (suspect tumor)
e. Recurrent paralysis
f. Bilateral paralysis
g. Association of hemifacial spasm
h. Associated deafness
i. Vestibular symptoms
j. Any eruptions on the pinna or the external canal.

Chapter 18

Ménière's Disease and Other Common Disorders of the Inner Ear

Ménière's Disease

This is a disease of the inner ear characterized by sudden and recurrent attacks of vertigo, often associated with nausea and vomiting together with deafness and tinnitus.

PATHOGENESIS

The basic histopathological change noted in these cases has been endolymphatic hydrops (gross distension of endolymphatic system). However, there has been difficulty in explaining its cause and in correlating it with the symptomatology. Generally, the theories of causation of endolymphatic hydrops are grouped as follows:

1. A theory suggests that the distension occurs because of disturbances of fluid formation, which occur due to local disturbances of capillary permeability or colloid osmotic disturbances. Factors like, retention of sodium, allergic edema and autonomic imbalance have been incriminated.
2. Another theory suggests that distension of the endolymphatic system occurs because of mechanical blockage and disturbed reabsorption. Proponents of this theory maintain that the endolymph traverses the endolymphatic duct and gets absorbed in the sac. In Ménière's disease, the defective absorption by the sac is regarded as the cause of hydrops.

CLINICAL FEATURES

Paroxysmal attacks of vertigo with deafness and tinnitus mark the acute stage. The acute attack typically starts with a feeling of aural fullness followed by vertigo which is accompanied by nausea, vomiting, deafness and tinnitus. The attack may last for a varying period of time and may recur at short intervals. Deafness is sensorineural in type, fluctuating, usually unilateral and progressive. As the disease progresses the deafness becomes more pronounced and speech discrimination worsens. The tinnitus is usually low-pitched. There are no other neurological symptoms and signs.

The remission or inactive phase: As the vertigo subsides, hearing loss and tinnitus may improve but with recurrent attacks, the patient's hearing deteriorates and tinnitus becomes a constant feature. Recent studies have shown a spontaneous remission rate of up to 71 percent of cases within 8 years of diagnosis.

Variations of the clinical picture may occur owing to the absence of one or more of the main features that constitute the disease.

INVESTIGATIONS

1. *Audiometry:* Pure tone audiometry reveals sensorineural deafness. The hearing loss is more for the lower frequencies in the early stages of the disease. Loudness recruitment is usually present. The short increment sensitivity index (SISI) test shows a high score. The tone decay test is near normal. Bekesy audiometer traces a type II curve.
2. *Vestibular function test:* Spontaneous nystagmus is absent except during an attack. Caloric tests show hypoactivity on the affected side. However, a normal caloric test does not rule out Ménière's disease as the vestibular system is capable of recovery in the early stages of the disorder.
3. *CT scan:* CT scan of the temporal bone helps to rule out internal acoustic meatus pathology.
4. *Glycerol test:* The glycerol test is regarded as valuable diagnostic tool. Glycerine makes blood hypertonic and reduces the hydrops.

   Ninety-five percent glycerine, 1.5 cc/kg of body weight with addition of the same amount of physiological saline is given orally on a fasting stomach. Pure tone audiometry and speech audiometry are done after intervals of one hour for 2 to 3 hours and compared with pretest records.

   Improvement in hearing signifies an endolymphatic hydrops in about 60 percent of cases. 15 db improvement on pure tone audiometry or 12 percent improvement in speech discrimination ability are taken as positive data. However, a negative test does not exclude Méniére's disease.The test is contraindicated in patients with cardiac and renal diseases as well as in diabetics.
5. *Electrocochleography:* This test is done to determine the SP/AP ratio which is normally 20 percent. More than 30 percent is suggestive of Ménière's disease.

TREATMENT

There is no definite treatment of this condition. Various methods (medical and surgical) have been adopted to alleviate the patient's symptoms. The general management of the patient is of prime importance. An understanding and sympathetic approach to the problem is essential. Strong reassurance and stressing the nonfatal nature of the disorder is necessary.

Treatment of the acute attack: The patient is put to bed rest. Any of the vestibular suppressants is given to control the vestibular symptoms. The following drugs are commonly used—prochlorperazine (Stemetil) 15 to 75 mg daily, orally or by injections; promethazine (Avomine, Phenergan); chlorpromazine (Largactil 25 mg thrice daily); or dimenhydrinate (Dramamine).

The dosage is adjusted according to the patient's needs. Sometimes the stellate ganglion block during an acute attack helps to relieve the symptoms. The long-term medical treatment has been based on various theories.

1. *Dietetic therapy:* It is suggested that low salt and limited water intake reduces the hydrops.
2. *Vitamin therapy:* All the vitamins, coenzymes and trace elements have been used. Favorable effects have resulted from the administration of nicotinic acid and vitamin A and D.
3. *Diuretic therapy:* Diuretics like acetazolamide have been used on the assumption that these drugs will reduce the hydrops.
4. *Vasodilators:* Such drugs have been used with an idea that they relieve the angiospastic vascular changes in the endarterial distribution of the labyrinthine artery.

   Recently betahistadine hydrochloride (Vertin, Serc) has shown good results.
5. *Streptomycin therapy:* Previously large doses of streptomycin were used particularly in bilateral cases to inducel labyrinthine damage (Chemical Labyrinthectomy).

Surgical treatment of Ménière's disease: Surgery is considered for those cases of Ménière's disease, which do not respond to medical therapy and where the disabling symptoms continue to occur.

The following procedures have been used:

1. *Cervical sympathectomy:* The operation is thought to correct the microcirculatory fault in the labyrinth and thus relieve the symptoms.
2. *Myringotomy with grommet insertion:* The exact mode of action is not clearly known.
3. *Operations on the endolymphatic sac:* The aim of the operation is to decompress and/or drain the sac (shunt operation) so that adequate absorption of endolymph occurs with resultant relief of the hydrops.
4. *Vestibular neurectomy:* This involves selective section of the vestibular division of the eighth nerve, particularly in cases with intractable vertigo but with a good hearing. The middle cranial fossa approach to the eighth nerve is chosen.
5. *Labyrinth destruction:* Total destruction of the labyrinth (labyrinthectomy) may be the last resort for cases with intractable symptoms and poor hearing levels. The transmastoid and transmeatal route can be used for labyrinthectomy.
6. *Selective destruction of vestibular labyrinth by cryosurgery or ultrasound:* These physical methods have recently been used for the treatment of Ménière's disease. This is accomplished by selective destruction of the vestibular end organs in the labyrinth without damaging the cochlea or facial nerve.
7. *Cryosurgical methods:* A cryoprobe is placed on the semicircular canal or promontory and subnormal temperature achieved which causes destruction of the adjacent labyrinthine tissue.
8. *Ultrasound:* Ultrasonic vibrations are passed to the semicircular canal by an applicator through the mastoid route.

Lermoyez's syndrome: This is a variant of Ménière's syndrome in which hearing loss and tinnitus occur first, followed by vertigo that appears suddenly and with it hearing and tinnitus improve.

DIFFERENTIAL DIAGNOSIS OF MÉNIÈRE'S DISEASE

The disease has to be differentiated from other conditions which produce paroxysmal attacks of vertigo, tinnitus or deafness.

1. *Eighth nerve tumor (acoustic neuroma):* Differentiation of this condition is difficult particularly in the early stages when it only gives otological symptoms.

   The main symptom is usually progressive unilateral sensorineural hearing loss associated with tinnitus and diminished caloric response. However, the vertigo is neither marked nor usually paroxysmal. Other neurological deficits occur. Audiometry shows a retrocochlear lesion. X-ray studies of internal auditory meatus and other tests like myelography, and scanning help in the final diagnosis.
2. *Vestibular neuronitis:* This disease is characterized by vertigo of sudden onset, sometimes occurring in small epidemics, often with a recent history of upper respiratory tract infection. The condition is usually unilateral but could be bilateral also.

   Caloric responses are diminished but hearing tests are normal.
3. *Benign positional vertigo:* The patient complains of recurring attacks of vertigo which are induced by change in position. Neurological examination is normal, hearing is unaffected and caloric tests are also usually normal. The only consistent physical finding is the vertigo and nystagmus that develop when the head is placed in a particular position. The nystagmus appears after a few seconds and is fatiguable.
4. *Epileptic vertigo:* Cases of epilepsy may present with an attack of vertigo but features-like loss of consciousness, fits, and normal hearing and caloric tests distinguish it from Ménière's disease.
5. *Vertebrobasilar insufficiency:* This condition in which transient episodes of ischemia occur in the distribution of the vertebrobasilar arterial system may present with vertigo and

tinnitus. However, other associated focal signs like diplopia, ipsilateral ataxia, facial paralysis and homonymous hemianopia indicate that the lesion is in the vascular system rather than in the inner ear.

Vertigo

Vertigo is the feeling that you or your environment is moving or spinning. It differs from dizziness in that vertigo describes a false or an illusion of movement. When you feel as if you yourself are moving, it's called *subjective vertigo*, and the perception that your surroundings are moving is called *objective vertigo*. In addition, the individual may have any or all of these symptoms: Nausea, vomiting, sweating and/or abnormal eye movements. The duration of symptoms can be from minutes to hours, and the symptoms can be constant or episodic.

Unlike nonspecific lightheadedness or dizziness, vertigo has relatively specific causes.

CAUSES OF VERTIGO

V—*Vascular*
- i. Vertebrobasilar insufficiency
- ii. Stroke
- iii. Migraine
- iv. Hypotension
- v. Anemia
- vi. Hypoglycemia
- vii. Ménière's disease

E—*Epilepsy*

R—*Receiving any treatment*
- i. Antibiotics
- ii. Cardiac drugs
- iii. Antihypertensive drugs
- iv. Sedatives and tranquilizers
- v. Aspirin
- vi. Quinine

T—1. *Tumor*
- a. Primary
  - i. Acoustic neuromas
  - ii. Glioma
  - iii. Intraventricular tumor
- b. Metastatic
  - i. Meningeal
  - ii. Carcinomatosis

2. *Trauma*
   - i. To labyrinth (temporal bone fractures)
   - ii. To brainstem (cervical vertebtrae fractures)
3. *Thyroid* Hypofunction

I—*Infections*
- i. Bacterial—labyrinthitis
- ii. Viral—vestibular neuronitis
- iii. Spirochetal—syphilis

G—*Glial diseases* Multiple sclerosis

O—*Ocular diseases or imbalance*

Vestibular Neuronitis

It is a viral infection of the vestibular nerve which may be preceded by upper respiratory tract infection. It is characterized by a sudden and severe attack of vertigo associated with nausea and vomiting. The vertigo gradually subsides. There is no deafness and no other neurological deficit. Examination reveals spontaneous nystagmus which gradually disappears within a few weeks.

The caloric tests show diminished response on the affected side. Hearing tests are normal.

TREATMENT

Bed rest is advised for a few weeks and vestibular suppressants like dimenhydrinate, chlorpromazine, prochlorperazine and betahistidine hydrochloride may be prescribed for a short period. The symptoms usually disappear over 3 to 4 weeks.

Benign Paroxysmal Positional Vertigo

This condition is characterized by sudden, severe attack of vertigo associated with nausea and vomiting which occurs when the head is placed in a particular position. The etiology of the condition is unknown but it is sometimes seen after head injury, ear operations or infections of the middle ear.

PATHOLOGY

There are two theories regarding the pathogenesis of this condition:
1. Cupulolithiasis hypothesis
2. Canalolithiasis hypothesis

It is postulated that calcium carbonate particles from the otolithic organs (of utricle and saccule) become detached and are displaced via gravity to the posterior semicircular canal since this is the most horizontal of the three canals. The displaced otoconia either become attached to the cupula of the posterior semicircular canal(cupulolithiasis) or remain as free floating particles in the posterior semicircular canal(canalolithiasis).

CLINICAL FEATURES

Vertigo is the main symptom. It occurs in episodes lasting usually less than a minute. Although brief, the episodes are severe, accompanied by nausea and vomiting and a characteristic nystagmus lasting 40 seconds and with a latency of up to 10 seconds which demonstrates fatiguability with repetitive testing.

Hallpike positional testing is diagnostic.

TREATMENT

Vestibular suppressants have been shown to be largely ineffective.

Habituation exercises may help. Epley maneuver and vestibular rehabilitation is the mainstay of treatment.The aim of Epley maneuver is to move the otoliths out of the posterior semicircular canals back to the utricle where they belong. Success rates of over 90 percent have been reported but recurrences do occur.

Chapter 19

Ototoxicity

Introduction

Ototoxicity may be defined as the tendency of certain therapeutic agents and other chemical substances to cause functional impairment and cellular degeneration of the tissues of the inner ear and especially of the end organs and neurons of the cochlear and vestibular divisions of the 8th cranial nerve. Important groups of ototoxic drugs can be classified as follows:

Quinine and salicylates: Tinnitus and/or hearing loss may occur with these drugs but the effects are reversible. These drugs probably induce vasoconstriction of the small vessels of the cochlear microvasculature.

Diuretics: Ethacrynic acid and frusemide are two potent diuretic agents. Both transient and permanent sensorineural hearing losses have been reported with these drugs especially when administered intravenously.

Permanent hearing loss may also occur when the patients being treated with an aminoglycoside are given either of these diuretics. The main histopathological changes have been found in the stria vascularis in which extensive edematous changes have been seen within minutes of injection of these drugs.

Antiheparinizing agents: Several cases of sensorineural hearing loss due to the drug hexadimethrine bromide (Polybrene) have been reported. This was formerly used in patients who were being treated for renal failure by hemodialysis, during the course of which heparin was given as an anticoagulant and Polybrene was given at the end of each dialysis as an antiheparinizing agent. Sensorineural deafness has been reported with this drug. There is degeneration of the organ of Corti and stria vascularis.

Cytotoxic agents: There have been several reports of sensorineural hearing loss following regional perfusion of nitrogen mustard; pathological changes have been demonstrated in the organ of Corti.

Antiepileptic drugs: Phenytoin over dosage may be associated with vestibular disorders. Ethosuximide is also vestibulotoxic.

Beta blocking agents: These drugs include propranolol, oxprenolol and practolol. All of them may produce adverse reactions but practolol appears to be unique in its ability to cause deafness. In a significant proportion of such cases, the deafness has presented clinically as mixed deafness.

Aminoglycoside antibiotics: In a dose exceeding 0.5 gm daily, streptomycin can damage both balance and hearing. Dihydrostreptomycin is more cochleotoxic than streptomycin. Kanamycin and neomycin are particularly toxic to the cochlea and rarely to the vestibular system but gentamycin and tobramycin are more vestibulotoxic. Sensorineural hearing loss also follows topical application of neomycin.

When aminoglycosides are applied topically to the middle ear, they may reach the perilymph by passing through either the round window membrane or the annular ligament, and hence to the organ of Corti by passing from the scala vestibuli, through Reissner's membrane, into the endolymphatic space.

Other antibiotics: These include vancomycin, capreomycin, viomicin, ampicillin and chloramphenicol. Minocycline is a new semisynthetic derivative of tetracycline which also has vestibulotoxic properties.

Clinical Features of Ototoxicity

The earliest symptom of ototoxicity is often high-pitched tinnitus. Hearing loss follows tinnitus. With those drugs which are mainly vestibulotoxic, the main symptom is disturbance of balance.

Pure tone audiogram shows a high tone loss. Recruitment can be demonstrated.

Prevention and Treatment of Ototoxicity

Although there are a few reports of spontaneous recovery of hearing, there is at present no effective treatment for ototoxicity. *Ozothine* (an aqueous preparation of oxidative products of oil of turpentine) with streptomycin has been found to reduce the toxicity of the latter, but it also reduces its antimicrobial activity.

Some authors have recommended certain maximum doses of ototoxic drugs and others have suggested regular monitoring of their serum levels.

Ototoxic drugs should be avoided unless they are essential to the survival and future wellbeing of the patient.

Serial audiograms should be done in all patients receiving these drugs, which should be withdrawn, if possible, as soon as any symptoms or signs of ototoxicity develop.

Patients with vestibular symptoms may be helped by labyrinthine sedatives and those with hearing problems may require a hearing aid.

Chapter

20

Tinnitus

Tinnitus Aurium

Tinnitus indicates hearing of adventitious sounds by the ear which are not attributed to any external sound. The word tinnitus is derived from the latin word 'tinnire' which means 'to ring'. It is usually described in terms of familiar monotonous sounds such as hissing, roaring, ringing, etc. Unlike hallucination which is a compound sound sensation such as hearing of voices.

CLASSIFICATION

Tinnitus indicates some disturbance of the auditory mechanism or its central connections. It is classified as central and peripheral.

Peripheral tinnitus may be *subjective*, which is audible only to the patient or *objective*, which is audible to others also. Peripheral tinnitus may be unilateral or bilateral.

Objective tinnitus: It may be caused by palatal myoclonus and is resistant to treatment. Sometimes, it responds to simple grommet insertion. The tensor tympani and stapedius muscle myoclonus also produces objective tinnitus. Other causes are arteriovenous shunts, glomus jugular tumor and aneurysms of the occipital or superficial temporal arteries and the aortic arch. This type of tinnitus is relieved by treatment of the cause.

Subjective tinnitus: Various causes of subjective tinnitus are as follows:

1. Wax in the external auditory canal.
2. Pathology in the middle ear stimulating the tympanic plexus.
3. Autonomic imbalance affecting the cochlear blood vessels.
4. Sensorineural hearing loss, which is usually associated with tinnitus.
5. Aspirin and other ototoxic drugs.
6. Otosclerosis.
7. *Poststapedectomy tinnitus:* It is one of the worst types of tinnitus which disappoints both the surgeon and the patient.
8. Acoustic neuroma.
9. Secretory otitis media.
10. Acoustic trauma.
11. Anemia.
12. Leukemia.
13. Renal disease.
14. Allergy.
15. Paget's disease.
16. Disseminated sclerosis.
17. Autoimmune involvement of the auditory end organ.

Idiopathic tinnitus: This is the most common form of tinnitus. Normally, the reflex pathway from the end organ to the cerebral cortex is through the auditory nerve, cochlear neurons and brainstem and back through the olivocochlear bundle. This controls the auditory apparatus. Some abnormality in this pathway which may be in the form of increased discharge from the cochlea or demyelination of the nerve fibers, etc. causes the patient to hear adventitious sounds. Patients who are tense and psychologically unbalanced are more prone to have tinnitus.

MANAGEMENT

In many cases, there is no specific treatment for tinnitus. It may simply go away on its own, or it may be a permanent disability that the patient will have to "live with". However, the patient is to be investigated thoroughly to rule out any organic cause for tinnitus and if present, treatment should be directed towards the basic cause. The underlying causes whose removal may relieve tinnitus include:

Earwax removal: Removing impacted earwax can decrease tinnitus symptoms.

Treating a vascular condition: Underlying vascular conditions may require medication, surgery or another treatment to address the problem.

Changing medication: If a medication appears to be the cause of tinnitus, recommend stopping or reducing the drug, or switching to a different medication.

NOISE SUPPRESSION

In some cases white noise may help suppress the sound so that it's less bothersome. Devices include:

White noise machines: These devices, which produce simulated environmental sounds such as falling rain or ocean waves, are often an effective treatment for tinnitus. A white noise machine with pillow speakers helps patients sleep. Fans, humidifiers, dehumidifiers and air conditioners in the bedroom may also help cover the internal noise at night.

Hearing aids: These can be especially helpful if patients have hearing problems as well as tinnitus.

Masking devices: Worn in the ear and similar to hearing aids, these devices produce a continuous, low-level white noise that suppresses tinnitus symptoms.

Tinnitus retraining: A wearable device delivers individually programmed tonal music to mask the specific frequencies of the tinnitus you experience. Over time, this technique may accustom you to the tinnitus, thereby helping patients not to focus on it. Counseling is often a component of tinnitus retraining.

MEDICATIONS

The intensity of tinnitus is measured by masking sounds. The intensity of the sound which masks the tinnitus is the intensity of the tinnitus and as such a *tinnitogram* can be plotted. After excluding all other causes, the following treatment is given.

1. *Lidocaine HCl* 100 mg infused rapidly intravenously acts as a local anesthetic and blocks multisynaptic junctions. It abolishes tinnitus in 70 percent of the cases but only for a short period. The drawback is that the treatment has to be given in a hospital under supervision and ECGs have to be done pre and post-treatment.
2. *Carbamazepine* 200 mg three times daily is effective but causes bone marrow depression and hepatotoxicity.

Besides these, tricyclic antidepressants, such as amitriptyline and nortriptyline, have been used with some success. However, these medications are generally used for only severe tinnitus, as they can cause troublesome side effects, including dry mouth, blurred vision, constipation and heart problems. Alprazolam (Niravam, Xanax) may help reduce tinnitus symptoms, but side effects can include drowsiness and nausea. It can also become habit-forming. Vasodilators like Nylidrine, etc. are also used.

SURGICAL TREATMENT

Operations usually undertaken for tinnitus include the following:

1. Stellate ganglion block
2. Cervical sympathectomy
3. Labyrinthectomy (in very severe cases)
4. Cochlear nerve section
5. Prefrontal leukotomy
6. Chorda tympani neurectomy

Newer forms of treatments also include the use of *low-power laser irradiation* given through the external acoustic meatus of the affected ear towards the cochlea. Varying results have been reported and none of the reported results would recommend a wider use for this form of therapy.

Chapter 21

Deafness

Deafness denotes loss of auditory function and depending upon the severity of hypoacusis, deafness may be mild, moderate, severe or total.

Classification

Deafness is classified into three groups (**Fig. 21.1**):

1. *Conductive deafness:* This occurs when the sound conducting mechanism of the ear is defective. The lesion could be anywhere from the external auditory canal to the footplate of stapes.
2. *Sensorineural deafness:* This type of deafness is due to abnormality in the cochlea, auditory nerve, neural pathway or their central connections with the auditory cortex.
3. *Mixed deafness:* It denotes that both conductive and sensorineural abnormality is present in the deaf person.

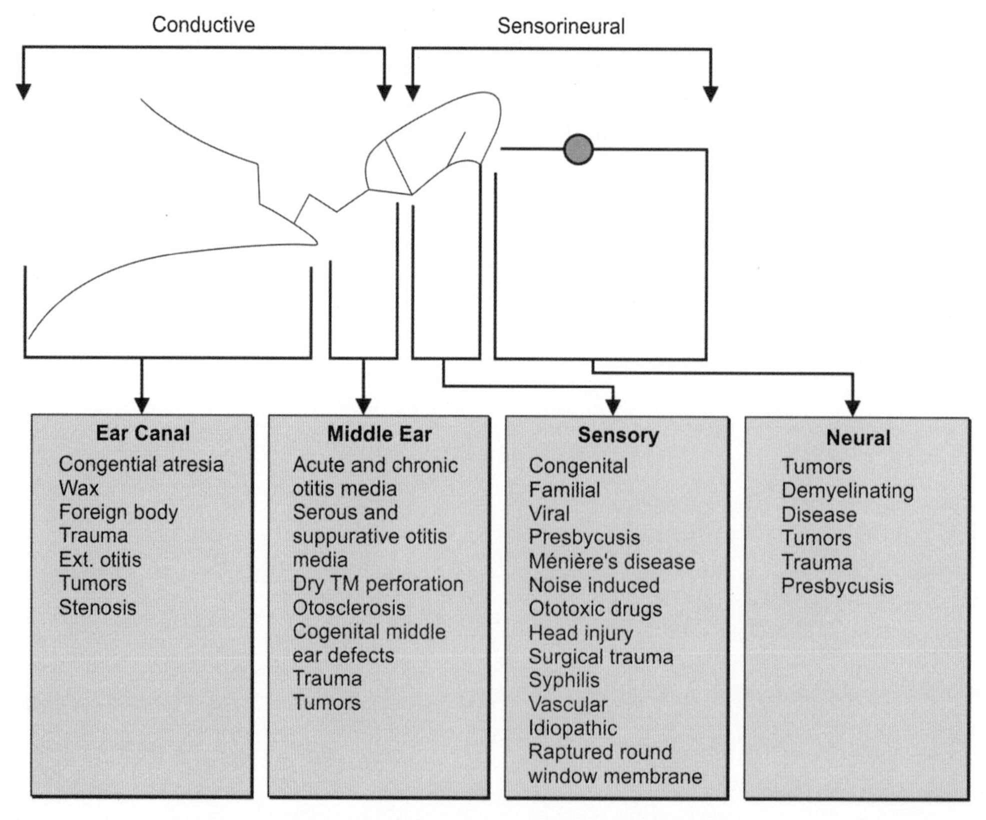

Fig. 21.1: Lesions producing conductive hearing loss (lesions of ear canal and middle ear) and sensorineural loss (lesions of sensory end organ and 8th cranial nerve)

CONDUCTIVE DEAFNESS

Etiology

Conductive deafness could be congenital or acquired.

Congenital abnormalities leading to conductive deafness include the following:

i. Atresia of the external auditory canal
ii. Ossicular anomalies like malformations, fixation, etc.
iii. Congenital absence of the oval window.

Acquired lesions causing conductive deafness are the following:

1. *External auditory canal* conditions
   a. Wax or foreign bodies in the external canal
   b. Inflammatory diseases like external otitis, otomycosis
   c. Traumatic stenosis
   d. Tumors of the external auditory canal causing blockage of the passage, like osteoma, exostosis.
2. *Acquired middle ear lesions*
   a. Inflammatory lesions like acute suppurative otitis media, chronic suppurative otitis media, secretory otitis media and adhesive otitis media.
   b. Traumatic causes like traumatic tympanic membrane perforations, ossicular disruption and hemotympanum.
   c. Tumors of the middle ear and mastoid, e.g. glomus jugular and carcinoma.
   d. Otosclerosis.

The treatment of conductive deafness depends upon the cause and such patients can usually be helped by modern microsurgical procedures. Alternatively a hearing aid can be fitted to overcome the hearing difficulty.

SENSORINEURAL DEAFNESS

Sensorineural deafness can be congenital or acquired.

Congenital Sensorineural Deafness

The causes are enumerated below:

1. *Genetic causes*
   a. Deafness occurring alone
      i. Michel's aplasia
      ii. Mondini-Alexander aplasia
      iii. Scheibe aplasia
      iv. Bing-Siebenmann aplasia.
   b. Deafness occurring with other abnormalities (syndromes)
      i. Waardenburg syndrome (deafness may be delayed)
      ii. Albinism
      iii. Hyperpigmentation
      iv. Onychodystrophy
      v. Pendred's syndrome
      vi. Jervell's syndrome
      vii. Usher's syndrome.
   c. Chromosomal abnormalities
      i. Trisomy 13, 15
      ii. Trisomy 21
2. *Nongenetic etiological factors*
   a. Deafness occurring alone.
      i. Ototoxic poisoning (streptomycin, aspirin, quinine, etc.).
   b. Deafness occurring with other abnormalities
      i. Viral infection (maternal rubella)
      ii. Bacterial infection
      iii. Ototoxic poisoning (thalidomide)
      iv. Metabolic disorders (cretinism)
      v. Erythroblastosis fetalis
      vi. Radiation (first trimester)
      vii. Prematurity
      viii. Birth trauma, anoxia.

Delayed Sensorineural Deafness

The causes are enumerated below.

1. *Genetic causes*
   a. Deafness occurring alone
      i. Familial progressive sensorineural deafness
      ii. Otosclerosis
      iii. Presbycusis
   b. Deafness occurring with other abnormalities (syndromes)
      i. Alport's disease
      ii. Hurler's syndrome (gargoylism)
      iii. Klippel-Feil syndrome
      iv. Refsum's disease
      v. Alstrom's disease
      vi. Paget's disease
      vii. Richard's Rundel syndrome
      viii. von Recklinghausen's disease
      ix. Crouzon's disease.
2. *Nongenetic causes*
   a. Inflammatory diseases
      i. Bacterial (labyrinthitis and otitis media)
      ii. Viral (measles, mumps, influenza labyrinthitis, etc.)
      iii. Spirochetal (congenital and acquired syphilis)
   b. Ototoxic poisoning
   c. Neoplastic disorders (leukemia, peripheral and CP angle tumors, etc.)
   d. Traumatic injury (acoustic trauma, temporal bone fractures)
   e. Metabolic disorders (hypothyroidism, allergies, Méniére's disease, etc.
   f. Vascular insufficiency (sudden deafness, presbycusis)
   g. Central nervous system disease (multiple sclerosis).

1. *Scheibe's (sacculocochlear type):* The whole bony labyrinth and membranous utricle and canals are fully formed while the cochlea and saccule show the early fetal type of sensory epithelium. It appears to be the most common type and is not associated with other developmental anomalies.
2. *Mondini-Alexander aplasia:* The cochlea is flattened with development of the basal coil only and underdevelopment of the vestibular structures.
3. *Bing-Siebenmann aplasia:* The bony cochlea and vestibule are fully formed but the membranous internal ear is malformed.
4. *Michel's type aplasia:* There is total lack of development of the internal ear.

Management of Congenital Sensorineural Deafness

Normal hearing is necessary for the development of speech, hence, patients with severe degrees of deafness fail to develop speech and thus remain deaf-mutes. Every effort should be made to detect these cases early.

Detection of Deafness

The babies who are at the risk, and the risk factors include(1) perinatal infections like toxoplasmosis, rubella, CMV, herpes and syphilis (2) Low birth weight (<1.5 Kg) (3) Neonatal bacterial meningiti (4) Kernicterus and hyperbilirubinemia (5) Congenital head and neck malformations (6) Family history of congenital deafness (7) Birth asphyxia, should be properly screened at 6 monthly intervals for hearing loss.

Similarly, if the parents suspect that the child is not responding to sounds properly or there is failure on the part of child to utter common words by 18 months to 2 years, a hearing handicap should be suspected and such patients should be properly investigated.

Startle Reflex Test

The newborn respond, to loud sound by moving its head, legs and arms.

Cochleopalpebral Reflex

Normally a loud sound made near a healthy infant causes blinking of its eyes.

Screening Test

A sound is made at 2 to 3 feet from the head of the baby. A baby with good hearing turns his head towards the sound source at the age of 7 to 9 months.

Objective audiological tests like evoked response audiometry are the most reliable method available at present.

The treatment of such patients is difficult. Depending upon the degree of deafness, hearing aids are fitted and auditory training given by the speech pathologist/therapist.

Deaf-Mute

EXAMINATION OF A DEAF-MUTE

History

1. *Family history*
   a. Is there any deafness in the family of either parent?
   b. Are the parents related to each other?
   c. How many children are in the family and is any of them deaf?
2. *Past history of the mother*
   a. Is there any history suggestive of syphilis?
   b. Is there a history of maternal rubella or other specific fever during pregnancy?
   c. Did the pregnancy go to full-term and was the confinement normal?
3. *Past history of the child's general health*
   a. Is there any history of neonatal jaundice?
   b. What illness has the child suffered to date?
4. *Speech*
   a. At what age, if at all did speech develop, did the child babble normally? If so, did he babble for a short time and then stopped?
   b. If the child is suspected of being partially deaf, is the tone defective or is there a difficulty in pronouncing consonants?
5. *Hearing*
   a. Does the mother communicate with the child by voice or by signs?
   b. Can the child hear when spoken to from another room?
   c. What is the greatest distance at which the child can hear when spoken to?
   d. Does he react to the noise of a motor car, the wireless, or the door bell?
6. *Age of onset*
   a. At what age was deafness first suspected?
7. *State of development*
   a. What standard of education has the child reached?
   b. At what age were the normal milestones, e.g. sitting up, learning to crawl, etc. reached?
   c. Is there any evidence of abnormalities of behavior such as triancy, lying, stealing or extreme introversion?
   d. A school report may give valuable information about the child's intelligence.

Assessing the Hearing

After watching and speaking to the child, Sheridan's test series is followed.

1. Test for babies (Play Audiometry)
   a. If 6 to 14 months—voice and noise-making instruments
   b. 15 to 18 months—same

c. 19 to 23 months—five toys test. Cup ball, toy motor car, a plastic doll and a toy bike. The child is given the toys one by one and they are named as they are given to him. 'Here is a cup. He is then asked to return them, e.g. give me the cup and so on.' Instructions are repeated at a distance.
2. Tests for 2 years old—six toys test and first cube test.
3. Test for 3 to 6 years children—seven toys test and second cube test. Training of deaf children is carried out in two ways.
   a. Auditory training or teaching the children to listen and hear to the fullest extent to which they are capable.
   b. *Speech training:* Teaching the child to speak properly.
   c. *Social and general training:* Teaching the child to act normally to his environment.

Acoustic Trauma

Acoustic trauma means noise induced hearing loss. It is directly proportional to civilization, i.e. more advanced a country is, more are the chances of noise induced hearing loss. The modern machineries, heavy industries, aeroplanes, fireworks, notorious old steam and diesel engines, pop music and above all modern warfare and so many other things which generate noise of high sound pressure level (SPL) produce injurious effects to the highly sensitive and delicate auditory end organ.

If the ear is exposed to explosive sounds for a short period only, there occurs a temporary shift in the hearing threshold, seen on audiometry as a steep dip at 4 kHz, called acoustic dip. If the person remains in a noisy atmosphere for a long time, the dip involves other frequencies and finally a flat curve is obtained on audiometry. 40 hours/week of 90 dB noise is safe for factory workers.

This 4 kHz area of basilar membrane is in basal turn of cochlea and is first exposed to noise and is first affected.

Histopathological studies have shown degenerative changes in the stria vascularis, hair cells as well as in the supporting cells in chronic acoustic trauma.

Noise induces vasospasm of the cochlear vessels and anoxia to the hair cells thus causing the damage.

Sociacusis: It is the hearing impairment because of noise of recreative places like pop music, snow mobiles, and car races, etc.

White noise: Like white light, it consists of a random mixture of all frequencies. The random movements of electrons in conducer and vacuum tubes also produce white noise which is audible as characteristic background "S-h-h-h" from a prolong vaph or radio. The sounds of speech form a constantly changing pattern of complex tones, noise and transients.

Presbycusis (Senile Deafness)

This is a type of sensorineural hearing loss which results due to the ageing process and is an auditory manifestation of senility. Degenerative changes occur in the cells of the organ of Corti and nerve fibres. The patient of an elderly age group presents with a slow, progressive deafness which may be associated with tinnitus. The deafness is bilateral and symmetrical, commonly affecting the high tones.

TREATMENT

The problem should be explained to the patients, sometimes a hearing aid may help.

Sudden Deafness

Sudden occurrence of hearing loss may be due to various known and unknown causes. Such a hearing loss may be conductive or sensorineural.

CONDUCTIVE TYPE OF SUDDEN DEAFNESS

This may be due to sudden impaction of wax in the canal, traumatic perforation of the tympanic membrane, foreign body in the external canal, hemotympanum, ossicular chain disruption or aero-otitis. Examination of the ear usually reveals the underlying disease and treatment is directed towards the cause.

SUDDEN SENSORINEURAL HEARING LOSS

Sensorineural hearing loss of sudden onset may be due to the following causes:

1. *Vascular lesions*
   a. Hemorrhage in the labyrinth as occurs in trauma, hypertension, leukemia, purpura, etc.
   b. Thromboembolism involving the internal auditory artery.
   c. Vascular spasm may be due to autonomic imbalance.
2. *Trauma*
   a. Acoustic trauma
   b. Fracture of the petrous part of temporal bone.
3. *Viral*
   a. Mumps
   b. Measles
   c. Herpes zoster
   d. Encephalitis.
4. *Miscellaneous*
   a. Functional
   b. Raised intracranial tension as might occur during straining, coughing and which may lead to rupture of the round window membrane producing sudden deafness.
5. *Idiopathic:* Majority of the cases of sudden deafness fall within this category.

Management

Attempts should be made to investigate the cause and treatment should be accordingly instituted. In those cases where the cause is unknown, following treatment may help:

1. Vasodilator drugs like nylidrin hydrochloride, beta-histidine and nicotinic acid should be given parenterally or orally in sufficient doses.
2. Steroid therapy with ACTH or oral steroids
3. Low molecular weight dextran
4. Intravenous histamine
5. Mixture of carbon dioxide and oxygen given under high pressure produces cerebral vasodilatation and thereby may help in such cases.
6. Stellate ganglion block may be done to correct the autonomic imbalance.
7. Intravenous conray.

Psychogenic Deafness

This is nonorganic hearing loss. It is classified into two types:

i. Malingering (feigned hearing loss).
ii. Hysterical deafness.

MALINGERING OR SIMULATED DEAFNESS

The deafness is due to conscious effort on the part of the subject to deceive. The subject tries to use hearing loss for the better circumstances, such as for legal, social or service compensation. The deafness is usually unilateral and of sensorineural type since it is difficult to feign conductive deafness.

The following factors help in arriving at the diagnosis:

1. History suggestive of a background motive.
2. Absence of ear disease.
3. Tricky remarks and test by examiner to elicit the response, such as dropping a coin or making a sound without the subject's knowledge and noting his response.
4. Inconsistency of response to various tuning forks and audiometric tests.
5. Various tests like Lombard's test, Stenger's test, Chimani Moose test, Erhard's test, Gault test, stethoscope test may be helpful in detecting a malingerer.

HYSTERICAL DEAFNESS

This type of deafness is a manifestation of hysteria. There is a subconscious wish to elevate the hearing threshold and is, therefore, outside the patient's control. The following features are suggestive:

1. Other evidence of hysteria such as tremors
2. Deafness is usually bilateral and persists during sleep
3. Repeated pure tone audiometry shows varying response
4. Definite improvement occurs with psychotherapy.

VARIOUS TESTS TO DETECT PSYCHOGENIC DEAFNESS

Stenger's Test

It is very useful and a reliable test. Two equal (512 or 256 Hz) and identical sounds strike each normal ear and the individual gets the impression in one ear only. The nearer the sounds, the impression in other ear is masked out by the nearer stimulus. If one ear is totally deaf from any organic cause, two identical tuning forks at the same distance from the two ears will lead to hearing of sound in the normal ear. With a suspected malingerer the eyes are blindfolded so that he has no idea that the tuning forks are being used. The tuning forks are struck with moderate intensity and held at 10 inches away from the each ear and the following procedure used. The patient is asked if he hears it, a malingerer will maintain one ear as deaf. The fork on the deaf side is advanced to 3 inches from the ear and on the other side to 6 inches. The malingerer will now deny hearing the fork with the normal ear though it is at less distance than before.

Weber's Test or Chimani Moose Test (Lateralization Test)

It is not a reliable test. A tuning fork of 256 cycles/sec is placed on the vertex. If true unilateral conductive deafness exists, the vibrations are localized in the deaf ear. If true perceptive deafness exists then vibrations are localized in the sound ear. The malingerer will also state that he hears from the sound ear. The meatus of the sound ear is then tightly occluded. If truly deaf he will hear either on the sound side or will be uncertain. The malingerer will state that he does not hear the fork at all.

Lombard's Test

It is a fairly reliable test. A barany noise box is placed in the sound ear and the patient is accustomed to the noise. He is then asked to count up to 100 or to read aloud from a book in his natural voice and not to stop when the noise starts. With true deafness, the voice is raised markedly, often to a shout, the malingerer (unless coached) continues in the same tone or only slightly raises his voice.

Loud Voice Test (Erhard's Test)

The sound ear is occluded by a finger in the meatus. This dampens reception but never completely cuts out loud sounds. The malingerer will often deny hearing even the loudest noises. He denies hearing the test sounds or words with the meatus of the sound ear lightly closed, when these were heard at double the distance with the meatus open.

Cochleopalpebral Test (Gault Test)

The sound ear is tightly occluded and a noise is made near the "deaf" ear. If a slight winking movement or contraction of the lid of the corresponding eye occurs, it indicates that the sound was heard in the ear. The pupil may also change in size, it usually contracts (auditory pupillary reaction). This test is more valuable in bilateral simulated deafness.

Stethoscope Test

One ear piece of the stethoscope is tightly occluded by wax, etc. A funnel replaces the chest piece. The malingerer becomes confused as not knowing whether the words spoken into the tunnel are being conducted to both ears or to one or other single ear.

Two Speaking Tubes

The examiner and his assistant react simultaneously short sentences from book of charts, each using a separate speaking tube which the patient holds one in each ear with unilateral organic deafness. The sentences spoken into the normal ear will be heard clearly and can be repeated. The malingerer will be confused by the two different voices and only occasional words from one or both speakers can be repeated.

Test During Sleep

A loud noise wakens a malingerer when he is asleep. In this respect it differs from a hysterical case.

Audiometric Tests

It is impossible to take constant audiograms, no matter how practised the audiometrist is.

Doerfler-Stewart Test

The feigned or functional deaf have usually adopted a subjective reference level for their hearing. By using a system of superimposed signals of speech and masking noise in measured amounts this reference level is disturbed, and on several counts, the test points to deviation from the finding on normal and on pathological ear. Psychogenic patients look more confused (upset) by masking noises than patients with organic lesions.

Hypnosis

Intravenous injection of a small dose of pentothal sodium is given. Tests with audiometer and with speech are made during hypnosis and results compared with those obtained before hand.

Chapter 22

Hearing Aids and Cochlear Implant

Hearing Aids

The hearing aid is a device that brings sound to the ear more effectively (**Fig. 22.1**). It is a miniature audioamplifier which is designed specifically for improving human communication.

The function of a hearing aid is to amplify sound and to couple the amplified sound to the ear. Since sound cannot be adequately amplified directly, it is necessary to change the acoustic signal to an electrical one. This electrical signal is then amplified and reconverted to acoustic energy at the ear. A hearing aid has three basic parts as mentioned below:

1. *Microphone:* Its function is to convert the sound signal into electric voltage.
2. *Amplifier:* This device amplifies the electric signal produced at the microphone.
3. *Receiver:* The receiver (earphone) reconverts the amplified electric signals into acoustic ones.

In addition to these basic components, most hearing aids have a gain control, tone control, off and on switch, a battery compartment, a cord and an ear mould.

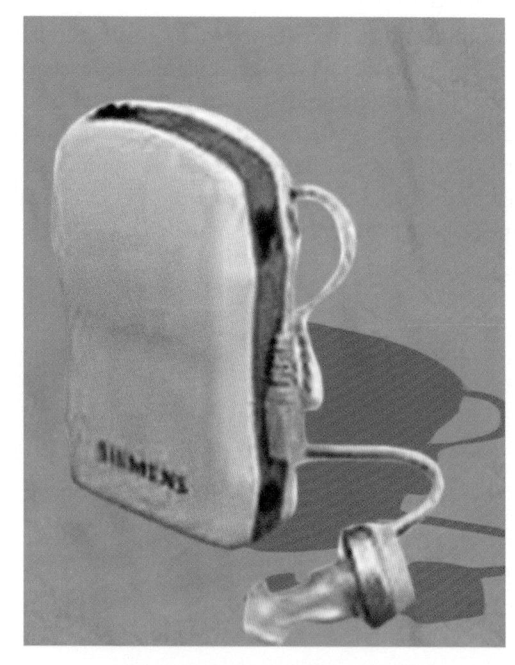

Fig. 22.2: Body worn hearing aid

DIFFERENT TYPES OF HEARING AIDS

1. Body worn hearing aids (**Fig. 22.2**).
2. Behind the ear hearing aid (postaural) (**Fig. 22.3**).

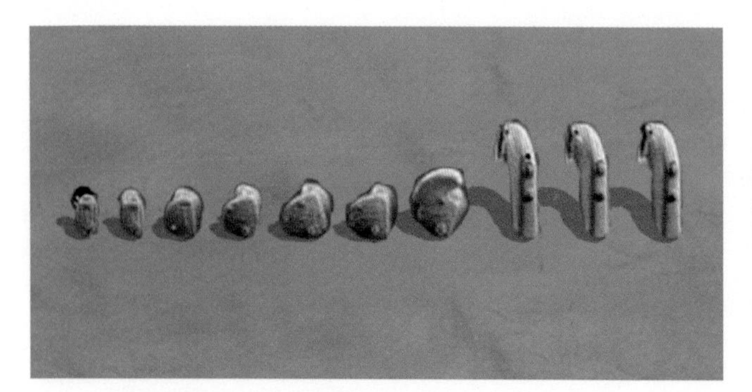

Fig. 22.1: Various types and sizes of hearing aids

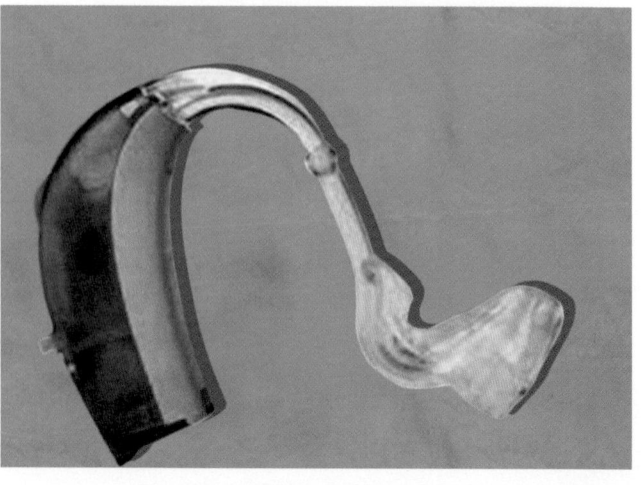

Fig. 22.3: Behind the ear hearing aid

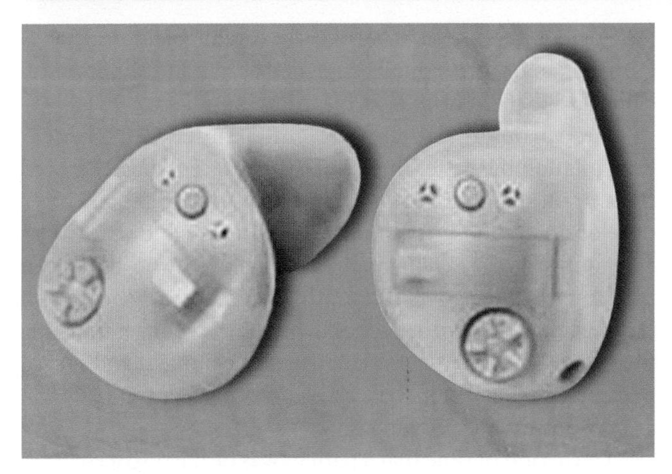

Fig. 22.4: In the ear canal aids, inside the canal (ITC) and completely in the canal (CIC)

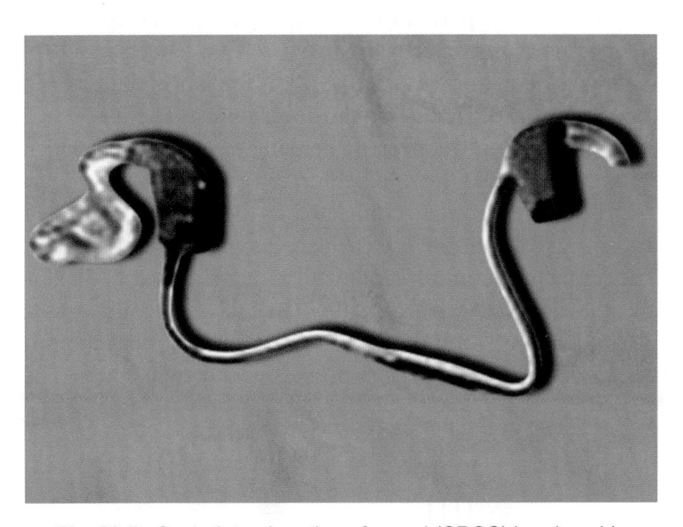

Fig. 22.5: Contralateral routing of sound (CROS) hearing aids

3. In the ear canal aids, inside the canal (ITC) and completely in the canal (CIC) (**Fig. 22.4**).
4. Contralateral routing of sound (CROS) hearing aids (**Fig. 22.5**).
5. Bone anchored hearing aid (BAHA) (**Fig. 22.6**).
6. Assistive listening devices.

GENERAL CONSIDERATIONS ABOUT HEARING AIDS

1. Use of a hearing aid is palliative. It does not cure deafness, nor does it arrest the disease producing the deafness. It only amplifies the sound and, therefore, may only alleviate the effects of deafness.
2. A hearing aid rarely restores the hearing acuity to 100 percent.

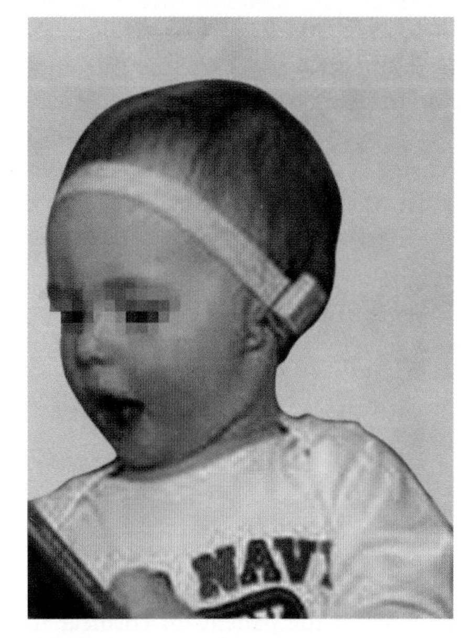

Fig. 22.6: Bone anchored hearing aid (BAHA)

3. A hearing aid simplifies to amplify all frequencies within its range, it does not select or emphasise certain frequencies over others as the ear does.

Audiological tests like pure tone audiometry and speech audiometry give an idea about the suitability of a hearing aid in the particular patient. Moreover, the hearing aid trials should be given to know whether it suits the patient's needs or not.

Cochlear Implant (Fig. 22.7)

It consists of stimulating the auditory system with electrical impulses as compared to a hearing aid which uses the surviving

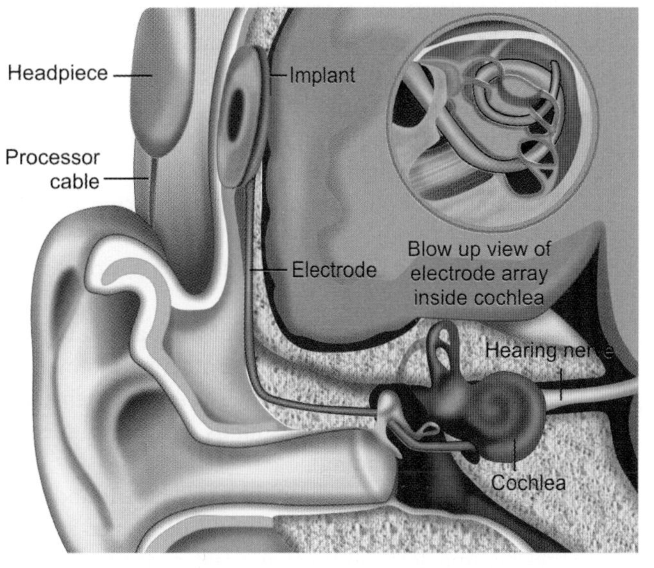

Fig. 22.7: Cochlear Implant

hair cells. It is indicated in patients with bilateral severe sensorineural deafness who do not respond to amplified sound stimuli. The electrical stimulation is used because it is easier to use and also because the cochlea itself acts as a transducer changing mechanical energy of sound vibration into electrical impulses. It is these impulses which are transmitted along the nerve.

The following disorders can cause severe or total hearing loss:

1. Congenital deafness
2. Trauma
   - Head injury
   - Surgical
3. Labyrinthitis
4. Ototoxic drugs
5. Ménière's disease
6. Meningitis
7. Idiopathic.

In order to select the patient for cochlear implant, the following tests are done to evaluate the degree of deafness and to assess the quality of the surviving neurons.

1. *Pure tone audiometry:* The patient should show no response on pure tone audiometry.
2. *Electrocochleography:* It can give direct indication as to whether a patient will or will not benefit from an implant.
3. *Promontory stimulation:* If a patient cannot hear on electrical stimulation, then the implant is of no value.

The various approaches are as follows:

1. Cortical stimulation
2. Acoustic nerve stimulation
3. Single channel intracochlear stimulation
4. Multiple channel intracochlear stimulation
5. Extracochlear stimulation.

Cochlear implants are more useful in postlingually deaf patients, i.e. who lost their hearing after acquisition of language.

Criteria for selection of patients for the implant are:

i. Bilateral deafness with average hearing threshold of 95 dB for speech frequencies of 500, 1000 and 2000 Hz.
ii. Physically and mentally normal person.
iii. There should be no improvement to hearing from a hearing aid.
iv. Patient should be ready and available for postoperative rehabilitation program.

It is an electronic device consisting of two parts, one part is surgically inserted into the ear, and the other part known as a speech processor is worn on the body. The implant helps the patient in hearing environmental sounds and allows speech discrimination (understanding).

Implant researchers throughout the world have found that people who became deaf late and had fully developed speech before they became deaf (postlingually deafened) usually gain more benefit from a cochlear implant than those who were born deaf or lost their hearing very early (prelingually deafened). However, many prelingually deafened adults and children still gain much benefit from a cochlear implant.

The earlier the prelingual child undergoes cochlear implantation the better the results. It has recently been proved from brain mapping that certain areas in the cerebral cortex develop in response to sound stimuli in a child as early as 10 months of age. Prelingually deaf children who have been implanted at the age of 10 months attain normal speech and are integrated into normal schools, hence, the younger the child, the greater the potential for language development and speech perception. The postlinguals excel after cochlear implantation as they possess auditory memory.

The period of time that a patient was deaf is also a factor in how much benefit is gained from a cochlear implant. Patients that have been deaf for less than six years usually gain more benefit than those who have been deaf for many years.

The internal part implanted at operation consists of a receiver, an active electrode and a reference electrode. All material used in the manufacture of the implant are fully tested for biological compatibility and durability. The electronic components of the receiver are held in a sealed housing which is implanted under the skin behind the ear (**Fig. 22.8**).

The active electrode connected to the receiver is inserted into the cochlea through a cochleostomy into the basal turn. The contacts (platinum-iridium alloy) are enclosed in silicone and the electrode cable is made in such a way that it can be inserted about 25 mm into the cochlea. The external components consists of the speech processor and transmitter. The

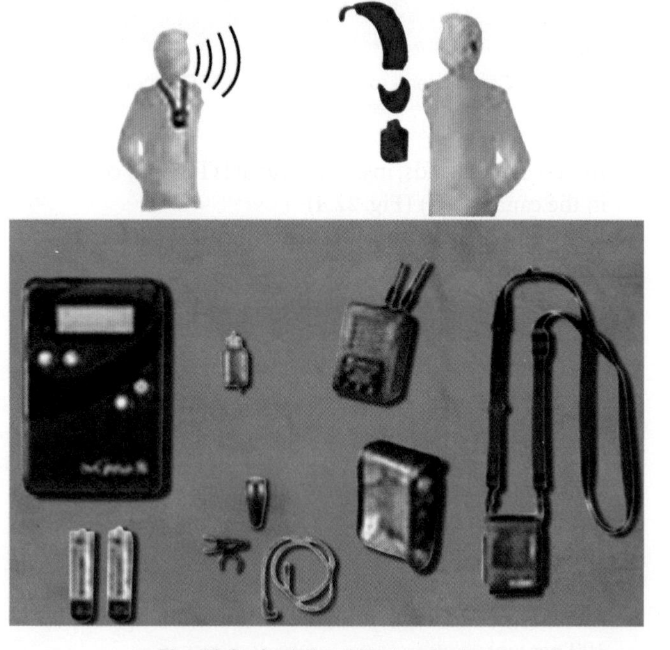

Fig. 22.8: Assistive listening devices

speech processor can be body worn or behind the ear. The speech processor powered by batteries converts incoming signals into the required electrical signals.

HOW DOES THE IMPLANT WORK?

1. Sound waves are received by the microphone.
2. The signal from the microphone is sent along the cable to the speech processor.
3. The speech processor acts on the signal according to coding strategies develop to enable optimal hearing with the cochlear implant.
4. The coded signal is sent through the cable to the transmitter.
5. The transmitter transfers the signal together with the energy required by the implanted electronic through the intact skin to the implanted receiver.
6. The implanted receiver and stimulator decodes the signal and sends a pattern of small electrical impulses to the electrodes in the cochlea.
7. The small pulses conducted by the electrode contacts stimulate the spinal ganglia at various sites and different parts of the auditory nerve are stimulated according to the pitch of the sound. In response the auditory nerve carries out its natural function and conducts nerve impulses to the brain.
8. The brain receives the nerve impulses and interprets them as sound, which the implant user hears.

The whole process takes place within a few milliseconds, corresponding to the processing time in the normally functioning ear.

HOW DOES THE IMPLANT BENEFIT THE PATIENT?

There is an improved level of auditory sensation and the ability to detect the presence of different sounds.

a. *Environmental sounds:* There is immediate detection of normal everyday sounds in the environment such as knock on the door or a door bell, horns of cars and motors, telephone ringing, dogs barking, background music and pleasurable sounds such as cooing of babies and rustling of leaves.
b. *Understanding of speech:* Implanted patients have limited speech discrimination (understanding). However, since the patient can hear his own voice with the implant he can improve his speech production because voice and articulation can be better controlled. An important gain which is usually observed by implant users is improvement with lip reading as the sound signal from the implant and visual information work together. The ability to lip read faster and better means people can take part in everyday conversation more easily and can avoid to write things down.

   Most implant users can tell the difference between a man and a woman's voice and they describe speech as sounding natural, mechanical, clangy or muffled (like a radio not tuned accurately to a station). Some patients enjoy the sound of music and some interpret music as noise. In adults with postlinguistic deafness, using the recent advanced fast stimulating cochlear implants 90 percent of the participants have improved communication abilities when using the implant without lip reading.
c. *Telephone communication:* Some postlingual patients can hear sounds of speech over the telephone but, in general are not able to understand words, and for this reason they are still denied easy access to the telephone for full communication. They are able to determine if there is a dial tone a busy signal, a ringing tone or whether someone has answered at the other end. Communication codes may be devised with family and friends to help in the use of the telephone.
d. *Tinnitus (Noises in the ear):* These usually diminish or decrease after implantation.
e. *Adult benefits:* Although the cochlear implant cannot fully restore normal hearing, adult clinical trials indicate 80 percent of average sentence recognition after six months with significant improvement in word and sentence recognition both in quiet and in noisy surroundings compared to their ability with hearing aids.
f. *Child benefits:* Children also show significant gains in sound awareness and speech uderstanding as reported by their parents. After six months of use, a majority of children respond to their names in quiet environment and spontaneously recognize common sounds in the classroom. Children implanted before the age of 3 years develop vocabulary within 3 months.

SELECTION OF PATIENTS FOR COCHLEAR IMPLANT SURGERY

The suitablity of a person for a cochlear implant is evaluated by several tests. The tests cover both medical and audiological aspect and test results are obtained and evaluated by the ENT surgeon and the audiologist. If there are no contraindications, the patient is invited to take part in further assessments.

a. *Otologic (ear) evaluation:* This forms part of the medical assessment so as to ensure that there are no middle or inner ear problems that can interfere with the implantation. A CT scan of the inner ear is taken to check that the cochlea is accessible and electrodes can be inserted.
b. *Audiologic (hearing) evaluation:* This includes standard hearing tests, hearing aid fitting and tests of speech understanding with hearing aids. The hearing loss should be profound and an aided audiogram should not show any significant hearing. BERA and if necessary electrocochleography are carried out as objective tests to establish the patients threshold and to confirm whether

the deafness is sensorineural or central. These tests provide a base line for comparison with average cochlear implant performance. In small children it is particularly important to evaluate if the child can be helped with a conventional hearing aid before considering a cochlear implant.

c. *Counseling:* This is carried out to ensure proper motivation and realistic expectations. The user must be willing and able to participate in regular programming and speech processor adjustment visits during the first couple of years after implantation. Deaf born children especially require intensive rehabilitation with the cochlear implant. The scope of these follow up activities must be fully understood by the candidate or the child's family before deciding for implantation.
d. *Psychological assessment:* This is carried out to ensure that the patient is well-motivated for this kind of treatment and has realistic expectations. He/she must also show willingness to take part in auditory and speech training after the operation.
e. *Other test:* If the above tests indicate that the person might be a candidate, then physical examination, vestibular tests, medical and other general tests to ensure that the individual can successfully undergo general anesthesia and surgery need to be done. Assessments of participation of patient's relatives in the cochlear implant program is also done prior to surgery.

At the beginning of the operation the hair behid the ear to be operated should be shaved off to prevent infection around the implant. While the patient is under general anesthesia the surgeon marks an incision in the skin above and behind the ear to allow access to the temporal bone and the cochlea. The surgeon forms a small depression in the mastoid bone behind the ear to hold the receiver/stimulator. The electrode array is inserted through an opening into the cochlea. The thin (0.6–0.4 mm) tapered and flexible construction of the electrode array helps it to be placed into the cochlea and conform to its curved shape. The ground electrode is placed on the bone under the muscle. When the incision is closed and the skin heals, the internal parts of the implant cannot be seen by the recipient or others. Some specific risks include possible strong interaction of strong magnetic fields used in magnetic resonance imaging (MRI) with the implant. Hence implant user should not undergo MRI of the skull.

SWITCH ON SPEECH THERAPY AND REHABILITATION

Four to six weeks after surgey the patient returns to the hospital for the initial switch on of the speech processor. In adults this usually takes about a day. In small children the initial switch on may require several days.

During the programming an audiologist presents signals through the implant that produce different pitched sounds and different levels of loudness. The user is asked to rank these signals from very soft to comfortably loud. At the end of the programming session the information will be stored in the speech processor, such that they can be used to convert everyday sounds into appropriately loud signals for the implant. In small children, an experienced audiologist will play a game with the child in order to make the switch on more fun and secure the child's cooperation. After switch on the rehabilitation sessions begins in which the patient learns to associate speech with the patterns of sound which come from the implant.

The program involves both the patient and the family. It is directed towards utilization of the new auditory clues available, as well as improvement in communication ability and speech production. The success of this therapy depends in large measure on the cooperation of the patient who should also be prepared to work between therapy sessions at home according to the instructions of the therapist. The initial benefit received from the implant can be increased by auditory verbal therapy at regular intervals usually a couple of hours a week. The time of therapy that is needed can vary widely from case-to-case. The least amount of speech therapy is generally required by people who have been deaf for only a short time. Many postlingually deaf adults with period of deafness of less than 5 years find speech therapy necessary only during the first few weeks following surgery.

Intensive initial habilitation and speech therapy is required for deaf born children, who had no spoken language before receiving the cochlear implant. The older a congenitally deaf child is at the time of implantation, the more therapy will be necessary in trying to make up for the time that was lost regarding speech and language acquisition.

The speech processors can store 3 maps so that the patient can have 3 different programs to use as the need arises in their listening environment. For example, one for noise, another for quiet and a third for music.

TRAINING OF DEAF-MUTES

i. *Speech reading or lipreading:* Here patient is trained to study the movements of lips facial expressions, gestures and hand movements.
ii. *Auditory training:* Through an auditory trainer the deaf person is exposed to various listening situations with different degrees of difficulty and are taught selectively to concentrate on speech sounds. It is very helful for persons using hearing aids or having cochlear implants.
iii. *Speech conservation:* It is useful in persons having sudden severe hearing loss who cannot monitor his own speech production. Here tactile and proprioceptive feedback is used to monitor the speech production.

Other facilities for severely deaf patients can be:

i. Hard wired system induction loops. Amplitude modulation or frequency modulation or infrared signals.
ii. Alerting devices to hear a telephone or door bell or baby cry. These devices produce extra loud signals.
iii. Telecommunication devices, where a telephone amplifier is attached to a telephone to increase the sound or a telecommunication device for deaf (TDD) which converts typed massage into sound that can be transmitted over the standard telephone lines and at the other end another TDD converts these sound signals back into type written messages.
iv. Closed caption television decoders can be attached to television sets to provide cues for news, dramas and other programs.

Chapter 23

Principles of Audiometry

Sound is a mechanical wave that is an oscillation of pressure transmitted through a solid, liquid, or gas, composed of frequencies within the range of hearing. Sound is a sensation and sound waves are a form of energy. Sound is made up of either simple harmonic motion (the pure tone) or complex harmonic motion in which there are several simple harmonic motions occurring simultaneously (such as the human voice) (**Fig. 23.1**).

Acoustics

Sound waves are often simplified to a description in terms of sinusoidal plane waves, which are characterized by these generic properties:

- Frequency, or its inverse, the period
- Wavelength
- Wavenumber
- Amplitude
- Sound pressure
- Sound intensity
- Speed of sound
- Direction

Acoustics involves the study of sound dealing with vibratory motion perceptible through the organ of hearing.

PARAMETERS OF SOUND

1. *Frequency:* A vibrating body produces sound waves at a particular rate per second (cycles/second), called frequency.

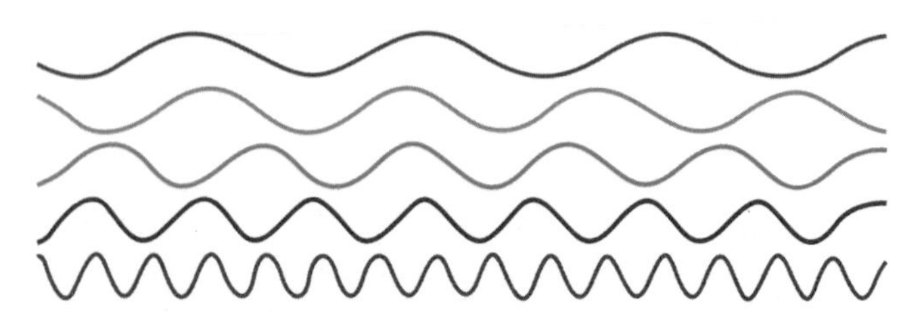

Fig. 23.1: Sinusoidal waves of various frequencies

   It confers upon a sound its apparent musical pitch. The range of frequencies to which the normal ear is sensitive is usually said to extend from 20 to 20,000 cycles/second covering approximately 10 octaves. The variation in the velocity of propogation of sound waves is very wide, varying with the density and elasticity of the medium through which it passes. In air at 0°C, it is 332 meter/sec and increases with temperature. In water, the velocity is over 1400 meter/sec and in a rigid solid, e.g. ivory (which has physical properties resembling those of petrous bone), it is 3000 meter/sec.
2. *Wave length:* It is the time duration of one complete cycle in a sinusoidal wave pattern representing vibratory motion (**Fig. 23.1**). It involves one positive and one negative excursion.
3. *Pitch:* It is the psychological counterpart of frequency. Faster the rate of vibration, higher the perceived pitch.
4. *Intensity:* It is the physical measure of amplitude of mass movement and is the measure of loudness of sound.
5. *Loudness:* It is the physiological counterpart of the intensity. The unit of loudness is called, decibel which is 1/10 of a bel, the unit called after Graham Bell, inventor of the telephone. In the decibel scale, the faintest audible sound is taken as the unit and called '0'.

The scale is as follows: 1 bel is 10^1, i.e. 10 times 0; 2 bel is 10^2, i.e. 100 times 0; 3 bel is 10^3, i.e. 1000 times 0 and so on.

When comparing intensities of two different sounds, it is often convenient to use in place of a simple ratio, decibel (dB) which is equal to 10 times the logarithm of a sound under consideration to a reference sound. The reference sound usually taken is an intensity which is very close to the normal threshold of hearing of the human ear at 1000 Hz.

The reason for notation is to reduce a rather larger ratio to a small usable number. This is necessary primarily because of the tremendous capability of the ear to hear over a large dynamic range.

In noting, the degree of hearing at two different frequencies, it would be a bit awkward to say that a person hears 1000 units at one frequency and 40000 units at another. Thus, dB notation is used to break a large number into small usable numbers.

The sound intensity can be expressed as sound pressure in dynes/cm^2, or as particle velocity is cm/s or as power in watts.

The formula for decibel (dB) estimation is as follows:

$$dB = 10 \log \frac{t_1}{t_2}$$

Where t_1 is the intensity in watts of the existing sound and t_2 the intensity in watts of a reference sound.

$$\text{Alternatively, } dB = 20 \log \frac{P_1}{P_2}$$

Where P_1 is the sound pressure in dynes/cm^2 of the existing sound and P_2 the sound pressure of a reference sound. A common reference pressure is 0.0002 dynes/cm^2.

The intensity of various noises in decibels is given below:

Jet plane with burner	160
Pain	140
Limit of endurance	130
Discomfort (thunder)	120
Boiler shop	100
Noisy street	80
Normal conversation	60
Average office	40
Quiet street	30
Whisper	20
Faintest audible sound	0

ROOM ACOUSTICS

It is by reflection on hard walls and by absorption in loose material that one can control the acoustic properties of a room. Reflective walls keep energy from spreading beyond the confinements of the room so that even low-intensity sounds are heard from one end to the other. However, such rooms are highly reverberant, that is, each signal causes multiple echoes which last for some time afterwards and tend to obscure subsequent signals. Walls covered with absorptive material "deaden" a room. There is little or no reverberation but sound does not "carry" either, so that low intensity sounds are lost in such rooms. Moreover, because of the stronger effect of absorption upon high frequencies, signals are deprived of their high frequency components and sound is muffled.

For these reasons, one must keep a compromise between reflection and absorption depending upon the purpose of the room.

Rooms in which audiometric tests are to be conducted must be reasonably quiet. Testing must be disturbed neither by sounds created within the room nor by those intruding from outside. Such rooms are known as sound-treated rooms. The outside walls of such rooms consist of heavy, hard-surfaced shell in order to keep out extraneous noises. The inside is lined with absorptive material to keep reverberation low.

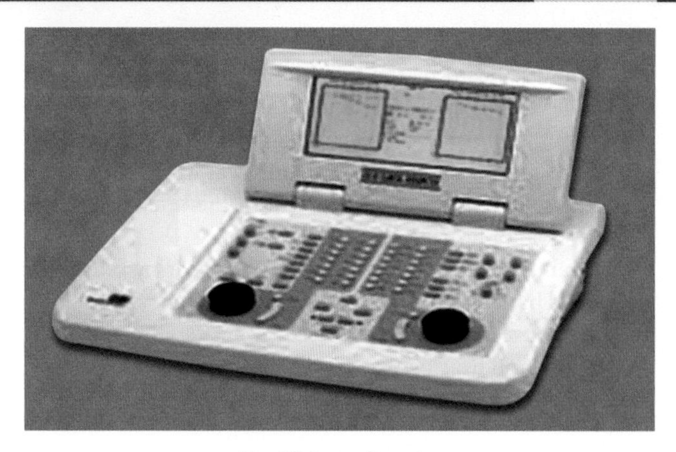

Fig. 23.2: Audiometer

Audiometry

It is an important investigation for auditory dysfunction. It not only gives us an idea about the handicap and degree of deafness that the patient is having but it is also a valuable method for diagnosing ear disease (**Fig. 23.2**).

Besides pure tone audiometry, a battery of other audiological tests is now being done for localization of the lesion.

PURE TONE AUDIOMETRY

Audiometer

It is an electronic device that consists of a pure tone generator, an amplifier and an attenuator.

It is an instrument for testing the intensity and frequency range of sound that is capable of detection by the human ear.

The frequencies can be selected from pure tone generator by the frequency selector switch. The attenuator or hearing level dial controls the intensity of the stimulus.

A noise generator unit in this device is used for masking. Besides, all audiometers have a set of earphones and bone-conduction receiver, for air and bone conduction tests.

The ear is not equally sensitive at all frequencies. Therefore, a system has been developed in standard audiometers to make all test frequencies equally loud at 0 dB approximating the normal threshold of hearing.

Method of Pure Tone Audiometry

In a soundproof room, the patient's ability to hear pure tones in the frequency range of about 125 to 8000 Hz is measured. The frequencies usually tested are 125, 250, 500, 1000, 2000, 4000, 6000 and 8000 Hz. Pure tone sensitivity can be measured by air conduction and by bone conduction.

The tester gradually increases the intensity of stimulus (pure tone), till it is heard by the subject or the tester may present a stimulus that is easily heard and then slowly decreases the intensity until the subject no longer hears the tone. The process is repeated several times and the intensity at which the subject hears the sound (tone) for 50 percent of the time, is taken as the threshold of hearing at that frequency.

The audiogram is a graph showing the hearing sensitivity for air and bone-conducted sounds. The frequency of the tone in cycles per second (CPS) or Hertz (Hz) is represented along the abscissa and hearing threshold level in decibels (dB) along the ordinate (**Figs 23.3 and 23.4**).

Symbols on Audiogram

Red "0" represents air conduction for the right ear while blue "X" represents air conduction for the left ear. The symbol of > is for bone conduction of the right ear and symbol < for bone conduction of the left ear.

The hearing threshold level numbers along the ordinate are read as "hearing loss in decibels" at a particular frequency.

Audiogram Interpretation

Normally, both air and bone conduction curves superimpose on the graph showing no hearing loss at 0 to 20 dB.

1. *Conductive deafness:* Conductive deafness occurs due to malfunction of the external or middle ear. The cochlea is not affected. Therefore, conductive loss shows a loss of hearing by air conduction tests and normal hearing by bone conduction test (airborne or AB gap).
2. *Sensorineural loss:* In this type of hearing loss, the defect lies in the cochlea and neural pathways. Therefore, thresholds for bone-conducted sounds are the same as thresholds for air-conducted sounds of the same frequency, and both show equal losses.
3. *Mixed hearing loss:* The hearing loss affects both air and bone conduction but the hearing loss for air conduction is more than the loss by bone conduction.

Advantages of Pure Tone Audiometry

1. It gives an idea about the type of hearing loss (quality).
2. It gives a measure of the degree of hearing loss (quantity).
3. It provides a base line for various reconstructive and rehabilitative procedures like tympanoplasty and hearing aids.
4. The method can be used to detect malingerers and is useful for medicolegal purposes.

Speech Audiometry

Speech audiometry is aimed at evaluating the listener's responses to speech. Speech audiometry is helpful in the following:

1. To evaluate the functional state of the auditory system at suprathreshold levels
2. To contribute to the localization of the specific lesions of the auditory tracts
3. To predict the outcome of the otologic surgery
4. To assess the value of therapeutic measures such as auditory training or selection of hearing aid.

Various parameters tested in speech audiometry are as follows:

Response			
Modality	Ear		
	Left	Unspecified	Right
Air conduction-earphones			
Unmasked	X		O
Masked	□		△
Bone conduction-mastoid			
Unmasked	>	↑	<
Masked	]		[
Bone conduction-forehead			
Unmasked		↓	
Masked	⌐		¬
Air conduction-sound field	*	S	Ø
Acoustic-reflex threshold			
Contralateral	≻		≺
Ipsilateral	⊢		⊣

Fig. 23.3: Symbols on audiogram

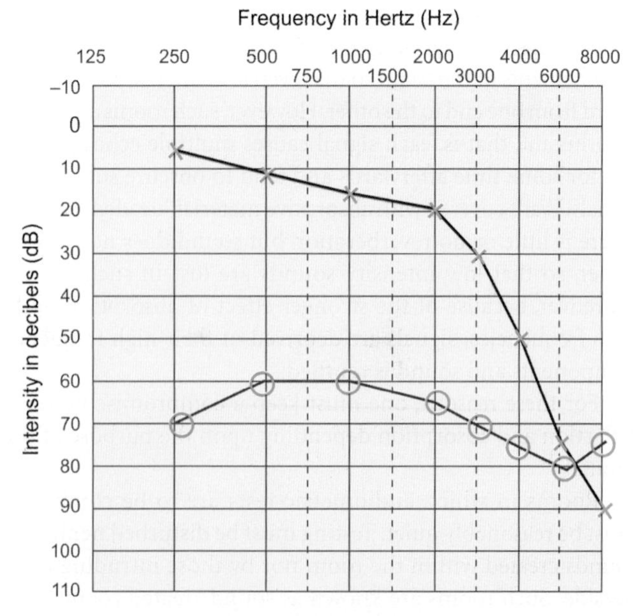

Fig. 23.4: Audiogram

1. *Speech reception threshold:* The test material is recorded live voice. Spondee words are used. Spondee is a word with two syllables, both pronounced with equal stress and effort like toothbrush, aeroplane, eardrum, sunset, farewell.

   The intensity, at which the patient identifies 50 percent of the words and repeats them correctly is called speech reception threshold (SRT).
2. *Most comfortable loudness (MCL):* It is the intensity at which the speech is most comfortable for the patient. The patient is instructed to signal when speech is comfortably loud for him, as the examiner varies the intensity at suprathreshold levels.
3. *Threshold of discomfort (uncomfortable loudness level, ULL):* It is a level at which the listener reports speech as being uncomfortable.
4. *Dynamic range:* The speech reception threshold level value subtracted from the uncomfortable loudness level gives the dynamic range of the patient's speech. It represents the amount of useful hearing that the patient has in each ear and is a useful parameter for fitting the hearing aid.

SPEECH DISCRIMINATION

The handicap of hearing loss may consist not only of decrease in sensitivity to sound but also of an impairment in understanding what is heard.

Speech discrimination function is usually measured by administering the so-called phonetically balanced (PB) word lists, at levels above the patient's speech reception threshold. These are monosyllablic words, which are presented at a level of about 40 dB greater than the individual's speech reception threshold.

The discrimination tests are scored in terms of the percentage of words heard correctly.

Uses of Speech Discrimination Test

1. It determines the extent of discrimination difficulty.
2. It aids in diagnosis of the site of pathology in the auditory system, e.g. it is poor in acoustic neuroma. The score is normal in conductive deafness.
3. It assists in rehabilitative measures like fitting of a hearing aid.

SOCIAL ADEQUACY INDEX (SAI)

It represents the patient's ability to understand phonetically balanced words at three standard levels of intensity (33, 48, and 63 dB). The average of scores made by patients on these levels is taken and the result called social adequacy index. The result gives the degree of handicap that the patient is suffering from.

Vocal index It is the relation between hearing loss for speech and whispered voice.

In conductive deafness, the index is small and there is little difference between the two.

In perceptive deafness in which the loss is mainly confined to high tones, there may be considerable discrepancy between the hearing for speech and whisper, so the vocal index is high.

SHORT INCREMENT SENSITIVITY INDEX TEST (SISI TEST OF JERGER)

The test is designed to test the ability of a patient to detect the presence of small increments in intensity at suprathreshold levels.

The tone is presented at 20 dB above the patient's threshold for that frequency. Every 5 seconds, 1 dB increment is superimposed. The tester presents 20 such 1 dB increments for each test.

The SISI test is scored in terms of the percentage of correctly identified 1 dB increments out of a possible 20 increments. The number obtained is multiplied by 5 for getting the percentage.

SISI score over 70 percent usually occurs in hearing loss due to inner ear damage, e.g. in Ménière's disease. This is called a positive test.

TONE DECAY TEST (AUDITORY ADAPTATION)

The tone is presented to the patient who is asked to listen and signal as soon as he hears a tone at threshold. A stop-watch is started, which should be stopped when the patient signals that the tone is no longer heard. The number of seconds for which the tone is heard at threshold is recorded. The stop-watch is reset and the level of tone raised by 5 dB without interrupting the tone. This procedure is continued until.

i. The patient can hear the tone for a full 60 seconds, and
ii. Increments up to 30 dB have been reached and the patient fails to hear the tone for at least 60 seconds at that level.

The amount of tone decay is expressed as the number of decibels above the threshold at which the tone can be heard for a full minute.

Interpretation

1. Normal 0-5 dB in 60 seconds	Suggestive of cochlear deafness (inner ear deafness)
2. Mild decay 10-15 dB/minute	
3. Moderate decay 20-25 dB/minutes	Suggestive of retrocochlear deafness like acoustic neuroma
4. Marked decay 30 dB or above in 60 seconds	

Recruitment

It is a phenomenon which occurs in some pathological diseases of the ear (like cochlear lesions) where there occurs rapid growth of loudness in the affected ear disproportionate to the sound stimulus given.

Loudness grows so rapidly that a tone sounds louder in the impaired ear than in a normal ear at the same intensity.

Procedure to Demonstrate Recruitment

Alternate binaural loudness balance test (ABLB test, *Fowler's test*) For this test, the hearing threshold for the poor ear should be at least 25 dB poorer than hearing in the better ear. A two-channel audiometer is used for alternating two tones of identical frequency from one ear to the other. The intensity of each tone must be individually controllable. The purpose of this test is to compare the growth of loudness in the deaf ear with the growth of loudness in the opposite (normal) ear. In this way, the degree of recruitment, if present, can be demonstrated.

The growth of loudness in the impaired ear as it is compared with the reference ear, can be illustrated in a graph (*Laddergram*).

Decruitment

This phenomenon denotes an abnormally slow growth of loudness and is considered as pathognomonic of retrocochlear lesion.

BEKESY AUDIOMETRY

It is an automatic audiometer which scans the patient's threshold to both continuous and alternating stimulus. Depending upon the curves traced, the graph is classified as under:

- Type I — The continuous and interrupted tracings overlap (normal and conductive deafness)
- Type II — The curves overlap at lower frequencies but at around 1000 Hz, the continuous tracing falls below the interrupted tracing and then runs parallel to it. Such a curve occurs in some cases of sensory hearing loss
- Type III — The continuous curve dips abruptly from the interrupted curve before 500 Hz. This type of graph signifies retrocochlear disease (acoustic neuroma)
- Type IV — Continuous tracing from the very beginning remains lower than the interrupted tracing (occurs in some cases of retrocochlear lesion)
- Type V — The continuous tracing lies above the interrupted tracing (suggestive of non-organic hearing loss).

IMPEDANCE AUDIOMETRY

This is a recent advance in audiometry which includes the measurement of middle ear pressure (tympanometry). Tympanometry measures the change in impedance of the middle ear. The air pressure in the external canal is varied from –200 mm H_2O to +200 mm of H_2O by an air pump attached to a manometer. The results are plotted and the graph is called a tympanogram. Automatic impedance audiometers are available these days which scan the patient's middle ear compliance on a graph paper.

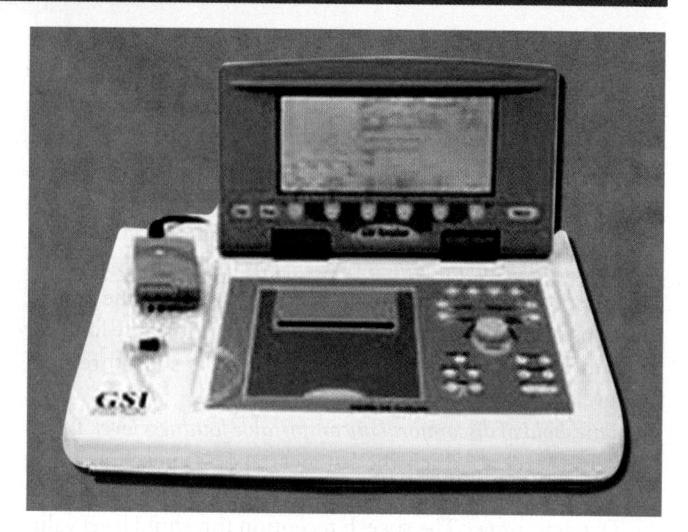

Fig. 23.5: Impedence audiometer

This type of audiometry is helpful in diagnosing various middle ear conditions like secretory otitis media, adhesive otitis media, ossicular chain disruption and also noting the results of their treatment. Eustachian tube functioning and acoustic reflexes are also elicited by this method (**Fig. 23.5**).

The acoustic stapedius reflex is an involuntary muscle contraction that occurs in the middle ear in response to high-intensity sound stimuli. When presented with a high-intensity sound stimulus, the stapedius and tensor tympani muscles of the ossicles contract. The stapedius pulls the stapes (stirr-up) of the middle ear away from the oval window of the cochlea and the tensor tympani muscle pulls the malleus (hammer) away from ear drum. The reflex decreases the transmission of vibrational energy to the cochlea.

Reflexes are ordinarily present for fairly loud sounds, relative to hearing ability.

- Ordinarily one needs an 70 to 90 dB sound to produce an AR in a normal hearing individual, or a person with a mild-to-moderate cochlear hearing loss.
- Reflexes may be absent even to louder inputs in persons with
  - Conductive hearing loss
    - Otosclerosis, or other middle ear disease
    - Stapes fixation in probe ear
  - Severe sensory hearing loss
  - 8th nerve hearing loss (such as due to an acoustic neuroma
  - 7th nerve injury on side being measured.

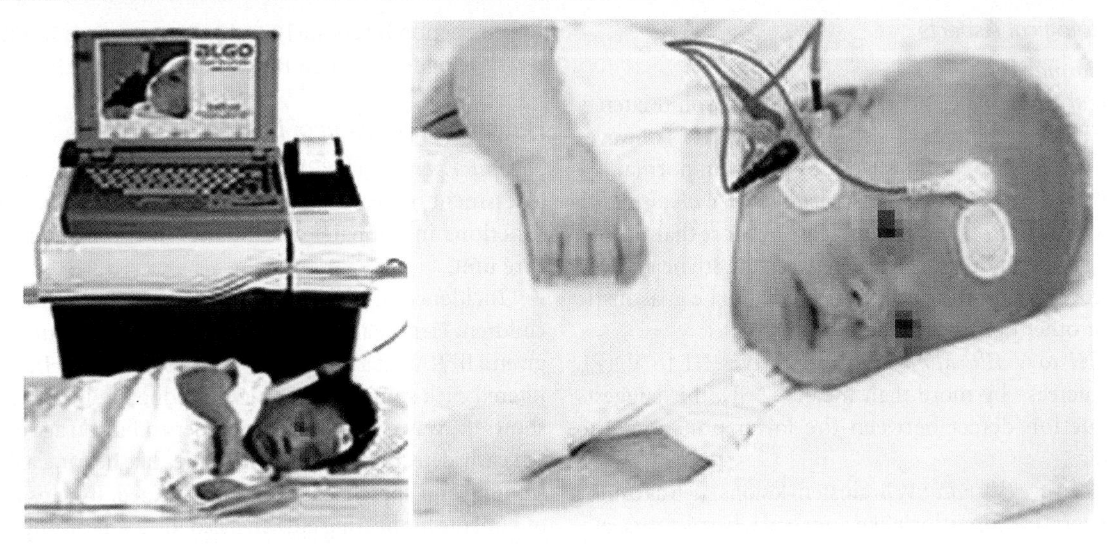

Fig. 23.6: Evoked response audiometry

ELECTROCOCHLEOGRAPHY AND EVOKED RESPONSE AUDIOMETRY (FIG. 23.6)

These are objective audiometric tests particularly useful in children who are not cooperative for the usual audiological tests. Brainstem auditory evoked responses, also known as auditory brainstem evoked response (ABR), test both the ear and the brain. They measure the timing of electrical waves from the brainstem in response to clicks or tone bursts in the ear. Computer averaging over time to filters background noise to generate an averaged response of the auditory pathway to an auditory stimulus.

The 8th nerve action potentials and cochlear microphonics are recorded by placing the electrodes in the canal or through the tympanic membrane on the promontory.

BRAINSTEM EVOKED RESPONSE AUDIOMETRY

This is a reliable diagnostic neuro-otological test which can be done even in infants.

A series of electrical waves generated at various points in the auditory apparatus (cochlea, cochlear-neurons, superior olive, lateral lemniscus and inferior colliculus) are recorded.

During the last decade, auditory brainstem evoked responses (BERA) have been used extensively in clinical medicine. It has greatly contributed in two major areas, viz. audiological evaluation in infants and children, especially in those with risk factors and neuroaudiological evaluation of the 8th nerve and brainstem function in variety of neurologic conditions. Presently, several other neurologic conditions have attracted its application, e.g. sudden infant death syndrome (SIDS) and near miss for sudden infant death episode (NMSID). The proximity of the respiratory centers to the auditory brainstem pathways is the basis for application of BERA in its early detection in suspect apneic infants (**Fig. 23.7**).

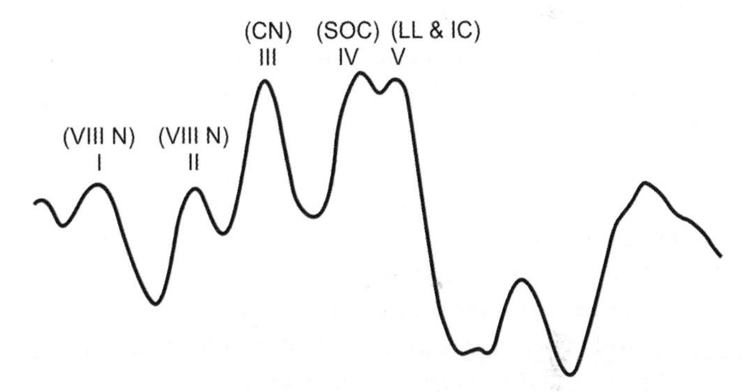

Fig. 23.7: Wave recordings on ERA

WAVE GENERATOR SITE

Sohmer and Feinmesser (1967) described electrical recording of the 8th nerve, it was Jewett (1971) who successfully demonstrated seven upward deflections of submicrovolt amplitude during the first 10 msec period following click stimulation. Such minute electrical responses were extracted, with the help of the computer at the scalp from the background electroencephalogram activity. With the newer generation of computer now, it is possible to have variety of far-field scalp averaging system for clinical use. Clinical studies have corroborated the location of the brainstem generation sites, described as follows:

1. *Auditory nerve:* Wave I (8th nerve action potential).
2. *Brainstem level:* Wave II—cochlear nucleus, Wave III—superior olivary nucleus, Wave IV—lateral lemniscus, Wave V—inferior colliculus, Wave VI—not well understood.

Pathophysiological Aspects

Latency abnormalities:

1. *Peripheral defect:* In peripheral hearing loss, absolute latency of wave I increases but the interpeak latencies (IPL) of waves I to III, waves III to V and waves I to V remain normal.
2. *Central conduction defects—interpeak latency abnormality (IPL):* Wave I to III IPL values increase by more than +2 SD, this suggests a conduction defect between the 8th nerve close to the cochlea and the lower pontine region, e.g. acoustic nerve or other pontine tumors.
3. *Waves III to V IPL abnormality:* If waves III to V IPL values increase by more than mean +2 SD, this suggests a conduction defect between the lower pons and the midbrain.
4. *Absence of wave IV and/or V:* Brainstem lesions such as tumor or degenerative conditions like anoxemia, kernicterus, etc. can produce such (BERA) abnormality ipsilaterally as well as contralaterally.

Amplitude abnormality:

1. *Loss of amplitude:* The loss of amplitude is assumed to be due to less number of fibers conducting the volley and desynchronization of the volley, secondary to widely different velocities.
2. *Wave V: Wave I amplitude ratio:* It is usually more than 1 in normal condition.
3. *Laterality of BERA abnormality: Unilateral or bilateral change:* Unilateral changes of BERA are usually more prominent as a result of unilateral disease. Even in intrinsic brainstem lesion, unilateral BERA change may be more discernible.
4. *Stimulus:* For audiologic evaluation, most commonly used stimuli are: (i) toneburst, and (ii) filtered clicks and for neurologic conditions, it is the clicks or the filtered clicks at 4 kHz.
5. *Stimulus rate:* Most commonly used stimulus rate is 10-20/sec. However for audiologic purposes in infants and children rate can be increased up to 30 to 50/sec.
6. *Polarity:* In noisy situation, an alternate condensation and rarefaction-stimulus helps to avoid noise stimulus artifact.
7. *Infant and newborn testing:* In infant testing, the head-phone should be kept near the side of the ear under test since it is painful to tightly keep a head-phone. This may result in reduction of about 5 to 10 dB intensity of the sound stimulus at the drum.
8. *Resolution of waveform:* To get better resolution of waveforms stimulus repetition may be given upto 2000, and stimulus intensity may be reduced from 80 dBSL.
9. *Interpretation of latency and amplitude:* It must be remembered while assessing the hearing threshold in children that the BERA threshold in response to a minimum intensity-stimulus is higher by about 20 dB than the one at conventional pure tone audiometry. Hence, a factor of correction by about 10 to 15 dB is required in interpreting hearing function on BERA in infants and children.

Pediatric Application of BERA

Neonatal period: The BERA has been extensively used in early assessment of hearing function and other possible neurologic functions in neonates and infants in the neonatal intensive care unit.

Incidence of sensorineural loss is very high in high-risk children. Hence, all infants in the intensive care unit should be given a BERA test. For screening purposes, a 40 dB HL, 2 and 4 kHz filtered click stimulus can be given monoaurally and it normally shows the wave V after 6 or 7 msec depending on age of gestation. On early detection, adequate measures like hearing aids auditory training and speech skills can be instituted. It helps in selection of patients for hearing aids and also for cochlear implantation.

Several conditions during newborn period may be subjected to BERA. They includes:

- Hyperbilirubinemia
- Kernicterus
- Perinatal anoxia
- Prematurity
- Cerebral palsy
- Suspected mental retardation
- Microcephaly
- Congenital rubella
- Several metabolic disorders like non-ketotic hyperglycemia, maple syrup urine disease, phenyl ketonuria and thiamine metabolism disorder.

Pediatric neurologic application: BERA is also employed in the following commonly seen neurologic conditions in children:

- Coma
- Epilepsy
- Drug effects and ototoxicity
- Adrenoleukodystrophy
- Sudden infant death syndrome and apnea (SIDS) head injury.
- Auditory neuropathy spectrum disorder

Neurologic conditions in adults: Evoked potentials give the most accurate and reproducible information in the diagnosis of: (a) acoustic neuromas, (b) non-acoustic lesions in the vicinity of the 8th nerve or in the cerebellopontine angle and in the brainstem or those tumors/lesions from the CP angle of cerebellum; pressing over the brainstem.

Evoked potentials provide excellent data on the contralateral effects of tumors of acoustic and non-acoustic origin in the cerebellopontine angle region.

Futhermore the technique is being used in the diagnosis of multiple sclerosis, brainstem stroke, comatose patients, herpes cephalicus, and several other neurologic conditions including head injury.

MCQs on Ear

Select the most appropriate answer:

1. In sudden hearing loss, all of the following are poor prognostic factors except:
   A. Old age
   B. Profound sensory neural hearing loss
   C. Absence of vestibular symptoms
   D. High frequency hearing loss
   E. Presence of vascular risk factor.
2. Rinne' test positive means that:
   A. Air conduction is better than bone conduction
   B. Bone conduction is better than air conduction
   C. Bone is equal to air conduction
   D. Cholesteatoma
   E. Sensorineural hearing loss
3. Innervation of the external auditory canal includes all except:
   A. Facial nerve
   B. Vagus nerve
   C. Vestibulocochlear nerve
   D. Glossopharyngeal nerve
   E. Greater auricular nerve.
4. A mother visits the ENT clinic with her 5-year-old daughter with complaints of fever and pain in the right ear for the last 2 days. On examination, the right tympanic membrane is congested and bulging. Rest of the examination is unremarkable. You diagnose the child as:
   A. Acute otitis externa
   B. Acute otitis media
   C. Serous otitis media
   D. Ramsay hunt syndrome
   E. Furunculosis.
5. External auditory meatus is cartilaginous in its:
   A. Outer one-third
   B. Outer two-third
   C. Outer one-fourth
   D. Outer half.
6. Greisinger's sign means:
   A. Pain over the temporomandibular joint
   B. Pain in the eye
   C. Pain and tenderness over the mastoid
   D. Pain and tenderness over the auricle.
7. Fistula sign may be positive in:
   A. Central drum perforation
   B. Atelectatic drum
   C. Cholesteatoma
   D. Otosclerosis.
8. A tympanogram with a dome-shaped or flat curve is indicative of:
   A. Ossicular discontinuity
   B. Stapedial fixation
   C. Fluid in the middle ear
   D. Malleus head fixation.
9. Ménière's disease is mainly characterized by:
   A. Sudden in onset
   B. Conductive hearing loss
   C. Episodic vertigo
   D. Brief vertigo with movement
   E. Bilateral hearing loss.
10. Cochlear implant is indicated to replace the:
    A. Function of the hair cells
    B. Function of the cochlear nerve
    C. Function of the middle ear
    D. a + b
    E. All of the above.
11. Sudden unilateral complete loss of vestibular function with hearing preservation is seen in:
    A. Acoustic neuroma
    B. Ménière's disease
    C. Vestibular neuritis
    D. Benign paroxysmal positional vertigo
    E. Perilymph fistula.

12. The sensory innervation of the ear doesn't include:
A. Hypoglossal nerve
B Glossopharyngeal nerve
C. Facial nerve
D. Trigeminal nerve
E. Vagus nerve.
13. An adult presented with unilateral acute otitis media with effusion. The first cause you have to think about is:
A. Serous otitis media
B. AIDS
C. Carcinoma of the nasopharynx
D. Adhesive otitis.
14. External ear canal exostoses are more common in:
A. Immunocompromised patients
B. Smokers
C. Old diabetics
D. Alcoholics
E. Swimmers.
15. Hematoma of the auricle should be drained to prevent:
A. Deformity of pinna
B. Stenosis of external canal
C. Development of conductive hearing loss
D. Development of sensorineural hearing loss.
16. CSF otorrhea following temporal bone fracture:
A. Should be treated surgically
B. Is self limiting in most cases
C. Is fatal in all cases
D. Should be treated with craniotomy.
17. In patients with otosclerosis, the tympanogram is of:
A. A type
B. Ad type
C. As type
D. B type.
18. Absolute contraindication for stapedectomy is:
A. > 80 dB air bone gap
B. Only hearing ear
C. < 40 dB air bone gap
D. Negative Rinne's test.
19. Cochlear otosclerosis causes deafness by:
A. Stapes fixation
B. Toxic enzymes released to inner ear
C. Malleus head fixation
D. Necrosis of the long process of incus.
20. Most common type of temporal bone fracture is:
A. Longitudinal
B. Transverse
C. Circular
D. Mixed.
21. Fluctuating deafness following temporal bone trauma is due to:
A. Middle ear injury
B. Perilymph fistula
C. Tympanic membrane perforation
D. Internal auditory meatal injury.
22. Battle's sign means:
A. Reddish blue discoloration over mastoid process
B. Reddish bulge over the tympanic membrane
C. Deformed pinna
D. Tympanic membrane perforation.
23. Gradenigo's syndrome features include:
A. Acute petrositis with 6th nerve palsy
B. Acute mastoiditis with 4th nerve palsy
C. Acute petrositis with 7th nerve palsy
D. Both A and C.
24. Cholesteatoma contains:
A. Mucoid material
B. Cholesterol crystal
C. Desquamated squamous epithelium
D. Cuboidal epithelial nests.
25. Surface marking for mastoid antrum is:
A. McEwen's triangle
B. Line joining the helix and the tragus
C. Line joining the antihelix and the tragus
D. Line joining the lobule with the tragus.
26. Schwartze's sign when seen in otosclerosis indicates:
A. Subclinical otosclerosis
B. Active disease
C. Cochlear otosclerosis
D. Obliterative otosclerosis.
27. In adult the average length of external auditory canal is:
A. 18 mm
B. 20 mm
C. 24 mm
D. 26 mm.
28. Most common cause of conductive deafness is:
A. Otosclerosis
B. Secretory otitis media
C. Congenital ossicular fixation
D. Collection of wax.
29. The human ear is capable of hearing the (frequency range from):
A. 500 to 5000 Hz
B. 100 to 10,000 Hz
C. 10 to 30,000 Hz
D. 20 to 20,000 Hz.
30. Uncontrolled diabetes in elderly patient may predispose to:
A. Cholesteatoma
B. Malignant otitis externa
C. Presbycusis
D. Vestibular.
31. The term Hertz (Hz) is a measure of:
A. Power
B. Intensity

C. Impedance
D. Frequency.

32. Tympanoplasty is an operation aimed at:
A. Correction of hearing in perceptive deafness
B. Eradication of infection and correction of hearing
C. Drainage of mastoid abscess
D. Correction of hearing in otosclerosis.

33. Stapedectomy is the operation of choice for:
A. Otosclerosis
B. Bell's palsy
C. Ménière's disease
D. Cholesteatoma.

34. Referred otalgia may be due to the following except:
A. Acute suppurative otitis media
B. Peritonsillar abscess
C. Dental infection
D. Maxillary sinusitis.

35. Otitic barotrauma is characterized by:
A. Attic perforation
B. Middle ear effusion
C. Mucopurulant discharge
D. Central drum perforation.

36. Severe headache, vomiting, dysphagia, and visual field defects in a patient with cholesteatoma indicate:
A. Secretory otitis media
B. Labyrinthitis
C. Distant metastasis
D. Temporal lobe abscess.

37. Ramsey-Hunt syndrome is:
A. Herpes-zoster affection of the geniculate ganglion of the facial nerve
B. Dysphagia in a middle aged female
C. Varicella affection of the abducent nerve
D. Sensory-neural deafness and choanal atresia in newly born.

38. Tobey-Ayer's test is a characteristic sign in:
A. Brain abscess
B. Lateral sinus thrombosis
C. Extradural abscess
D. Meningitis.

39. Pain in acute tonsillitis is referred to the ear through:
A. The 7th nerve
B. The 9th nerve
C. The 10th nerve
D. The 12th nerve.

40. Bell's palsy:
A. Is mainly caused by trauma
B. Majority of cases resolves spontaneously
C. Causes conductive hearing loss
D. Needs surgical intervention.

41. All are present in the medial wall of tympanic cavity except:
A. Oval window
B. Round window
C. Pyramid
D. Promontory.

42. 40 years old male presented with unilateral slowly progressive sensorineural hearing loss, most likely diagnosis is:
A. Acoustic neuroma
B. Viral labyrinthitis
C. Presbycusis
D. Otosclerosis.

43. Otoacoustic emissions:
A. Cannot be used in infants
B. Are a measure of outer hair cell function
C. Are a measure of inner hair cell function
D. Are high intensity sounds produced by the cochlea without an acoustic stimulus.

44. Hair follicles in the external auditory canal are seen in:
A. Its whole length
B. Bony part
C. Cartilaginous part
D. Junction of the bony and cartilaginous part.

45. Marginal perforation in the tympanic membrane is usually due to:
A. Acute otitis media
B. Barotrauma
C. Tuberculous otitis media
D. Atticoantral chronic suppurative otitis media.

46. Patients with sensorineural hearing loss will have:
A. Normal air conduction and abnormal air conduction
B. Normal bone conduction and abnormal air conduction
C. Both air and bone conductions are abnormal
D. Air bone gap.

47. Intracranial venous sinus thrombosis due to chronic suppurative otitis media is more likely to affect:
A. Cavernous sinus
B. Superior sagittal sinus
C. Lateral sinus
D. Superior petrosal sinus.

48. Perilymphatic fistula:
A. Is always acquired in origin
B. Presents with conductive hearing loss
C. Is never seen as a complication of stapedectomy
D. Can develop as a result of direct trauma to temporal bone.

49. Bullous myringitis:
A. Occurs exclusively in adults
B. Occurs only in children
C. Pain is an outstanding feature
D. Pain is relieved by opening the bullae.

50. A 50-year-old man presents with a six months history of right pulsatile tinnitus and progressive hearing loss. He has no past history of ear problems and denies trauma to his head or ears. He recently developed some difficulty swallowing. Examination reveals a large red mass behind an intact tympanic membrane. His audiogram shows mostly conductive hearing loss. What is the most likely diagnosis?
    A. Otospongiosis
    B. Acoustic neuroma
    C. Glomus jugulare
    D. Congenital cholesteatoma.

ANSWERS

1. D	9. C	17. C	25. A	33. A	41. C	49. C
2. A	10. A	18. B	26. B	34. D	42. A	50. C
3. C	11. C	19. B	27. C	35. B	43. B	
4. B	12. A	20. A	28. D	36. D	44. C	
5. A	13. C	21. B	29. D	37. A	45. D	
6. C	14. E	22. A	30. B	38. B	46. C	
7. C	15. A	23. A	31. D	39. B	47. C	
8. C	16. B	24. C	32. A	40. B	48. D	

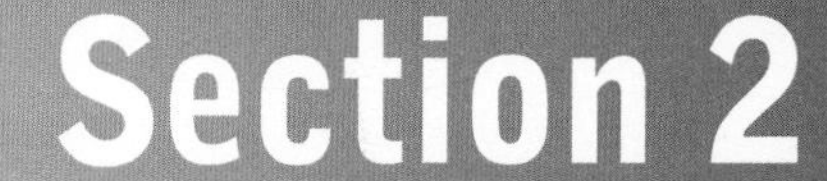

NOSE

Section Outline

Chapter 24

Development and Anatomy of the Nose and Paranasal Sinuses

Development

At about the fourth week of fetal life, two epithelial thickenings known as nasal placodes develop on the head. These nasal placodes get depressed due to proliferation of surrounding mesoderm and form olfactory pits. The raised areas of mesoderm are known as *medial and lateral nasal folds.* With further proliferation, the olfactory pits get depressed to form *nasal sacs.* The maxillary processes grow medially underneath the eyes and come in contact with the lateral nasal process (**Fig. 24.1**). The nasal sac thus forms the primitive nasal cavity. The medial nasal folds fuse together to form the frontonasal process, the upper and anterior end of which forms the primitive nasal septum while the free lower surface forms the primitive palate. The primitive nasal cavities are closed posteriorly by the bucconasal membrane which ruptures and thus each side of the nasal sac communicates with the roof of mouth behind the primitive palate and the communication forms the primitive posterior naris.

A ridge of mesoderm extends from the site of *Rathke's pouch* to the level of the posterior edge of the frontonasal process. This is called the tectoseptal expansion and forms the definitive nasal septum.

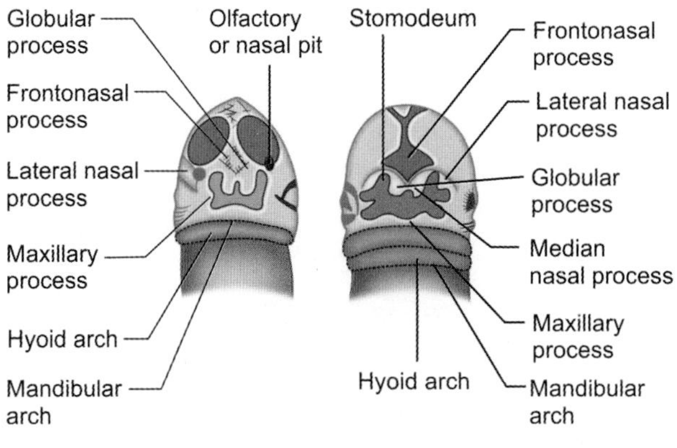

Globular process
Olfactory or nasal pit
Stomodeum
Frontonasal process
Frontonasal process
Lateral nasal process
Lateral nasal process
Globular process
Median nasal process
Maxillary process
Maxillary process
Hyoid arch
Hyoid arch
Mandibular arch
Mandibular arch

Fig. 24.1: Development of the nose and oral cavity

Each mass of maxillary mesoderm provides a medially directed extension (palatal process) towards the definitive septum. These palatal processes fuse with the primitive palate as well as with each other to form the hard and soft palates.

A small opening, nasopalatine canal is the fusion site of the primitive palate with the maxillary processes. This canal is represented in the adult life in hard palate by a foramen known as *incisive foramen.*

Failure of fusion of maxillary processes results in cleft palate and harelip.

DEVELOPMENT OF THE PARANASAL SINUSES

Three ectodermal elevations appear in the primitive nasal cavity on its lateral surface. The mesenchyme migrates into these elevations which form the turbinates. **Figure 24.2** shows the development of nasal sinuses from 3 months to 11 years.

The sinuses develop in late embryonic life and some develop during the early postnatal life and appear as extensions of mucosal pouches into the surrounding bone.

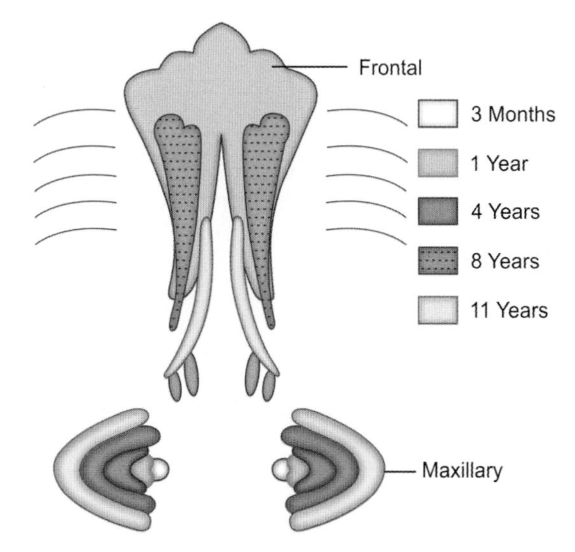

Fig. 24.2: Development of the nasal sinuses from 3 months to 11 years

The maxillary sinus develops as a mucosal depression below the middle turbinate, which invades the maxilla. Its growth is complete by about nine years of age.

The sphenoid sinus is present at birth but reaches adult size at puberty.

The frontal and ethmoid sinuses are represented by diverticula at birth. The frontal sinus develops as an extension of the mucosal pouch that forms the anterior ethmoid cells. The sinus invades the frontal bone by the first year of life and reaches the adult size at puberty. The ethmoid cells develop from grooves between ethmoturbinates.

Anatomy

EXTERNAL NOSE

External nose has a bony and cartilaginous structure. The bony framework is formed by a pair of nasal bones, the frontal processes of maxillae and the nasal spine of the frontal bone (**Fig. 24.3**).

Cartilages of the Nose

1. Paired upper lateral nasal cartilages
2. Paired lower nasal cartilages (greater alar cartilage)
3. Accessory alar cartilages
4. Septal cartilage.

The upper lateral cartilages are triangular in shape and are attached above to the lower borders of the nasal bones. Medially these are attached to the dorsum of the septal cartilage. The lower nasal cartilage or the greater alar cartilage bends around to form the contour of the ala and the nasal tip. The medial crus of this cartilage joins with its opposite process to form the columella. Small alar cartilages are situated posterior to the lateral crus of the lower nasal cartilage.

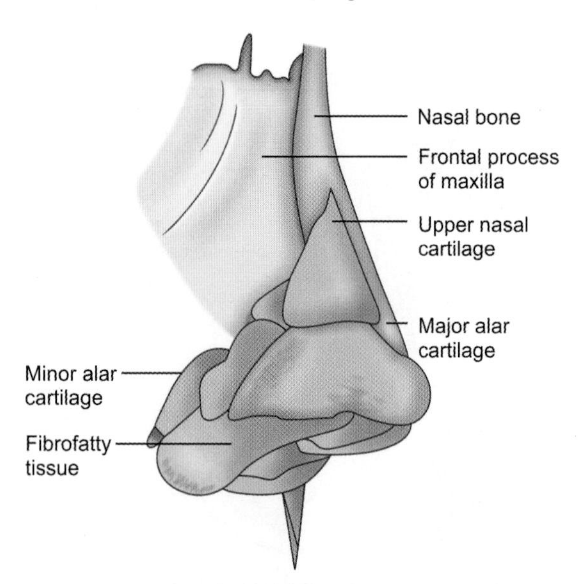

Fig. 24.3: Skeletal structure of the external nose

NASAL CAVITIES

The interior of the nasal cavity is divided into two halves by a central septum.

The anterior and posterior apertures of the nose are called the anterior and posterior choanae respectively. The nasal cavity has a roof, floor, and medial and lateral walls.

The floor is formed by the palatine processes of maxillae and horizontal plates of the two palatine bones.

The roof is made of nasal bones, under surface of the nasal spine of the frontal bone, cribriform plate of the ethmoid and undersurface of the body of sphenoid bone.

The *medial wall* of the nasal cavity is formed by the nasal septum.

The lateral wall of the nose has ridges and depressions. The ridges are formed by *turbinates.* There are three turbinates—superior, middle and inferior. While the inferior turbinate is a separate bone, the middle and superior turbinates are parts of the ethmoid bone (**Figs 24.4 and 24.5**).

The anterior part of the lateral wall is formed by the inner aspect of the nasal bone, anterior part of the body of maxilla, frontal process of the maxilla and a portion of the inferior turbinate. The middle part of the lateral wall is formed by the medial surface of the ethmoid labyrinth, superior and middle turbinates and the pterygoid plates. In the upper part is the sphenopalatine foramen.

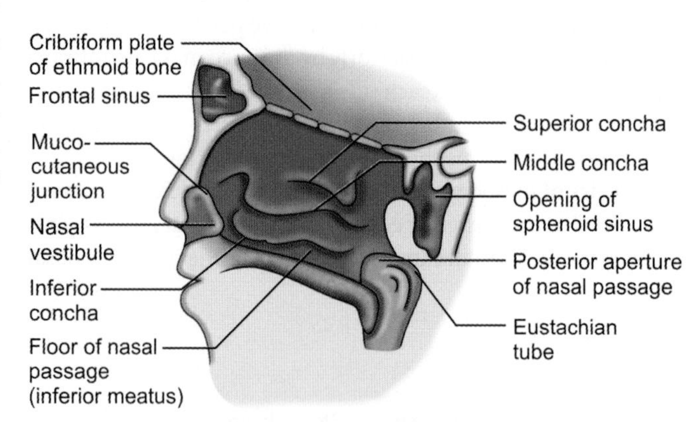

Fig. 24.4: Lateral wall of the nose

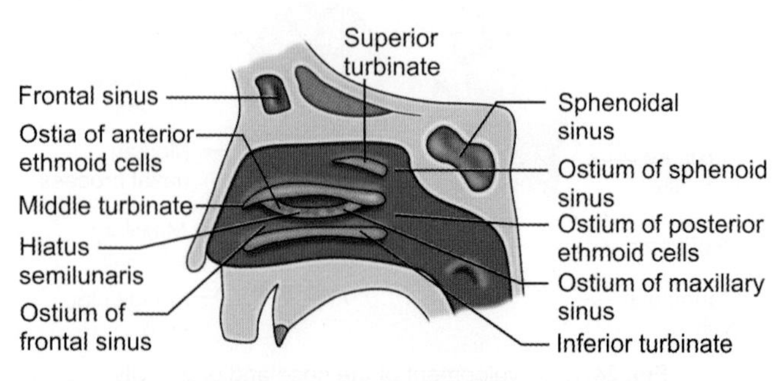

Fig. 24.5: Lateral wall of the nose revealing ostia of sinuses

The area below the turbinate is called the *meatus*. Each meatus is named after the turbinate under which it lies, that is, superior meatus, middle meatus and inferior meatus.

In the meati, various ducts and sinuses open. In the inferior meatus opens the nasolacrimal duct.

The following sinuses open in the middle meatus.

1. Anterior ethmoidal cells and the frontal sinus open in the anterior part of the meatus
2. Middle ethmoidal cells open above the bulla ethmoidalis or hiatus semilunaris
3. Maxillary sinuses open in the posterior part of the hiatus semilunaris.

In the middle meatus, there is a bulge called *bulla ethmoidalis* due to middle ethmoidal cells. Below this bulge, the uncinate process of the ethmoid projects backwards. The posterosuperior surface of the uncinate process forms the lower boundary of a fissure called hiatus semilunaris. The upper boundary of the fissure is formed by bulla ethmoidalis.

The area above the middle turbinate is the superior meatus. In this area, open the posterior ethmoid cells. Above and behind the superior turbinate is a small depression called, the sphenoethmoidal recess in which the sphenoid sinus opens.

NASAL SEPTUM

The nasal septum has cartilaginous and bony parts (**Fig. 24.6**). The bony parts of the septum is formed by the following:

1. Posteroinferiorly by the vomer.
2. Posterosuperiorly by the perpendicular plate of ethmoid.
3. The nasal spine of the frontal bone joins the ethmoid plate.
4. Rostrum of sphenoid between the vomer and ethmoidal plate.
5. Nasal crest of the two maxillae and palatine bones.

Cartilaginous Part of Nasal Septum

This is formed by a quadrilateral cartilage. It is attached to the perpendicular plate of the ethmoid bone posterosuperiorly, to the anterior border of vomer posteriorly, to the internasal crest superiorly, and to the nasal crest of the maxilla and anterior nasal spine inferiorly.

The upper nasal cartilages are attached to the anterosuperior border of the septal cartilage.

Membranous Septum

This is formed by the juxtaposition of two mucocutaneous flaps. These flaps extend forwards from the free margins of the septal cartilage to cutaneous coverings of the medial crurae of the lower lateral cartilages which form cartilaginous support of the columella. The cartilage is enveloped by a perichondrial and submucosal fascial sheath. The perichondrium of the cartilage is not in continuity with the periosteum of the perpendicular plate of ethmoid. The perichondrium of the quadrilateral cartilage of one side is continuous with the perichondrium of the opposite side. The premaxillary and maxillary crests are similarly covered by periosteum separately (**Fig. 24.7**). This fiber arrangement is kept in mind while elevating the flaps in septal operations to avoid tearing of the flaps.

Blood Supply of the Septum

The nasal septum derives its blood supply from the following sources:

1. Long sphenopalatine branch of the internal maxillary artery (main blood supply to the septum).
2. Anterior and posterior ethmoid branches of the ophthalmic artery (supply the septum in the upper and posterior part).
3. Terminal branches of the greater palatine artery through the incisive canal.
4. Septal branches of the superior labial artery (coronary artery of the nose), a branch of facial artery.

The ramifications of these blood vessels form an anastomosis (*Keissel-Bach's plexus*) at the anteroinferior portion of

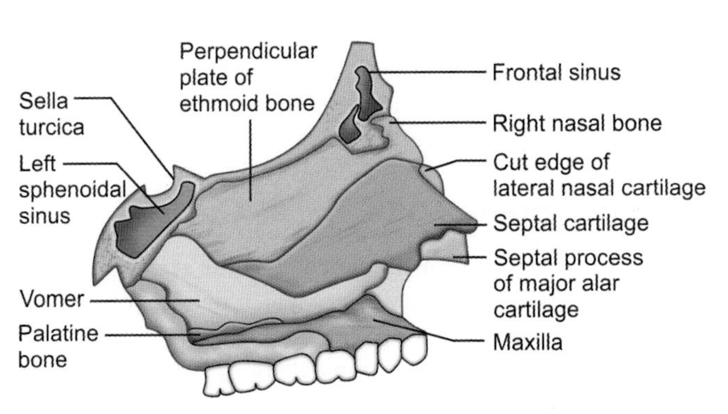

Fig. 24.6: Medial wall of the nose

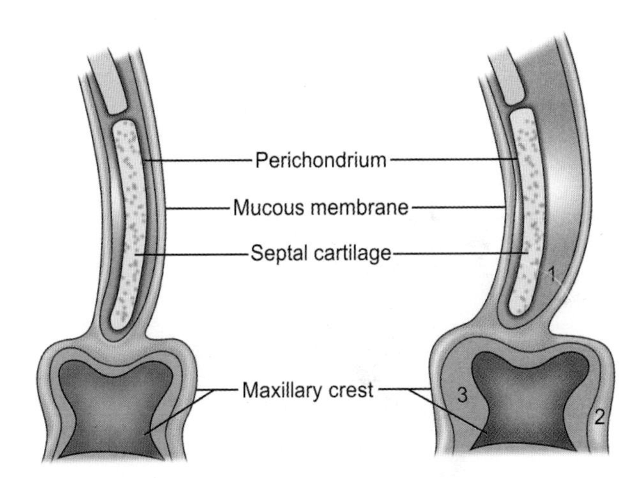

Fig. 24.7: Mucoperichondrial and mucoperiosteal layers in the septum, septal cartilage (dotted area), ethmoid and maxillary crest (black): (1) Left anterior tunnel, (2) Left inferior tunnel, (3) Right inferior tunnel

the septum called *Little's area* (see Fig. 32.1). This is a frequent site of bleeding.

MUCOSA OF NOSE

1. The anterior vestibular region has stratified squamous epithelium. It ends at the mucocutaneous junction.
2. *Respiratory portion* of the nasal mucosa is lined by pseudostratified columnar ciliated epithelium. The mucosa is firmly adherent to the perichondrium and periosteum.
3. *Olfactory mucosa:* This part of the mucosa occupies the olfactory portion of the nose which extends over the upper part of septum and adjacent lateral wall up to the superior turbinate. This mucosa has a yellowish color and consists of olfactory receptor cells among basal cells and supporting cells.

Paranasal Sinuses

A diagrammatic representation of the sinuses is given in **Figure 24.8**.

MAXILLARY SINUS (ANTRUM OF HIGHMORE)

This is a pyramidal cavity in the maxilla. The sinus cavity may be divided into small spaces by bony septa.

The roof of the sinus is formed by the floor of the orbit. The floor of the sinus lies about 1 cm below the level of the nasal cavity in adults and is formed by the alveolar process of maxilla.

The anteriolateral wall is formed by the anterior part of the body of maxilla. It contains the anterior superior dental vessels and nerves.

The medial wall is formed by the nasal surface of maxilla, the perpendicular plate of palatine bone, maxillary process of inferior turbinate and the uncinate process of ethmoid.

The posterior wall is formed by the posterior surface of maxilla.

The opening of the maxillary sinus is in the posterior part of the hiatus semilunaris between bulla ethmoidalis and the uncinate process of the ethmoid bone, on the lateral wall of the nose below the middle turbinate. The capacity of sinus varies between 15 ml to 30 ml.

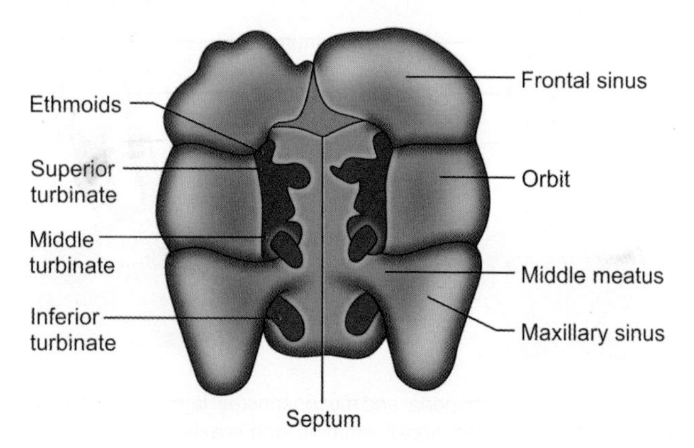

Fig. 24.8: Diagrammatic representation of the paranasal sinuses

The roots of the premolar and molar teeth may project into the sinus cavity. The marrow containing bone may be present up to 18 months of age and, therefore, osteomyelitis of the maxilla may occur during this period. The posterosuperior dental vessels and nerves supply the sinus mucosa.

FRONTAL SINUS

Frontal sinuses are two in number and develop in the frontal bone. The two sinuses are usually unequal in size. The anterior wall and floor of the sinus have marrow containing bone, hence, osteomyelitis can develop in this region at any age. The floor of the sinus forms parts of the roof of orbit. The posterior wall forms the anterior boundary of the anterior cranial fossa, hence infection of the sinus can travel to the anterior cranial fossa and orbit. The frontal sinus is drained by the frontonasal duct which opens in the anterior part of the middle meatus. The average capacity of the sinus is about 7 ml in adults. The sinus is supplied by the supraorbital nerve and vessels.

ETHMOID SINUSES

These are multiple air-containing cells situated in the ethmoidal labyrinth. These are arranged in three main groups. Anterior group, middle group and the posterior group.

The anterior group of cells drain into the anterior part of the middle meatus. The middle ethmoidal cells drain in the middle meatus on the ethmoid bulla or above it while the posterior ethmoid cells drain into the superior meatus.

The ethmoid air cells are related laterally to the orbit and are separated from it by a thin bone lamina papyracea. Posteriorly the ethmoids are related to the optic foramina. Superiorly the ethmoid air cells may reach to a level above the cribriform plate. These sinuses are supplied by the anterior and posterior ethmoid nerves and vessels.

SPHENOID SINUS

Sphenoid sinuses develop in the body of the sphenoid bone. The two sinuses are unequally divided by a septum.

Superiorly, the sinus is related to the frontal lobe and olfactory tracts. Above and posteriorly lies the pituitary gland in the sella turcica. Laterally, the sinus is related to the optic nerve and cavernous sinus. The sinus opens through the anterior wall in the sphenoethmoidal recess.

Blood Supply of the Nasal Cavity

1. The main supply is by the sphenopalatine artery, a branch of the internal maxillary artery which divides into lateral nasal branches and a long septal branch.
2. Anterior and posterior ethmoidal arteries, branches of the ophthalmic artery supply the upper part of the lateral wall and upper posterior part of the septum.

3. The greater palatine artery enters through the incisive canal into the nose and supplies the anteroinferior part of the septum and adjacent areas of the floor and lateral wall.
4. The superior labial branch of the facial artery supplies the septum and nasal alae.

VENOUS DRAINAGE

Veins form a plexus which drains anteriorly into the facial vein, posteriorly into the pharyngeal plexus of veins and from the middle part to the pterygoid plexus of veins.

Nerve Supply of the Nose

The respiratory portion of the nose is supplied by the following nerves:

1. Anterior ethmoidal branch of the nasociliary nerve, supplying the upper part of the lateral wall and the septum.
2. Sphenopalatine nerves (long and short), branches from the sphenopalatine ganglion.
3. Greater palatine nerve.
4. Anterior superior dental nerve.

From the olfactory portion of the nose, nerve filaments pass through the foramina in the cribriform plate of ethmoid and end up in the olfactory bulb in which they form synapses.

SYMPATHETIC SUPPLY

The preganglionic fibers arise from the first and second thoracic segments of the spinal cord and end in the corresponding sympathetic ganglia. These fibers ascend in the cervical sympathetic chain to synapse in the superior cervical ganglion. The postganglionic fibers pass from this ganglion around the internal carotid artery. The fibers pass from the internal carotid as the deep petrosal nerve.

PARASYMPATHETIC SUPPLY

The preganglionic fibers arise in the superior salivary nucleus in the brainstem and pass in the nervus intermedius to the geniculate ganglion.

The fibers from this ganglion pass in the greater superficial petrosal nerve.

The deep petrosal nerve and greater superficial petrosal nerves join together to form the nerve of pterygoid canal (Vidian nerve) which joins the sphenopalatine ganglion. The fibers in the greater superficial petrosal nerve end in the sphenopalatine ganglion. Postganglionic fibers arise from this ganglion and both sympathetic and parasympathetic fibers are distributed through the sphenopalatine nerves to the nasal mucosa.

Lymphatic Drainage of Nose and Paranasal Sinuses

Submandibular lymph nodes collect lymph from the external and anterior parts of the nasal cavity.

Upper deep cervical nodes drain the rest of the nasal cavity either directly or through the retropharyngeal nodes.

Chapter 25

Physiology of the Nose and Paranasal Sinuses

The nose forms the gateway of the respiratory system and serves the following important functions:

1. *Respiratory passage:* Normally, breathing takes place through the nose. The inspired air passes upwards in a narrow stream medial to the middle turbinate and then downwards and backwards in the form of an arc, and thus respiratory air currents are restricted to the central part of the nasal chambers. Any anatomical or pathological obstructive lesion in this region is important, as this disturbs the air flow.
2. *Filtration:* The nose serves as an effective filter for the inspired air.
   a. Vibrissae (nasal hair) in the nasal vestibule arrest large particulate matter of the inspired air.
   b. The fine particulate matter and bacteria are deposited on the mucus blanket which covers the nasal mucosa. The mucus contains various enzymes like lysozymes having antibacterial properties.
   c. The mucus with the particulate matter is carried by the ciliary movements posteriorly to the oropharynx to be swallowed.
3. *Airconditioning and humidification:* The highly vascular mucosa of the nose maintains constancy of the temperature of air and thus, prevents the delicate mucosa of the respiratory tract from any damage due to temperature variations. The humidified air is necessary for proper functioning and integrity of the ciliated epithelium.
4. *Vocal resonance:* The nose and paranasal sinuses serve as vocal resonators and nasal passages are concerned with production of nasal consonants like M and N. Thus, obstructions of the nasopharynx and nose alter the tone of voice (rhinolalia clausa).
5. *Nasal reflex functions:* The receptive fields of various reflexes lie in the nose. These include sneezing, and nasopulmonary, nasobronchial and olfactory reflexes. These protect the mucosa and regulate the vasomotor tone of the blood vessels. Olfactory reflexes influence salivary, gastric and pancreatic glands.
6. The nasal cavity serves as an outlet for lacrimal and sinus secretions.
7. *Olfaction:* This function of the nose is less developed in human beings. This sensation plays the most important role in behavior and reflex responses of lower animals.

The olfactory mucosa is located in the roof of nasal cavity and adjacent area of superior turbinate and upper part of septum. The olfactory cells are distributed in the olfactory mucosa.

The mechanism of olfactory stimulation is uncertain. Various theories have been propagated. The odoriferous substance reaches the olfactory cells by air, probably by diffusion. The olfactory sensitivity differs in individuals and is influenced by many physiological factors and pathological changes in the nose.

Olfactometry (Odor Measurement)

Various methods have been used to assess the olfactory function in man.

QUALITATIVE OLFACTOMETRY

The olfactory sense is assessed by taking a solution or extract before the patient's nose.

The following primary odors are usually tested:

1. Etherial—Ether
2. Camphoraceous—Camphor
3. Flora(l)—Salicyldehyde
4. Musky—Phenyl acetic acid
5. Minty—Mint
6. Pungent—Formalin
7. Putrid—Thiophenol.

QUANTITATIVE OLFACTOMETRY

The measurement of olfactory sense can be done by an olfactometer. This instrument gives an idea about the qualitative defects of olfaction. The reading is taken as the number of olfacts. Normally, the olfactory sense smells one olfact.

Olfactometry gives information about the following:

1. The extent of the field of smell.
2. It gives an idea about the patient's acuity of smell.
3. Possible parosmia (perverted smell).

Disturbances of Olfaction

Hyposmi: Diminished sense of smell is termed hyposmia. Its causative factors are the following:

i. Old age (Presbyosmia)
ii. Hypogonadal women, menopause
iii. Tobacco smoker, radiation therapy of nose
iv. Surgical removal of the mucosa.

Parosmia: It is a qualitative change. There occurs an unpleasant change in sense of smell.

It may occur in the following conditions:

i. Skull fractures
ii. Injury to uncus of the temporal lobe
iii. May follow administration of streptomycin or tyrothricin.

Anosmia: Anosmia is the loss of the sense of smell. Its causes are the following:

i. Obstructive lesions in the nose and nasopharynx
ii. Lesions of mucosa
iii. Trauma—surgical or accidental
iv. Neuritis
v. Central lesions in the brain.

Hyperosmia: Exaggeration of the olfactory sensitivity is termed as hyperosmia and it occurs with the following:

i. Epilepsy
ii. Pregnancy, hunger, strychnine poisoning
iii. General paralysis of insane
iv. Cystic fibrosis.

Functions of the Paranasal Sinuses

The paranasal sinuses are thought to serve the following functions:

1. Warming and moistening of inspired air may be partly done by the large mucosal surfaces of these adjacent sinuses.
2. The air filled sinus cavities probably add resonance to the laryngeal voice.
3. The temperature buffers: It is regarded that these chambers probably protect the contents of orbits and cranial fossae from the intranasal temperature variations.
4. Probably, sinus formation in the cranial bones helps in reducing the weight of the facial bones.
5. The sinus mucosa may act as a donor site for reconstructive procedures, e.g. for subglottic stenosis and implantation of maxillary sinus mucosa into the nasal cavity in atrophic rhinitis.
6. They act as shock buffers.

Multifarious Functions of Nose

The nature has provided nose in almost all the animals, but function varies from species to species. As is evident from the appearance of the different animals, nature has provided nose as such a place and in such a form as the concerned species needs it for its survival.

In the Crocodile and Hippopotamus, the anterior nares are placed high up on the snout, so that the animal may breathe when under water with the snout projecting and the mouth open.

The Curlew (Numenius arquatus) has a long nose to seek food in marshy ground.

Echidna (Echidna aculeata), Aard-vark (Orycteropus capensis) and Tree Shrew (Tupaia), have long noses with which to seek for insects.

Wart Hog (Phacochoerus), Moose (Alces) and Tapir (Tapirus) have a long proboscis for grubbing in soft ground.

The Elephant Seal (Macrohinus leoninus) has nostrils that can be closed under water.

The snout of a Greyhound (Canis familiaris) is long for seizing prey.

In the Chimpanzee (Anthropopithectus troglodytes), the nose is very short in relation to snout. In man, recession of the jaws causes the nose to project slightly. The nose of the Crested Seal (Crystophora cristata) can be inflated for purposes of respiration under water. The Elephant (Elephas) has a long trunk for prehension. The function of the projecting nostrils of the Tube-Nosed Bar (Harpyiocephalus) is not ascertainable that of the proboscis monkey (Nasatis laryatus) is said to be for attraction of the female, the male alone being so adorned.

Chapter 26

Common Symptoms of Nasal and Paranasal Sinus Diseases

The nose and paranasal sinuses are closely related anatomically, so are their presenting symptoms. The following symptoms may be present alone or in combination depending upon the disease process.

Nasal Discharge

The discharge from the nose may be unilateral or bilateral and further it could be watery, mucoid, mucopurulent, purulent or blood-stained.

Watery discharge is usually found in the early stages of common cold, vasomotor rhinitis and CSF rhinorrhea. Mucoid discharge is usually a feature of allergic rhinitis while mucopurulent discharge occurs in infective rhinitis and sinusitis.

Purulent discharge is a feature of atrophic rhinitis, foreign bodies in the nose, furunculosis and longstanding sinusitis.

Blood-stained nasal discharge usually indicates an underlying malignant process, foreign body or nonhealing granulomas, etc.

Nasal Obstruction

Obstruction to the passage of air through the nose may be unilateral or bilateral. The obstruction may be alternating on the two sides and may be progressive and persistent. The common conditions of the nose and paranasal sinuses which result in nasal obstruction include deviated nasal septum, ethmoidal and antrochoanal polypi, hypertrophied turbinates, septal hematoma, foreign bodies in nose, nasal and paranasal sinus tumors, and granulomatous diseases.

Besides the lesions in the nose and paranasal sinuses, adenoids, tumors and cysts of the nasopharynx can also cause nasal obstruction.

The symptom of nasal obstruction is often associated with a history of breathing through the mouth, and dryness of the throat due to lack of the humidifying action of the nose.

Facial Pain and Headache

Nasal and paranasal sinuses are frequently blamed for headaches and facial pain. Pain due to involvement of different sinuses has different characteristics.

FRONTAL SINUS HEADACHE

Pain due to inflammation of the frontal sinus is usually localized over the forehead. The pain is more during early hours of the day and subsides or diminishes in intensity by afternoon as by that time drainage of the infected discharge occurs.

MAXILLARY SINUS HEADACHE

Pain due to the involvement of the maxillary sinus is more over the maxillary region. It may be referred to the upper alveolus. Ethmoid sinus pain usually occurs along sides of the nose or in the orbits.

SPHENOID SINUS HEADACHE

The pain is referred to the vertex or occiput or may be present behind the eyes.

Facial pain due to other nasal and paranasal lesions may occur as in furunculosis, syphilis, due to nerve infiltration as in sinus tumors and trigeminal neuralgias.

Epistaxis

Bleeding from the nose may be unilateral or bilateral and may be due to a variety of lesions of the nose, paranasal sinuses and the nasopharynx. The etiology of epistaxis has been discussed in Chapter 32.

Disorders of Olfaction

Various olfactory derangements have already been discussed.

Postnasal Drip

Normally, the secretions from the nose and nasopharynx are carried to the oropharynx by the mucociliary mechanism of the nose, where from these are swallowed. Many times the patient complains of excessive nasal discharge coming into the oropharynx causing various pharyngeal symptoms.

Postnasal drip occurs commonly in allergic and infective diseases of the nose and paranasal sinuses, due to adenoids or in Thornwaldt's disease (bursitis).

Speech Defect

Disorders of the nose and nasal sinuses may result in loss of the resonating function and this may give a nasal tone to voice like a closed nose speech as occurs in obstructive lesions.

Symptoms due to Extension of the Disease to the Adjacent Regions

Diseases of the nose or paranasal sinuses may involve adjacent structures like the orbit, cranial cavity, cavernous sinus, etc. and produce symptoms of their involvement.

Sneezing

Sneezing is the normal nasal reflex to clear secretion from the nose and is of great importance in young children who have yet not learnt to blow their nose. It is stimulated by irritation within the nose by infection or allergy or following inhalation of noxious gases or polluted air. The sensory side of the reflex is transmitted through the trigeminal nerve, and stimulation of the skin supplied by the maxillary division of this nerve by cold, strong light, pain or heat can also stimulate this reflex.

Snoring

Abnormal sound produced through nose during sleep is called snoring. It has many causes like adenoids in children or polypi or growth in nose, too much hypertrophied turbinates, edematous mucosa of nose or soft palate. While the treatment of all pathological conditions relieves snoring but some people have habitual snoring making others difficult to sleep or concentrate on studies if they are in same room. For such patients, recent laser technique has been devised to treat the snoring. Under local anesthesia, a small needle connected to a radio-frequency generator is inserted into the soft palate junction of oronasopharyngeal mucosa. The radiofrequency energy is directed through shaking and disruption. Over few weeks, the body naturally reabsorbs some of the loose tissue thus relieving snoring.

Sleep Apnea

Normal respiration requires air to be displaced from external environment to alveolar membrane to make oxygen available for gas exchange. This simple looking involuntary act is extraordinarily complex. Crucial in this process is the ability of upper airway to permit the unimpeded transport of air to tracheobronchial tree. Apnea results when this process is partially or completely interrupted. The supralaryngeal airway is most susceptible to obstruction during the skeletal muscle hypotonicity associated with sleep. This resulting in sleep apnea which is defined as intermittent cessation of airway during sleep. Sleep apnea is divided into obstructive, central and mixed types. The obstructive apnea is preceded by upper respiratory obstruction with increasing respiratory effort.

During sleep, there is reduced activity and tone in the muscles of tongue, soft palate and pharynx which results in collapse of airway due to suction effect and as respiratory effort increases, the resulting apnea causes progressive asphyxia, which results in arousal from sleep, with restoration of patency and airflow. In most of the patients, the patency of airway is also compromised structurally, which include obvious anatomic disturbance like DNS, adenotonsillar hypertrophy, macroglossia, retrognathia in a minority of patients, and a subtle reduction in airway size in a majority of patients. This subtle reduction can be usually demonstrated by imaging and acoustic reflection techniques.

In central sleep apnea, there is transient abolition of central drive to ventilatory muscles. Purely central apnea without obstructive element is very rare. Mixed apnea is a combination of failure of central control and upper airway obstruction.

CLINICAL MANIFESTATION

The narrowing of airway during sleep inevitably results in snoring. In most pateints snoring antedates the development of obstructive events by many years.

The nocturnal asphyxia and frequent arousal from sleep lead to day-time sleepiness, intellectual impairment, memory loss, personality disturbance and impotence.

OTHER MANIFESTATIONS

Cardiorespiratory in nature. Obstructive sleep apnea (OSA) is considered to be risk factor for the development of systemic hypertension, myocardial ischemia, infarction, stroke and premature death.

The clinical manifestations are aggravated by obesity and alcohol intake.

MANAGEMENT

Investigations

The investigatory part includes:

1. Detailed history and clinical examinations.
2. Observation of patient during sleep.
3. Polysomnography, which is detailed examination during sleep with monitoring of sleep stages.

4. Transcutaneous monitoring of (oxygen) O_2 saturation during sleep.
5. Measurement of airflow.
6. Continuous ECG monitoring.
7. Radiology for identification of adenoid obstruction of nasopharynx and tonsillar obstruction of oropharynx.
8. CT of pharyngeal airway.
9. Nasal endoscopy.

Treatment

It can be medical or surgical. Medical treatment includes continuous positive airway pressure. This has the disadvantage that it cannot be used for long-term management.

Surgical treatment includes adenotonsillectomy, velopalato pharyngoplasty. In severely affected patients, who are unsuitable for surgery, tracheostomy may be done to at least partially reverse the gross cardiopulmonary abnormalities.

Chapter 27

Examination of the Nose, Paranasal Sinuses and Nasopharynx

The examination of these regions includes general examination of the face and nose, anterior rhinoscopy, oropharyngeal examination, posterior rhinoscopy and various other investigative procedures.

Inspection and Palpation

This is done to detect any deformity, asymmetry or swelling of the nose and face. Depression or deviation of the nasal bridge due to injury or disease may be present. A sinus in the midline of the nasal dorsum is usually congenital. Rarely a sebaceous horn may be present. Gentle palpation of the nose may detect crepitus in fractured nasal bones.

Dislocated anterior end of the septum may be projecting into the vestibule. The nose must also be observed by standing above and behind the patient.

Anterior Rhinoscopy

This procedure is carried out using a head mirror and a light source.

Examination of the nasal vestibule is usually done without a nasal speculum. The tip of the nose is raised up and the nostrils inspected for redness or swelling as in furunculosis. A dislocated anterior end of the septum may be visible.

An assessment of the nasal airway is done by keeping a cold glass slide or a metallic tongue depressor just in front of the nostrils. On expiration, the warm air produces an area of condensation on the surface. The difference on the two sides is an indication of nasal obstruction. Alternatively, degree of displacement, on expiration, of a cotton wick held near the nostrils also gives an idea about the degree of nasal obstruction.

This initial examination of the nasal vestibule without nasal speculum is necessary as otherwise blades of the speculum may obscure papillomas, cysts and bleeding points in this region.

EXAMINATION WITH A NASAL SPECULUM

A Thudicum's speculum or a St. Clair-Thompson's speculum with a handle are commonly used for examination. These are available in many sizes. The speculum must be held in the left hand, keeping the right hand free for manipulations.

The Thudicum's speculum is held with the thumb and forefinger of the left hand. The middle finger rests on one side and ring finger on the other side to control the spring of the speculum. The closed speculum is introduced into the nasal vestibule and blades of the speculum directed in line of opening of the nostrils. The blades are opened to permit proper examination of the nose but not so wide as to cause discomfort. Care is taken in introducing and opening of blades in inflammatory lesions of the vestibule. The nasal cavities are properly examined. The floor, lateral wall, septum and posterior portions of nasal cavities are viewed. The color of the nasal mucosa is noted. Normally, it is dull red. Variations from normal are observed. A congested mucosa is seen in inflammatory lesions while pale or bluish mucosa is seen in allergic conditions. Septal deviations or spurs are noted. Prominence of vessels or crusting is often seen in the Little's area. Perforations of the septum may be present.

The nasal cavity may be widened as in atrophic rhinitis. Dryness of the nasal mucosa and crust formation inside the nasal cavity may be seen.

The anterior ends of the inferior and middle turbinates are visible on anterior rhinoscopy. These appear as prominent fleshy, firm and red projections on the lateral wall. These do not move on probing. The turbinates may appear atrophic and shrivelled up as in atrophic rhinitis. They may be grossly hypertrophied in chronic rhinitis, vasomotor rhinitis and in allergic rhinitis.

The meati are mostly covered by the turbinates and hardly visible on anterior rhinoscopy.

The view of inside of the nose in general is improved by using a vasoconstrictor spray in the nose. Any manipulation of the nose is facilitated by spraying the mucosa with topical xylocaine four percent.

A suction apparatus is a valuable asset for proper examination.

The meati are noted for discharge, local edema or redness. The middle meatus is a common site for polypi. The type of discharge is noted and a postural test may be done to note its probable site of origin.

POSTURAL TEST

If discharge is seen in the middle meatus, it usually means an infection of the anterior group of sinuses; when discharge in this region accumulates immediately on its removal, it indicates that it is coming from the frontal sinus.

If the discharge does not immediately reaccumulate, the patient's head is turned to the side of the normal maxillary sinus and the patient kept in this position for some time. The patient is made to sit upright again and reaccumulation of discharge in the middle meatus indicates involvement of the maxillary sinus.

EXAMINATION OF THE ORAL CAVITY AND OROPHARYNX

On examination of the oral cavity in relation to nasal and paranasal sinus disease, it is important to note following:

The gingivobuccal sulcus is inspected for any fulness or discharge. The anterolateral surface of the maxilla is palpated sublabially.

Carious teeth, loose teeth or widening of an alveolus are looked for. Any bulge of the hard palate is noted and palpated. Oroantral fistula is a communication between the maxillary sinus and the oral cavity. This may be the result or an etiological factor of maxillary sinus disease. A probe is used to note the extent and direction of any discharging sinus.

The soft palate may appear bulging down because of a mass in the nasopharynx, like an antrochoanal polypus, tumor, etc.

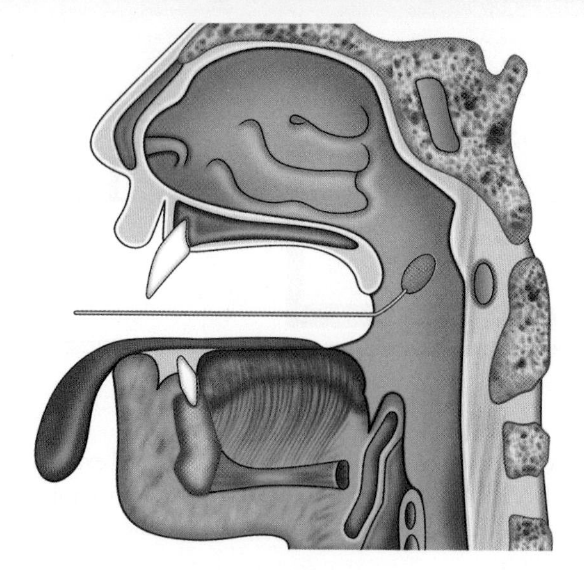

Fig. 27.1: Method of performing posterior rhinoscopy

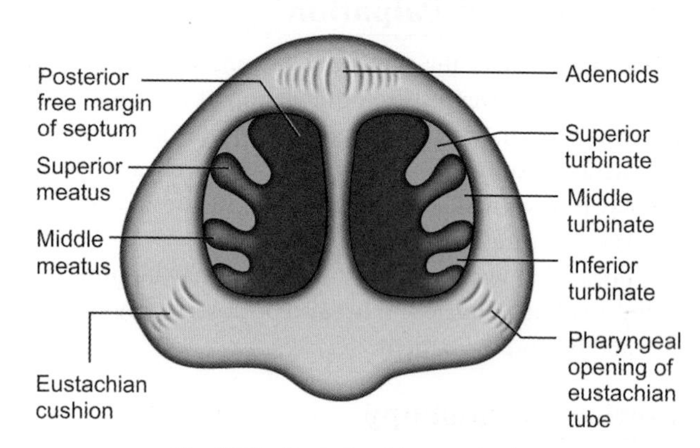

Fig. 27.2: Posterior rhinoscopic view

Posterior Rhinoscopy

This procedure permits the examination of the posterior aspects of nose and nasopharynx. The examination is a slightly difficult procedure and needs some experience. The procedure is explained to the patient.

The patient is asked to open the mouth. A tongue depressor is used with left hand to depress the anterior two-thirds of the tongue. The patient is advised to breathe quietly through the nose, and relax. A warmed postnasal mirror is held in the right hand and passed into the oropharynx between the posterior pharyngeal wall and soft palate without touching either.

Topical xylocaine may be needed to prevent gagging and allowing proper examination. The nasopharynx is examined in a systematic way using the head mirror and a light source (**Fig. 27.1**).

The posterior end of septum is seen as a vertical edge. On each side of posterior end of the septum are seen posterior choanae. The posterior edges of the inferior, middle and superior turbinates are seen on the lateral side of the nasal cavity. Hypertrophied posterior ends of the inferior turbinates appear as rounded, mulberry swelling on each side in the posterior choanae (**Fig. 27.2**). Discharge may be seen trickling from the meati over the turbinate ends. Discharge from the maxillary sinus may be seen over the inferior turbinate while discharge from posterior ethmoidal sinuses and the sphenoid sinuses appear above the superior turbinate. Antrochoanal polyp may be seen as a grayish, pale, smooth swelling, coming out of posterior choana into the nasopharynx.

A lateral tilt of the mirror, brings the lateral wall of the nasopharynx into view. The nasopharyngeal opening of the eustachian tube and a recess above and behind this (*fossa of Rossenmuller*) is noted. The fossa of Rossenmuller is frequently a site of malignancy.

The roof and posterior walls of the nasopharynx are examined next. Adenoid tissue is seen as a pinkish mass at the junction of roof and posterior wall of the nasopharynx up to early adult life. The surface shows clefts.

A nasopharyngeal angiofibroma appears as a red, firm lobulated mass with prominent vessels unlike the grayish pale, smooth antrochoanal polyp.

Nasopharyngeal cancer may appear as a proliferative or ulcerative lesion. Sometimes only fulness of nasopharynx is visible.

Rhinomanometry

Measurement of nasal air flow in studying nasal obstruction and its role in the production of some respiratory and cardiac changes is still in the research stage.

Digital Palpation of the Nasopharynx

This is an unpleasant procedure for the patient if not done under general anesthesia. The examiner stands on the right side of the seated patient and holds the patient's head against his left hip. The patient is asked to open the mouth and his cheek is pressed between his teeth by the left hand fingers of the examiner to prevent closure of the jaw.

The examiner passes the fingers of the right hand behind the soft palate into the nasopharynx.

Palpation may be needed in doubtful cases of malignancy of the nasopharynx. In children it may be done for adenoids.

Nasopharyngoscopy

Examination of the nasopharynx may be done under topical anesthesia using a nasopharyngoscope with a distal light source or by a fiberoptic nasopharyngoscope. The nasopharyngoscope is passed along the inferior turbinate and examination of the nasopharynx done through its window. This is useful for evaluating cases of suspected cancer and may also be used for guiding the tip of the eustachian catheter inside the eustachian orifice.

EXAMINATION OF NASOPHARYNX WITH RETRACTED SOFT PALATE

In patients, who do not allow proper examination of the naso-pharynx, the soft palate may be retracted. Rubber catheters are passed from the nose into the oropharynx. The end of the catheter is brought out from the oropharynx and the two ends tied together. This retracts the soft palate and thus allows a direct view of the nasopharynx (**Fig. 27.3**).

Transillumination of the Sinuses

This procedure is done in a darkroom. The light source (the sinus transilluminator) is placed in the oral cavity for testing the maxillary sinuses. The light transmitted through the sinus is seen as glowing of pupils and the infraorbital crescent. For

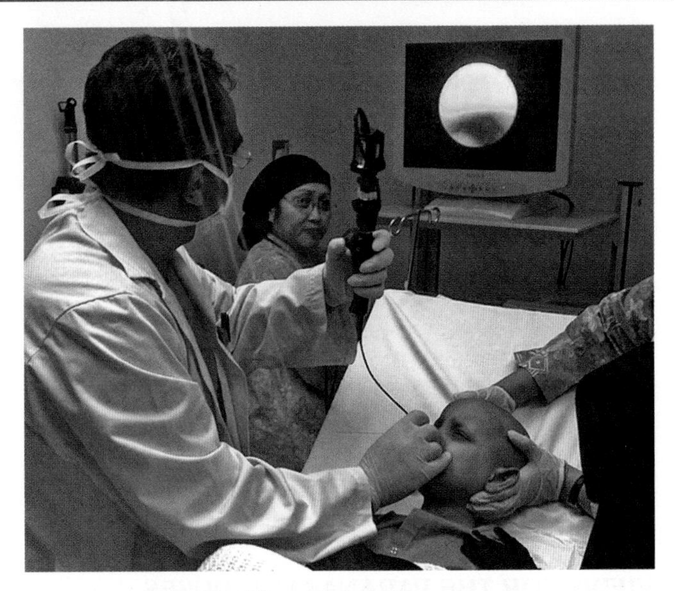

Fig. 27.3: Fiberoptic nasopharyngoscope

the frontal sinus, the light source is placed against the floor of the sinus. The light transmitted is seen as a glow on the anterior wall of the sinus.

The test is not of much help as thickened mucosa, mucopus, pus or tumor, all show an opaque sinus. The test is not possible for sphenoids and is not helpful for multiple ethmoid cells.

Sinoscopy

It is the direct visualization of the interior of the maxillary sinus by means of a fiberoptic endoscope called maxillary antrumscope. The endoscope is introduced through a cannula which is introduced into the maxillary sinus after the usual antrum puncture technique, either through the inferior meatus route or through the canine fossa. This diagnostic method is specific and accurate as compared to radiological examination of the maxillary sinus. It markedly reduces indications for the Caldwell-Luc operation.

Radiological Examination of the Nose and Paranasal Sinuses

The following radiological procedures may be needed for evaluation of diseases of the nose and paranasal sinuses.

PLAIN X-RAYS

Plain X-rays of the nasal bones may be required after injury to determine fractures or displacement.

The film is taken with the patient's head in the lateral position. This view projects the nose and adjacent areas of the face. A shadow of the nasal cartilages may also appear.

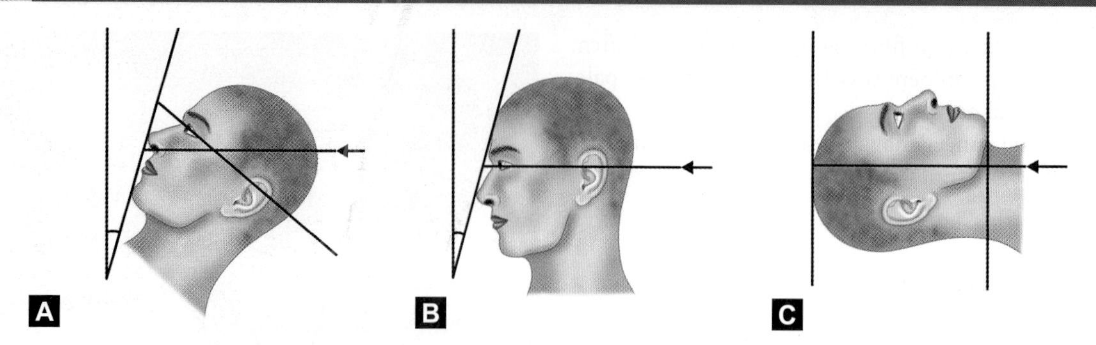

Figs 27.4A to C: Radiology of nasal structures: (A) Occipitomental view; (B) Occipitofrontal view; (C) Submentovertical view

In the superoinferior view, the patient holds a dental occlusal film in between the teeth. The rays pass from above through the roof of the nose to the center of the film.

VIEWS FOR THE PARANASAL SINUSES

It is difficult to examine all the paranasal sinuses on one projection, so the examination of individual sinus requires many views. The few standard views that are taken, which give an adequate idea about the condition of paranasal sinuses are as follows:

1. *Occipitomental view (Waters view):* The X-ray is taken in the nose-chin position with an open mouth. The film demonstrates mainly the maxillary sinuses, nasal cavity, septum, frontal sinuses and few cells of the ethmoids. The view taken in the standing position may show fluid level in the antrum **(Fig. 27.4A)**.
2. *Occipitofrontal view (Caldwell view):* The patient's forehead and tip of the nose are kept in contact with the film. This view is particularly useful for frontal sinuses. A portion of the maxillary antrum and nasal cavity are also shown **(Fig. 27.4B)**.
3. *X-ray, the base of the skull (Submentovertical view):* The neck and head are fully extended so that vertex faces the film and the rays are directed beneath the mandible. The view is useful for demonstrating sphenoid sinuses, ethmoids, nasopharynx, petrous apex, posterior wall of the maxillary sinus and fractures of the zygomatic arch **(Fig. 27.4C)**.
4. *Lateral view:* The patient's head is placed in a lateral position against the film and the ray is directed behind the outer canthus of the eye towards the film.

   The maxillary, ethmoidal and frontal sinuses superimpose each other but this film is useful for the following purposes:

   i. To demonstrate the extent of pneumatization of the sphenoid and frontal sinuses.
   ii. To demonstrate the position of a radiopaque foreign body in the nasal cavity or nasopharynx.
   iii. To demonstrate the thickness of soft tissues of the nasopharynx which should not normally be more than 5 mm.
   iv. To show the nasopharyngeal airway.
   v. To demonstrate the adenoid mass or a tumor in the nasopharynx.

Lateral oblique view for ethmoids: If the disease involves the ethmoids, a special lateral oblique view provides an idea about the ethmoidal air cells, being relatively free of superimposition by other structures.

On plain radiography, the normal sinuses appear as air filled translucent cavities. Opacity of the sinuses can be caused by fluid, thickened mucosa or tumors. Bony erosion can occur because of tumors, osteomyelitis or mucoceles.

CT Scan of the Nose, Paranasal Sinuses and Nasopharynx

CT scanning gives excellent details especially in case of early lesions which are not otherwise visible on plain radiography and is particularly useful in demonstrating the early tumors and fractures. CT is the most sensitive technique for evaluating sinus disease. It is very useful in defining bony landmarks and sinus abnormalities.

Angiography

External carotid angiography may be helpful in nasopharyngeal angiofibromas and other vascular lesions of the nose and paranasal sinuses.

Chapter 28

Congenital Diseases of the Nose

Choanal Atresia

Congenital atresia of the anterior apertures of the nasal passage is seldom seen. This fault occurs when the original epithelial plugs between the developing medial and lateral nasal folds fail to get absorbed during embryonic life.

Posterior choanal atresia (**Fig. 28.1**) is a more common congenital disease, though its incidence is also rare. Choanal atresia can be unilateral or bilateral, bony or membranous, and complete or incomplete. Various opinions have been expressed to explain its occurrence. While some authors believe that this anomaly is due to persistence of the bucconasal membrane, others think that atresia results from persistence of another membrane, the buccopharyngeal membrane from the foregut. Choanal atresia may also be present with other anomalies the so called 'CHARGE' association: C-coloboma of eyes, H-heart disease, A-atresia, R-mental retardation, G-genital hypoplasia, E-ear anomalies or deafness (**Fig. 28.2**).

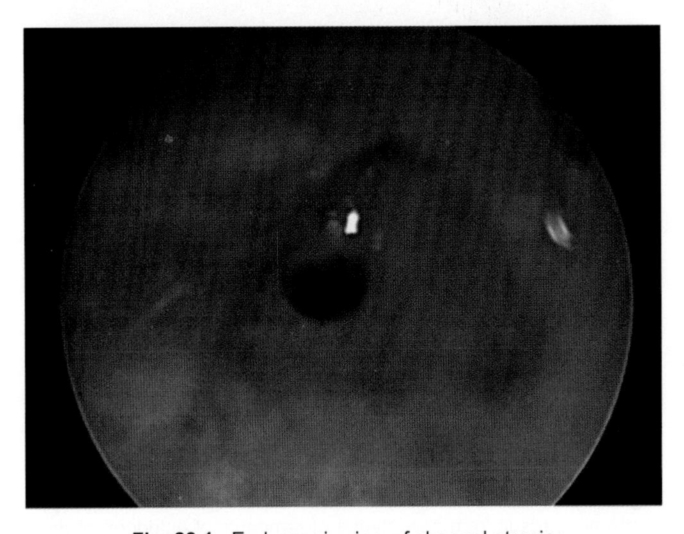

Fig. 28.1: Endoscopic view of choanal atresia

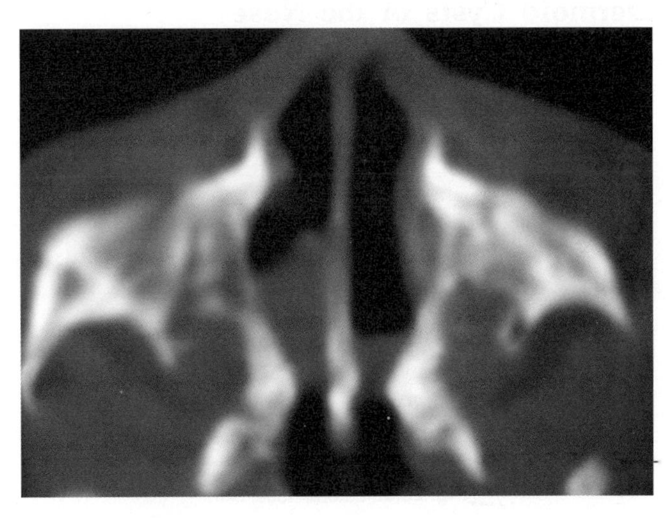

Fig. 28.2: Choanal atresia (membranous)

CLINICAL FEATURES

Bilateral atresia of the posterior nares, though not always a life threatening airway emergency, produces symptoms of high airway obstruction and the infant shows considerable difficulty in breathing immediately after birth.

There is marked difficulty in swallowing feeds due to the inability to coordinate breathing and swallowing. Tracheostomy may be needed.

Unilateral choanal atresia is usually not diagnosed early. Such patients present with a history of nasal obstruction with a mucoid discharge and the patient is unable to blow the nose on affected side.

DIAGNOSIS

Atresia should be suspected if there is evidence of persistent nasal obstruction which does not respond to cleaning, suction or decongestants. The diagnosis is clinched if a catheter passed through the nose, fails to appear in the pharynx. A contrast nasogram in the lateral position may confirm the diagnosis. CT scan is diagnostic.

TREATMENT

Bilateral choanal atresia in the newborn is an emergency. Rubber, plastic or metal airway tubes have been used to overcome the initial respiratory difficulty. A rubber teat (McGovern type) with holes for breathing and feeding is very useful. Several surgical procedures (transnasal and transpalatine) are done to expose the posterior nares and remove the atresia. The intranasal route involves a simpler procedure than the transpalatine route, though the latter gives the best exposure of the site of obstruction under direct vision. **Figures 28.3 and 28.4** show lateral and median nasal clefts.

Dermoid Cysts of the Nose

Dermoid cysts of the nose occur almost always in the midline between the alar cartilages on the bridge of the nose. Frequently, a sinus tract exposes itself as a pimple on the dorsum of the nose with a tuft of hair. The cysts arise as a result of ectopic ectodermal inclusions during development. Treatment is surgical excision of the cyst and the sinus tract (**Figs 28.5A to C**).

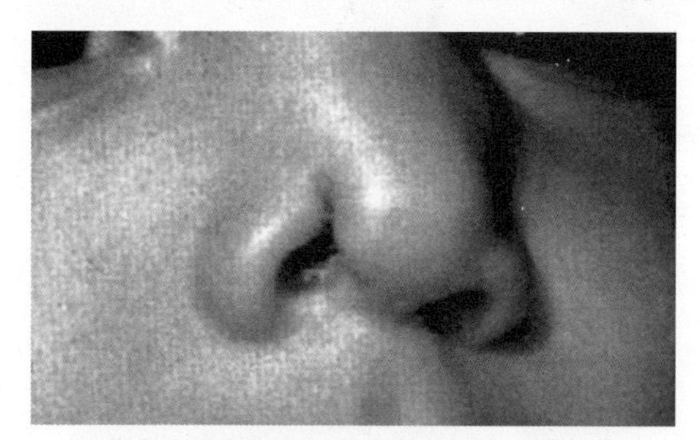

Fig. 28.3: Lateral nasal cleft

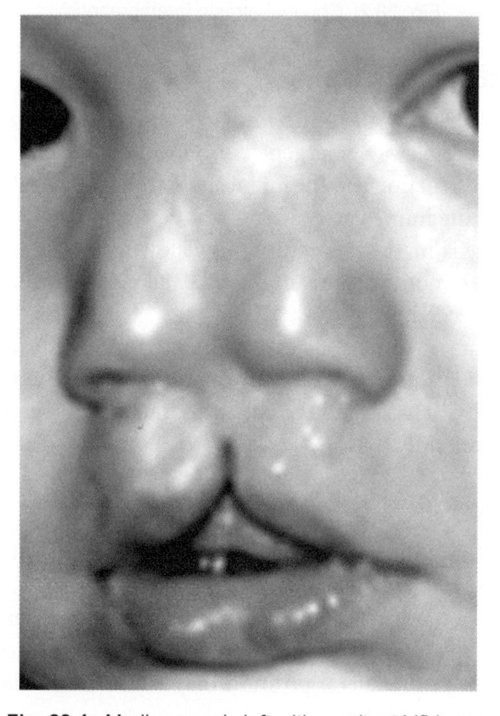

Fig. 28.4: Median nasal cleft with resultant bifid nose

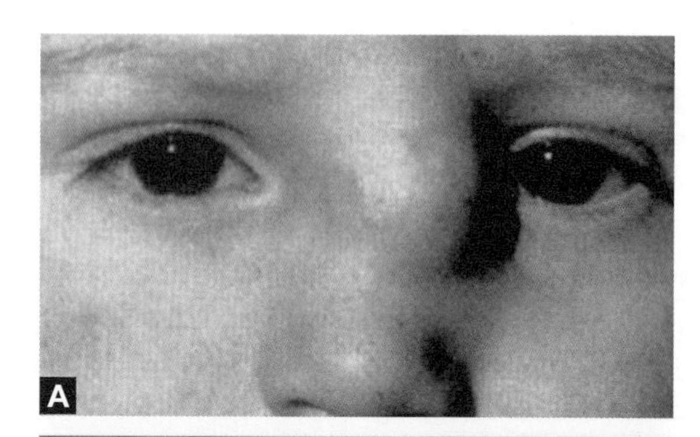

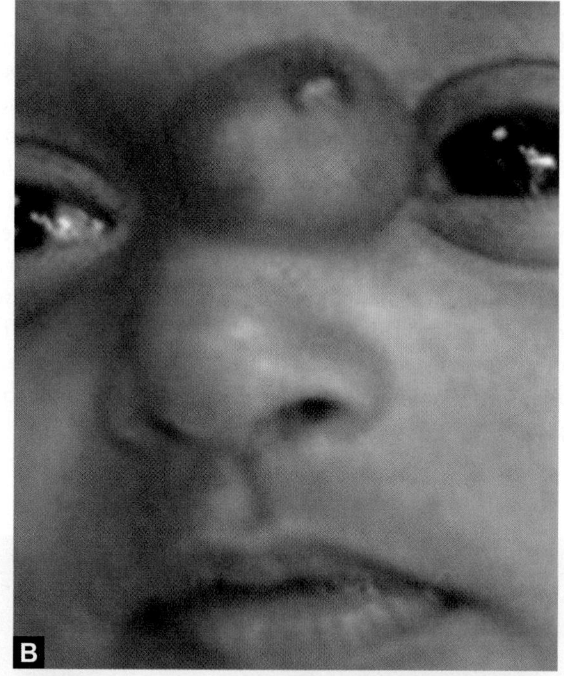

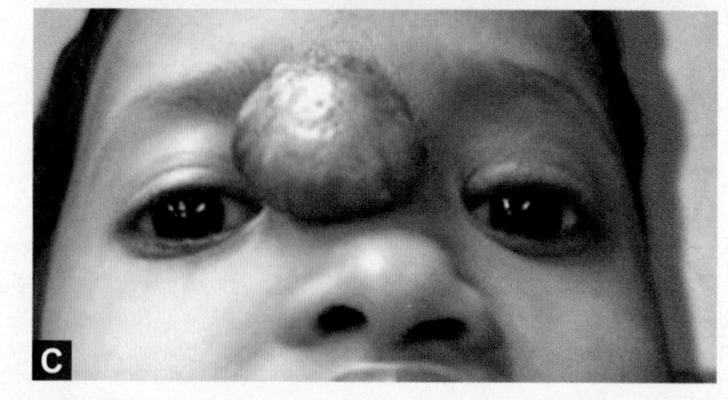

Figs 28.5A to C: Dermoid cyst and sinus. Congenital dermoid cysts of the nose result from persistence of remnants of ectoderm of dural origin in the prenasal space

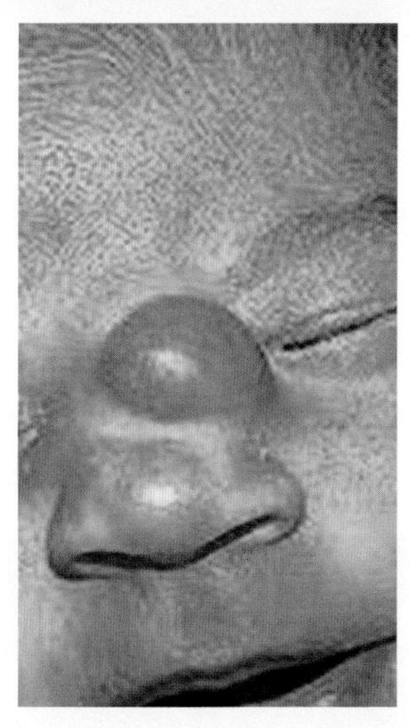

Fig. 28.6: Extranasal glioma

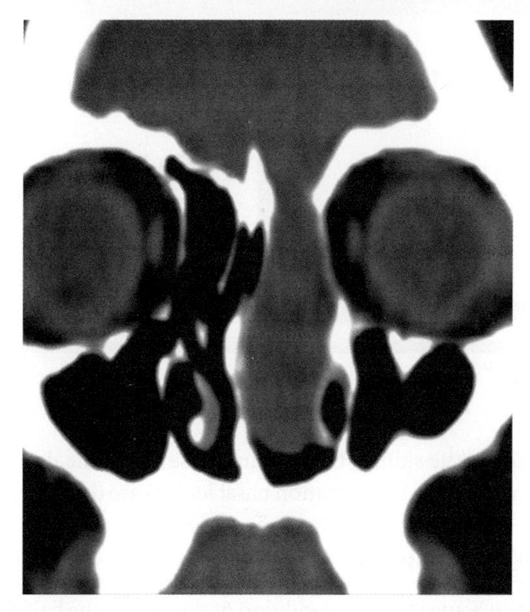

Fig. 28.7: CT image of left ethmoidal meningoencephalocele

Nasal Glioma

Nasal glioma (**Fig. 28.6**) is a congenital condition unlike the intracranial gliomas. It presents as a solid tumor which may produce a swelling on the bridge of nose (extranasal glioma) or may present as a nasal polyp (intranasal glioma). It does not contain any brain tissue but may be connected by a stalk to the meninges. It does not increase in size on coughing, i.e. the cough impulse is negative. Treatment is by excision.

Encephalocele

This is a rare congenital condition which can present as a herniation of meninges and brain tissue (**Fig. 28.7**) through a dehiscence in the frontal bone. The cough impulse is positive, i.e. the swelling increases on straining and coughing. Treatment lies in closing the bony defect. If the defect is larger, the patient should be referred to a neurosurgeon.

Chapter

29

Diseases of the External Nose

Diseases of the skin of the face and nose fall in the domain of a dermatologist. The common nasal lesions are described here.

Furunculosis of the Nose

This is an acute infective condition of the root of the hair follicle or sebaceous gland in the nasal vestibule, caused by *Staphylococcus aureus*. Trauma as in nose picking or pulling of hair are the usual predisposing factors.

The condition is very painful and these tissues are very tender. Clinically, there occurs localized redness with swelling of the nasal vestibule and adjacent columella (**Fig. 29.1**).

Furunculosis of the nose is a potentially dangerous condition as the infection can spread to adjacent tissues of face and upper lip causing cellulitis of the face (**Fig. 29.2**). The infective process can cause cavernous sinus thrombosis as the veins of the nose and face which have no valves communicate through the ophthalmic veins and pterygoid plexus with the cavernous sinus.

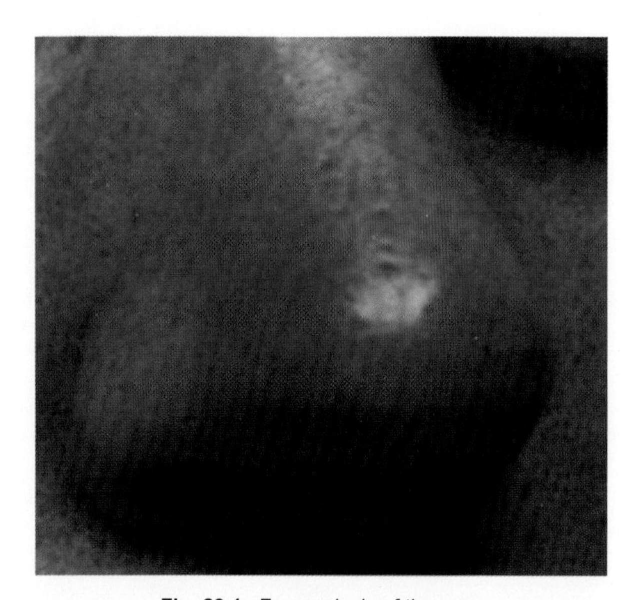

Fig. 29.1: Furunculosis of the nose

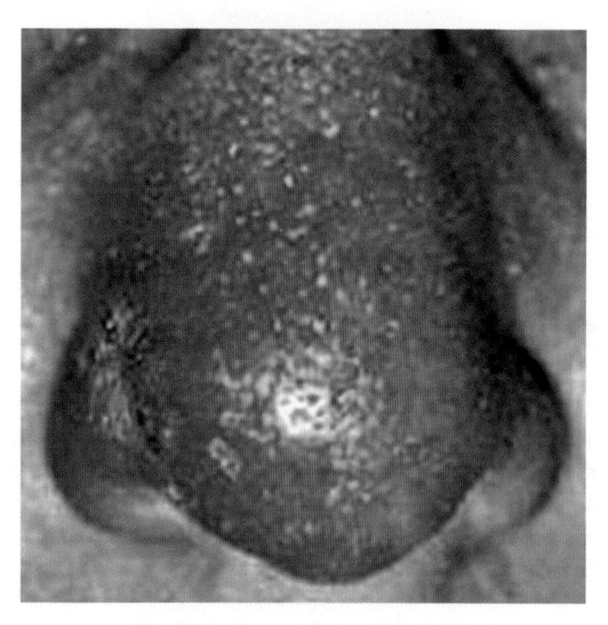

Fig. 29.2: Furunculosis with cellulitis

TREATMENT

Majority of the boils in the nose resolve spontaneously. Treatment involves application of local heat and antibiotic ointment, and analgesics to relieve the pain. Antibiotics like penicillin and cloxacillin may be needed in severe cases.

Squeezing or incising the furuncle should be avoided as this can lead to dissemination of the infection.

Recurrent boils in the nose occur either due to frequent trauma like in nose picking or suggest an underlying debilitating disease like diabetes.

Cavernous Sinus Thrombosis

This can result secondary to nasal infections especially nasal furuncles as veins of the nose are connected with the cavernous sinus through two routes, viz. (i) through facial veins communicating with ophthalmic veins (both having no valves), and (ii) through the pterygoid plexus of veins which communicate with facial veins on one hand and the cavernous sinus through emissary veins on the other hand. If a patient of nasal furunculosis complains of malaise, headache and pyrexia, cavernous sinus thrombosis should be suspected. Later, there is lid edema, chemosis of the conjunctivae and proptosis of the eye with restricted eye movements. Heavy doses of broad-spectrum antibiotics should be given after hospitalizing the patient.

Vestibulitis

Diffuse infection of the skin of the anterior nares may result from frequent trauma as in nosepicking. This produces traumatic ulceration and crusting, thus giving a foothold to the infection. Similarly, persistent nasal discharge leads to excoriation and infection of the skin of the nasal vestibule. Sometimes, the projecting end of a dislocated septal cartilage stretches the skin of the vestibule, which gets easily traumatized (**Fig. 29.3**).

TREATMENT

Local applications of neomycin or polymyxin-B with hydrocortisone ointments are advised. The underlying predisposing factor should be looked into and properly dealt with.

Erysipelas

This is an acute streptococcal inflammation of the skin and subcutaneous tissues of the nose. The skin becomes red, raised hot and surrounded by vesicles. It is associated with local pain, headache, fever and malaise. There are no intranasal symptoms and signs. Sinuses are normal on X-ray. Penicillin is treatment of choice.

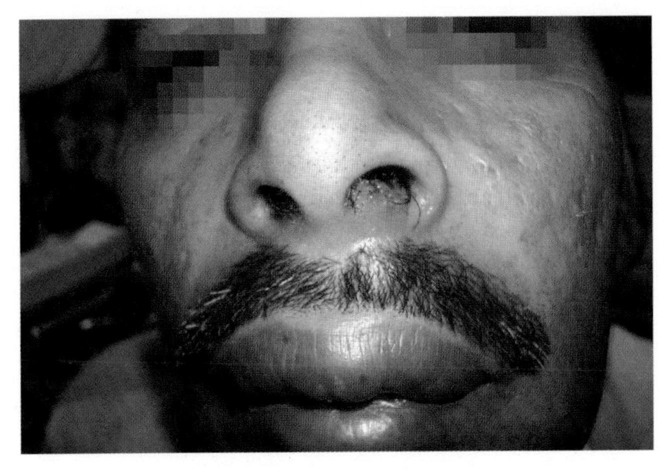

Fig. 29.3: Nasal vestibulitis

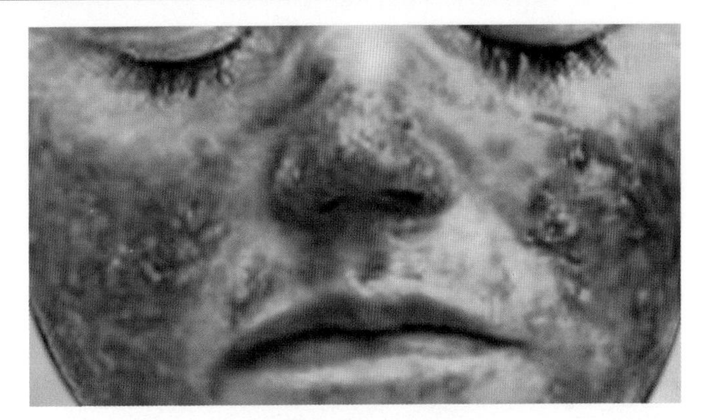

Fig. 29.4: Acne rosacea

Acne Rosacea

This condition, seen more commonly in women at menopause, is characterized by enlarged superficial blood vessels in the skin of the nose and cheek, giving the skin a dusky red and shining appearance. Secondary hypertrophy of the sebaceous glands may be superimposed (**Fig. 29.4**).

Lupus Erythematosus

This skin lesion affects the nose and cheeks in a butterfly distribution. It is characterized by patches of erythema and scaling followed by thin atrophic scars. The orifices of the sweat gland may get plugged by horny material. In five percent cases the condition may become systemic with malaise, arthritis and kidney lesions.

Herpes Simplex

This is an infection caused by the herpes simplex virus, which manifests as a vesicular eruption around the nasal vestibule and lips. The eruption usually occurs following an attack of cold or an acute debilitating illness. There is no specific treatment, however, local applications of acyclovir, neomycin or polymyxin with hydrocortisone are advised.

Herpes Zoster

It is characterized by vesicular eruptions along the cutaneous nerves which cause severe pain. The eruptions leave scars on the face on healing (**Fig. 29.5**). The condition is the result of reactivation of varicella zoster virus. The virus affects one or more branches of the trigeminal nerve unilaterally.

Rhinophyma

This condition is caused by hypertrophy of the sebaceous glands of the tip of the nose. The thickening of the skin produces a bulbous projection called potato nose or rhinophyma.

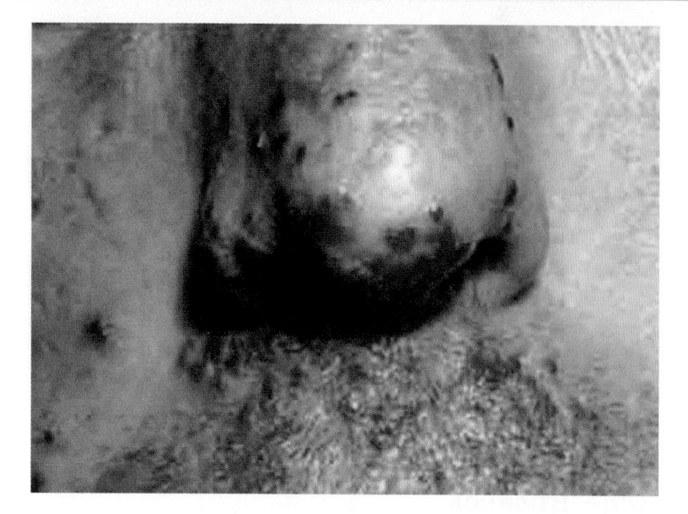

Fig. 29.5: Herpes zoster

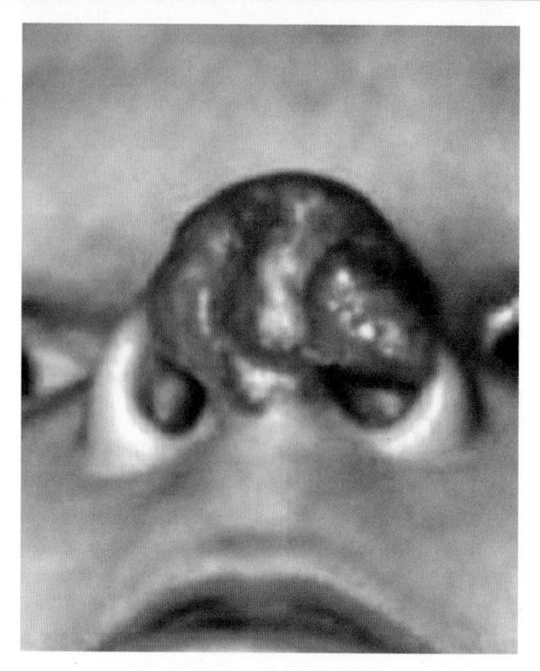

Fig. 29.6: Hemangioma destroying the nasal pyramid

Treatment is surgical excision by shaving down the excessive sebaceous tissue without traumatizing the underlying nasal cartilages. The remnants of the sebaceous glands help in reepithelization.

Neoplasms of the External Nose

Neoplasms of the external nose can be benign or malignant.

Benign tumors include papillomas that occur frequently in the nasal vestibule and require surgical excision, and *hemangiomas.* Capillary or cavernous type of hemangiomas may occur on the skin of the nose and cause cosmetic disfigurement (**Fig. 29.6**). These may need diathermy coagulation, injection of sclerotic fluids, surgical excision or cryosurgery.

Malignant tumors include basal and squamous cell carcinoma.

RODENT ULCER

Basal cell carcinomas occur commonly on the skin of the nose, usually over the alae nasi. The lesion presents as a raised pigmented nodule which ulcerates and refuses to heal (**Fig. 29.7**). The ulcer gradually burrows and causes destruction of the nasal cartilages and adjacent facial tissues and bones. Diagnosis is made by biopsy.

Treatment

Small lesions are excised with surrounding healthy area. A large defect may need skin grafting. Alternatively radiotherapy is given.

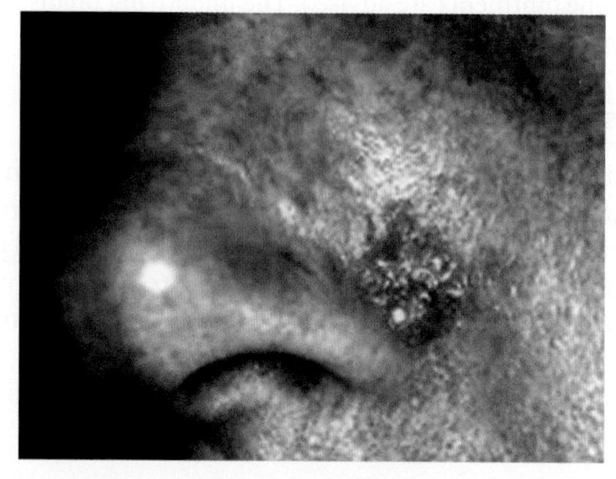

Fig. 29.7: Rodent ulcer

SQUAMOUS CELL CARCINOMA

This lesion may occur in the nasal vestibule or on the skin of the external nose. The condition presents as a progressive bleeding ulcer with raised margins. Biopsy is confirmatory.

Early cases are treated by radiotherapy and advanced ones with lymph node metastasis require surgery.

Chapter

30

Bony Injuries of the Face

Fracture of the Nasal Bones

This is a common traumatic injury. The fracture may give rise to swelling, displacement and deformity of the nasal bridge besides causing epistaxis and nasal obstruction. The degree of displacement depends upon the force and direction of blow. A lateral blow causes displacement of the nasal bridge to the opposite side. The fractured bone on the side of blow overrides the frontal process of maxilla, while it gets impacted under the frontal process of the maxilla of the opposite side. The septum may also get displaced (**Fig. 30.1**).

A frontal blow to the nose may lead to flattening and widening of the bridge which varies, depending upon the severity of trauma. In severe forms, fracture of the nasal bones may be associated with fracture of the frontal process of maxillae and of ethmoid and lacrimal bones producing a flat profile of face (dish face deformity).

X-rays are of help for medicolegal purposes and to note the degree of deformity and displacement.

TREATMENT

A fracture causing displacement, deformity or obstruction needs reduction. If the patient reports early before the onset of edema, the deformity can be corrected manually or under general anesthesia. The fractured fragments are disimpacted by Walsham's forceps on each side. Asch's septal forceps help to relocate the septum in the midline (**Fig. 30.2**). The fractured fragments are repositioned in proper alignment using forehead as a horizon. An external nasal splint or plaster of paris cast may be placed particularly in children to avoid displacement of the repositioned bones.

In frontal type of injury, which has caused flattening of the bridge line, the fractured bones are elevated and may require external support to remain in the midline. This may be done by passing wires through the nose which are then tied over lead plates on either side of the nose.

If the patient reports with swelling and ecchymosis, no intervention is made until the smelling subsides (7 to 14 days)

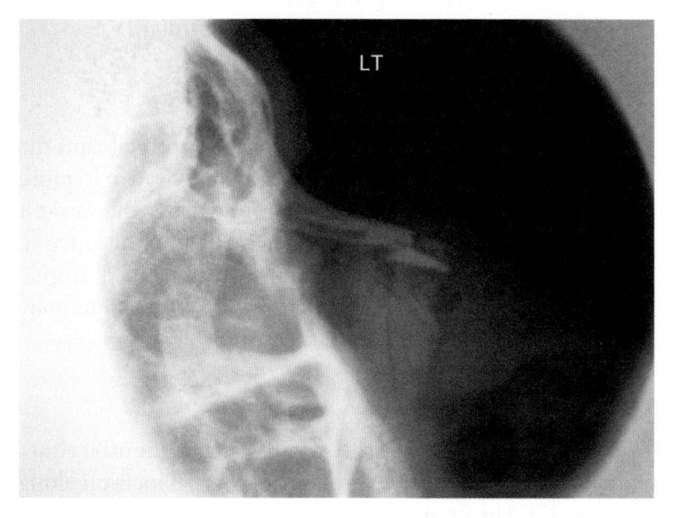

Fig. 30.1: Fracture of nasal bones

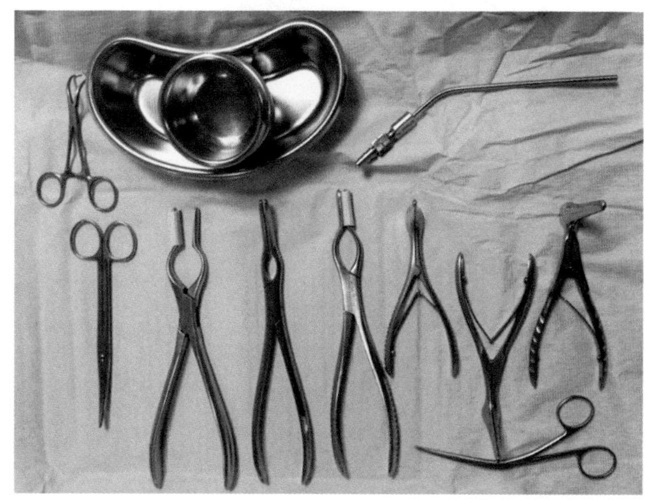

Fig. 30.2: Nasal fracture reduction set

when reduction under local or general anesthesia may be undertaken.

Fractures of the Maxilla

LeFort of Paris, in 1901 classified maxillary fractures into three types (**Figs 30.3A to C**).

LeFort I fracture (Guerin's fracture): It is a lower maxillary fracture where the fracture line passes through the alveolar process, palate and pterygoid process. It is a fracture of the tooth bearing segment of the maxilla.

LeFort II fracture: It involves both sides of the face. The fracture line passes through nasal bones, frontal process of maxilla, lacrimal bones, orbital plate, infraorbital margin, anterior wall of the maxilla and pterygoid processes in the middle also involving the posterior wall of antrum on each side.

LeFort III fracture: This injury causes a craniofacial dissociation and the fracture line separates the bones of the middle portion of the face from the cranium.

The fracture line passes through the zygomatic arches, zygomatic process of frontal bones, back of orbit, ethmoids, lacrimal bone, frontal process of maxillae and nasal bones. Posteriorly the fracture line passes through the pterygoid plates.

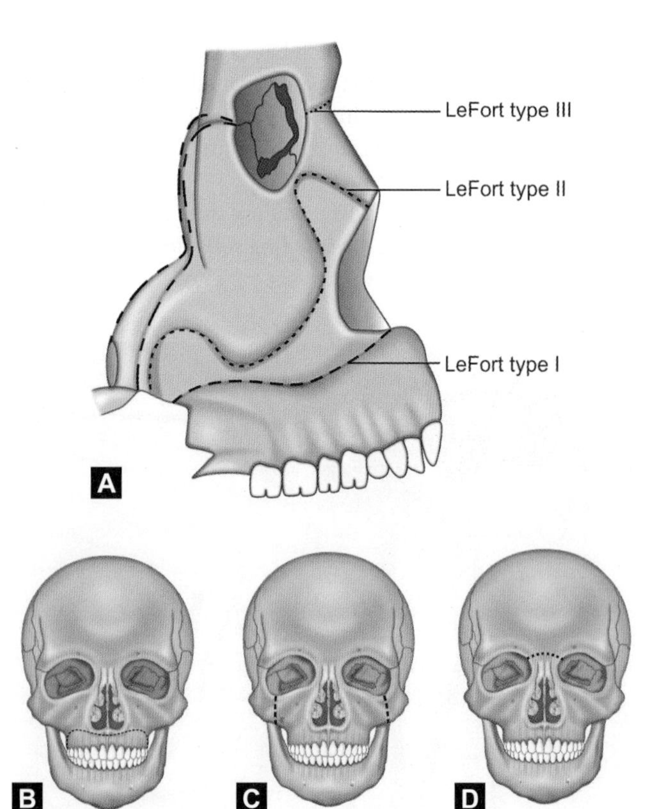

Figs 30.3A to D: (A) Maxillary fractures; (B) LeFort I fracture; (C) LeFort II fracture; (D) LeFort III fracture

In this way the maxilla, the nasomaxillary and malar-zygomatic complex on both sides are separated from the cranium. Depending upon the severity of trauma, the patient's complaints can be epistaxis, nasal obstruction, deformity of face, improper bite and diplopia.

Treatment of maxillary fractures depends upon the severity and degree of displacement. Immediate attention should be given to restore a proper airway and control the bleeding. The principles of treatment include proper reduction of displaced fragments maintaining the useful bite of teeth. The fragments are kept in position by interdental wiring, plaster of paris head cap or crossbars passed through the mandible or cranium till union occurs.

Fractures of the Malar-Zygomatic Complex

External trauma leading to fracture of the malar-zygomatic complex produces flattening of the malar prominence, swelling of the cheek, ecchymosis of lower eyelid, unilateral epistaxis and numbness over the infraorbital part of the face. Diplopia may be present. Fracture of the zygomatic arch may produce trismus. External deformity may be visible and the fracture line can be palpated.

X-ray examination of the paranasal sinuses (occipitomental and occipitofrontal views) is done to note the condition of antra and infraorbital margins. The submentovertical view projects the zygomatic arch. Fracture reduction is done through the antrum. The fractured portions are elevated and maintained over an antral pack, which is removed after 10 to 14 days.

The fractured segments may be elevated through the temporal route also when an elevator is passed deep to the temporalis fascia to the zygomatic arch. It is then elevated into position. Sometimes, an open reduction is done which is then maintained by passing a wire through the segments.

Blow-out Fracture of the Orbit

With the impact of a rounded object on the orbital rim, the contents of the orbit are pushed backwards and lead to fracture and collapse of the inferior wall of orbit which is the weakest area. The orbital contents may thus herniate into the antrum. The clinical features include enophthalmos and diplopia. Radiological investigation particularly scan and tomography are helpful in such fractures.

TREATMENT

The contents of the eyeball are replaced back into the orbit either by the transantral route or through an external incision along the lower lid. The floor can be supplemented by a polythene or silastic sheet or by using a septal cartilage graft.

Cerebrospinal Rhinorrhea

Trauma to the anterior base of the skull and dura may be associated with fracture of the nasal bones which leads to CSF leak from the nose. It is diagnosed by the characteristic feature that the fluid "does not stiffen the handkerchief (since the fluid does not contain any mucus or albumin)". The fluid tests positive for sugar as it reduces Fehling's solution. Although a CSF leak usually seals spontaneously, it may form a tract for recurrent meningitis. The leak can be closed by craniotomy and fascial graft insertion after localizing it with radioactive tracer or fluorescent testing. The patient is treated first conservatively and kept in the sitting position. He is advised not to blow the nose. No nasal packing should be done. Heavy doses of antibiotics should be given and the patient watched for 14 to 21 days.

Chapter 31

Foreign Bodies in the Nose

Foreign bodies in the nasal passages are not uncommon especially in children, mentally retarded adults. The most common route by which a foreign body enters the nose is the anterior nares. Sometimes contents from the mouth or stomach may enter the nasopharynx and nose during vomiting or coughing. Rarely a foreign body like gauze pack, injecting needle or a small instrument may be left in the nose during nasal surgery.

Inanimate Foreign Bodies

Inanimate foreign bodies found in the nose include glass beads, buttons, pieces of pencil, paper, peas and beans, metal, plastic pieces and button cells.

PATHOLOGY

A foreign body retained in the nose produces an inflammatory reaction and stagnation. This leads to the formation of granulation tissue and ulceration. Sometimes, a rhinolith may form. Sinusitis and soft-tissue infection of the nose and adjacent face may occur.

DIAGNOSIS

The history is suggestive but many a time children do not report after the mishap. In such cases, complaints of nasal obstruction and unilateral blood-stained, foul smelling discharge should make the clinician suspicious of a foreign body in the nose.

A foreign body may be visible on anterior rhinoscopy or may be obscured by mucopurulent discharge and granulations in long-standing cases. The foreign body is felt on probing. Radiological examination of the nasal cavities and nasopharynx is helpful in demonstrating a radiopaque foreign body (**Fig. 31.1**).

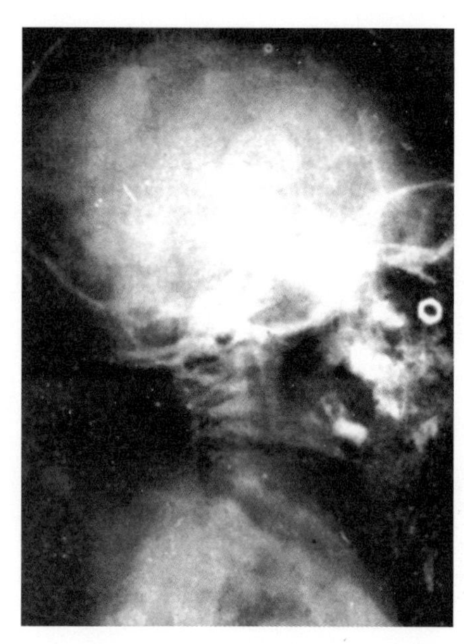

Fig. 31.1: A radiopaque foreign body in the nose of a child

MANAGEMENT

The patient is usually held in an upright position and the nasal fossae illuminated. A curved hook is passed beyond the foreign body which is then gently pulled forward. A eustachian catheter usually serves this purpose. When the patient is uncooperative and the foreign body is impacted or deeply seated, general anesthesia may be needed.

Animate Foreign Bodies

Animate foreign bodies include maggots, leeches and other insects. Leech can be removed by putting pinch of salt, or hypertonic saline or a few drops of oxalic acid on their body surface.

Maggots in the nose are asphyxiated with a ribbon gauze pack soaked in terpentine oil, kept in the nasal cavity for some time and then removed with a forceps as maggots crawl out for want of oxygen.

Rhinolith

Concretion formation in the nose results if a foreign body gets burried in granulations and remains neglected. This forms a nucleus around which a coating of calcium and magnesium phosphate and carbonate occurs and thus a rhinolith forms. Sometimes inspissated mucopus or a blood clot may be a nidus around which such a change takes place.

A rhinolith increases in size slowly and is symptomless at the onset. When large, it produces nasal obstruction. Examination shows a brown or grayish irregular mass near the floor of the nose. It feels stony hard and gritty on probing. X-ray shows a radiopaque shadow. It is surgically removed under general anesthesia. It may be necessary to break it in the nasal fossa and then remove it piecemeal. Sometimes, a large rhinolith may necessitate a lateral rhinotomy procedure for its removal.

Chapter

32

Epistaxis

Epistaxis (from Greek meaning a dripping) is blood flow from the nasal cavity, nasal sinuses or postnasal space. Epistaxis is a commonly occurring phenomenon. It is estimated that approximately 60 percent of the population at 1 time or another their lifetime will suffer from varying degrees of epistaxis. Fortunately, only 6 percent of these people will require medical treatment to control and stop the hemorrhage. Although epistaxis may occur at any age, bimodal incidence exists, with peaks in those aged 2 to 10 years and 50 to 80 years. It is relatively uncommon in children younger than 2 years.

Epistaxis is a common problem that ranges from a minor nuisance to a life-threatening emergency, especially in elderly patients and in those with underlying medical problems.

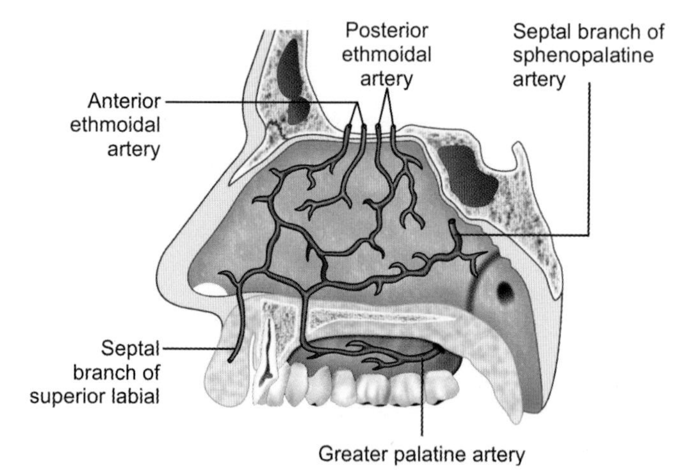

Fig. 32.1: Anastomosis at Little's area

Applied Anatomy

The blood supply of the nasal cavity comes from the internal and external carotid arteries **(Fig. 32.1)**.

- The internal carotid artery gives two branches:
  1. *Anterior ethmoidal artery (AEA):* It arises in the posterior orbit from the ophthalmic artery. It supplies the lateral wall of the nose, part of the nasal septum, and nasal tip.
  2. *Posterior ethmoidal artery (PEA):* It arises in the posterior orbit from the ophthalmic artery. It supplies the posterior wall of the nose, including the superior turbinate and the superior aspect of the septum.
- The external carotid artery gives three branches:
  1. *Sphenopalatine artery (SPA):* It is the largest and most significant. Arise from the internal maxillary artery (IMA), in the pterygomaxillary fossa exiting through the sphenopalatine foramen. It supplies the lateral wall and most of the septum.
  2. *Greater palatine artery:* Also from the internal maxillary artery. Supply the lower midseptum.
  3. *Superior labial artery:* A branch from facial artery. Supply the anterior tip of the septum.

The anteroinferior part of the septum is the most common site of bleeding in majority of the cases. This is a highly vascular area marking the anastomosis between the branches of various blood vessels supplying the nose. Branches from the anterior ethmoid, sphenopalatine, greater palatine and superior labial arteries take part in this anastomosis *(Kiesselbach's plexus)* **(Fig. 32.1)**.

There is a venous plexus near the posterior end of the inferior turbinate called *Woodruff's* area, which is another common site of bleeding in the nose.

ETIOLOGY

The main causes of epistaxis are grouped as under:

Local

- Idiopathic
- Trauma
  - Dry air (especially in winter months)
  - Foreign body
  - Patient induced (nose picking)

- Facial fracture, blunt trauma
- Sudden barometric pressure change
- Cocaine abuse.

- Inflammatory
  - Upper respiratory tract infection
  - Allergic rhinitis
  - atrophic rhinitis
  - Vestibulitis (furuncolosis)
  - Nonallergic rhinitis with eosinophilia
  - Granulomatous diseases such as sarcoidosis, Wegener granulomatosis, tuberculosis, syphilis, and rhinoscleroma.
- Neoplastic
  - *Benign:* Nasopharyngeal angiofibroma, pyogenic granuloma, polyps, papillomas.
  - *Malignant:* Rhabdomyosarcoma, lymphoma, nasopharyngeal carcinoma.
- Vascular
  - Internal carotid pseudoaneurysm
  - Hemangioma.
- Structural
  - Severe septal deviation.
- Congenital
  - Vascular anomalies
  - Telangiectasia (Osler-Weber-Rendu syndrome).
- Iatrogenic
  - Nasal O_2 cannulation, nasal steroid spray, Postsurgical adhesions.

Systemic Diseases

Hypertension

- Hematological
  - Platelet abnormalities;
    - Primary (idiopathic thrombocytopenic purpura).
    - Acquired (aspirin, NSAIDs, leukemia, and renal failure).
  - Coagulation defects;
    - Primary (von Willebrand, hemophilia).
    - Acquired (Warfarin, liver disease).
  - Thrombocytopenia, Vitamin C deficiency "scurvy", vitamin K deficiency and uremia.
- Inflammation
  - Rheumatic fever
  - Exanthematous fevers like measles, mumps, typhoid
  - Cirrhosis of the liver.
- Vascular
  Hereditary hemorrhagic telangiectasia (Osler-Rendu-Weber disease
  - Hormonal factors
    - Puberty
    - Pregnancy
    - Granuloma gravidarum
    - Vicarious menstruation.

Management

History of the presenting illness:

- A quick and concise history of present illness is essential. Ask specific questions about the severity, frequency, duration, and laterality of the nosebleed. Local trauma, and drug or alcohol abuse. Inquire about precipitating and aggravating factors and methods used to stop the bleeding.
- In most cases, anterior bleeding is clinically obvious. In contrast, posterior bleeding may be asymptomatic or may present insidiously as nausea, hematemesis, anemia, hemoptysis, or melena. Sometimes, larger vessels are involved in posterior epistaxis and can result in sudden, massive bleeding.

History to detect the underlying causes:

- History of URTI (e.g. rhinitis, sinusitis)
- Ask about symptoms that suggest nasopharyngeal tumor (e.g. angiofibroma, polyps, papillomas, rhabdomyosarcoma, granulomatous diseases).
  - *Nasal symptoms:* Nasal obstruction, discharge, rhinolalia clausa, hyposmia, snoring.
  - *Aural symptoms (due to ET dysfunction):* Otalgia, middle ear effusion, deafness.
- Suspect a foreign body when bleeding is minimal and accompanied by foul or purulent discharge.
- A history of recurrent nosebleeds (and how were treated), easy bruising, or other bleeding episodes give rise to suspicious regarding a systemic cause and prompt a hematologic workup.
- *Drug history:* Use of medications, especially aspirin, nonsteroidal anti-inflammatory drugs (NSAIDs), warfarin, heparin, ticlopidine, and dipyridamole should be documented, as these not only predispose to epistaxis but also make treatment more difficult.
- *Social history:* Smoking, cocaine and drinking habits.
- *Family history:* Obtain any family history of bleeding disorders or leukemia.

Examination

General assessment of the patient's condition is essential. The pulse and blood pressure are monitored and resuscitative measures like intravenous infusions or blood transfusion started if thought necessary. In majority of the cases of epistaxis, the bleeding is minor and stops spontaneously. When a patient is seen during a bleed, he is asked to clean the nose which is then pinched for about 10 minutes. This stops the bleeding by pressure. Once the bleeding is controlled, the nose is examined and the site located.

Treatment

Cauterization: The bleeding point can be cauterized by electric, chemical or thermal cautery. The area is anesthetized by local xylocaine pack and cauterization done. Chemicals used for cauterization include silver nitrate (freshly prepared solution, a bead or a crystal) or dilute solutions of carbolic acid and trichloroacetic acid.

Lubricating ointments and liquid paraffin help to prevent crusting.

Nasal packing: Every attempt should be made to control the bleeding without packing the nose, as this causes further trauma to the nasal mucosa, is troublesome for the patient, and delays recovery.

1. *Anterior nasal packing:* Anterior nasal packing is needed when bleeding is profuse and does not stop on pinching the nose. A lubricated or medicated gauze is used for this purpose although nowadays merocel packs are preferred. Packing should never be done with dry gauze. Nasal packing should be tight, starting from the floor upwards. The pack is usually removed after 24 to 48 hours. Subsequently after pack removal, the nose is again examined and bleeding points cauterized.
2. *Posterior nasal packing:* If bleeding is continuous in spite of proper anterior nasal packing, then posterior nasal pack may be necessary. This can be done under general or local anesthesia supplemented by sedation. Rubber catheters are passed from the nose to the oropharynx. The threads of the pack are attached to the ends of the catheters which are then withdrawn into the nasopharynx, pulling a gauze pack along with it. The pack is guided by fingers behind the soft palate. The threads on the rubber catheter are tied on a rubber piece at the columella. Tight anterior packing is done. A separate thread attached to the gauze pack is brought out through the mouth.

Adjuvant therapy: Bed rest and sedation are important. Antibiotics are prescribed if the nose is packed, as packing disturbs the nasal physiology and leads to stagnation of the secretions with resultant infection. Various hemostatic preparations like adenochrome, vitamin C and K, and calcium preparations play only an adjuvant role in stopping the bleeding.

Alternatively, nasal packing may be replaced by a specially devised (Brighton) balloon which has a fixed nasopharyngeal and sliding anterior nasal balloon. Pressure on the bleeding vessels is exerted by inflating the balloons.

Ligation of blood vessels: Rarely a situation may arise when bleeding does not stop by an efficient nasal packing. In such cases ligation of the blood vessels supplying the nose may be the only alternative.

The nose is mostly supplied by the external carotid artery through its sphenopalatine branches. Thus ligation of the external carotid artery in the neck or the internal maxillary artery in the sphenopalatine fossa arrests bleeding.

Sometimes, bleeding is high up in the nose from the area supplied by the anterior ethmoid artery. The ligation of ethmoid vessels is done through a periorbital incision in the medial canthus of the eye.

Besides these measures of controlling bleeding from the nose, attention should be paid to the underlying cause like hypertension, blood dyscrasia, local pathology in the nose and the treatment accordingly instituted.

Chapter 33

Diseases of the Nasal Septum

Deviated Nasal Septum

Deviations of the nasal septum are commonly found and often responsible for various anatomical, physiological and pathological changes in the nose (**Fig. 33.1**).

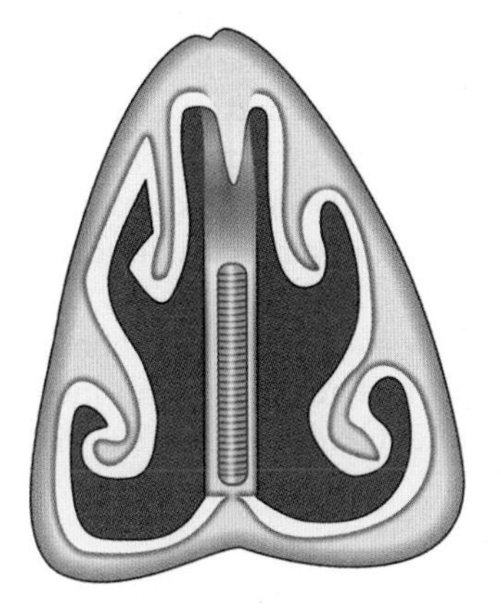

Normal septum

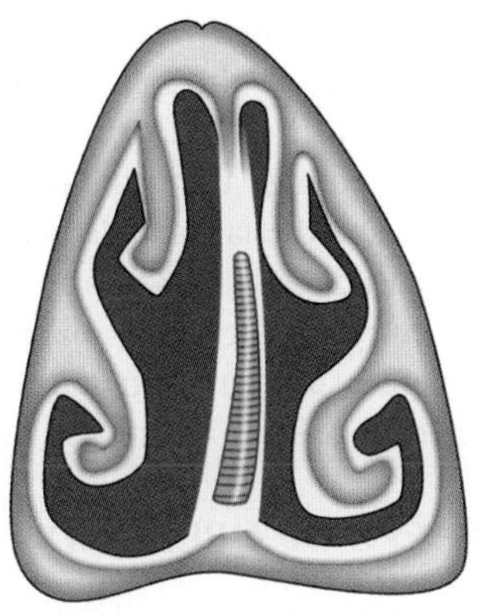

Unilateral cartilaginous deformity

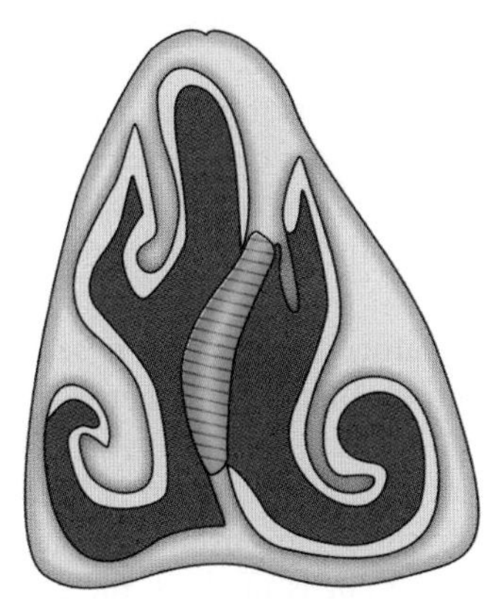

S-shaped deformity

Fig. 33.1: Nasal septum—normal and deformed

ETIOLOGICAL CONSIDERATIONS

Various theories and factors have been put forward to explain the septal deflections.

1. *Racial:* The deflections are more common in Europeans than in Asian or African races.
2. *Age:* Deflections are uncommon in children.
3. *Sex:* They are found more commonly in males.
4. *Hereditary:* Heredity may be a factor in its causation.
5. *High arched palate:* Lack of descent or broadening of the palate as occurs normally during infancy may be a factor. This might cause buckling of the developing septum.
6. *Trauma:* Trauma is the most important factor. Injury ruptures the chondro-osseous joint capsule of the septum and causes dislocations and fracture of the premaxillary wings.
7. *Birth moulding theory:* Prolonged and forceful stress during the birth process affects the nose and causes dislocations and deformations.

CLINICAL FEATURES

Many of us have varying degrees of septal deviations but only a few are symptomatic. The common symptoms produced are the following:

1. Nasal obstruction, which may be unilateral or bilateral and can be continuous or intermittent.
2. Dryness of the mouth and pharynx.
3. Recurrent attacks of cold.
4. Headache and facial pains.
5. Epistaxis.
6. *Cosmetic deformity:* The dislocated anterior end may project out into the nasal vestibule or cause deformity of the tip.
7. Anosmia may be a complaint of some patients.
8. Pain due to pressure on the anterior ethmoidal nerve.

An external nasal deformity affecting the cartilaginous part of the nose may be present. The anterior end of the cartilaginous septum may project into one of the nasal vestibules (called

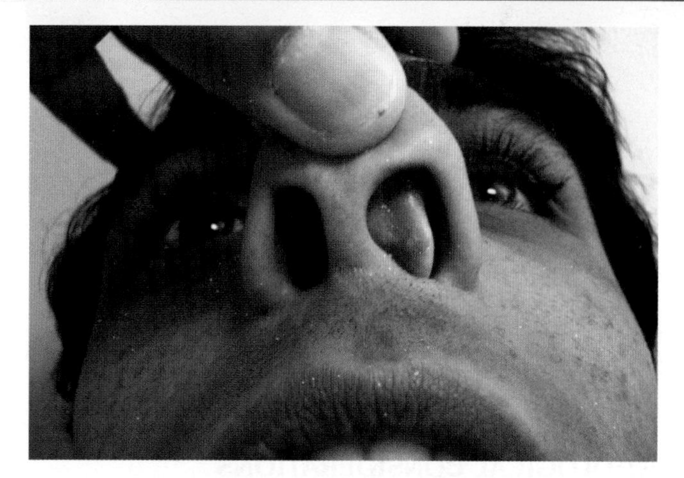

Fig. 33.2: Anterior septal deviation

dislocation of anterior end of the septum) (Fig. 33.2). Anterior rhinoscopy shows deflection of the cartilaginous or bony septum or combination of both.

The deflection may be confined to one (C-shaped deflection) or both the sides (S-shaped deflection).

A cartilaginous or a bony projection (septal spur) may protrude from the septum. Compensatory hypertrophy of the turbinates may be present.

PATHOPHYSIOLOGY OF SEPTAL DEVIATIONS

The deviated septum, depending on its location and degree, is the most common cause of nasal obstruction. Associated factors like infection and allergy perpetuate the effects. Nasal obstruction in turn leads to mouth breathing with consequent dryness of the mouth, pharynx and larynx. These predispose to recurrent attacks of sore throat, common cold, tonsillitis and bronchitis. Impairment of drainage of the sinuses may occur due to mechanical obstruction of septal deviations or by compensatory hypertrophy of turbinates. Headache and facial neuralgia might occur because of defective aeration and impingement of the septum over the turbinates. Nose bleeding may also occur. This occurs because of stretching the mucosal vessels complicated with dryness of the mucosa and associated nose picking.

Nasal obstruction is thought to produce pulmonary and cardiac effects too. Severe degrees of deflected septum may produce anosmia.

TREATMENT OF DEVIATED NASAL SEPTUM

Surgical correction is done to relieve the patient of symptoms. The conventional operation is called submucous resection (SMR) of the septum.

Submucous Resection of Septum

INDICATION

1. Deviated nasal septum producing symptoms like nasal obstruction.
2. When the deviated septum is a predisposing factor for sinusitis or recurrent colds, and if the obstruction is contributing to the poor development of the teeth and mouth.
3. Deviated septum causing epistaxis.
4. Deviated septum preventing access for removal of polypi or ethmoidectomy. SMR operation may be needed for complete removal of the polypi.
5. For taking septal cartilage for graft purposes.
6. To gain, access for other intranasal operations, for example, trans-sphenoidal hypophysectomy, vidian neurectomy.
7. To reduce the roominess in unilateral atrophic rhinitis.

The operation can be performed under local or general anesthesia.

After xylocaine sensitivity is ruled out, the patient's nose is sprayed with 4 percent topical xylocaine. A ribbon gauze pack soaked in xylocaine is packed into the nose with an idea to anesthetize the sphenopalatine ganglion and its emerging nerves at the posterior end of the middle turbinate. The pack is carried high up in the nose to block the ethmoidal nerves. Local anesthesia is supplemented by an intramuscular injection of pethidine and diazepam.

Surgery starts half an hour later after local infiltration of 2 percent xylocaine and adrenaline that helps further to anesthetize the septum and also to reduce bleeding during surgery.

STEPS OF OPERATION

1. A curved incision is made at the mucocutaneous junction, usually on the convex side of the deflection.
2. With an elevator the mucoperichondrial flap is elevated and the cartilage exposed.
3. Using a knife an incision is made in the cartilage anteriorly leaving a strip for columellar support. The incision is made to the subperichondrial space of the other side without cutting the mucoperichondrium of the other side.
4. With an elevator, the cartilage is separated from the mucoperichondrium of the other side without tearing the flap.
5. A long bladed nasal speculum is used to retract two mucoperichondrial flaps from the central cartilage.
6. With scissors, a cut is made in the cartilage along the dorsum, keeping a strut for dorsal support to prevent the fall of the bridge. Deflected cartilage is then removed with Ballenger's knife or Luc's forceps. The mucoperio-

steum may need elevation from the perpendicular plate of ethmoid, vomer and maxillary crest, if there is an associated bony deviation which is then removed.
7. Cartilaginous and bony spurs are removed.
8. The flaps are approximated and may be stitched.
9. The nose is packed using merocel pack to prevent mucosal trauma.
10. The patient is given antibiotics and analgesics. The pack is removed after 24 to 48 hours. Subsequently the nose is cleaned of the clots and discharge and ointment is applied. Liquid paraffin drops are used to lubricate the nose.

COMPLICATIONS

1. *Hemorrhage:* The bleeding may be *primary, reactionary* or *secondary. Secondary hemorrhage* may occur after 5 to 6 days and is due to infection. Septal hematoma or abscess may occur.
2. *Perforation:* Septal perforation may occur if tears in the mucoperichondrial flaps superimpose on each other.
3. *Flapping septum:* Excessive removal of the septal structure results in a weak septum which yields to inspiratory negative pressure in the nose. This causes flapping of the septum and may lead to nasal obstruction.
4. Depression of the cartilaginous dorsum may occur if an adequate strip of the cartilage is not kept superiorly.
5. Drooping of the tip and recession of the columella might occur if the anterior strip of the cartilage is not preserved.
6. Adhesions may develop between the septum and turbinates because of the trauma at the time of surgery.

DRAWBACKS OF SUBMUCOUS RESECTION OPERATION

Since the anterior and dorsal strips are preserved to maintain the normal contour of the nose, this operation, therefore, is not feasible for dislocations of the anterior end of the septum or for deviations involving dorsum of the septum.

This operation is not advocated for children up to the age of 18 years. The resection operation if performed in young age may interfere with the development of the facial bones.

Septoplasty

This is an advance over the conventional submucous resection operation. The principle of septoplasty is the correction of the deviated septum with minimal sacrifice of its structure. Septoplasty is indicated when the deviation lies anterior to a vertical line drawn from nasal process of the frontal bone to nasal spine of the maxilla. In children under 18 years of age, septoplasty is preferrable to SMR. The instruments used are shown in **Figure 33.3**.

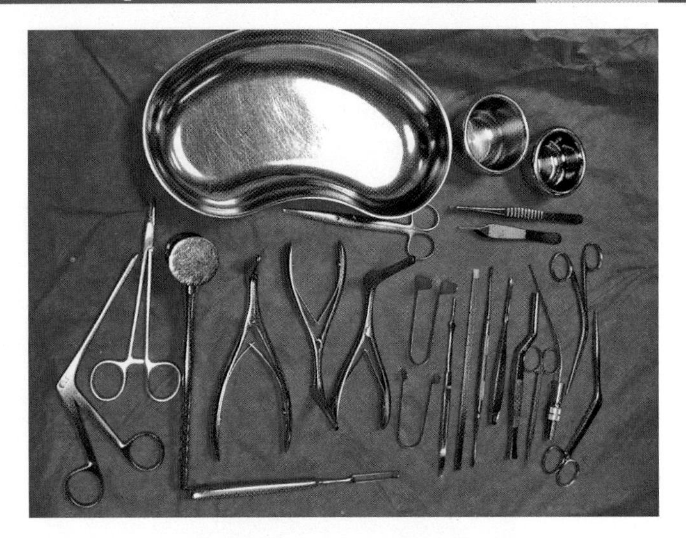

Fig. 33.3: Septoplasty-set

The main steps of operation are as follows (**Figs 33.4A to D**):

1. A unilateral (hemitransfixation) incision is made in the mucoperichondrial flap at the lower border of the septal cartilage on the left side for right-handed persons.
2. The mucoperichondrial flap is elevated on one side making an anterior tunnel. Another incision is made in the mucoperiosteum over the nasal spine on the same side, elevating the mucoperiosteum from the nasal spine on both sides thus making two more tunnels called inferior tunnels. The two tunnels are joined by sharp dissection.
3. The septal cartilage is then separated from the vomero-ethmoid bones posteriorly and the nasal spine inferiorly.
4. Minor deviations of the septal cartilage can be corrected by making criss-cross incisions through the whole thickness of the cartilage thus breaking its spring action. If this does not straighten the septum, a small strip of cartilage may be removed along the inferior border.
5. In case of superior deviation of the septal cartilage, it is to be separated from the alar cartilage through an intercartilaginous incision. This makes the septal cartilage free on all sides. This method of septoplasty is called Cottle's maxilla-premaxilla approach.

ADVANTAGES OF SEPTOPLASTY

1. Since the septal structure is preserved, this operation can be done in children.
2. There is minimal resection of the septum, and undesirable changes in the nasal contour, like columella recession, drooping of the nasal tip, depression of the bridge, widening of nostrils and broadening of the cartilaginous half of the nose are avoided.
3. Flapping of the septum and perforation do not usually occur.

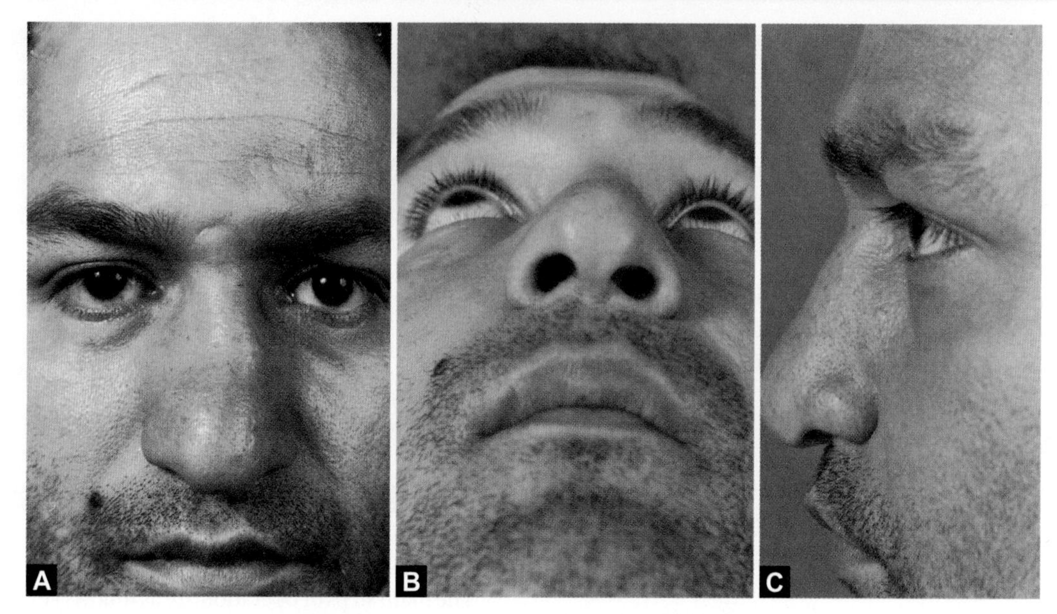

Figs 33.4A to C: Preoperative photographs for rhinoplasty

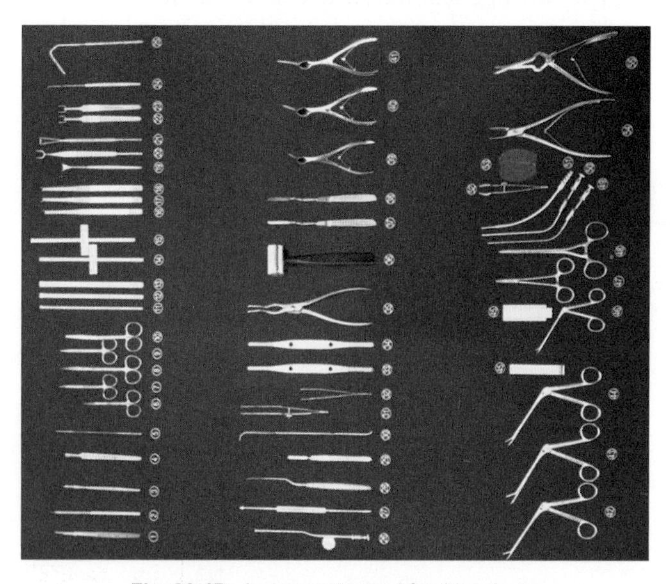
Fig. 33.4D: Instruments used for rhinoplasty

4. Revision surgery, if needed, is easy as compared to SMR operation.

Septorhinoplasty

This includes correction of the nasal pyramid in addition to septal correction. The various deformities of the nasal pyramid include depressed nasal bridge, wide nose, nasal humps, crooked nose (laterally deviated nose), bulbous tip and drooping tip, etc.

GENERAL PRINCIPLES OF SEPTORHINOPLASTY

1. *Assessment of the external nose:* The nasal pyramid should be assessed before taking the patient for surgery. Various nasal angles are measured deformity noted and the type of correction decided. Preoperative photographs are essential for this purpose.
2. *Septal correction:* This should be done in the first stage as a straight septum is a must on which external nasal pyramid can be reconstructed.

STEPS OF OPERATION FOR RHINOPLASTY

1. The procedure can be performed done under local or general anesthesia.
2. An intercartilaginous incision is made between the alar cartilages on the inner aspect.
3. The skin and soft tissues are elevated from the cartilaginous and bony framework of the nasal pyramid (deskeletonisation), using sharp dissectors and Knapp scissors.
4. The nasal hump should be removed *reduction rhinoplasty* before osteotomy is done. The excessive bone of hump is chiselled off.
5. The nasal bones are separated from the ascending process of maxilla (lateral osteotomy) on both sides and from each other (median osteotomy). The nasal bones then become free and can be kept in the desired position.
6. In case of the depressed nasal bridge (**Figs 33.5 and 33.6**), the nasal bridge is elevated by using either autograft or

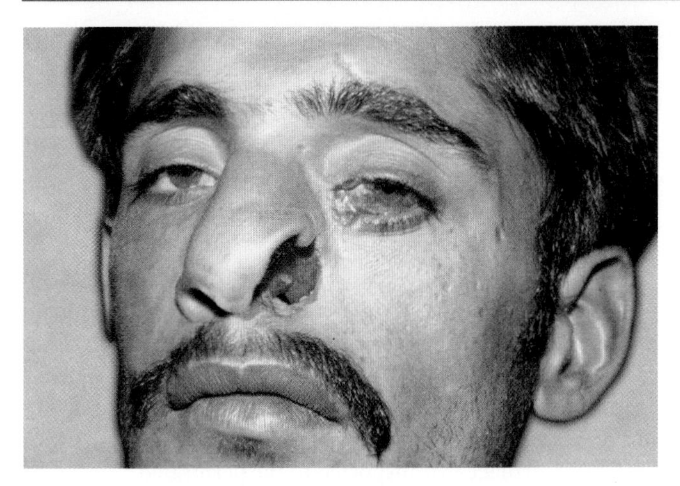

Fig. 33.5: Traumatic deformity of the nose

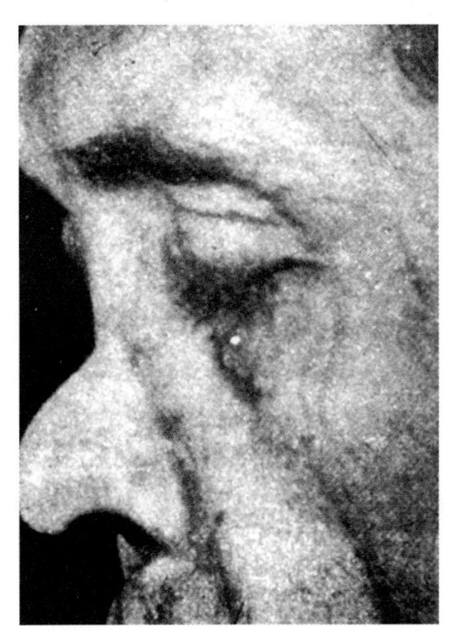

Fig. 33.6: Saddle nose

homograft bone or cartilage. Silastic sheets are also used. The procedure is known as augmentation rhinoplasty.

Septal Hematoma

Collection of blood in the subperichondrial plane of the septum may occur because of external trauma to the nose or after surgery for the deviated nasal septum.

The main symptoms of the patient are nasal obstruction and pain. On examination, a boggy swelling of the septum is seen blocking the nostril on one or both sides.

TREATMENT

Incision drainage is done under aseptic precautions. After drainage the nose is packed and a gauze wick kept in the incisions line to prevent reaccumulation of blood. Antibiotics are given to prevent infections.

Septal Abscess

This is usually a complication of septal hematoma. The patient presents with pain, fever and nasal obstruction. Septal swelling is seen on examination. The abscess is drained in the same way as the hematoma and the patient is put on heavy doses of antibiotics. Cartilage necrosis may occur with external deformity. Sometimes infection may lead to facial cellulitis or cavernous sinus thrombosis.

Perforation of the Nasal Septum

The septum being a midline structure divides the nose into two halves and thus helps in regulating the normal nasal cycle and physiology. Its perforation may, therefore, alter the physiology of the nose (**Figs 33.7 and 33.8**).

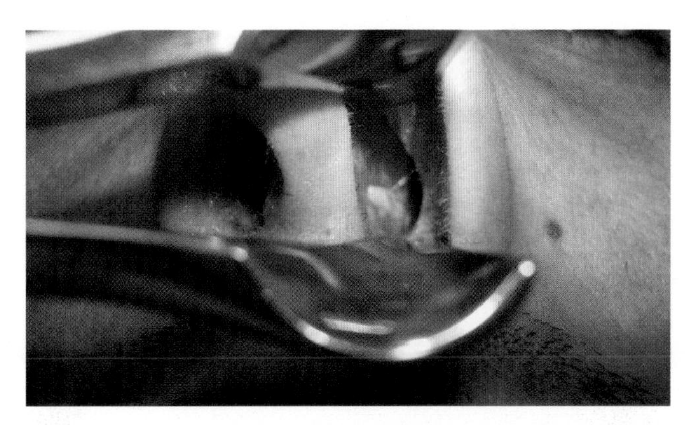

Fig. 33.7: Deviated nasal septum

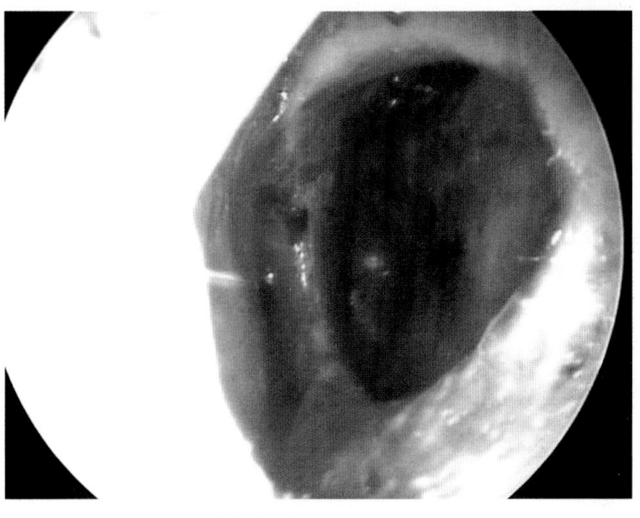

Fig. 33.8: Perforated nasal septum

ETIOLOGY

The causes of perforation are enumerated below:

1. Trauma:
   a. Surgical (during and after SMR) or accidental
   b. Constant habit of nose picking
   c. Tight nasal packing
   d. Repeated cauterization
   e. Hematoma and abscess formation due to necrosis of the septal cartilage.
2. Disease like tuberculosis, syphilis, midline granuloma, atrophic rhinitis, and lupus vulgaris.
3. Irritants like tobacco or cocaine snuff and fumes such as those of chromic acid and mercury.
4. Tumors of the septum, e.g. chondrosarcoma, granuloma.
5. Idiopathic.

CLINICAL FEATURES

The perforation may remain asymptomatic. Dryness and crusting of nose may occur and bleeding may be the presenting feature. Small perforations can give rise to a whistling sound on inspiration.

TREATMENT

Local application of ointments helps to prevent crusting. Sometimes surgical treatment is needed. The repair is difficult and is suitable for smaller perforations only.

Various surgical methods have been tried. Mucosal flaps can be rotated from the floor or lateral wall of the nose and from the undersurface of the upper lip and stitched to the margins of the perforation.

Grafts may be taken from the middle turbinate and skin of the nasal vestibule and stitched in position. A segment of the septal cartilage is transported to the perforated area by the hinge-graft technique and covered by skin graft on either side. Simple flat splints are kept in both the nostrils for 24 to 48 hours. The pericranium has also been used for the repair and synthetic material like silastic buttons have also been used to seal the perforation site.

Chapter 34

Acute Rhinitis

Acute inflammation of the nasal mucosa is called acute rhinitis. It is an exceedingly common infection prevalent in all ages, particularly in children.

Etiology

Acute rhinitis, primarily a viral infection, is followed by secondary infection with bacteria. Various types of viruses which may be responsible include influenza viruses, coxsackievirus, reovirus, Echovirus, and rhinovirus.

Pathology

In the initial stage, there occurs a transient vasoconstriction which is followed by vasodilation, edema and increased secretions that contain epithelial cells.

Initially the cultures are sterile but after a few days, secondary invading organisms like *Micrococcus catarrhalis,* streptococci, pneumococci, *Haemophilus influenzae* and staphylococci can be grown on culture.

CLINICAL FEATURES

At the onset of invasion, the patient feels an irritation in the nose with a burning sensation followed by sneezing, watery nasal discharge and obstruction. Fever, malaise and generalized aches and pains may be present.

Within a day or two, the nasal secretion becomes mucopurulent. Symptoms of toxemia are marked. Subsequently after 5 to 10 days resolution takes place and recovery sets in. The following complications may occur: (i) nasopharyngitis, (ii) pharyngitis, (iii) sinusitis, (iv) acute otitis media, (v) tonsillitis, (vi) laryngitis, (vii) laryngotracheobronchitis, (viii) bronchitis, and (ix) pneumonia.

TREATMENT

There is no specific treatment for the disease. Certain local and general measures can be taken up to relieve the symptoms. These include bed rest, analgesics and antipyretics for the fever and pain. Systemic and local decongestants reduce the nasal obstruction. Antihistaminic preparations help to reduce the irritation, sneezing and secretions. Steam or menthol vapor produce a soothing effect on the nasal mucosa.

Antibiotics do not influence the course of the disease but help in controlling secondary infection. Vitamin C supplements have proved effective.

Nasal Diphtheria

Corynebacterium diphtheriae may invade the nasal mucosa and produce a picture of acute or chronic rhinitis. The disease may be primary or secondary to faucial diphtheria. In the acute form of rhinitis, there occur general toxemia, fever, and catarrhal symptoms which subside within a few days. Complications are less common with nasal diphtheria. This is probably due to less absorption of toxins from a membrane on the columnar epithelium. The disease itself may pass unnoticed. Sometimes, the disease takes a chronic course when it manifests as fibrinous rhinitis. There occurs extensive necrosis of the epithelium with formation of a grayish-white membrane which is adherent to the underlying mucosa and bleeds on its removal.

The local symptoms include nasal obstruction and nasal discharge which may be blood-stained and mucopurulent. The anterior nares may show excoriation. This variety of infection takes a slow course. Treatment includes nasal cleaning, adequate doses of systemic antibiotics and antitoxin. The patient should be isolated.

Pneumococcal infection of the nasal mucosa may also produce an adherent membrane. The bacteriological examination helps to differentiate this condition.

Nonadherent superficial membrane formation may also occur because of staphylococcal and streptococcal infections, candidiasis and irritant fumes.

Other Causes of Rhinorrhea

The following are the lesions which cause nasal discharge.

1. Acute rhinitis
2. Chronic rhinitis
3. Vasomotor rhinitis
4. Allergic rhinitis
5. Rhinoscleroma (catarrhal stage)
6. Choanal atresia
7. Malignant granulomas
8. Acute sinusitis
9. Rhinitis medicamentosa
10. Chronic sinusitis
11. Foreign body
12. CSF rhinorrhea, trauma and tumors
13. Atrophic rhinitis
14. Syphilis, leprosy, tuberculosis and fungal infections
15. Tumors of the nose and paranasal sinuses
16. Furunculosis.

Chapter 35

Chronic Rhinitis

Chronic inflammation of the nasal mucosa may occur in various nonspecific and specific infections and are grouped as under:

1. *Nonspecific*
   a. Chronic hypertrophic rhinitis
   b. Atrophic rhinitis
   c. Rhinitis caseosa (nasal cholesteatoma)
   d. Rhinitis sicca
   e. Allergic rhinitis
   f. Vasomotor rhinitis
   g. Midline granuloma.
2. *Specific infections*
   a. Lupus vulgaris of nose
   b. Tuberculosis of nose
   c. Syphilitic rhinitis
   d. Leprosy of nose
   e. Rhinosporidiosis
   f. Rhinoscleroma.

Chronic Hypertrophic Rhinitis

Hypertrophic rhinitis may arise as a result of chronic infection in the nose or paranasal sinuses. The condition may also result from chronic nasal allergy.

The patient's main problem is a stuffy nose. He may also complain of anosmia.

Examination reveals hypertrophied and congested mucosa and enlarged turbinates. Local application of vasoconstrictors may not result in shrinkage of the mucosa denoting the presence of excessive fibrous tissue.

Treatment of this condition is not usually satisfactory. Conservative methods like systemic decongestants, antihistaminics may prove of some help. Surgical procedures required to relieve the nasal obstruction include partial turbinectomy, submucosal diathermy of enlarged turbinates or cryosurgery of the turbinates.

Rhinitis Caseosa (Nasal Cholesteatoma)

This is a rare chronic inflammation of the nose associated with formation of granulation tissue and a cheesy epithelial debris in the nose. The condition may result from chronic sinusitis, presence of a foreign body or disintegration of nasal polypi. There is an unpleasant smell.

The mucosa shows chronic inflammatory changes and examination of the debris shows keratinous material, cholesterol crystals and numerous organisms. Anterior rhinoscopy shows granulation tissue in the nose alongwith whitish debris. Treatment is to find and treat the underlying causative factors in the nose and cleaning the nose by removing the debris.

Atrophic Rhinitis (Ozena)

This is a chronic inflammatory condition of the nose characterized by atrophic changes of the mucosa of the nose and the turbinates. It is called ozena when associated with fetor.

There are two forms of the disease, primary atrophic rhinitis and secondary atrophic rhinitis.

PRIMARY ATROPHIC RHINITIS

The condition is common in young adolescent females of poor socioeconomic status. Various theories have been put forward to explain the causation.

1. *Infective theory:* Various organisms like *Coccobacillus foetidus ozaenae, Klebsiella ozaenae,* and diphtheroids have been isolated from the nose of such patients but it is thought that these are secondary invaders rather than the primary etiological agents.
2. *Endocrine theory:* The disease is common in females particularly at puberty. The higher incidence in females and improvement with estrogen therapy has given rise to speculations that endocrine imbalance has a part to play in its causation.
3. *Deficient diet theory:* According to this theory, deficiency of iron and fat soluble vitamins especially A and D, results in atrophic changes.
4. *Developmental factors:* Factors like wide breadth of the nasal cavities and small antra have been blamed for the atrophic changes that result in the nose.

SECONDARY ATROPHIC RHINITIS

The atrophic changes in the nose occur as a result of underlying nasal disease like chronic sinusitis, lupus, tuberculosis, syphilis, leprosy or as a result of extensive tissue destruction from surgery or accidents.

Pathology

As a result of chronic inflammatory changes, the ciliated columnar epithelium of the nasal cavity and turbinates atrophies and shows squamous metaplasia. Glands and goblet cells become fewer. The endarteritis of blood vessels causes diminished blood supply to the mucosa. There occurs submucous infiltration by round cells. The bone of the turbinates also show atrophic changes.

As a result of the loss of ciliated epithelium, thick viscid secretions of the nose get stagnated and result in secondary infection and crust formation. The fetor and loss of mucosal sensation attracts flies which lay eggs that hatch out into larvae and pupae called maggots.

Clinical Features

The main presenting features include dryness of nose, nasal obstruction, headache and sometimes epistaxis. Though the nasal cavities are widened, the patient has a feeling of nasal obstruction because of the crusts. Sometimes fetor is a very marked feature noted by the examiner of which the patient is unaware because of atrophic changes and anosmia.

Such patients present with a broadened nose and widened nostrils. The nasal cavities are filled up with crusts. The mucosa looks congested and atrophic, turbinates look atrophic and shrivelled up and the nasal cavities are more roomy. Sometimes even the nasopharynx may be visible on anterior rhinoscopy.

Investigations

Various radiological, hematological, and serological tests may be needed to rule out disease like tuberculosis, syphilis, lupus and leprosy.

Management

There is no definite treatment of the disease, however, the symptoms can be relieved to a great extent by various medical and surgical methods.

Conservative Treatment

Nasal hygiene is improved by alkaline douching of the nose. This removes the stagnant discharge and crusts. Gauze packs soaked in liquid paraffin may be kept in the nasal cavities to lubricate the nose and loosen crusts.

A solution of 25 percent anhydrous glucose in glycerine used locally in the nose, prevents the growth of saprophytic proteolytic organisms and helps to retain moisture in the mucosa. Local application of estrogen to the nasal mucosa may prove helpful. Weekly injection of placental extract (Placentrex) in the turbinates has shown beneficial results. Placental extracts act as local biogenic stimulants and helps in regeneration of the epithelium and glandular tissue. Iron and vitamins are also helpful.

Surgical methods: The aim of various surgical procedures (endonasal microplasty) is to narrow the internal dimensions of the nose. This has been achieved by submucosal implantations in the floor, septum and lateral wall of the nose, of various materials like autogenous bone graft pieces, cartilage pieces, dermofat grafts, silicon, paraffin paste, teflon in glycerine paste, porcelain pellets, etc.

Partial or complete closure of the nostrils (Young's operation) for a period of six months to a few years has been performed with better results. The closure is done by raising the skin flaps from inside the nasal vestibules and stitching them together. The closure gives rest to the nose and thus sets up conditions for epithelial regeneration.

Transplantation of the Stenson's duct into the maxillary sinus for the moisture of nasal mucosa, and stellate ganglion block to relieve autonomic dysfunction are the other procedures performed for this distressing malady.

Nasal submucosal implantation of pieces of placenta has lately been done with varying results.

Sequelae and Complications of Atrophic Rhinitis

1. Consequent to atrophy, septal perforations occur and deformity of the nose might occur.
2. Due to unhygienic conditions in the nose, maggot formation might occur causing extensive destruction of tissues.

RHINITIS SICCA

This is a mild form of atrophic rhinitis in which dryness of nasal mucosa and crusting occurs, particularly in the anterior portion. This condition is usually seen in people working in dusty surroundings.

Anthrax

It is an acute infectious disease caused by *Bacillus anthracis* and affects usually cattle, sheep, goats and horses. Human beings contract it by contact with animal hair, hides or waste. The disease may affect lungs (wool sorter diseases) or loose connective tissue giving rise to malignant edema, necrosis of mediastinal lymph nodes and pleural effusion, followed by respiratory distress, cyanosis, shock, coma and death.

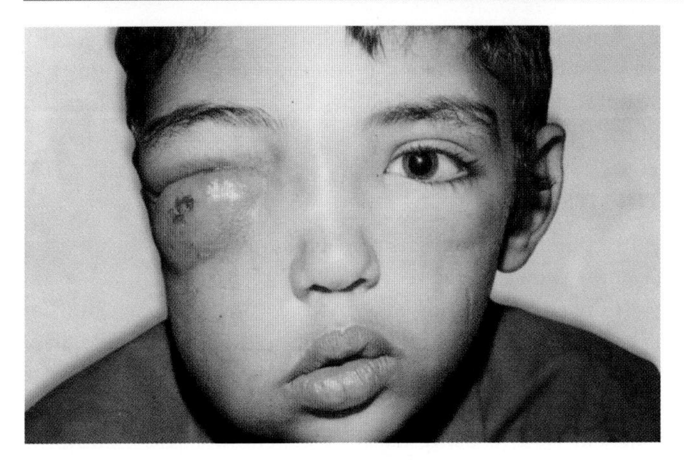

Fig. 35.1: Anthrax pustule

More commonly anthrax occurs in the form of a pustule called anthrax boil or malignant pustule (**Fig. 35.1**). This cutaneous form exhibits redness, induration, vesiculation with central ulceration and a black eschar. Rarely anthrax may occur in intestinal tract.

TREATMENT

Preventive measures are a must for inhalation. Anthrax, high doses of antibiotics, respiratory support and attention to vital signs is essential. For cutaneous anthrax, lesion is kept clean and covered with sterile dressings, frequent oral hygiene and skin care, plenty of fluid intake, and small nutritious meals. Isolation precautions are to be observed like use of mask, gown, hand washing and incineration of contaminated material.

Xeroderma Pigmentosa

It is a rare disease of skin starting in childhood and marked by disseminated pigment discolorations, cutaneous ulcers, muscular atrophy and death. There is roughness and dryness of skin with ichthyosis (**Fig. 35.2**).

GRANULOMATOUS LESIONS OF NOSE

Lupus Vulgaris of Nose

Lupus vulgaris is a chronic form of tuberculosis which affects the skin and mucosa. This condition is common in females particularly in early adult life. In the nose, it starts at the mucocutaneous junction of the septum. The typical early lesion is a reddish nodule which gradually ulcerates and the lesions spread over the floor of the nose, turbinates, skin of upper lip and the adjacent face. The ulceration may be followed by fibrosis and contraction of tissue with distortion of alae nasi (**Fig. 35.3**). The septum gets destroyed and perforation occurs in the cartilaginous septum. Pinkish, firm apple-jelly nodules, particularly prominent on applying pressure by a glass slide, appear on the skin and mucosa. These are the diagnostic features of lupus. Another characteristic feature of lupus is that areas of active ulcerations are associated with healing and scarring (**Fig. 35.4**). Histology shows features of tubercle formation. The symptoms are nasal discharge, obstruction with occasional epistaxis.

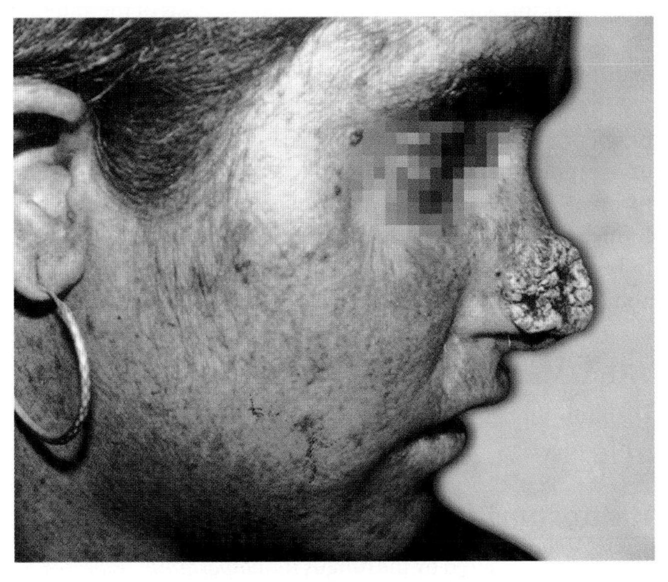

Fig. 35.2: Xeroderma pigmentosa

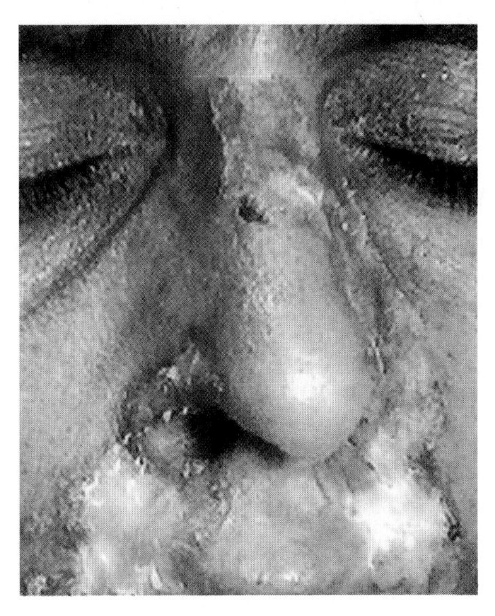

Fig. 35.3: Lupus of nose

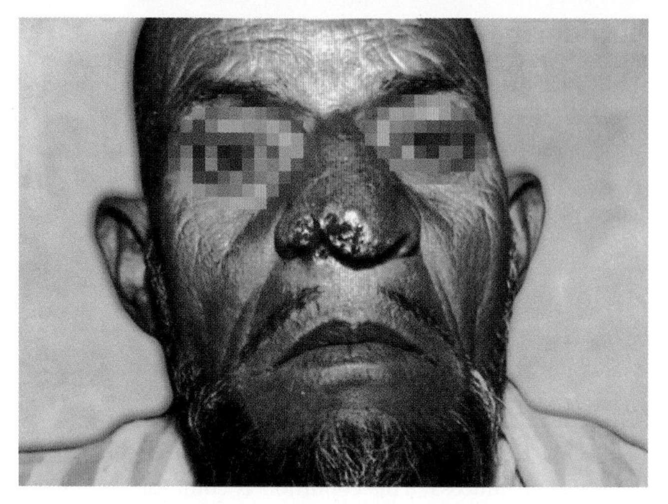

Fig. 35.4: Scarring of right nasal ala following lupus

The disease may spread to the pharynx and larynx. Pulmonary tuberculosis may develop in some cases. Destruction of the nasal mucosa and septum results in atrophic rhinitis.

TREATMENT

The disease is treated by antitubercular therapy.

Tuberculosis of the Nose

Tuberculosis of the nasal cavity occurs secondary to pulmonary tuberculosis. It may rarely be a primary infection. It affects the cartilaginous part of the nose. Symptoms include nasal discharge, pain in the nose, crusting and nasal obstruction.

Local examination reveals ulcerative or nodular type of granulomatous lesions in the nose. The cartilaginous septum shows perforation. Tuberculoma may occur on the nasal septum.

Biopsy confirms the tuberculosis pathology.

TREATMENT

Antitubercular treatment is given along with local douching and cleaning of the nose.

Syphilis of the Nose

The nose is commonly affected in the tertiary stage of syphilis. The lesion is a gumma. The bony portion of the nose is commonly involved. The main symptoms include offensive nasal discharge, nasal obstruction, pain and headache particularly during night.

Examination reveals a diffuse firm swelling of the bony septum which may show perforation. A gummatous ulcer may be visible. There occurs marked tenderness of the nasal bridge.

Serological tests for syphilis are usually positive and biopsy shows syphilitic histological appearance. Complications like atrophic rhinitis, collapse of the nasal framework, perforation of the palate and stenosis of the nasal passages may occur.

TREATMENT

Antisyphilitic treatment by systemic penicillin is given local cleaning done and sequestrated bone removed.

Congenital syphilis may manifest in the nose. Snuffles is the most common nasal manifestation in infants where catarrhal symptoms are followed by purulent discharge with excoriation and fissuring of the nasal vestibules and adjacent skin, causing nasal obstruction. These symptoms interfere with suckling and nutrition of the infant. In latent cases of congenital syphilis gummatous lesions appear in the nose at puberty. These lead to destruction of the mucosa and supportive framework of the nose with resultant sinking of the nasal bridge *(Saddle deformity)*. The other stigmata of congenital syphilis like Hutchinson's teeth, and interstitial keratitis may be present.

Leprosy

This type of chronic granulomatous lesion of the nose is caused by *Mycobacterium leprae.* Nasal lesions are commonly seen in lepromatous leprosy. The patient complains of nasal obstruction, crust formation and blood-stained discharge. On examination, a nodular thickening of the nasal mucosa, particularly at the anterior end of the inferior turbinate is seen. The nasal mucosa appears pale. The infective process may involve the septum and cause septal perforation. Changes of atrophic rhinitis may be evident. Fibrotic stenosis of the anterior nares and deformity occurs in the late stages. Other systemic features of the disease are visible.

Erosion or destruction of the anterior nasal spine is frequently seen on radiography. Smear of the nasal discharge or scrapings of nasal mucosa particularly from the inferior turbinate usually demonstrate acid-fast bacilli on microscopy. Biopsy shows a granulomatous lesion of the mucosa with infiltration of lymphocytes, mononuclear cells, macrophages and fibroblasts. Lepra bacilli may be seen in macrophages.

TREATMENT

Diamino diphenyl sulphone (Dapsone) is the standard drug for leprosy.

Rhinosporidiosis (Fig. 35.5)

The disease is caused by the fungus *Rhinosporidium seeberi* or *R. kinealyi*. The disease in India is usually limited to coastal states like Kerala, Tamil Nadu, Karnataka, Maharashtra and Orissa.

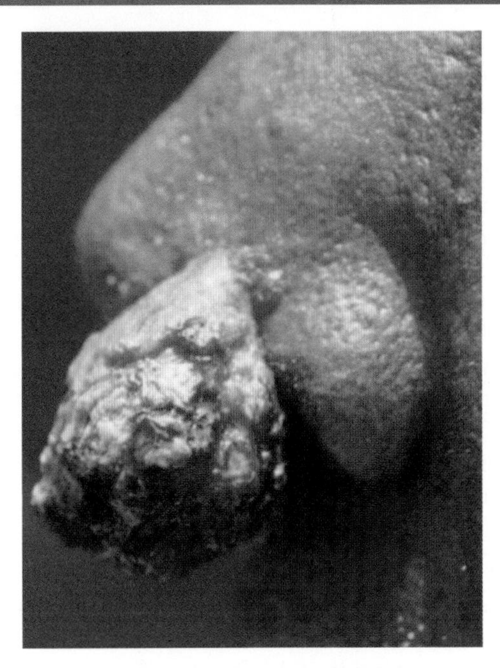

Fig. 35.5: Rhinosporidiosis

The disease is endemic in some parts of Africa and Sri Lanka as well. The mode of infection is thought to be dust from the dung of infected cattle. It principally affects the mucosa of the nose but the lesion can occur in other areas like the nasopharynx, pharynx, bronchi, skin, etc. The disease is clinically characterized by formation of bleeding papillomatous and polypoidal lesions arising from the septum or the nasal vestibule which have a strawberry appearance.

Histology shows vascular fibromyxomatous structure, in which are found large cells containing sporangia.

TREATMENT

These growths are removed by wide excision and cauterization of the base. Systemic therapy with amphotericin-B may be useful for patients with widespread lesions.

Other fungal infections like rhinophycomycosis, aspergillosis, blastomycosis, cryptococcosis, actinomycosis and candidiasis may be rarely encountered in the nose.

Rhinoscleroma

This is a progressive granulomatous disease of the respiratory tract caused by *Klebsiella rhinoscleromatis* (Frisch bacillus). The disease has a worldwide distribution and in India is usually seen in Madhya Pradesh, Mumbai, Delhi, Uttar Pradesh and Punjab. Central and eastern Europe and central and south America are other endemic areas of this disease. The disease starts in the nose and may spread to the nasopharynx, larynx, and bronchi. Histology of the lesion shows a picture of granuloma characterized by plasma cells, lymphocytes and eosinophils among which are scattered large foam cells *(Mikulicz cells)* with vacuolated cytoplasm, and mononuclear cells with nucleus *(Russell bodies)* having an eosinophilic cytoplasm and enveloping large quantities of Frisch organisms.

CLINICAL FEATURES

Four stages of disease may be clinically seen:

1. *Prodromal stage* or *catarrhal stage*: This stage passes with symptoms and signs of nasal catarrh.
2. *Atrophic stage:* Changes occur in the mucosa of the nose which resemble atrophic rhinitis. Anosmia is not a usual feature in such cases.
3. *Nodular stage:* Bluish red nodules appear at the mucocutaneous junction of the septum. These have initially a rubbery consistency but later on become pale and hard. A cartilaginous feel of the nose is typical.
4. *Stenotic or cicatrising stage:* As the disease progresses, adhesions develop and the nostrils get stenosed. Stenosis of the nasopharynx may also occur.

Diagnosis of the disease is by its typical lesions in the nose and its cartilaginous feel. Biopsy is confirmatory.

TREATMENT

Streptomycin is the drug of choice at present. It should be prescribed for a period of two to three months depending upon the response. Rifampicin, cotrimoxazole, tetracycline and ampicillin may prove helpful.

Surgery may be required to re-establish the airway.

Midline Nasal Granulomas

Two separate entities have been demonstrated within this group:

i. Stewart's granuloma
ii. Wegener's granuloma.

STEWART'S GRANULOMA (MALIGNANT NASAL LYMPHOMA)

A disease characterized by apparent chronic inflammatory granulation tissue in the nose with rather rapid destruction of the nose and midfacial region with little systemic disturbance and no evidence of pulmonary or nasal involvement is now considered to be malignant lymphoma (**Fig. 35.6**). Microscopy of the lesion shows necrosis with atypical cellular exudate (NACE) and is considered to be consistent with histiocytic lymphoma.

The disease is treated by full dose radiotherapy to the midfacial region and regional lymph nodes. Surgical debridement and reconstruction can be undertaken to minimize the deformity. Steroids and cytotoxic drugs have no role in the treatment.

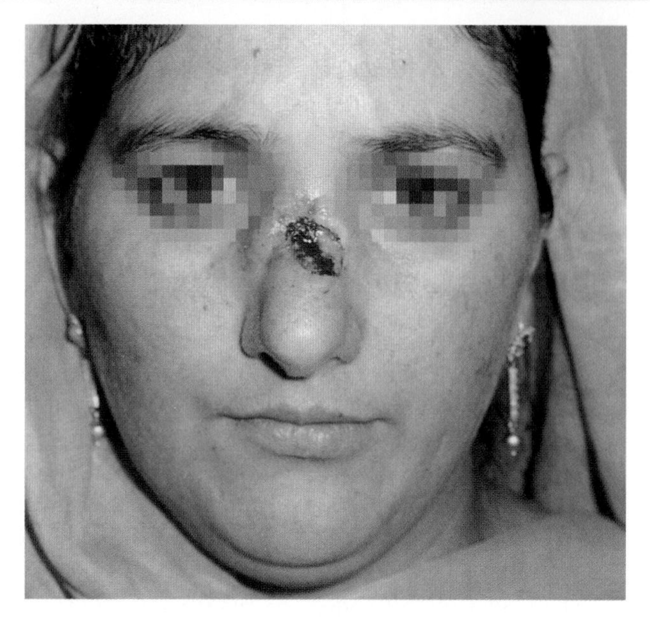

Fig. 35.6: Midline nasal granuloma

WEGENER'S GRANULOMA

The disease is of unknown etiology, however, it is currently thought to be an autoimmune disease. The mechanism is probably based on delayed hypersensitivity.

It is characterized by necrotizing granulomatous lesions of the upper respiratory tract. The lesions are smaller and have less tendency to involve the cartilage and bone in contrast to Stewart's type. Besides lesions in the upper respiratory tract, the Wegener's type is characterized by generalized vasculitis and focal glomerulitis.

The clinical picture is of insidious onset of nonspecific upper respiratory infection. The patient complains of fever, malaise and blood-stained nasal discharge. Granulomatous lesions may be seen in the nose.

Urine analysis shows red cells, casts and proteinuria. ESR is raised and serum proteins show increase in gamma globulins. Biopsy from the nose or even renal biopsy may be needed for confirming the diagnosis. Histological picture reveals giant cell granuloma and features of vasculitis.

TREATMENT

Previously this group of diseases had poor prognosis and patients died within a few months from kidney failure. Treatment by steroids and immunosuppressive drugs like azathioprine, cyclophosphomide (Fauci regime), has proved useful with better prognosis.

Local treatment consists of frequent nasal irrigations and glucose-in-glycerine drops for prevention of crusting. Associated sinus infection is also to be taken care of.

Chapter 36

Nasal Allergy, Vasomotor Rhinitis and Nasal Polyposis

Nasal Allergy

Nasal allergy occurs as a result of altered reactivity of the nasal mucosa to an antigen (allergen). It is a Ige mediated type I hypersensitivity response. It can occur due to a variety of substances and changes affect the mucosa of the nose, paranasal sinuses and sometimes the mucosa of the lower respiratory tract also. There are two types of nasal allergy, seasonal and perennial.

Seasonal nasal allergy (hay fever, pollinosis): Seasonal nasal allergy is due to inhalant allergens like pollens of flowers, trees, fungi grasses and weeds. Depending upon the climate and environment, the peak months of seasonal allergy vary from place to place.

Besides the nose, conjunctiva and bronchial mucosa may also be involved. The patient during an attack presents with intense irritation in the nose and eyes associated with sneezing, nasal obstruction, profuse discharge and excessive watering of the eyes.

On examination, the nasal mucosa appears swollen and pale or may have a bluish tinge. There is watery nasal discharge and diminished nasal airway. The conjunctiva may appear red and the patient may present with an attack of bronchospasm.

Perennial nasal allergy: This type of allergy can occur any time during the year and the symptomatology is similar but not so marked as in the seasonal type of allergic rhinitis. Perennial allergic rhinitis may be due to inhalant substances like house dust, smoke, spores, etc. or ingestants like milk, egg, fish and cheese. This type can also be due to certain drugs, bacteria and contactants like clothes and perfumes.

PATHOLOGY

When the allergen comes in contact with the sensitized mucosa, there occurs release of histamine and other kinins producing vasodilatation, increased capillary permeability and copious secretions from the mucosal glands. This results in congestion, edema and swelling of the mucosa. Cellular infiltration of the mucosa by eosinophils, plasma cells and lymphocytes takes place. Because of edema and blockage secondary bacterial infection may occur. Polyp formation in the nose and sinuses and frank sinusitis may occur as the disease progresses. Complications like serous otitis media, suppurative otitis media and bronchial asthma may occur.

INVESTIGATIONS

A detailed history is helpful in pinpointing the causative substance. Blood picture and nasal smears reveal increase in eosinophils. Skin tests with various allergens are carried out to identify the underlying causative agent. Sometimes provocative tests by the allergens are done to note the response.

There are certain diagnostic clues to allergy found in the children or young adults suffering from chronic allergic rhinitis which can often be recognized as such by keen clinicians:

i. The allergic shiners found as dark areas under the eyes as a result of discoloration in the lower orbitopalperbral grooves caused by venous stasis.

   An additional factor is spasm of Muller's muscle, a smooth muscle that is the only involuntary eyelid muscle. This muscle impedes venous return in the skin and subcutaneous alveolar tissues of the lower eyelids so that in addition to discoloration, edema occurs, resulting in 'bags' under the eyes.

ii. The transverse nasal crease is another visual sign. This appears in children as a horizontal hypopigmented or hyperpigmented groove across the lower third of the nose, where the bulbous, soft portion meets the more rigid nasal bridge. It results from constant rubbing of the itching obstructed nose and takes at least two years of develop. The allergic crease disappears when the tip of the nose is pulled downward. This fact differentiates it from the familial transverse nasal groove.

iii. *The allergic salute:* The often dripping nose is being wiped off by the children with hand. The thenar eminence is rubbed against the tip of the nose with rest of the hand stretched out as in salute.

iv. Long, thin, silky eye lashes are usually seen in young girls suffering from chronic allergic rhinitis.

TREATMENT

Treatment is based on avoidance of the allergen if possible, pharmacotherapy and immunotherapy. Pharmacotherapy includes the use of antihistaminic drugs alongwith nasal decongestants to improve the nasal airway.

Local application of drugs like silver nitrate 15 percent solution on anterior part of inferior turbinate on opposite area of septal mucosa for several days after application of local anesthesia (xylocaine 4%), and through steroid nasal sprays and injections of steroid preparation into the turbinates may reduce inflammation though the last mentioned treatment method has been reported to cause sudden blindness. Local spray of sodium cromoglycate preparations which prevent the release of histamine from the mast cells is useful in some patients.

If the allergen is identified, the subject should avoid contact with it. Ingestant allergens can be eliminated from the diet. Immunotherapy involves desensitization by increasing the doses of the allergen injected intradermally. This restores IgE serum levels and increases IgG antibody levels.

The superimposed bacterial infection is treated by antibiotics. Surgery is required to remove the nasal polypi to improve the airway and for drainage of sinuses.

Vasomotor Rhinitis

This is a noninfective condition which is due to vasomotor disturbances consequent to autonomic dysfunction. The nose is supplied by both parasympathetic and sympathetic fibers. Normally, an autonomic balance is maintained but sometimes alterations occur producing a clinical condition called vasomotor rhinitis. Various factors may play a part in its causation. Psychogenic instability and emotional conditions, hormonal changes as during pregnancy, menstruation and puberty, climatic conditions like extremes of temperature and humidity, and drugs like antihypertensive agents, local decongestants, and antidepressants are some such factors.

CLINICAL FEATURES

The disease is more common in females than males particularly during adolescent years of life.

The main symptoms are nasal obstruction and excessive nasal discharge. These symptoms may be associated with sneezing, headache, facial pains and generalized fatigue. The nose shows changes like marked hypertrophy of the turbinates, turgescent dusky red mucosa and watery discharge. Posterior rhinoscopy may show hypertrophied posterior ends of the inferior turbinates.

The history differentiates the condition from allergic rhinitis. The conjunctivae are not usually involved. X-ray and CT may show hypertrophied mucosa of the sinuses.

TREATMENT

Antihistaminics and nasal decongestants help in controlling symptoms in the majority of patients. Hypertrophied turbinates causing obstruction may require surgery. Submucosal diathermy, cryosurgery, somnoplasty or partial turbinectomy may be needed to relieve the obstruction.

Those cases where excessive nasal discharge is the main problem can be helped by performing vidian neurectomy. This nerve is exposed in the sphenopalatine fossa by removing the posterior wall of the maxillary sinus. The nerve is traced from the sphenopalatine ganglion to the opening of the pterygoid canal and is sectioned.

Nasal Polyposis

Polyp formation in nose is quite common. A polyp is pedunculated hypertrophied edematous mucosa (**Figs 36.1A and B**).

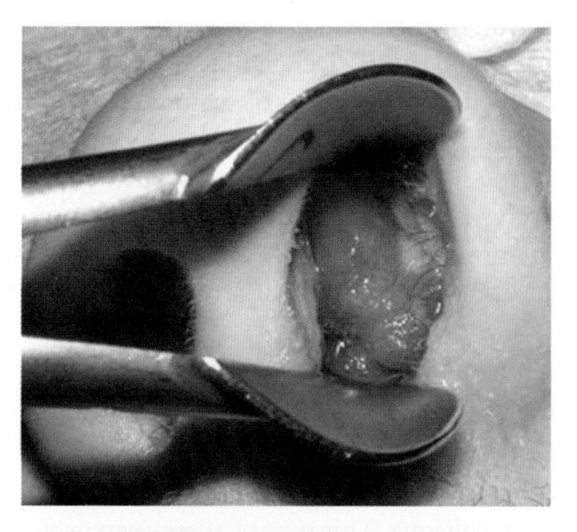

Fig. 36.1A: Antrochoanal polyp

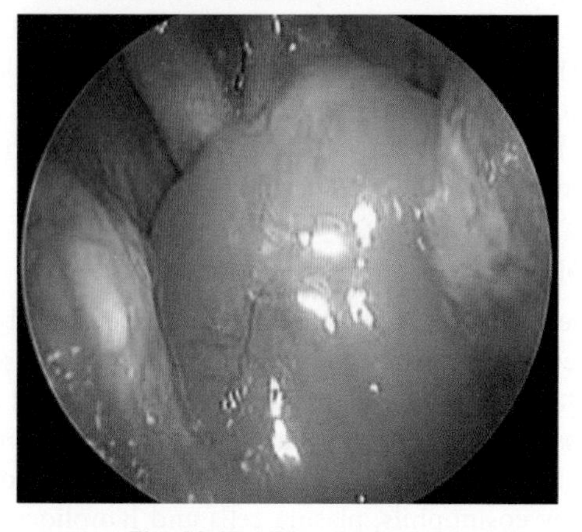

Fig. 36.1B: Ethmoidal polyp

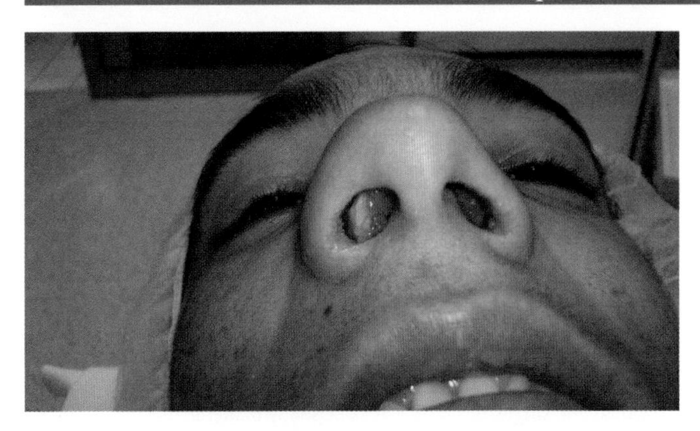

Fig. 36.2A: Bilateral ethmoidal polypi

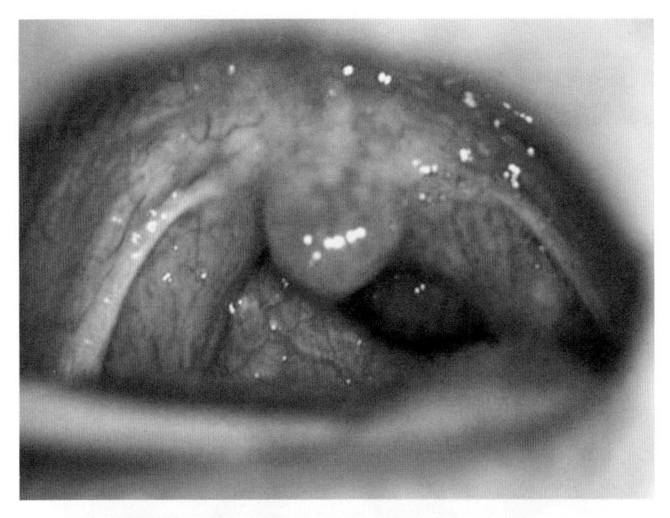

Fig. 36.2B: Antrochoanal polyp protruding into the oropharynx

Polypi commonly arise from the ethmoid labyrinth and sometimes may arise from the maxillary antrum. When this projects posteriorly in the nasopharynx, it is called an antrochoanal polyp.

ETIOLOGY

Etiology of polyposis is uncertain. Various views have been put forward to explain the causation.

1. *Bernoulli phenomenon:* Refers to a pressure drop next to a constriction which sucks the mucosa of the ethmoids into the nose with subsequent polyp formation.
2. *Polysaccharide changes:* It is postulated that alteration in the polysaccharides of the ground substance results in polyp formation.
3. *Vasomotor imbalance:* Polyposis may occur due to an imbalance between the sympathetic and the parasympathetic tone.
4. *Role of allergy:* Allergic reactions of the nasal mucosa produce vasodilatation and increased permeability of the vessels as a result of which fluid moves out of the intravascular compartment and causes water logging of the tissues. This edematous mucosa subsequently presents as a polypoidal mass.
5. *Infection:* It is also believed that longstanding infection gives rise to perilymphangitis and periphlebitis resulting in poor absorption of tissue fluid in the mucosa and thus this water-logged mucosa leads to polyp formation.
6. *Mixed etiology:* Allergy predisposes the tissues to infection and the allergy itself may be to bacterial proteins, hence it is contended that both allergy and infection are in etiological factors.

PATHOLOGY

Macroscopically, the polypi appear as pale, soft smooth masses. Sometimes these are opaque and fleshy. Histologically, the polypoidal tissue shows fibrillar stroma with wide spaces filled with intercellular fluid in the submucosa. The blood vessels and nerve fibers are scanty. Epithelium may be of the ciliated columnar type or may have undergone squamous metaplasia. IgA, IgG, eosinophilic and round cell infiltration of tissues is seen. There is an association between nasal polyposis, bronchial asthma and aspirin allergy and this is known as Samter's triad.

CLINICAL FEATURES

The main symptoms are nasal obstruction, hyposmia and postnasal drip. Associated with these are symptoms of rhinorrhea, sneezing and sometimes headache. Ethmoidal polypi are seen on anterior rhinoscopy as pale, smooth, soft masses. These are usually bilateral and multiple and are seen in all ages but are more commonly in adults. In children, these are invariably associated with cystic fibrosis.

The differences between the ethmoidal (**Fig. 36.2A**) and antrochoanal (**Fig. 36.2B**) polypi are summarized in a table form at the end of the chapter. Antrochoanal polyp arising from the antrum goes towards the posterior choana and is seen on posterior rhinoscopy as a pale, polypoidal mass in the nasopharynx. The soft palate is sometimes displaced downwards and the polyp may present in the oropharynx. Anterior rhinoscopy may not reveal any abnormality in the nose. This condition is mostly unilateral and the polyp is usually single. Antrochoanal polyps occur in the young, commonly during the second decade of life.

X-ray examination of the paranasal sinuses helps in diagnosis.

CT scan clinches the diagnosis and shows the exact extent of the polyp.

TREATMENT OF NASAL POLYP

A. *Medical treatment:* This involves the use of local and systemic corticosteroids, antihistamines, decongestants and/or antibiotics.

B. *Surgical treatment:*
   1. Functional endoscopic sinus surgery (FESS) is the surgical treatment of choice. In this procedure, all polypi are removed under endoscopic control especially from the key area of the osteomeatal complex. This procedure helps to preserve the normal function of the sinuses. FESS can be done under local analgesia although general anesthesia is preferred.
2. *Nasal polypectomy:* Ethmoidal polypi are removed under general or local anesthesia with the help of a nasal snare or a Luc's forceps. More than one sitting may be necessary for complete removal of the polypi.

Postoperatively, antihistaminics are given for a prolonged period and lavage of the antrum if needed may be done to clear the infection as recurrence is common. Recurrent ethmoidal polypi are dealt with by performing ethmoidectomy either via an endoscopic or an external approach.

The exenteration of the ethmoid air cells and diseased mucosa (ethmoidectomy) can be done either by the intranasal route, external approach or through the transantral approach. Ethmoidectomy should be done carefully to avoid damage to the orbital contents, optic nerve and cribriform plate.

Treatment of antrochoanal polyp: Polypectomy is done either using a long-bladed nasal speculum and visualizing the pedicle under endoscopic vision, which is then grasped and avulsed, or alternatively the soft palate is retracted and the polyp is grasped, avulsed and delivered orally.

In the postoperative period, antrum lavage may be necessary to clear the antrum of infected material. Recurrent antrochoanal polypi were treated by the Caldwell-Luc approach previously and that the diseased mucosa of the antrum was removed along with the polyp but this procedure is now largely out of favor.

Table 36.1: Difference between antrochoanal and ethmoidal polyps

Antrochoanal polypi	Ethmoidal polypi
Etiology	
Unknown	Bernoulli phenomenon,
Accessory ostium	polysaccharide changes, Vasomotor imbalance, allergy, infection, mixed
Age	
Children and adolescents	Adults
Origin	
Maxillary antrum	Ethmoids
Appearance	
Unilateral, single	Usually bilateral and multiple
Site	
Posteriorly (choana)	Anteriorly

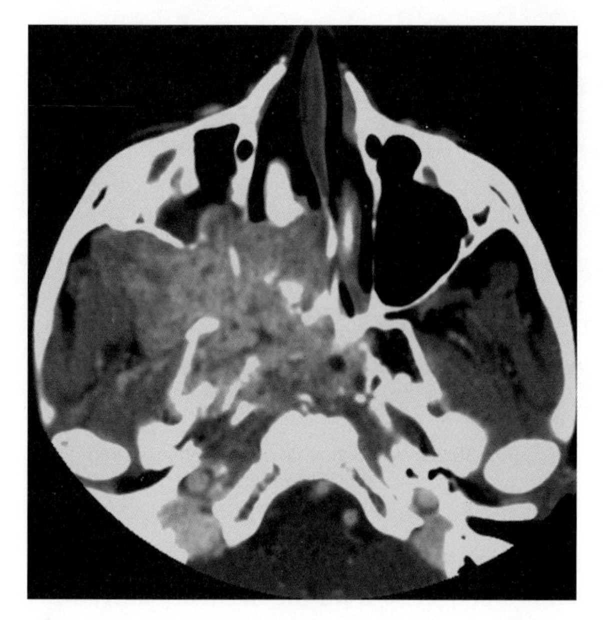

Fig. 36.3: CT image of nasopharyngeal angiofibroma expanding into the infratemporal fossa and extending intracranially

DIFFERENTIAL DIAGNOSIS OF NASAL POLYP

A variety of lesions may present as polypoidal masses in the nose. Ethmoidal and antrochoanal polyps have already been described in **Table 36.1**.

1. *Hypertrophied turbinate*: A hypertrophied turbinate may sometimes be mistaken for a polyp. The turbinate is pink in color, sensitive to touch as compared to an ethmoidal polyp and is firm to feel unlike the softness of a simple polyp. A probe cannot be passed around the turbinate as it is attached laterally and has no pedicle like an ethmoidal polyp.
2. *Rhinosporiodiosis*: This fungal infection of the nose produces a bleeding polypoidal mass in the nose usually arising from the septum and is strawberry like in appearance. It is common in people living in coastal areas of India. Histology is confirmatory.
3. *Angiofibroma of septum*: It presents as a bleeding polypoidal mass in the nose. A careful examination reveals its site of origin.
4. *Transitional cell or squamous papilloma*: Papilloma arising from the lateral wall in the region of the middle meatus may present as a polypoidal mass. This is usually single and has an opaque and fleshy look.
5. *Meningocele*: A prolongation of meninges may occur in the nasal cavity and appear as soft, cystic polyp-like swelling particularly in young children. Hence, it is always advisable

to aspirate a polypoidal swelling in a younger patient for cerebrospinal fluid.

6. *Malignancy of nose*: A malignant lesion in the nose (carcinomatous, sarcomatous or melanotic) may present as a polypoidal mass. However, it is usually friable and bleeds easily on touch. Sometimes polypoidal changes are associated features of malignancy. Therefore, all polyps removed from the nose should be examined histologically.
7. *Nasopharyngeal angiofibroma*: Nasopharyngeal angiofibroma **(Fig 36.3)**, particularly a less vascular variety, may be confused with an antrochoanal polyp. A history of epistaxis in an adolescent male with a lobulated mass in the nasopharynx indicates a nasopharyngeal lesion rather than antrochoanal polyp. Sometimes prominent vessels are visible on the tumor surface.
8. *Hamartoma*: Hamartoma means "fault" or "misfire" (Greek). It is a developmental malformation consisting of a tumor-like growth of tissue. It is a benign lesion but may become large enough to cause trouble according to size and location and but it rarely becomes malignant.

Chapter 37

Rhinosinusitis

Rhinosinusitis, the inflammation of the mucosal lining of the nose and paranasal sinuses, has replaced the previously used term sinusitis because the mucosal lining of the nose and paranasal sinuses is both continuous and contiguous hence inflammation of the nasal mucosa invariably involves the mucosa of the paranasal sinuses as well and vice versa. It is usually the maxillary sinus which gets involved, however, other sinuses can get involved as well; sometimes all the sinuses are involved, resulting in pansinusitis.

Traditionally classified as acute and chronic, rhinosinusitis is now classified as:

- *Acute:* Lasting up to 4 weeks, with total resolution of symptoms
- *Subacute:* Persisting more than 4 weeks, but less than 12 weeks, with total resolution of symptoms
- *Chronic:* Twelve weeks or more of signs/symptoms with or without acute exacerbation
- *Recurrent acute*: Four or more episodes per year, with resolution of symptoms between attacks.

Acute Rhinosinusitis

The acute inflammation of the sinus mucosa commonly follows an attack of acute rhinitis caused by viral infections as in common cold or influenza when the bacteria invade as secondary organisms, usually ten days or more after the onset of upper respiratory symptoms. Inflammation of the maxillary sinus may follow dental infections, particularly of the molar and premolar teeth. The sinus may get infected after trauma or through a blood-borne infection. Adenoids and infected tonsils may be predisposing factors responsible for the rhinosinusitis. Other contributory factors which play a role in the development of sinusitis include a deflected nasal septum, nasal polypi and other benign tumors of the nose. Patients of chronic suppurative lung disease constantly expectorate infected sputum that often leads to sinus infection.

The causative organisms for acute bacterial rhinosinusitis include *Pneumococcus, Haemophilus influenzae, Moraxella catarrhalis* and *Streptococcus pyogenes, Staphylococcus* and anaerobic bacteria have also been isolated.

CLINICAL FEATURES

Acute inflammation of the paranasal sinuses may produce various systemic effects like malaise, bodyache, fever and shivering. The local symptoms depend upon the sinus involved, the most important feature being pain. In maxillary sinusitis the pain is felt in the cheeks below the eyes, it may be referred to the teeth or along the distribution of the superior orbital nerve. Pain is aggravated on stooping or coughing.

In ethmoiditis, the pain is localized over the nasal bridge, inner canthus and behind the eye.

In frontal sinusitis the pain is localized over the forehead and the patient complains of headache. The pain is severe in the morning and gradually subsides towards noon as the infected material gets drained out from the sinus.

In sphenoidal sinusitis, the pain is usually referred to the vertex or occiput. Inflammation of more than one sinus is marked by pain over all the sinuses. Besides the pain, other symptoms of acute sinusitis include nasal blockage, and excessive mucopurulent nasal discharge.

SIGNS

Usually no external signs are present except in fulminating cases where, there may be redness and edema of the soft tissues of the face over the involved sinus (**Figs 37.1A and B**).

Tenderness on applying pressure over the sinus indicates underlying inflammation.

Anterior rhinoscopy reveals generalized congestion of the nasal mucosa, and localized edematous mucosa in the neighborhood of the ostium of the sinus. Presence of mucopus in the nose is suggestive of sinus infection and its position determines the sinus involved.

Posterior rhinoscopy also reveals the presence of mucopus and congestion. Fiberoptic examination of the nose using a fiberoptic nasolaryngoscope gives excellent visualization of the nasal cavity and the nasopharynx.

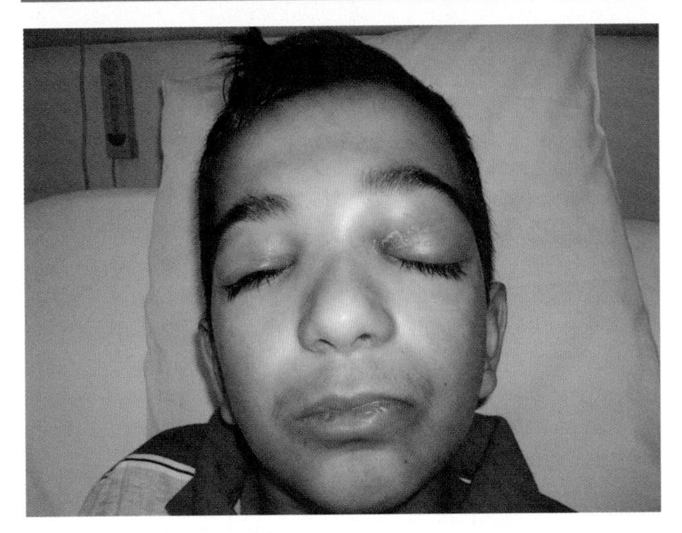

Fig. 37.1A: Acute frontal sinusitis causing cellulitis of the both eyelids

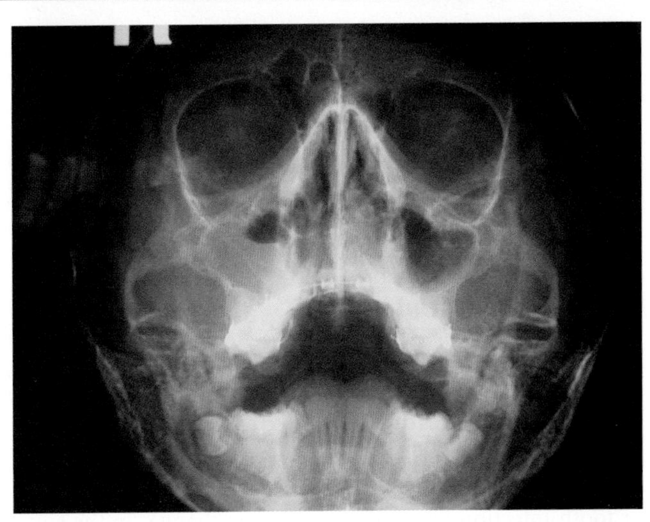

Fig. 37.2A: X-ray PNS (Water's view) showing haziness of the right maxillary sinus (maxillary sinusitis)

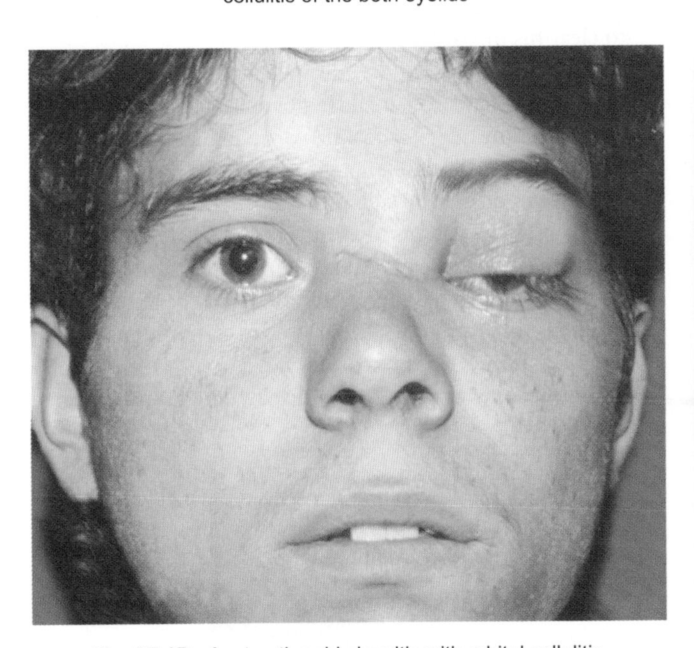

Fig. 37.1B: Acute ethmoid sinusitis with orbital cellulitis

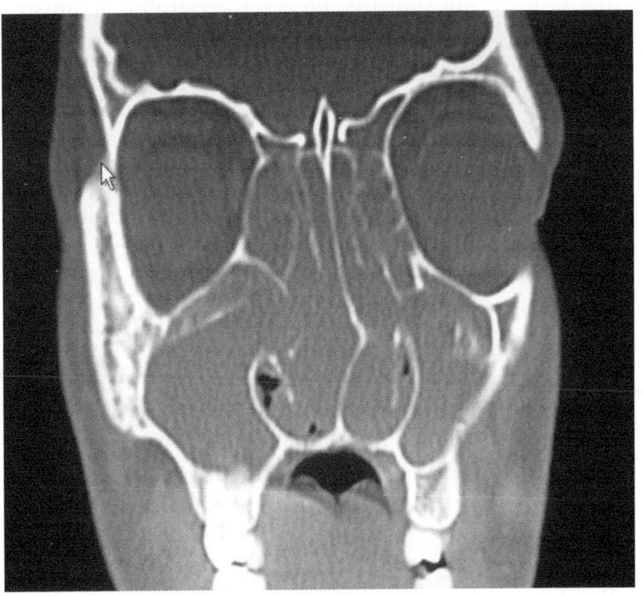

Fig. 37.2B: CT scans of mass: Sinuses showing allergic fungal sinusitis with extensive polyposis

INVESTIGATIONS

The X-ray examination of paranasal sinuses, occipitomental view (Water's view), is helpful in revealing the condition of the sinuses (**Figs 37.2A and B**). The sinuses appear as hazy and may show a fluid level. CT sinuses is diagnostic.

TREATMENT

Bed rest is important in the acute stages. Antibiotics are given to patients with moderate to severe symptoms and those whose symptoms are progressively worsening for more than 5 to 7 days of a common cold. High dose amoxycillin, or amoxycillin-clavulinic acid are the antibiotics of first choice, while cefuroxime and ceftriaxone are the second choice antibiotics used in acute bacterial rhinosinusitis. Nasal decongestants, help in relieving the nasal obstruction as well as reducing edema of the sinus opening and thus help in drainage of the sinus. Medicated steam inhalations through the nose are soothing. Analgesic and antipyretic drugs are prescribed to combat the pain and pyrexia. Surgery is avoided in acute sinusitis. However, if the symptoms do not subside, particularly in ethmoidal sinusitis with complications like unresolving orbital cellulitis/

abscess, then FESS (functional endoscopic sinus surgery) with drainage of the sinus and the abscess is performed. Previously, in patients having frontal sinusitis with cellulitis, the frontal sinus was drained through the floor of frontal sinus above the inner canthus. This procedure was known as *trephining of the frontal sinus,* however, nowadays the frontal sinus is drained endoscopically as part of the FESS procedure.

Chronic Rhinosinusitis

Chronic inflammation of the nasal and sinus mucosa is a common disease. The maxillary sinus is mostly involved; however, other sinuses can be involved as well. Chronic sinusitis is usually the result of incompletely resolved acute sinusitis. It may follow insidiously after repeated attacks of common cold or tooth infection which induce chronic changes in the sinus mucosa.

The bacteriological and etiological factors are usually the same as for acute sinusitis, however, anaerobic organisms predominate and *Pseudomonas* has also been implicated. Occasionally chronic sinusitis may even be fungal in origin.

PATHOPHYSIOLOGY

Allergy, infection, and chronic inflammation (aggravated by anatomical abnormalities) lead to mucosal congestion with subsequent obstruction of the sinus ostia in general and the key area of the osteomeatal complex (OMC) in particular. Obstruction of the sinus ostia results in anoxia within the sinuses resulting in mucosal hypoxia, edema and fluid leakage into the sinus cavity. The ensuing outflow obstruction leads to damage to the cilia resultanting in inadequate drainage of the sinus cavity leading to stasis, particularly of the maxillary sinus where the ostium is situated high up in the medial wall. Anoxia and stasis create excellent conditions for bacterial growth leading to reinfection. Periphlebitis and perilymphangitis may occur, leading to edema and polyp formation, the so-called *hypertrophic* or *polypoidal sinusitis.* Sometimes, there occurs metaplasia of the ciliated columnar epithelium to the stratified squamous type with intersperced papillary hyperplastic epithelial and inflammatory cells producing a picture of *papillary hypertrophic sinusitis.* Occasionally the chronic inflammatory process may induce atrophic changes in the sinus mucosa with increase in submucosal fibrous tissue (*atrophic sinusitis*).

CLINICAL FEATURES

The symptoms are variable and may be general or localized to the ear, nose and throat. The main symptoms are as follows:

- "Major" symptoms
  - Facial pain/pressure
  - Nasal obstruction
  - Hyposmia/anosmia
  - Purulence(discharge) on examination—nasal and/or postnasal
  - Fever
- "Minor" symptoms
  - Headache
  - Fatigue
  - Dental pain
  - Cough

1. *Nasal obstruction:* It may be the result of an underlying obstructive pathology of the nose like a deviated septum, polyposis or hypertrophied turbinates, or because of chronic turgescence of the nasal mucosa which results in a stuffy nose.
2. *Nasal discharge:* The patient frequently complains of excessive nasal discharge which could be mucoid, muco-purulent or purulent. Postnasal discharge is a common symptom which causes irritation and compels the patient to clear his throat frequently (**Fig. 37.3**).
3. *Abnormalities of smell:* The patient may complain of diminished acuity of smell (hyposmia). He may complain of unpleasant odor (cacosmia) or may have distortion of smell perception (parosmia).
4. *Facial pain or presssure:* It is the most common symptom with which the patient presents.
5. *Headache:* The cause of headache in sinusitis is not clear but the retained infected secretions are probably responsible.
6. *Epistaxis:* Inflammatory hyperemia in the nose may result in epistaxis but this is uncommon.
7. Symptoms like dryness of the throat, cough and repeated sore throat may occur.

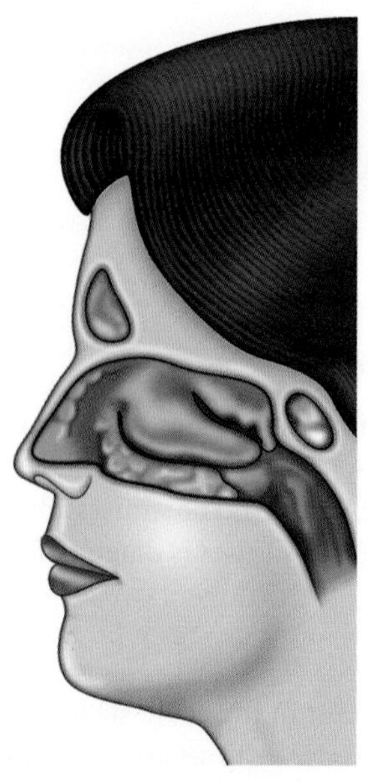

Fig. 37.3: Pus discharge from various paranasal sinuses

The general symptoms of chronic sinusitis include a sense of tiredness, low grade fever and a feeling of being unwell. Chronic sinusitis may produce effects on other systems like gastrointestinal upsets and chronic bronchitis, etc.

There may be excoriation of the skin of the nasal vestibule. Nasal mucosa appears red with turgescent mucosa. Crusting of the mucosa may be present. In maxillary sinusitis pus is seen in the middle meatus, particularly when the head is kept down with the infected sinus uppermost (**Fig. 37.3**).

In frontal sinusitis, the pus is usually seen in the middle meatus.

In sphenoidal sinusitis, pus may be visible in the olfactory cleft. Posterior rhinoscopy may show pus coming from the nose. If pus is seen trickling over the posterior end of the inferior turbinate, it indicates that the anterior group of sinuses is involved while pus above the middle turbinate indicates involvement of the posterior group of sinuses.

Tenderness of the sinuses may be present.

INVESTIGATION

Plain X-ray examination of the paranasal sinuses, though not specific, may reveal the condition of the sinuses which appear hazy and may show a fluid level or polypoidal changes. CT sinuses remains the radiographic investigation of choice.

Proof puncture: If pus can be obtained from the sinus cavity, it is a direct evidence of sinusitis. Besides, it can be cultured and its sensitivity tests done. The test used to be performed in the past particularly in chronic maxillary sinusitis.

TREATMENT OF CHRONIC SINUSITIS

The goal of treatment of chronic rhinosinusitis is three fold:

1. To control infection
2. To diminish tissue edema
3. To reverse sinus ostial obstruction, thereby aiding in the drainage of discharge from the sinus cavities, thus making the circumstances favorable for the recovery of the sinus mucosa. However, if the sinus mucosa is damaged beyond recovery, then radical surgery is undertaken and the diseased mucosa removed.

Medical therapy: Antibiotics, generally broad-spectrum ones like amoxicillin-clavilanic acid or respiratory quinolones like levofloxacin/moxifloxacin with either metronidazole or clindamycin to cover anaerobes, are given preferably after the culture sensitivity test for at least 3 weeks (4–6 weeks). Local and systemic decongestants, and analgesics help to relieve the symptoms. Topical steroid nasal sprays by virtue of reducing edema and inflammation constitute an essential part of the treatment. Antihistamines and antileukotrienes may also be prescribed.

Previously, surgical procedures like antrum washout for maxillary sinusitis to clear the sinus cavity off the discharge were performed. However, nowadays FESS is the preferred surgical treatment modality.

Antrum puncture: The procedure is mentioned here only for the sake of knowledge. Under local anesthesia, the trocar and cannula are placed under the inferior turbinate about half inch from the anterior end of the turbinate. The trocar is directed towards the outer canthus of eye of the same side. With firm and steady pressure, the nasoantral wall is pierced and antral cavity entered. The trocar is withdrawn and cannula placed properly in the sinus cavity (**Figs 37.4 and 37.5**).

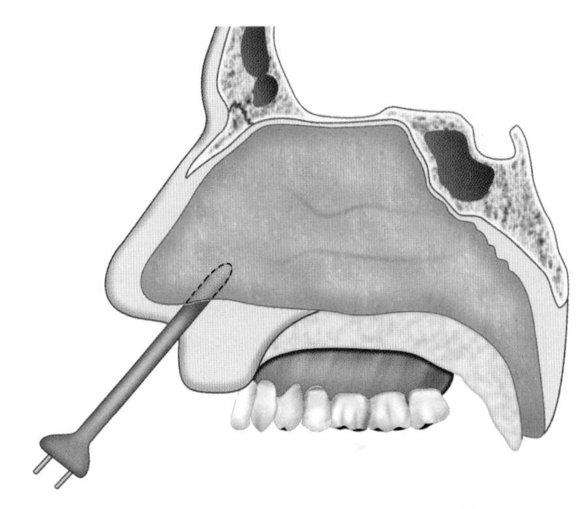

Fig. 37.4: Trocar and cannula in the maxillary antrum

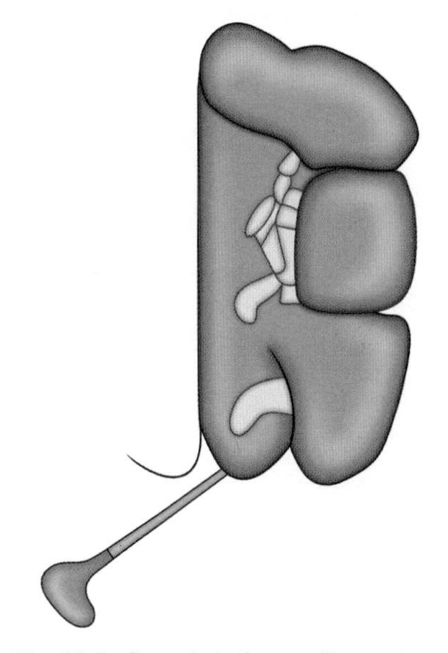

Fig. 37.5: Cannula in the maxillary antrum

The sinus is irrigated with sterile normal saline at body temperature and the patient is told to breath through the mouth with the head down. The discharge comes out through the natural ostium of the sinus. If the ostium is closed by edema, then a second cannula can be inserted through the inferior meatus. The washings are noted for the character of discharge and can be sent for cytological or bacteriological examination. At the end of the procedure, local medication may be instilled into the sinus cavity, the cannula is withdrawn and nose cleaned.

DIFFICULTIES AND DANGERS OF ANTRAL LAVAGE PROCEDURE

1. The trocar may slip under the inferior turbinate and cause laceration of the mucosa.
2. The trocar may enter the soft tissues of the cheek.
3. If too much force is applied, the trocar may slip through the antrum and might damage the orbit. Hence during a washout, the eyes and cheek should be closely observed to note any swelling or emphysema.
4. Air should not be injected into the sinus as there is a danger of air embolism through damaged vessels.
5. The procedure should not be undertaken during acute rhinitis or acute sinusitis as there is risk of spread of infection.

Puncture of the maxillary sinus through the middle meatus is avoided as it may damage the orbit and lead to reactionary edema of the natural ostium.

The puncture can also be done through the canine fossa.

INTRANASAL ANTROSTOMY

This is a drainage operation performed on the maxillary sinus. The purpose is to create a permanent window near the floor of antrum so as to facilitate drainage of the discharge. **Figure 37.6** shows the instruments used for the procedure.

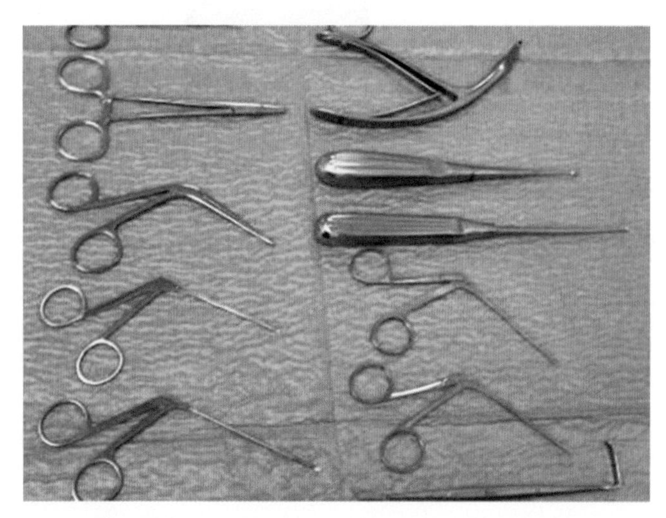

Fig. 37.6: Instruments used for intranasal antrostomy

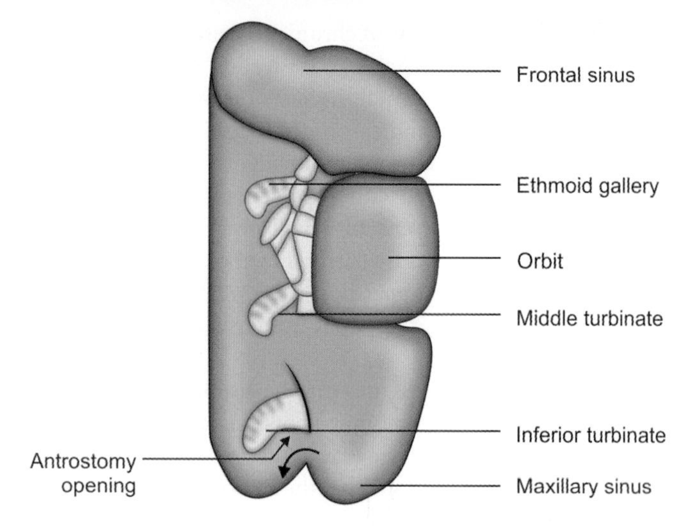

Fig. 37.7: Site for intranasal antrostomy

Under local or general anesthesia, the inferior meatus is exposed and then a harpoon or Myle's gouge is passed through the nasoantral wall, under the inferior turbinate. The opening is enlarged and made closer to the floor of the antrum. Subsequently antral washes are given. This is a simple and less radical procedure with less risk of damage to blood vessels and nerves of the teeth. However, there may occur permanent dribbling from the nose.

This procedure has now fallen out of favour because it has been demonstrated that the cilia of the maxillary antrum beat towards the natural ostium even in the presence of inferior meatal antrostomy.

More recently, intranasal antrostomy (INA) (**Fig. 37.7**) has been replaced by endoscopic middle meatal antrostomy (MMA) which is an endoscopic surgical procedure aimed at enlarging the natural ostium of the maxillary sinus.

CALDWELL-LUC OPERATION

With the advent of FESS, this procedure has fallen out of favor as well.

Indications

1. It is a radical operation for those cases of chronic maxillary sinusitis where the mucosa is permanently damaged and shows no chances of recovery.
2. Inspection and biopsy of suspected tumor of the sinus.
3. Surgery for dental or dentigerous cysts.
4. Recurrent antrochoanal polyp.
5. As an approach to reduce fracture of the orbital floor or zygoma.
6. As an approach to sphenopalatine fossa for maxillary artery ligation and vidian neurectomy.
7. Approach to transantral ethmoidectomy, sphenoidectomy and hypophysectomy.

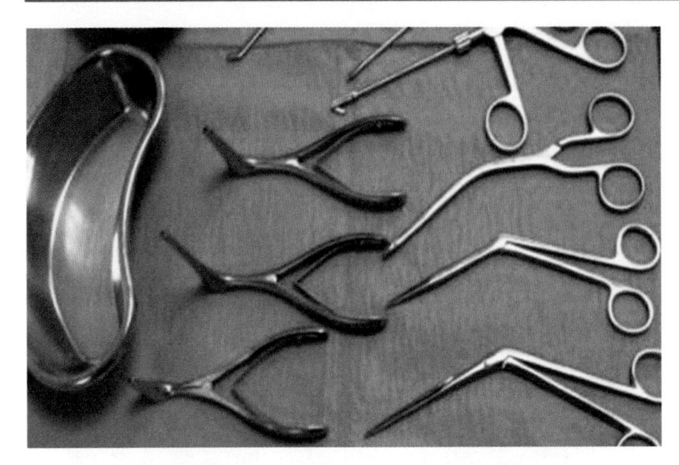

Fig. 37.8: Instruments for Caldwell-Luc operation

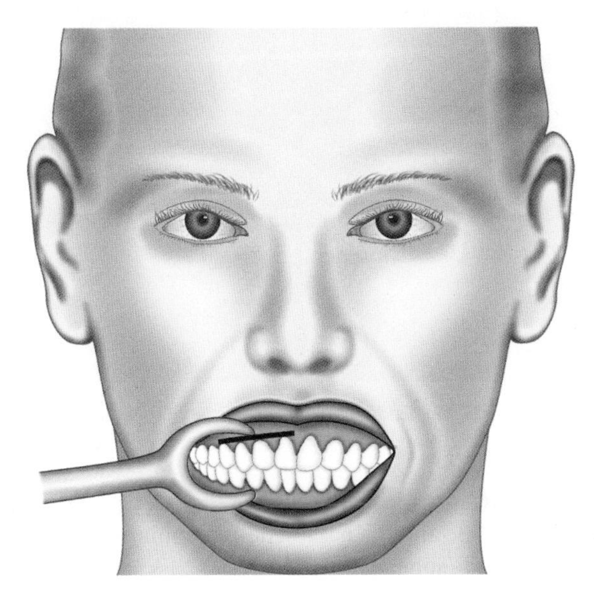

Fig. 37.9: Sublabial incision for Caldwell-Luc operation

8. Oroantral fistula.
9. Foreign body in maxillary antrum.

Steps of Operation

There are three main steps of the operation. **Figure 37.8** shows the instruments used for Caldwell-Luc's operation.

1. A sublabial incision is made and the anterolateral surface of the maxilla exposed (**Figs 37.9 and 37.10**).
2. Through the canine fossa, an opening is made in the anterolateral wall of the maxillary sinus and the sinus cavity explored. The diseased mucosa and polypi are removed.
3. A permanent opening is made in the nasoantral wall by performing an intranasal antrostomy.

The complications which can arise include hemorrhage from the branches of the sphenopalatine artery, damage to blood supply and nerves of the teeth, and sometimes a sublabial fistula.

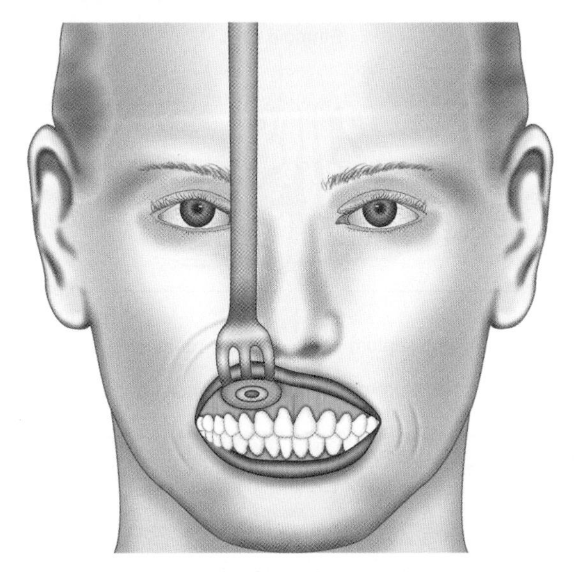

Fig. 37.10: Opening in anterolateral wall of maxillary sinus

FUNCTIONAL ENDOSCOPIC SINUS SURGERY

This procedure is a recent advance in the treatment of sinus diseases.

Concept of FESS: It has been clearly established that surgically unblocking the ostium of the diseased sinus, especially by removal of diseased ethmoidal air cells, leads to reestablishment of the normal drainage and ventilation of the sinuses, consequently the diseased mucosa, over a period of time, reverts back to normalcy. There is no need to remove all the diseased mucosa as used to be done previously. The mucociliary transport in the paranasal sinuses occurs in a definite genetically predetermined pattern and mucus is always transported by the cilia towards the natural ostium and creating a dependent opening such as in inferior meatus antrostomy, does not necessarily result in adequate drainage, as the secretions circumvent the antrostomy opening and track towards natural ostium.

Functional endoscopic sinus surgery (FESS) is a minimally invasive surgical procedure. It is called functional because the aim is to restore the function of the sinuses by providing drainage and aeration, by relieving the obstruction at the natural ostia of the sinuses. This has been made possible by advances in technology including :

i. *Rigid and fiberoptic endoscopes:* Which provide better illumination with magnification to visualize whole area from different angles.
ii. *Microsurgical instruments:* Which facilitate accurate and to the point surgery desired at particular sites to eradicate pathology and remove obstruction to the ostia.

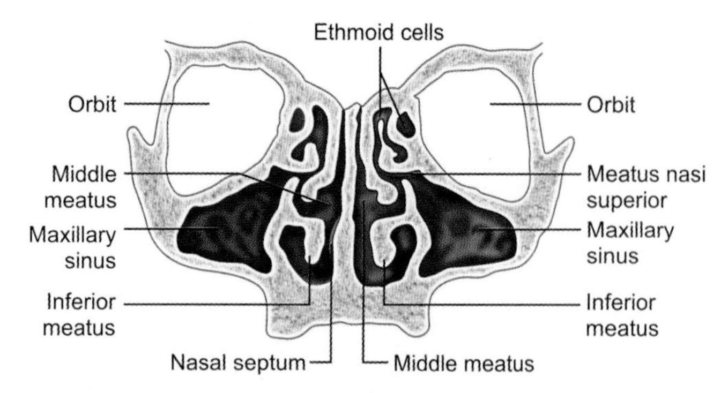

Fig. 37.11A: Coronal section through nose and sinuses

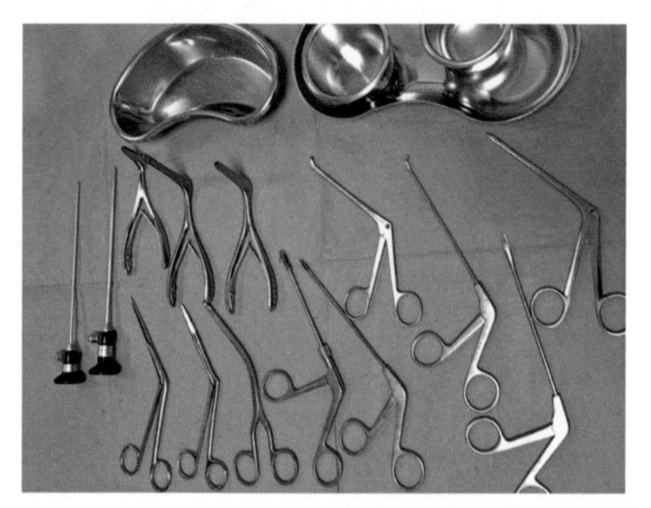

Fig. 37.11B: Instruments used for FESS

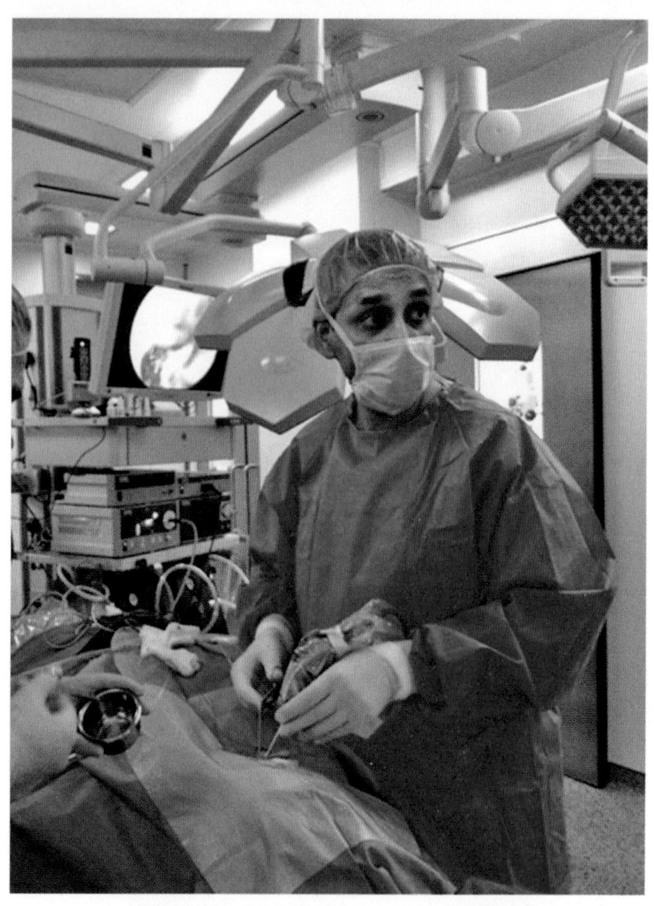

Fig. 37.12: Endoscopic sinus surgery procedure

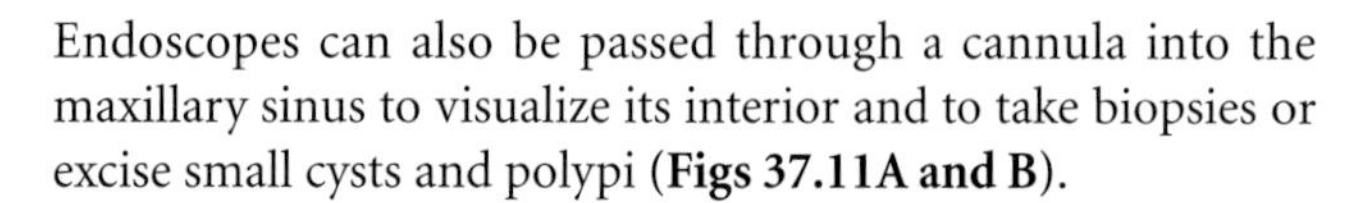

Endoscopes can also be passed through a cannula into the maxillary sinus to visualize its interior and to take biopsies or excise small cysts and polypi (**Figs 37.11A and B**).

Technique

Functional endoscopic sinus surgery (FESS) can be performed under local anesthesia, however, it is usually performed under general anesthesia with controlled hypotension. The nose is prepared by spraying with 4 percent xylocaine with adrenaline and packed with 2 percent xylocaine with adrenaline and/or decongestant nasal drops, this will cause adequate decongestion. A thorough endoscopic examination of the nasal cavity is then done by using 0° and 30° rigid nasal endoscopes. Three passes are usually made:

First pass is made by passing a zero degree rigid nasal endoscope below the inferior turbinate examining thoroughly the whole area upto the choana, visualizing both eustachian tube openings and the nasopharynx.

Second pass is made by passing the endoscope lateral to the middle turbinate to examine the osteomeatal complex in the middle meatus.

Third pass is made by passing the endoscope between the middle turbinate and the nasal septum examining the roof of the nose and the sphenoethmoidal recess.

Surgical procedure of FESS (**Fig. 37.12**)*:* The lateral wall of nose is infiltrated with 2 percent xylocaine with adrenaline at various points on uncinate process and in the axilla of the middle turbinate. In case of canine fossa puncture a sublabial injection of 2 percent xylocaine is also done.

Using 0° telescope, an incision is made with a sickle knife on the anterior margin of the uncinate process from the level of middle turbinate downwards along the curve of the uncinate process till just above the inferior turbinate and then carry it backward in an anterior to posterior direction. The uncinate process is grasped firmly with Blakesley's forceps and removed with a twisting movement, exposing the infundibulum. This procedure is known as *infundibulotomy.* The natural ostium of the maxillary sinus is then identified and widened. In case an accessory ostium is present it is combined with the natural ostium to prevent recirculation.

Next the bulla ethmoidalis and middle ethmoidal cells are removed with Blakesley's forceps. Here the dissection must stop on reaching the ethmoidal roof superiorly, as there is anterior ethmoidal artery and any injury to roof may expose the dura; also medially a thin bone separates it from cribriform plate. Laterally, the lamina papyracea is the limit of dissection. Here only the side of the forceps, and not the tip, should be used to prevent accidental perforation, posteriorly the limit of dissection is a bony partition called the ground lamella. *Ground lamella* or basal lamella is the bony attachment of middle turbinate to the lateral wall; it also separates the middle ethmoidal cells from posterior group of cells.

The anterior ethmoidal cells being situated around the frontal recess and anterior to anterior ethmoidal artery, are removed by using 30° endoscope and upward biting forceps. It is necessary to open the agar nasi cells to gain access to the frontal recess. *Agar nasi* are the anterior most anterior etmoidal air cells. Once identified the frontal recess is widened, if indicated by CT findings, only in one direction never circumferentially to prevent postoperative stenosis.

The posterior ethmoidal cells and the sphenoid sinus should be opened only if the CT scan has indicated presence of any disease in this area. The posterior ethmoidal cells are reached by gently perforating the basal lamella with tip of Blakesley's forceps and the cells are carefully removed up to the anterior wall of sphenoid. In this area, posterior ethmoidal cells form a very close relationship to the sphenoid ostium.

The sphenoid ostium lies approximately 1 to 1.5 cm above the superior border of the choana close to the nasal septum, approximately 5 to 6 cm from the anterior nasal spine at an angle of 30 degrees. The sphenoid sinus anterior wall is perforated and the ostium widened. Any pathology in the sphenoid sinus should only be removed under direct vision especially towards lateral wall which is having close relation to optic nerve and internal carotid artery.

Indications of FESS

Common indications:

i. Chronic rhinosinusitis not responding to medical treatment.
ii. Sinonasal polyposis.
iii. Extramucosal fungal sinusitis.
iv. Mucoceles.
v. Osteomas and other benign tumors.

Uncommon indications:

i. Recurrent acute sinusitis.
ii. Headache and facial pain.

Complications of FESS

Due to close relation to vital structures like orbit, brain, optic nerve and internal carotid artery the FESS procedure carries the risk of certain complications like:

i. Bleeding
ii. Orbital hematoma
iii. CSF leak
iv. Blindness
v. Diplopia
vi. Subcutaneous and orbital emphysema
vii. Synechiae
viii. Epiphora
ix. Closure of antrostomy
x. Pneumocephalus

These can be minimized by prior study of surgical anatomy of dry skull and cadaver dissections. CT scans both in axial and coronal planes act as road maps to guide the surgeon through the previously inaccessible areas of nose and paranasal sinuses.

TREATMENT OF ETHMOIDITIS

The acute or chronic inflammatory condition of the ethmoids may demand an operative procedure. As the cells are small and multiple, no drainage operation or lavage is possible. The only feasible procedure is exenteration of the ethmoid cells called *ethmoidectomy*. Nowadays a complete ethmoidectomy is performed as part of the FESS procedure.

Ethmoidectomy

This procedure as was done in the past is mentioned here for the sake of knowledge. The operation is indicated in chronic ethmoiditis which usually manifests as polyposis, particularly when simple polypectomy does not help.

The ethmoidectomy could be done through the nose or by an external route. The ethmoids can also be exenterated through the transantral route.

Under local or general anesthesia, the middle turbinate is gently pushed medially and may be fractured, thus exposing the ethmoid bulla.

The ethmoid bulla is opened, ethmoidal labyrinth exposed, and ethmoidal cells are exenterated. Laterally the exenteration is carried to the lamina papyracea and posteriorly up to the sphenoid sinus. Superiorly the smooth, white bone signifies the floor of the anterior cranial fossa. The roof of the ethmoidal labyrinth is higher than the cribriform plate. Anteriorly the exenteration is difficult. The operation on ethmoids can lead to damage to orbital contents, optic nerve or the anterior cranial fossa.

External ethmoidectomy: This procedure allows exenteration of the ethmoid cells under direct vision via an external incision but it leaves an external scar.

SURGERY FOR CHRONIC FRONTAL SINUSITIS

Drainage from the frontal sinus can be facilitated by treating the associated obstructive pathology in the nose like correcting the deflected septum or polypi. Usually opening the frontal recess and approaching the frontal sinus endoscopically as part of the FESS procedure is all that is required. However, if these procedures are not helpful, more radical procedures are undertaken, the diseased mucosa removed and sinus obliterated.

External Frontoethmoidectomy

The procedure is done to remove the disease from the ethmoids and frontal sinus. Through an external incision near the inner canthus, the bone is exposed and ethmoid labyrinth exenterated. The floor of the frontal sinus is removed and the diseased mucosa removed. Thus the frontal sinus and ethmoids are converted into a cavity communicating with the middle meatus.

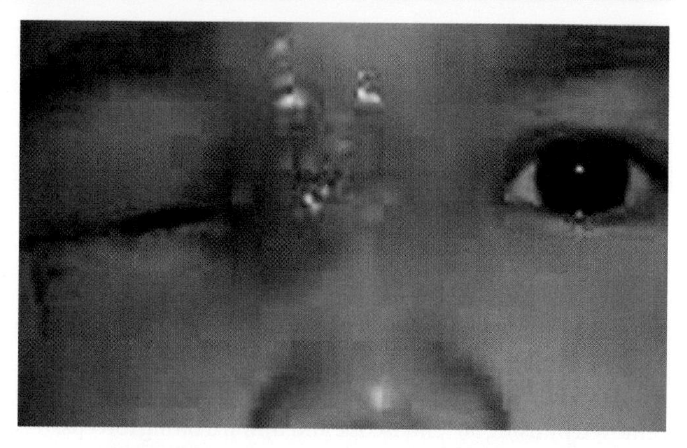

Fig. 37.13A: Osteomyelitis of the right frontal sinus

Osteoplastic Flap Operation on the Frontal Sinus

This is an obliterative operation performed on the frontal sinus which allows exenteration of the disease from the frontal sinus, without causing an external deformity of the forehead. The frontal sinus is exposed by raising a bony lid, hinged on the outer periosteum.

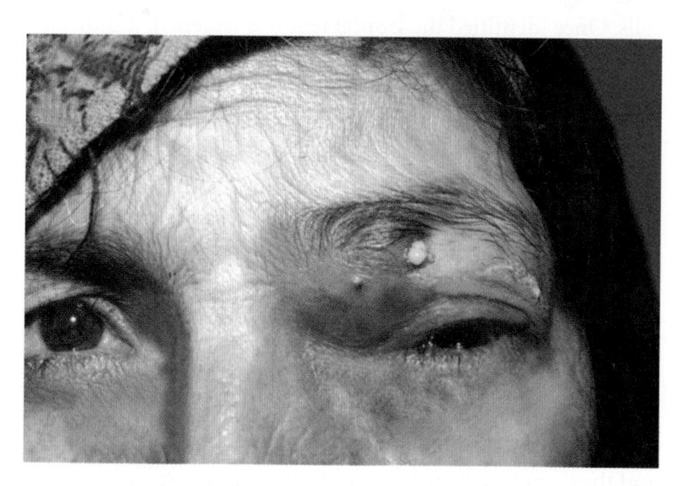

Fig. 37.13B: Frontal mucopyocele with fistula

Operations on the Sphenoid Sinus

Sphenoid sinusotomy as part of the FESS procedure is the surgical procedure of choice for sphenoid sinus disease. In the past sphenoid sinus lavage was sometimes done through its anterior wall using a trocar and cannula. The sinus can also be explored while performing ethmoidectomy when its anterior wall is removed and sinus explored.

COMPLICATIONS OF SINUSITIS

Osteomyelitis: Infection from the sinus can lead to osteitis in compact bone and osteomyelitis in cancellous or diploic bone (**Figs 37.13A and B**). Acute infection of the frontal sinus or ethmoid labyrinth may lead to osteomyelitis with resultant orbital cellulitis and proptosis. It may also be complicated by cavernous sinus thrombosis and cerebral abscess in the frontal lobe.

Pathology

Infection spreads either directly from mucous membrane to the diploe or through thrombophlebitis of veins of the sinus to the veins of dura (dura being internal periosteum of *culvarium* and responsible for the nutrition of skull through it nearly all the vessels are conveyed to the cranial vault). Retrograde thrombosis takes place from the dural veins to the veins of diploe. There the pus forms and the thin boneplates are destroyed and eventually perforation takes place through either the outer or the inner bony tables of the skull. If infection is not controlled, spread to the meninges may take place with consequent meningitis and brain abscess, or to sagittal and cavernous sinuses with resulting septicemia and cases end fatally. Osteomyelitis of maxilla is rarely a complication of maxillary sinusitis. It usually occurs in infants (almost unknown in adults) from infection in one of tooth buds. Begins with febrile illness. Swelling and redness develop over the cheeks. Soft parts are indurated. Later there is discharge of pus from the alveolus or into the nose or abscess may point about the lower orbital margin. Many cases of osteomyelitis skull result from exacerbation of a chronic infection of frontal sinus which has followed swimming.

Symptoms

1. Febrile illness with headache
2. Edema and tenderness over the infected bone—soft, 'doughy' swelling.

In 1 to 2 days, another patch of edema developes at a distance from the first and an area of healthy skin in between (Spreading osteomyelitis).

Treatment: Intensive course of antibiotics and localized abscesses are drained and sequestra removed.

INTRACRANIAL COMPLICATIONS

Meningitis: Most common complication of acute ethmoidal and sphenoidal sinusitis.

Symptoms

1. Severe headache
2. Photophobia
3. High temperature
4. Constipation
5. Convulsion
6. Paralysis of some cranial nerves
7. Unconsciousness
8. Febrile delirium.

Signs

1. Persistent and gradually increasing headache.
2. Drowsiness.
3. Neck rigidity less severe than in cases when meningitis follows lesions adjacent to posterior cranial fossa.
4. Temperature persistently elevated with slow pulse.
5. Kernig's sign positive.
6. Abdominal reflexes disappear early.
7. Moderate leukocytosis.
8. CSF examination shows increased pressure may be clear turbid or frankly purulent.

Pneumococci type II and IV and streptococci may be found. Cell count is increased. Chlorides are decreased, sugar decreased or absent and protein is increased.

Treatment

1. High doses of broad spectrum antibiotics.
2. Injection Cefatraxone 1 gm. IV b.i.d till symptoms subside.

CEREBRAL ABSCESS

It may result from infection of any of paranasal sinus but most common after chronic frontal sinus infection. Anterior pole of homolateral frontal lobe is most common site of abscess, usually secondary to osteitis of posterior wall of sinus.

Symptoms

1. Persistent frontal pain or headache after drainage of infected frontal sinus.
2. Nausea and vomiting.
3. Anorexia and loss of weight.

Signs

Tongue coated, breath foul. Bowels—constipated. Other signs of meningitis. Frontal lobe lesion symptoms, e.g. marked change in character, defects in memory and unilateral anosmia. Some motor disturbance of contralateral face and extremities due to pressure on internal capsule. Optic neuritis (Papilledema) is common. Pupil on affected side is commonly widely dilated. CSF examination may show increased pressure cell count increased polymorphs predominate but when encapsulation occurs lymphocytes predominant.

Treatment

If during operation, a defect is seen in posterior wall. Wall should be removed and dura exposed. Dura may be unduly tense and pulsations of brain absent then exploration of brain may be necessary.

Carotid angiography or ventriculography may help by showing displacement of blood vessels or deformity of ventricle. If abscess is found, it should be drained or excised if its capsule is firm sufficiently.

CAVERNOUS SINUS THROMBOSIS

It is more with acute exacerbation of a chronic infection of posterior ethmoidal or sphenoidal sinuses.

Pathology

i. Degenerative changes in the vessel wall
ii. Sluggishness of blood flow
iii. Pathological changes in blood.

Symptoms

High fever about 105°F, pain around the eye, proptosis, progressive edema and ecchymosis of eyelids and finally ophthalmoplegia.

The chronic inflammation may lead to scarring of the ostium with resultant mucocele or pyocele.

Mucocele: This is a cystic swelling commonly affecting the frontal and ethmoid sinuses (**Fig. 37.14**). The swelling contains tenacious mucus. It causes expansion of the sinus and thinning of the bony wall. It may also cause displacement of the orbit. Its contents may get infected.

It is thought to be due to trauma causing damage to the duct or because of inflammatory scarring of the duct. Clinically it presents as a slowly growing painless cystic swelling causing downward and outward displacement of the orbital contents. Sometimes egg shell crackling may be felt. The treatment is surgical. FESS, external frontoethmoidectomy or osteoplastic flap operation are the procedures of choice.

Oroantral fistula: The communication between the oral cavity and maxillary sinus usually occurs after dental extraction particularly of premolars and molars. The roots of these teeth are separated by thin bone which can easily get broken at the time of extraction and thus result in a fistula (**Fig. 37.15**).

Though in the majority of cases the fistula gets sealed off, but in some this leads to infection of the sinus which does not allow the fistula to heal. Other causes for oroantral fistula include

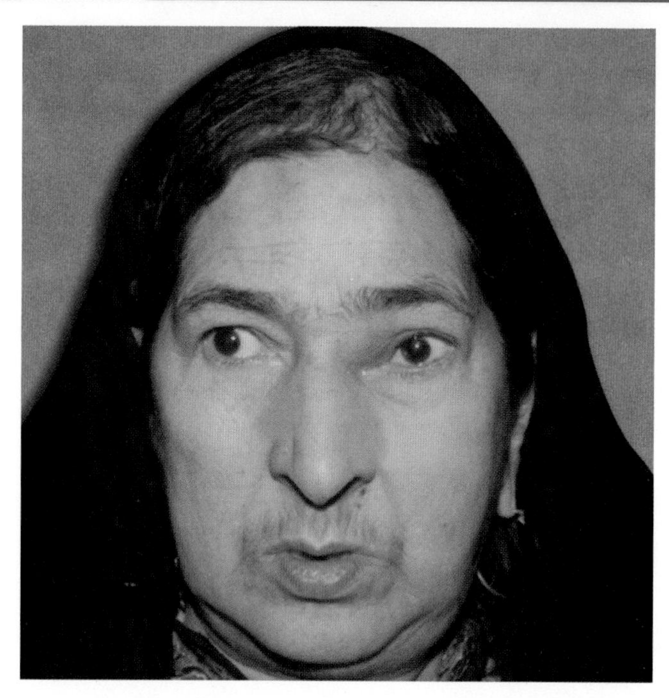

Fig. 37.14: Frontoethmoidal mucocele (left)

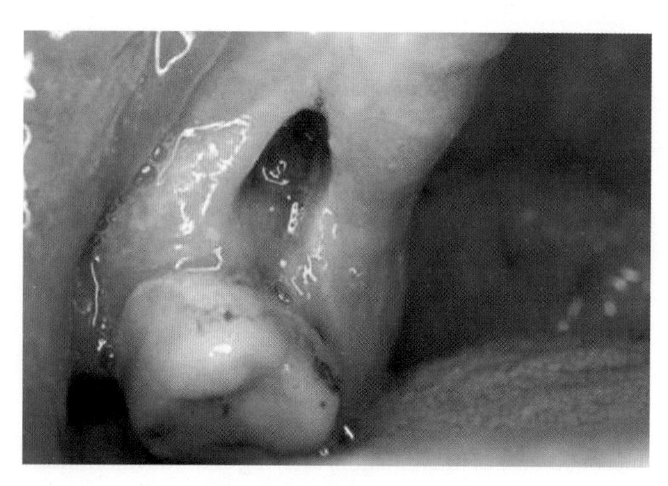

Fig. 37.15: Oroantral fistula

malignancy, granulomatous diseases of the nose and maxillary sinus, and trauma.

The common symptoms include passage of fluids or food particles into the nose and blowing of air from nose into the mouth. The patient may suffer from symptoms of recurrent sinusitis.

Proper treatment of sinus infection may allow a small fistula to heal up but a persistent large fistula requires surgery. The adjacent flaps can be rotated from the buccal mucosa or the palate and the fistula site closed. This procedure may or may not be combined with Caldwell-Luc operation.

For large fistulae or those in which the above measures have failed, usual methods of closing are: (i) by a palatal flap, (ii) by a buccal flap.

i. *Palatal flap:* It is made from the mucosa of hard palate and must be large enough to swing right across the fistulous opening to form the buccal flap as the sutures must not be immediately over the fistula, but well lateral to it.
ii. *The buccal flap:* It has advantage of being more mobile flap with no denuded area and a more satisfactory result for fitting dentures but the constant tension and movements of the lips and cheek prejudice the result and the palatal flap is generally accepted as a more certain method of closure. If buccal flap is used, best results are obtained by an incision along the given margin of two teeth on each side of the alveolar fistula. A mucoperiosteal flap is raised up to the canine fossa where the periosteum is incised to free the flap. It gives a mobile flap which can be carried medially over the area of the fistula after curetting.

SECONDARY EFFECTS OF SINUSITIS

Secondary changes include hypertrophy of lateral pharyngeal bands, persistent laryngitis, recurring attacks of bronchitis or bronchiectasis, etc.

Sinusitis may produce focal sepsis elsewhere. Arthritis, fibrositis, dermatological disorders may also be associated.

Kartagener's Syndrome

The association of sinusitis, bronchiectasis and dextrocardia is known as Kartagener's syndrome.

Sinusitis and bronchiectasis may be associated with keratosis in the external ear.

CYSTIC SWELLING OF THE NOSE AND PARANASAL SINUS

Dentigerous Cyst

The cyst arises from the follicle around an unerupted tooth (**Fig. 37.16A**). The tooth is seen in the cyst cavity on X-ray. Treatment is to remove the cyst along with the unerupted tooth.

Dental Cyst

The cyst arises around an infected tooth (**Fig. 37.16B**). The infection produces a granulomatous reaction at its apex and this leads to proliferation of the epithelium of the cyst wall. Treatment is enucleation of the cyst along with the infected tooth.

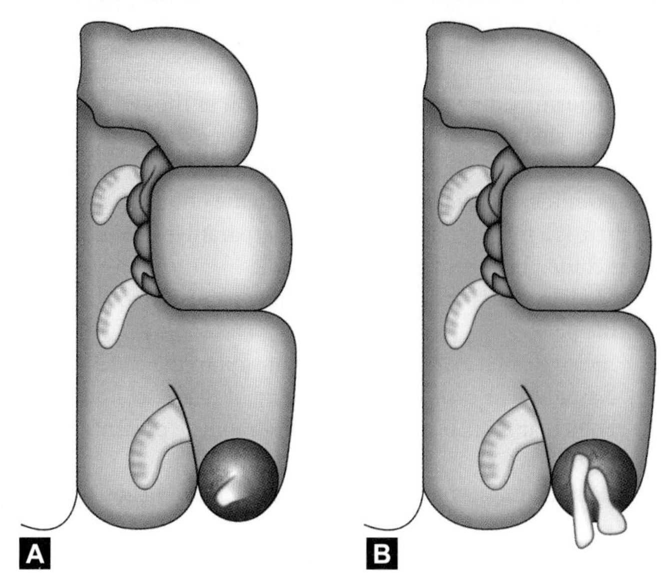

Figs 37.16A and B: Cysts: (A) Dentigerous; (B) Dental

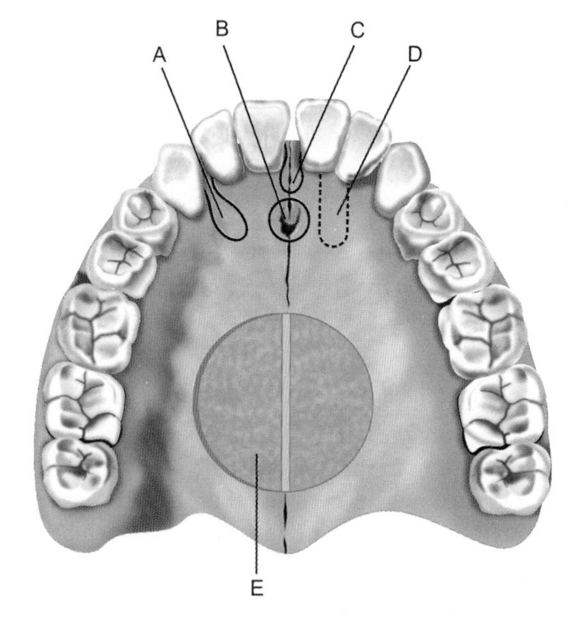

Fig. 37.17: Cysts associated with fusion of embryological elements forming the maxilla: (A) Lateral alveolar cyst; (B) Nasopalatine (incisive canal) cyst; (C) Median alveolar cyst; (D) Nasoalveolar cyst, and (E) Median palatal cyst

Cysts in the Maxillary Region

PATHOLOGICAL TYPES

1. Cysts associated with fusion of embryological elements forming the maxilla (**Fig. 37.17**) may be separated into the following:
   a. Medial group in which there are three forms:
      i. Median alveolar cyst which separates the upper central incisor teeth.
      ii. Median palatal cyst which lies between the palatine processes of the developing maxillae.
      iii. Nasopalatine cyst arising from tissue in the incisive canal or nests in the papilla palatine and present either on the palate or on the nasal floor.
   b. Lateral group in which there are two forms:
      i. Lateral alveolar cysts sited at the line of fusion of the maxillary and premaxillary elements of the palate, so as to cause separation of the canine and lateral incisor teeth.
      ii. Nasoalveolar cysts occurring in the lateral half of the nasal floor, anterior to the inferior turbinate. They enlarge to splay the nostril and to cause a fullness of the upper lip (**Fig. 37.18**). Because they are developed from the nasal mucosa they are lined by columnar (respiratory) epithelium but may show metaplasia to squamous epithelium in the presence of infection. When large they cause nasal obstruction and may thin the bony nasal floor. They are sometimes mistakenly incised as furuncles, only to recur later.

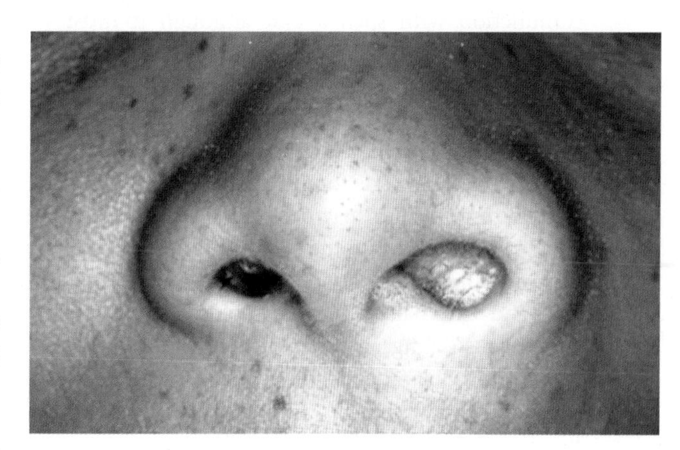

Fig. 37.18: Nasoalveolar cyst

2. *Cysts of dental origin* (**Fig. 37.19**)**:** These are derived from the epithelium that has been connected with the development of the tooth concerned.
   a. Primordial cysts arise from the epithelium of the enamel origin before the formation of the dental tissue. They occur in young people and the most common site is in the third molar region of the mandible.
   b. Cysts of eruption arise over a tooth that has not erupted from the remains of the dental lamina. They occur in young people and may appear over a deciduous or permanent molar tooth, appearing as small bluish swellings.

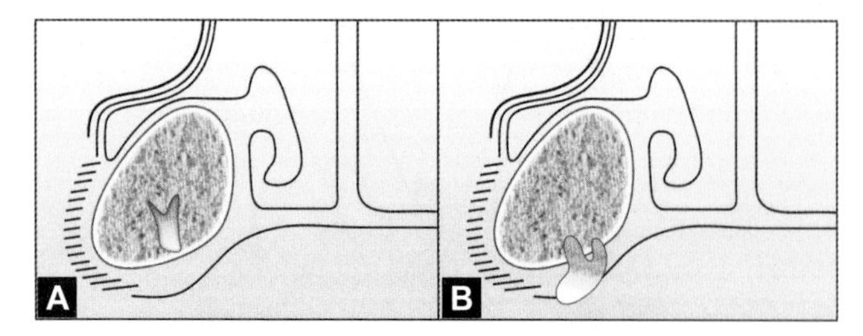

Figs 37.19A and B: Cysts of dental origin: (A) Follicular or dentigerous; (B) Radicular or dental

   c. Dentigerous (follicular) cysts (**Fig. 37.19A**) usually arise from the follicle around an unerupted tooth. The tooth projects into the cavity.
   d. Dental (radicular) cysts (**Fig. 37.19B**) arise from epithelial remains in the periodontal membrane and are the most common cysts that occur in the jaws. Chronically infected dead teeth or roots produce a granulomatous reaction at the apex. This granuloma contains epithelium and it is this epithelium that proliferates initially to produce the cyst lining. Therefore, the dead tooth or root is usually seen in conjunction with such a cyst although it must be remembered that teeth or roots might have been removed, the cyst remaining (residual cyst). Any of these cysts may be thin-walled and histologically show keratinization. Such cysts have a tendency to recur.
3. *Dermoid cysts:* They are found at the surface lines of embryonic fusion. They may occur in the midline of the nose and may extend into the septum; others may occur at the inner and outer parts of the orbital margins, *viz.* internal and external angular dermoids. Dermoid cysts form external swellings, with or without fistula.
4. Mucoceles of the paranasal sinuses may be caused by the following:
   a. Blockage of a mucous gland duct.
   b. Cystic formation of the mucosa undergoing polyposis.
   c. Atresia or stenosis of a sinus ostium. Mucoceles occur most commonly in the frontal sinus and enlarge to bulge into the orbit.
5. *Cherubism:* It is a rare familial multilocular cystic disease. Radiographic examination shows multiple radiolucent areas which are symmetrical and widespread throughout the lower and/or upper jaws. The radiolucent areas in fact contain mainly fibrous tissue and the condition seems to regress after adolescence.
6. *Hemorrhagic bone cysts:* These are found in the mandible and it is thought that the cause is related to trauma which may have occurred several years ago. It is probable that an intraosseous hemorrhage leads to excessive osteoclastic activity which slowly regresses, leaving the cyst behind.

CLINICAL FEATURES

All cysts tend to expand gradually without pain unless infected. The deformity depends upon the position of the cyst.

'Egg-shell crackling' can be elicited when the bone is thin.

Radiographic appearance is usually diagnostic in showing a clear outline in typical positions. When the outline is not clear or there is a multiple appearance, hyperparathyroidism should be excluded by serum electrolyte studies.

1. Median palatal cysts show a complete central dehiscence of the palate.
2. Incisive canal cysts cause an expansion of the canal.
3. Nasoalveolar cysts cause a thinning of the nasal floor.
4. Follicular cysts usually have a tooth follicle present within them.
5. Radicular cysts have an infected dental root below them.

DIFFERENTIAL DIAGNOSIS

Differential diagnosis is from any lesion which can produce a clearly defined radiolucent area in the bone, e.g. osteoclastoma, hemangioma, eosinophil granuloma, myeloma, etc.

TREATMENT

Complete removal or marsupialization is the treatment of choice.

FUNGAL INFECTION OF NOSE AND PARANASAL SINUSES

Fungal infections commence in the nose and can progress to involve paranasal sinuses.

Etiology

Most common type of fungal infection of nose and paranasal sinuses, are due to *Aspergillus*.

A. fumigatus, A. niger and *A. flavus* and dametaceous fungi are the most frequent offenders. Dry and hot climate acts as a predisposing factor.

Clinical Features

Fungal rhinosinusitis can be classified into *invasive form* and *non-invasive form:*

Invasive form is further classified as *acute fulminant type* and *chronic indolent form.*

Noninvasive is further classified as *allergic fungal sinusitis* and *fungal mycetoma.*

1. *Acute fulminant form:* This is the most serious and potentially fatal form, usually caused by *Rhizopus, Rhizomucor, Absidia,* and *Mucor or Aspergillus.* There is widespread hematological and intracranial spread. It is seen in patients who have uncontrolled diabetes mellitus or immunocompromised patients who are on systemic steroids or immunosuppressive therapy.

2. *Chronic indolent form:* In this form, there is history of chronic rhinosinusitis, the disease is usually persistent and recurrent. Progression is slow over months to years; with fungal organisms invading mucosa, submucosa, blood vessels, and bony walls leading to maxillofacial soft tissue swelling, orbital invasion with proptosis, cranial neuropathies, decreased vision, invasion of the cribriform plate causing headaches, seizures and decreased mental status.
3. *Fungal mycetoma or fungal ball:* This form occurs in immunocompetent individuals. It is usually asymptomatic or may cause minimal symptoms like nasal discharge or chronic pressure over the involved sinus, and cacosmia. There is a mass within the lumen of paranasal sinus which is usually limited to one sinus. Frontal sinus is most commonly involved followed by sphenoid sinus. CT scan reveals a hyperattenuating mass often with punctate calcifications.
4. *Allergic fungal sinusitis (AFS):* This is the most common form of fungal sinusitis. It occurs in immunocompetent young adults with history of asthma or polyps and produces pansinusitis without soft tissue or bone invasion, it may however, cause remodeling of the bone. Histologically there is no angioinvasion as opposed to invasive fungal sinusitis. Nasal secretions show marked eosinophilia. The sinus are filled with allergic (eosiophilic) mucin which has a characteristic peanut butter consistency. CT findings show characteristic hyperattenuation or heterogenicitiy due to accumulation of heavy metals (e.g. iron and manganese) and calcium within inspissated allergic fungal mucin.

Treatment

Functional endoscopic sinus surgery is the main stay of treatment. Systemic antifungal therapy is indicated in invasive fungal sinusitis; where as systemic steroids alongwith topical steroid nasal sprays are prescribed for AFS. Exenteration and craniofacial resection may be needed in acute fulminant forms.

Chapter 38

Tumors of the Nose and Paranasal Sinuses

The nose and paranasal sinuses are uncommon sites for the growth of tumors. The close anatomical relationship between nasal passages and the adjacent sinuses results in rapid involvement of one from the other. The etiology is uncertain. Wood dust, tobacco, snuff or nickle may have some role to play.

Tumors of the Nasal Cavity

Tumors of the nasal cavity are classified as follows:

1. *Benign:* Papilloma, inverted papilloma, hemangiomas, fibroma, adenoma, osteoma, and chondroma.
2. *Malignant*
   a. Squamous cell carcinoma
   b. Adenoid cystic carcinoma
   c. Malignant melanoma
   d. Olfactory neuroblastoma
   e. Chondrosarcoma
   f. Malignant lymphomas (Stewart's granuloma).

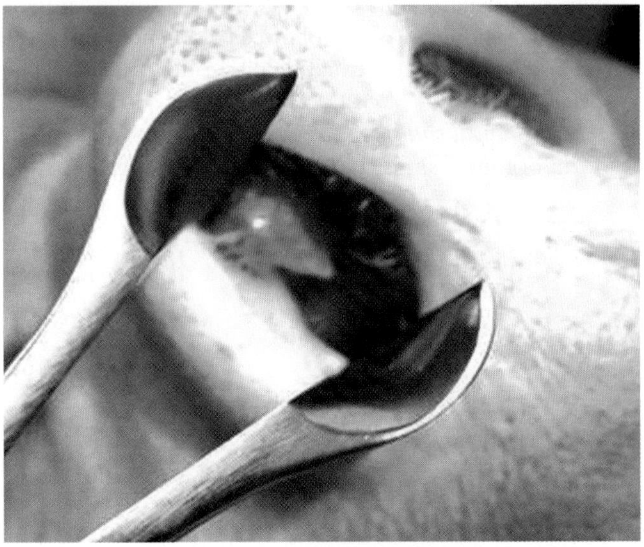

Fig. 38.1: Papilloma of nasal vestibule

PAPILLOMA

Squamous papilloma may arise from the nasal vestibule (**Fig. 38.1**) or from the anterior part of the septum and present as a keratinizing exophytic masses like elsewhere in the body. Surgical excision is the treatment of choice.

INVERTED PAPILLOMA (RINGERTZ TUMOR, SCHINELARIAN PAPILLOMA)

The tumor shows inversion of the epithelium into the underlying stroma instead of growing outwards as in other papillomas; the surface of the tumor being covered by alternating layers of squamous and columnar epithelium. Hence, the tumor is also called transitional cell papilloma.

It is commonly found in males, is mostly unilateral and spreads to adjacent sinuses (**Fig. 38.2**). It arises from the lateral wall of the nose and presents as a firm red or gray mass. Treatment is wide surgical excision through lateral rhinotomy approach. Sometimes it may undergo malignant change.

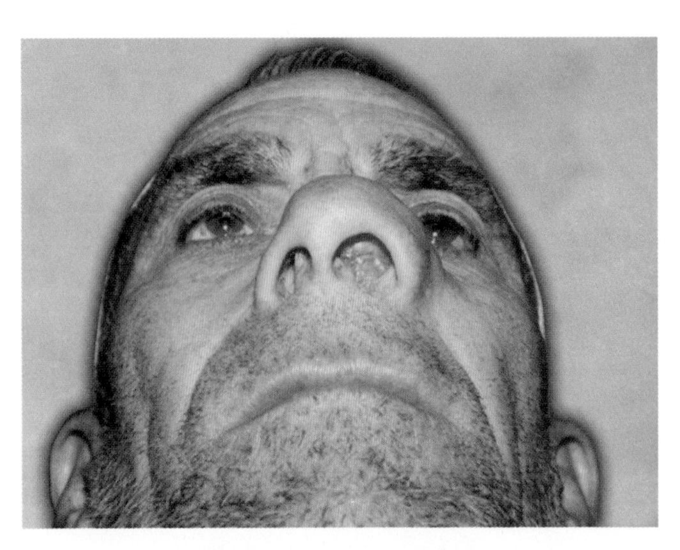

Fig. 38.2: Inverted papilloma

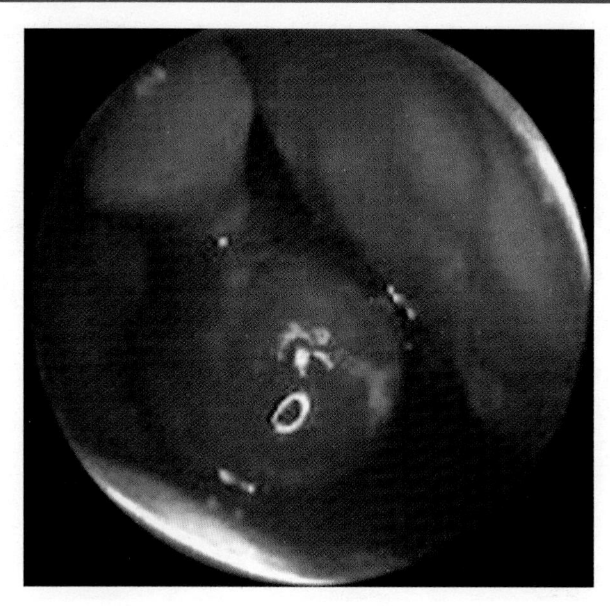

Fig. 38.3: Hemangioma of the nasal vestibule

HEMANGIOMAS

Vascular tumors may arise in the nose (**Fig. 38.3**). The commonly found lesion is capillary hemangioma of the septum. It presents as a pedunculated mass from the anterior part of the septum. Nasal obstruction and epistaxis are the common symptoms.

Surgical excision with healthy margins of the mucoperichondrium is done to prevent recurrence. Cryoapplication is another modality of treatment available for this disease.

FIBROMA

Pure fibromas are rare. When it occurs, it arises from posterior end of middle or inferior turbinate and hangs back into nasopharynx. It is of darker appearance, denser than polypus, and of firmer texture on probing or palpation. May arise from septum or floor of nose. They differ from nasopharyngeal fibromas—by occurring later in life, much less vascular and in their site of origin.

OSTEOMA

Origin is near epiphyseal center line (as in long bones) and ceases to grow when the affected bone ceases to grow (as in long bones).

Histopathologist Fetiss in 1929 discussed theories:

a. Arnold's osteoma develops in remnants of cartilage remaining unossified in ethmoid.
b. That they arise in the periosteum, in areas either torn of by trauma or by the initiation of chronic inflammation. He came to conclusion:
   i. That the growth is from within outwards by metaplasia of fibrous into bony tissue.
   ii. That the ossification at the periphery performs secondary role.
   iii. The fibrous tissue filling the interstitious space—of the spongiose bone is a direct continuation of periosteum covering the osteoma.
   iv. That the theory of origin from the periosteum split off during the period of development is the most probable.

Symptoms: Pressure with increasing obstruction, pressure-atrophy and destruction of neighboring bone and neuralgia.

Causse (1934) describes: (a) a period of subjective phenomena (b) early objective phenomena (c) advanced objective phenomena with compression of neighboring parts.

Treatment

If no symptoms, leave alone or removal, by removing bone around the base and whole tumor detached.

Section shows—typical osteitis fibrosa with increased vascularity and a few giant cells.

Diagnosis—smooth, solid, hard and ill-defined inflammation or other physical signs makes the diagnosis obvious.

ADENOMA

Histologically they contain cavities lined with cuboid or cylindrical epithelium and filled with mucoid material.

Cysts: Due to blockage of mouth of a gland and gradual expansion of gland by retained secretion. Usually occur in floor of nose just behind the vestibule of nose. Often small.

Treatment

Not necessary if no symptoms. Excision can be done.

CHONDROMA

Pure chondroma is very rare and may occur in ethmoid.

SQUAMOUS CELL CARCINOMA OF THE NOSE

It is the most common type of malignancy involving the nose. It may present as a bleeding polypoidal or sessile mass in the nose, in older age group, with symptoms of nasal obstruction and epistaxis.

Squamous cell carcinoma may arise from the vestibule, lateral wall, and nasal septum and extend to the adjacent columella, upper lip and face (**Figs 38.4 to 38.9**). Metastasis may occur to the facial or parotid nodes.

Radiotherapy is the treatment of choice. Advanced tumors need radiotherapy with wide surgical excision followed by reconstruction.

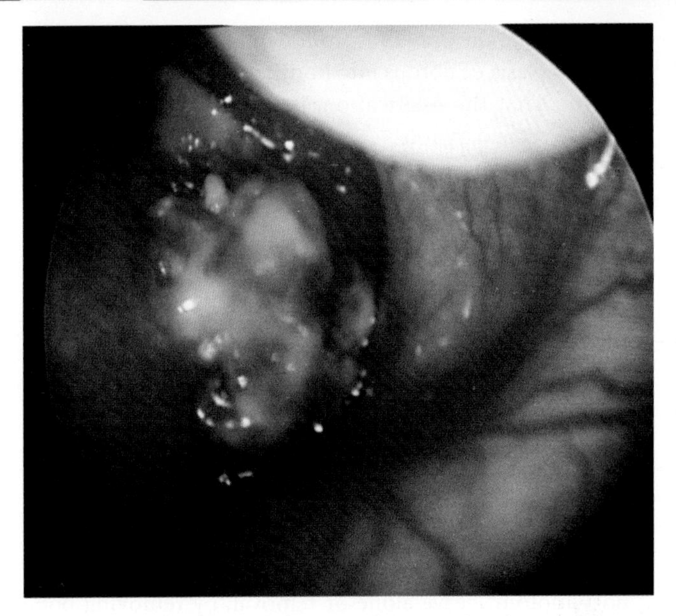

Fig. 38.4: Malignancy of the nasal cavity

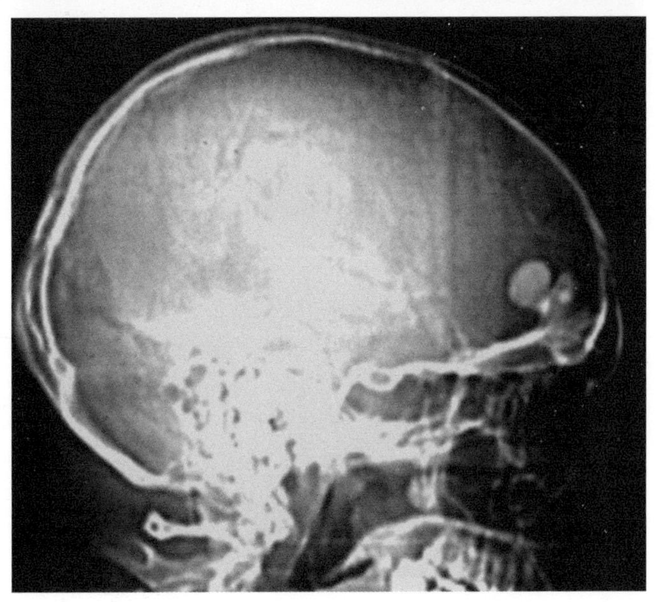

Fig. 38.5: Osteoma right frontal sinus

OLFACTORY NEUROBLASTOMA

This is a neuroectodermal tumor and may arise from the cribriform plate of the olfactory area. It consists of varying proportions of neuroblasts. Surgery is the treatment of choice. Prognosis is poor.

MALIGNANT MELANOMA

These are rare tumors arising from the melanocytes present in the nasal mucosa. Most patients are over the age of 50 years. The most common symptoms are nasal obstruction and epistaxis with a blackish mass inside the nose. Bone erosion and regional and systemic metastasis are uncommon. Treatment consists of wide surgical excision by the lateral rhinotomy approach. Radiotherapy and chemotherapy have no role in the treatment.

Adenoid cystic carcinoma and chondrosarcomas are very rare nasal tumors.

Tumors of the Paranasal Sinuses

The most common benign tumor is an osteoma. It occurs most frequently in the frontal sinus followed by ethmoids and maxillary sinus. It may be composed of compact or cancellous bone. The etiology is not clear, but embryonal, infective or traumatic factors may be involved.

Symptoms are produced by pressure on the nerves or extension of the tumor into surrounding tissues. Headache and nasal obstruction may result. X-ray shows dense, sclerotic bony swelling (**Fig. 38.5**). Treatment is surgical excision.

FIBROUS DYSPLASIA

It is a condition in which normal bone is replaced by collagen, fibroblasts and varying amounts of osteoid tissue. The condition may affect the facial bones and present as facial swelling or alveolar deformity. It presents as a bony hard, diffuse and painless swelling usually at puberty. The swelling may cause proptosis.

The growth ceases at 20 to 25 years of age. Two clinical types are generally recognized, viz. monostotic and polyostotic. Radiology shows ground glass appearance of the bone depending upon the relative amount of connective tissue to bone. Biopsy shows fibrous and osseous tissue. Treatment is surgical removal of the abnormal bone. Sometimes partial maxillectomy may be needed.

CARCINOMA OF PARANASAL SINUSES

Though the paranasal sinuses are lined by ciliated columnar epithelium, yet the most common malignant neoplasm of the paranasal sinuses is squamous cell carcinoma. It is believed that metaplasia of the epithelium precedes the malignant change.

Etiology of cancer of the paranasal sinuses is not clear. Factors like wood dust, snuff, and chronic suppurative disease of the sinuses may be playing some role.

Carcinoma is more common in the maxillary sinus than in ethmoids and frontal sinuses (**Figs 38.6 and 38.8**).

Classification

There has been no agreement on classifying tumors at these sites because of late diagnosis of the disease in these inaccessible deep recesses of the nasal cavities.

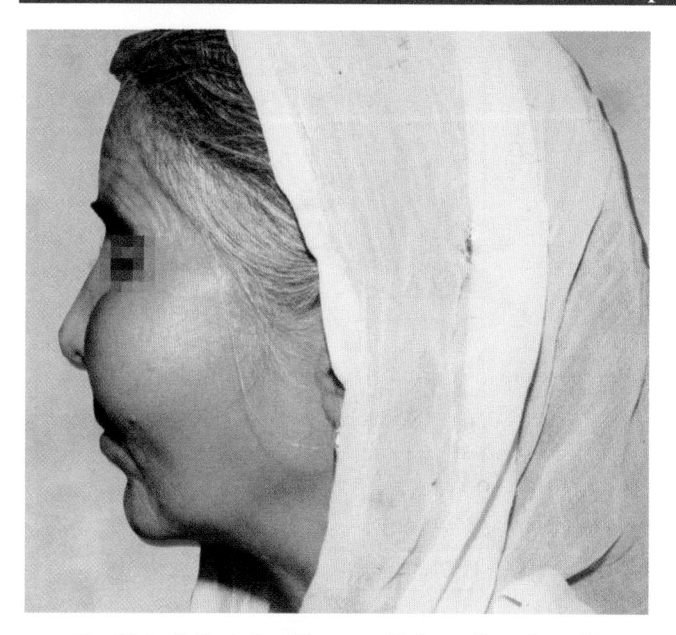

Fig. 38.6: Patient of malignancy of left maxillary sinus (1)

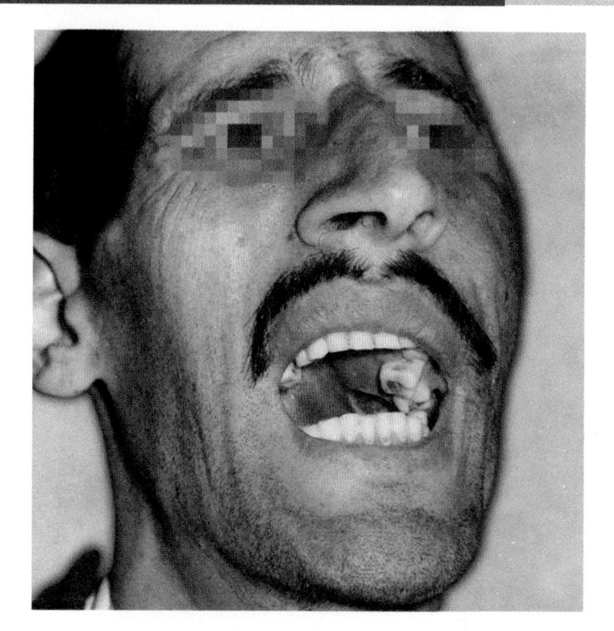

Fig. 38.7: Growth left maxilla involving palate and left alveolar border

Ohngren's classification: An imaginary line is drawn from the medial canthus to the angle of the mandible and a vertical line drawn through the pupils downwards, thus dividing the maxilla into four quadrants, namely anterosuperior, anteroinferior, posteroinferior, and posterosuperior.

It is thus appreciated that the tumors of the posterosuperior region carry worse prognosis as such tumors are difficult to resect than those situated inferiorly and anteriorly.

Lederman's classification: Lederman suggested two horizontal lines, one through the floor of the orbits and another through the floor of the antra, thus dividing the nose and paranasal sinuses into three compartments, i.e. infrastructure, mesostructure, and suprastructure (**Fig. 38.10**).

Two vertical lines are drawn through the medial canthi, which separate the ethmoid and nasal fossa from the maxillary sinus, the nasal septum separates the ethmoid and nasal fossa into right and left sides.

1. *Infrastructure sites (inferior region)*
   a. Floor of the antrum
   b. Floor of the nose
   c. Tumors simultaneously involving the hard palate and antrum or hard palate and floor of nose
   d. Dental tumors.
2. *Mesostructure (middle region)*
   a. Maxillary antrum
   b. Respiratory portion of the nasal fossa
   c. Vestibule of the nose
   d. Nasal septum
   e. Lateral nasal wall (including inferior turbinate).

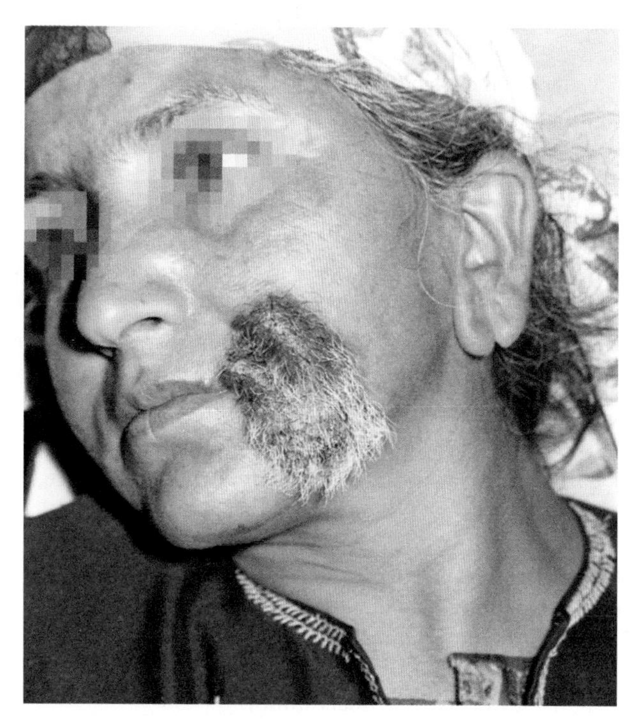

Fig. 38.8: Patient of malignancy of the right maxillary sinus showing palatal and alveolar involvement

3. *Suprastructure (superior region)*
   a. Ethmoid labyrinth
   b. Frontal sinus
   c. Sphenoid sinus (without nasopharyngeal involvement)
   d. Olfactory portion of the nose, i.e. above the middle turbinate.

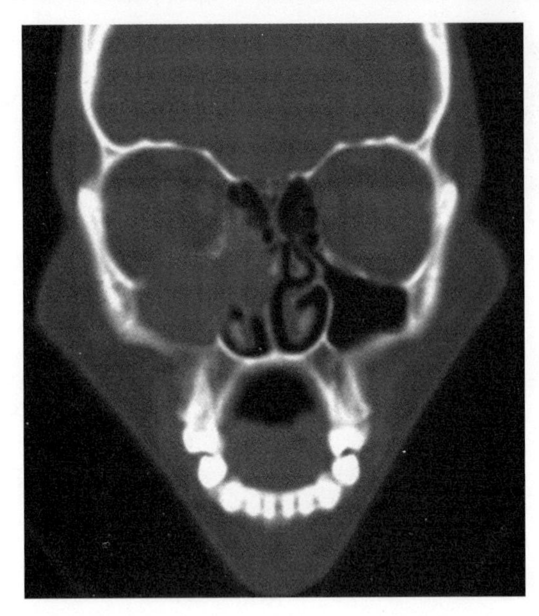

Fig. 38.9: CT image of right maxillary tumor with orbit involvement

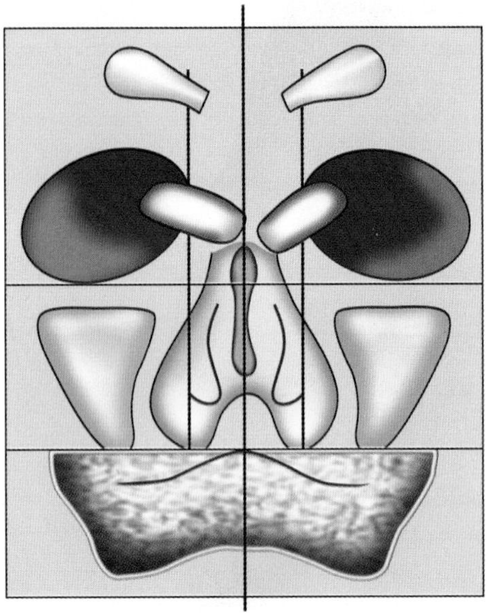

Suprastructure

Mesostructure

Infrastructure

Fig. 38.10: Lederman's classification for neoplasm of the nose and paranasal sinuses

Lederman's classification is based on the above mentioned regions and sites.

- T_1 Tumor limited to one sinus or tissue of origin, e.g. septum, turbinate or nasal vestibule.
- T_2 Tumor having limited spread to the same region or two adjacent horizontally or vertically related regions.
- T_3 i. Tumor involving three regions or compartments with or without orbital involvement.
  - ii. Extension of the tumor beyond the sinuses, i.e. nasopharynx, cranial cavity, buccal cavity, pterygopalatine fossa or involvement of the skin.

The N and M categories are the same as elsewhere.

Lederman's classification did not find wide acceptance.

TNM Classification

Maxillary sinus tumors:

Primary tumor (T)

- T_x Minimum requirements to assess the primary tumor cannot be met.
- T_0 No evidence of primary tumor.
- T_{is} Carcinoma *in situ.*
- T_1 Tumor confined to antral mucosa of infrastructure with no bone erosion or destruction.
- T_2 Tumor confined to the suprastructure mucosa with no bone erosion or to infrastructure with destruction of the medial or inferior bony walls only.
- T_3 More extensive tumor involving the skin of cheek, orbit, anterior ethmoid cells, or pterygoid muscles.
- T_4 Massive tumor with invasion of the cribriform plate, posterior ethmoids, sphenoid, nasopharynx, pterygoid plates or the base of skull.

Ethmoid tumors:

- T_1 Tumor confined to ethmoid with or without bone erosion
- T_2 Tumor extends into nasal cavity.
- T_3 Tumor extends into anterior orbit and/or maxillary antrum
- T_4 Tumor with intracranial extension.

Nodal involvement (N)

- N_x Minimum requirements to assess the regional nodes cannot be met.
- N_0 No clinically positive nodes.
- N_1 Single clinically positive homolateral node 3 cm or less in diameter.
- N_2 Single clinically positive homolateral node more than 3 cm but less than 6 cm in diameter or more than one homolateral lymph nodes, none more than 6 cm in diameter.
- N_3 Massive homolateral nodes, one more than 6 cm in diameter, bilateral nodes or contralateral nodes.

Distant metastasis

- M_x Minimum requirements to assess the distant metastasis cannot be met.
- M_0 No distant metastasis.
- M_1 Distant metastasis present.

Clinical Features

Malignancy of the paranasal sinuses usually presents in the late stages. Many patients present with facial swelling, when the growth has already extended beyond the sinus.

Nasal obstruction and blood-stained discharge or frank epistaxis may be the presenting features of a mass in the nasal cavity.

Dental pain is common and many times such patients land in dental clinics for extractions, without any relief. Palatal swelling and loosening of teeth may occur. Proptosis, orbital pain and epiphora may be complained or areas of paraesthesia or anesthesia over the cheek may be detected by such patients.

Diagnosis

The disease occurs mostly after 40 years of age. Visible facial swelling, a bleeding friable mass in the nose, fulness of the gingivobuccal region, palatal and alveolar swelling, proptosis and facial neuralgia should raise suspicion of malignancy in the nose and paranasal sinuses. An unresolving acute or chronic sinusitis may occur as a result of an underlying malignant process.

Spread of Malignant Lesions of the Paranasal Sinuses

Local spread: After filling the cavity, the growth causes bone destruction and may involve facial surface of the maxilla and skin over the face. Medially, the growth initially pushing out the lateral wall of nose, may present in the nose, wherefrom it may involve the ethmoids and nasopharynx.

The growth may spread to the cranial cavity from the nose and nasopharynx.

Posteriorly the spread occurs to the pterygopalatine fossa and infratemporal fossa resulting in trismus because of involvement of the pterygoids.

Superiorly the orbit gets involved resulting in proptosis or blindness.

Inferiorly the growth involves the oral cavity and palate.

Lymphatic spread: Lymphatics of the nose and paranasal sinuses drain first to retropharyngeal nodes, wherefrom these drain into the submandibular group of nodes. The retropharyngeal nodes are not palpable clinically. Blood spread may occur to the lungs and long bones of the body.

Investigation

Detailed examination of the nose and nasopharynx should be supplemented by radiology and proof puncture.

1. *Radiological examinations:* Plain views of the paranasal sinuses like occipitomental view, occipitofrontal view, oblique view of the ethmoid and base of the skull are of limited value in diagnosis showing any bony destruction and the rough extent of tumor (**Fig. 38.11**). CT sinuses gives better assessment of the base of the skull and posterior extension of the tumor alongwith a clear idea of the bony destruction.

   Magnetic resonance imaging (MRI) can help in distinguishing tumors from sinus inflammations. It is also useful to depict swellings arising from deeper soft tissues of the face, intracranial compartment and the orbit.

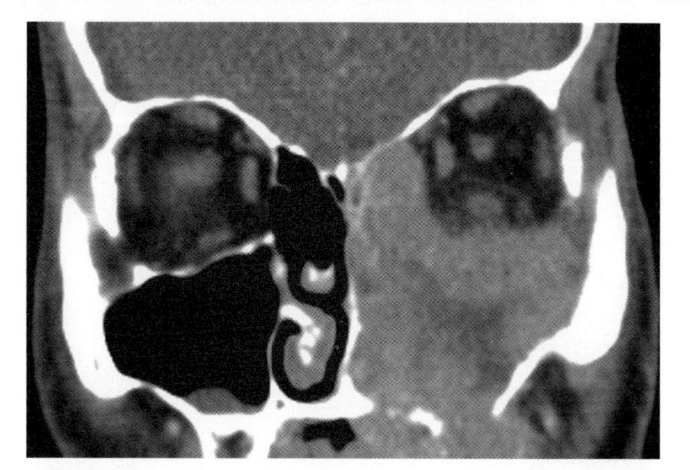

Fig. 38.11: CT scan showing malignancy of the left maxillary sinus

2. *Biopsy:* Tissue is taken for histopathological examination if growth is seen in the nose or oral cavity. Exploration of the antrum and biopsy may be undertaken by the sublabial route in suspicious cases. Preliminary antrumscopy has now proved to be of value in such cases.

Treatment

Because of late diagnosis and involvement of adjacent structures, treatment of cancer of the paranasal sinuses is difficult and prognosis is bad.

Surgery or radiotherapy alone have not shown good results. Combined therapy (surgery and radiotherapy) is the treatment of choice at present. Usually a preoperative dose of 5,500 to 6,000 rads of cobalt-60 is given over 5 to 6 weeks, followed by surgical excision. Sometimes the growth is removed surgically followed by postoperative radiotherapy.

Surgical procedures: The type of surgery performed depends upon the extent of involvement of the sinus and adjacent structures.

1. Total maxillectomy is done for an operable tumor involving the maxilla. The facial surface of the maxilla is exposed by Weber-Fergusson incision (**Fig. 38.12**) and the skin and soft tissues of the face are elevated. The soft palate is separated and the hard palate divided in the center. The bony attachments of the maxilla are broken and maxilla removed. For

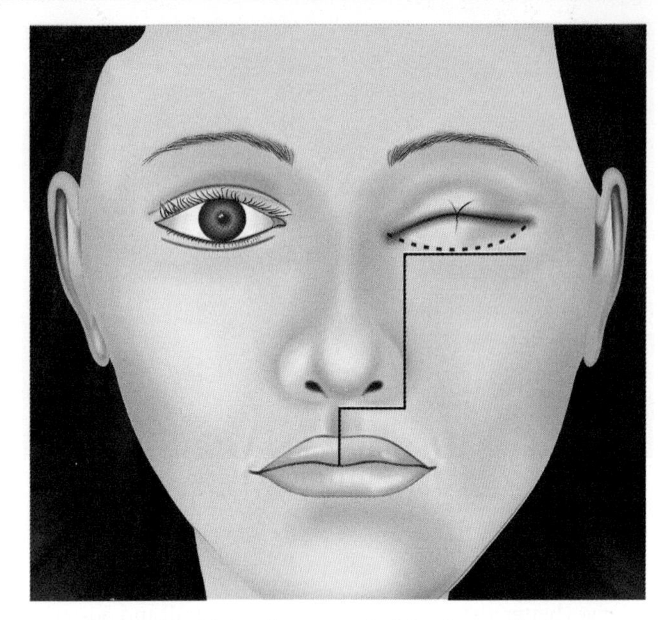

Fig. 38.12: Weber-Fergusson incision for maxillectomy

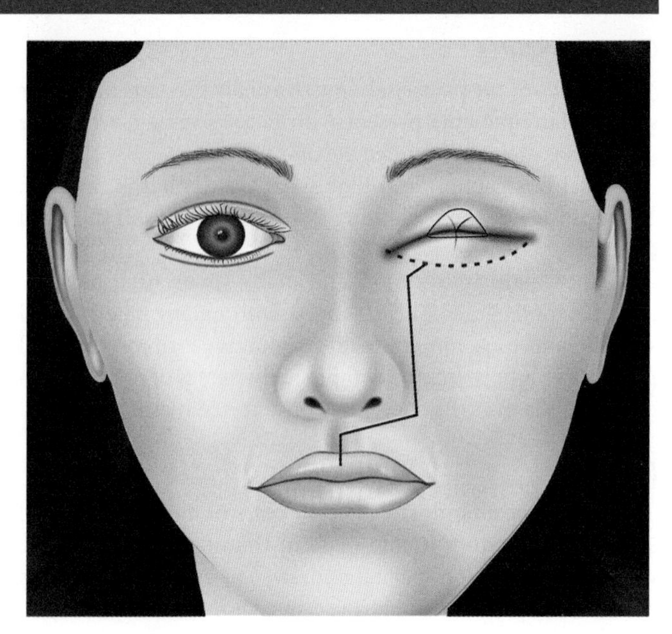

Fig. 38.13: Trotter's incision for maxillectomy

small limited tumors, partial maxillectomy may suffice. **Figure 38.13** shows the Trotter's incision.

2. *Extended maxillectomy:* Maxillectomy may be done along with orbital exentration, excision of the skin, face or the soft tissues in the infratemporal fossa if the growth involves these structures.
3. *Lateral rhinotomy:* This operation is done for tumors limited to the nasal cavity and ethmoids. An incision from the medial canthus follows the side of the nose into the nasal vestibule. The periosteum is elevated lateral bony wall of the nose broken and eradication of disease is done under direct vision.
4. *Neck dissection:* When metastasis is suspected in neck nodes, maxillectomy may be done along with block dissection of the neck nodes on that side.

Distant metastasis, inoperable metastatic nodes, involvement of the base of skull or nasopharynx are contraindications to surgical treatment.

Chemotherapy: Systemic anticancer drugs or intra-arterial chemotherapy through the external carotid artery may be given as adjuvant therapy and have only a palliative role.

Primary malignant tumors of the frontal sinus and ethmoids are rare and when present are also treated by the combined regime.

Chapter 39

Headache

Classification of Headache

The International Headache Society has classified headaches into the following types.

1. *Tension headache:* Tension headache is about five times more common than migraine, and these are the types of headaches most usually seen in general practice.
2. *Migraine:* Affects 10 percent of women and 2.5 percent of men.
3. Cluster headache.
4. *Miscellaneous:* Such as sinus headache, cold-induced headache, glaucoma-associated headache, drug-induced headache.

Other less common types of headache include:

i. Post-traumatic headache following severe head injury.
ii. *Cervicogenic headache:* Due to cervical spondylosis and causing pain on one or both sides of the neck radiating to the occiput, temples and frontal region.
iii. *Toxic headache:* After exposure to polluted environment, allergens, volatile chemicals and fumes.

DIAGNOSIS OF HEADACHES

Diagnosis should begin with a detailed medical history. The history taking session often provides enough information to yield a clear diagnosis, because many types of headaches have well-defined patterns of symptoms. Typical questions should be frequency of the headache—location of the pain, type of pain, duration of the headaches, time of the first episode, history of OTC medicines and history of head injury or surgery.

MANAGEMENT

In tension headache prompt and convincing reassurance is vital. Relaxation exercises, psychotherapy and biofeedback training are occasionally successful. Antidepressants and anxiolytics have a limited role, and all drugs including analgesics should be given for short periods under supervision, to prevent habituation and drug-induced headache.

MIGRAINE

Migraine is due to a vasomotor disturbance of arteries of the head. It is classically heralded by ocular prodromal symptoms; the pain is unilateral and of a throbbing, vascular type, and there may be associated nausea and vomiting. Migraine is easily diagnosed when presenting in this form, but it should be remembered that it is the most common cause of facial pain and is unlikely to have this classical presentation. Swelling and redness of the eyes and cheek, nasal obstruction and rhinorrhea are common accompaniments of pure migraine, and should not lure the otolaryngologist into thinking that nasal or sinus disease must be present.

Management of migraine is divided into abortive or symptomatic treatment for immediate relief of symptoms and prephylactic therapy for prevention of attacks.

SYMPTOMATIC TREATMENT

Analgesics (paracetamol, naproxen or aspirin) should be taken immediately when the attack begins and then repeated every 4 to 6 hours as necessary. Absorption is improved by ingestion of antiemetics such as domperidone, 10 to 20 mg. In recent years, serotonin (5th) receptor agonists have been introduced for the management of acute migraine. They act by reversing the dilation of cranial vessels seen during migraine. Sumatriptan is the prototype 5th receptor agonist. However, it is limited by its low oral bioavailability, high incidence of headache recurrence and contraindication in patients with coronary artery disease. Hence, the new 5th receptor agonists such as zelmitriptan, rizatriptan and nartriptan have become increasingly popular due to their better safety profiles.

PROPHYLAXIS

If the attacks occur more than twice each month, prophylactic agents such as calcium-channel blocker (flunarizine), beta blockers (propranolol) or cyproheptadine should be given.

CLUSTER HEADACHE

Treatment is with ergotamine, or sumatriptan given in anticipation of attacks or with methysergide or verapamil for the duration of cluster. In case of severe clusters, patients may require hospitalization. Oxygen, given at a rate of 6 to 8 liters/minute, often affords relief within 10 minutes. Lithium may be of value in chronic cluster headache.

Chapter 40

Facial Neuralgia (Pain in the Face)

The tissues of the face which contain pain-sensitive nerve endings are skin, mucosa, teeth, periosteum, blood vessels and the articular fat pads within the temporomandibular joints.

Pain in the face is a common presenting feature, and in history taking it is important to find out about the type of pain, its distribution, the duration of attacks, what stimulates them, and about any features which make the pain worse.

Pain caused by skin or mucosal lesions should be fairly easily excluded by examination of these tissues. Skin pain is caused by boils, cuts, bruises and burns which should be obvious. The well-known pain within the nose associated with acute viral infections is diagnosed by rhinoscopy, when an acutely infected mucosa will be apparent.

Pain due to periosteal disease in the face is caused by acute inflammation, cysts and tumors. Much of the periosteal area can be palpated, for example, the anterior walls of the sinuses, and the palate, and there will be evidence of swelling or tenderness on pressure.

Dental pain is associated with dental caries. The characteristic story that it is stimulated by change of temperature, as in drinking hot liquids, or by ingestion of sweet or spicy foods, suggests an origin in the teeth. Where dental disease is not obvious, but this story is present, percussion of the teeth is a useful clinical exercise.

Temporomandibular joint strain is common, and is due to the patient developing an abnormal biting pattern, frequently secondary to orthodontic problems, or due to ill-fitting or absent dentures. The pain is centralized in the temporal region, but may spread to the ear, and along the skin over the mandible. The temporomandibular joints are tender when the mouth is opened and closed, and some sideways deviation of the jaw on full opening is apparent. If the patient is seen during an acute episode, slight spasm of the masticatory muscles will be apparent. Radiography demonstrates that this is a functional abnormality, as signs of joint degeneration are absent, but there can be limitation of opening of the joint on one side. Treatment is orthodontic.

Vascular pain is characterized by the description of the pain as throbbing in character, and it is made worse by stooping or straining or by increase in the temperature of the face. Infective pains have a vascular component, for example, the pain of acute sinusitis and a tooth pulp infection are throbbing in character. In the absence of signs of infection, one should think of migraine, migrainous neuralgia and temporal arteritis.

Migrainous neuralgia is sufficiently different from migraine to be identified as a separate clinical entity. The patient is commonly male, aged between 25 and 40, and the attacks of pain, which last for a short period varying from a few minutes to an hour or two, are excruciating in degree, unilateral in distribution, centered around or deep to the eye, and accompanied by ipsilateral nasal obstruction with rhinorrhea. Attacks can occur once or more in 24 hours, and typically waken the patient about 3 am. A group of very similar attacks can occur over several weeks or months, and disappear, only to return in a similar fashion, perhaps years later. The pain is frequently precipitated by alcohol ingestion. Treatment is with clonidine hydrochloride (Dixarit).

Temporal arteritis always occurs after the age of 55 and gives rise to acute throbbing vascular-type pain in the temporal region. It is part of a giant-cell arteritis affecting many of the vessels of the head and neck, and is accompanied by lassitude and slight fever. The temporal arteries are tender to touch and feel thickened, and the overlying skin can be red. Temporal arteritis is an important disease to diagnose because although it is uncommon, its complications are serious, and it is amenable to treatment with systemic steroids.

Neuralgic pain is sharp and burning in character, and is interspersed with periods which are either free from pain or with a background ache. It occurs in disease affecting the nerves, when there will be evidence of altered sensation either to light touch or to a sharp pinprick. Neuralgic pain arising in the absence of evidence of neurological disease occurs in postherpetic neuralgia, when there will be a history of previous shingles, and in trigeminal neuralgia.

Trigeminal neuralgia rarely occurs before the age of 40. The trigeminal sensory dermatome always encloses the painful parts, and the ophthalmic area is least often affected. The pain is frequently stimulated by touching a specific part of the face—the trigger area—and initially consists of a series of short sharp spasms of pain, each one lasting a few minutes, but it can progress to a period of pain lasting several hours. The pain is severe, and if the patient is seen during an acute attack, spasm of the muscles of the ipsilateral side of the face will be noted. Treatment is with carbamazepine (Tegretol) starting with a dose of 100 mg twice a day, and increasing the dose until relief is obtained. The natural history of this condition is very variable, and the symptoms can disappear for a long period of time, only to recur. Surgical treatment with radiofrequency rhizotomy may be required in patients uncontrolled by medical therapy.

Atypical facial neuralgia is a rather unsatisfactory label applied to patients who have long-standing, often deep-seated, pain in the face in the absence of any clinical signs or of any characteristic history. These patients have often consulted many specialists and have had innumerable unsuccessful trials of medical or surgical treatment. They are often depressed, but this can be as much a function of their unremitting ailment as of psychological imbalance. Treatment is unsatisfactory, a combination of psychotropic drugs and psychotherapy giving the greatest chance of success.

MCQs on Nose

Select the most appropriate answer:

1. Nose is developed from:
   A. 1st branchial arch
   B. Second branchial arch
   C. Both A and B
   D. None of the above.
2. Inferior turbinate is:
   A. Separate bone
   B. Part of ethmoid bone
   C. Part of maxillary bone
   D. None of the above.
3. Middle turbinate is:
   A. Separate bone
   B. Part of ethmoid bone
   C. Part of maxillary bone
   D. None of the above.
4. Bulla ethmoidalis is situated on:
   A. Inferior meatus
   B. Middle meatus
   C. Superior meatus
   D. All of the above.
5. Maxillary sinus opening is situated on:
   A. Sphenoethmoidal recess
   B. Inferior meatus
   C. Superior meatus
   D. Middle meatus.
6. Posterior ethmoidal sinuses open in:
   A. Superior meatus
   B. Inferior meatus
   C. Middle meatus
   D. Sphenoethmoidal recess.
7. Keisselbach's plexus is formed by all of the following, except:
   A. Sphenopalatine artery
   B. Anterior and posterior ethmoidal arteries
   C. Infraorbital artery
   D. Septal branch of the superior labial artery.
8. Blood supply of the external nose is from all of the following, except:
   A. Infraorbital artery
   B. Dorsal nasal artery
   C. Supratrochlear artery
   D. Sphenopalatine artery.
9. Antral wash out:
   A. Is usually performed through the middle meatus
   B. The opening created in the sinus is permanent
   C. In children, it is best performed through the canine fossa
   D. May be carried out as a diagnostic or as a therapeutic procedure.
10. Infraorbital nerve is a branch of:
    A. Maxillary nerve
    B. Mandibular nerve
    C. Ophthalmic nerve
    D. None of the above.
11. Mucosa of nasal cavity is:
    A. Stratified squamous type
    B. Columnar type
    C. Pseudostratified ciliated columnar type
    D. Squamous type.
12. Cribriform plate is a part of:
    A. Frontal bone
    B. Ethmoid bone
    C. Sphenoid bone
    D. Nasal bone.
13. Upper limit of ethmoid cells is:
    A. Above the cribriform plate
    B. At the level of cribriform plate
    C. Below the cribriform plate
    D. None of the above.
14. Olfactory area is situated:
    A. In front of middle turbinate
    B. Above the middle turbinate
    C. Below the middle turbinate
    D. None of the above.

15. Infection of nose and paranasal sinuses mostly travels to intracranial compartment via:
    A. Blood vessels
    B. Direct extension
    C. Neural sheaths
    D. All of the above.
16. Color of olfactory area is:
    A. Grayish white
    B. Golden yellow
    C. Pinkish hue
    D. None of the above.
17. Sphenoid sinus drains in:
    A. Superior meatus
    B. Sphenoethmoid recess
    C. Middle meatus
    D. Inferior meatus.
18. Fibroma of the nasopharynx:
    A. Is most common in young boys
    B. May extend into the cranial fossa
    C. Bleeds excessively at biopsy
    D. All of the above.
19. Allergic rhinitis:
    A. Is usually associated with a pale nasal mucosa
    B. Is frequently associated with eosinophilia on nasal smear
    C. May be associated with clouding of the sinuses on X-ray in lime absence of infection
    D. All of the above.
20. Sepsis, chemosis and proptosis following an ENT infection suggest:
    A. Lateral sinus thrombosis
    B. Frontal osteomyelitis
    C. Brain abscess
    D. Cavernous sinus thrombosis.
21. A case of closed fracture of nasal bones with deformity comes after a fortnight. What should be the line of treatment?
    A. Closed reduction immediately
    B. Closed reduction after one week
    C. Closed reduction after one month
    D. No treatment is required if the air way is adequate.
22. Perforation of nasal septum occurs in:
    A. Tuberculosis
    B. Syphilis
    C. Trauma
    D. All of the above.
23. In ethmoidal nasal polypi:
    A. Recurrence occurs as a rule
    B. Recurrence does not occur on total removal and proper prophylaxis
    C. Rate of recurrence is very high
    D. Rate of recurrence is very low.
24. Antrochoanal polypi are usually:
    A. Single and unilateral
    B. Multiple and unilateral
    C. Multiple and bilateral
    D. Single and bilateral.
25. Little's area is supplied by all except:
    A. Anterior ethmoidal artery
    B. Mandibular artery
    C. Sphenopalatine artery
    D. Labial artery.
26. Saddle shaped nose is most commonly seen in:
    A. Tuberculosis
    B. Leprosy
    C. Trauma
    D. Syphilis.
27. Rhinosporodiosis is:
    A. Bacterial infection
    B. Viral infection
    C. Allergic disorder
    D. Fungal infection.
28. Rhinophyma is a complication of:
    A. Acne volgaris
    B. Psoriasis
    C. Seborrhic dermatitis.
    D. Acne rosacea.
29. Origin of nasopharyngeal fibroma is from:
    A. Penosteum of roof of nasopharynx
    B. Choanal borders
    C. Eustachian tube openings
    D. Fossa of rosenmullar.
30. The drug of choice in rhinoscleroma is:
    A. Sulpha drugs
    B. Penicillin
    C. Streptomycin
    D. Tetracycline.
31. Ethmoidal nasal polypi are of:
    A. Infective origin
    B. Allergic origin
    C. Neoplastic origin
    D. Idiopathic origin.
32. Ethmoidal nasal polypi are usually:
    A. Single
    B. Multiple and bilateral
    C. Unilateral
    D. None of the above.
33. Adenoidectomy is indicated in:
    A. Recurring attack of earache, deafness and acute otitis media.
    B. Adenoid facies
    C. Along with tonsillectomy
    D. All of the above.

34. The treatment of rhinoscieroma is mainly:
    A. Medical
    B. Surgical
    C. Radio therapy
    D. None of the above.
35. Karatagener's syndrome is characterized by each of the following, except:
    A. Mental retardation
    B. Dextrocardia
    C. Bronchiectasis
    D. Sinusitis.
36. Mulbery appearance of nasal mucous membrane is in:
    A. Coryza
    B. Chronic hypertrophic rhinitis
    C. Atrophic rhinitis
    D. Maxillary sinusitis
    E. None of the above.
37. Ozena is characterized by:
    A. Female patients
    B. Anosmia
    C. Fetid smell from nose
    D. All of the above.
38. The main presenting symptoms of ethmoidal nasal polypo persenting at the level of inferior turbinate are all, except:
    A. Repeated attacks of epistaxis
    B. Continuous nasal blockage
    C. Rhinorrhea
    D. Headache.
39. A rhinolith is a:
    A. Foreign body in nose
    B. Stone in nose
    C. Deposition of calcium over some foreign body in the nose
    D. Misnomer.
40. In malignancies of nasal cavity, the chief symptom is:
    A. Repeated epistaxis
    B. Continuous purulent and sangui nous discharge
    C. Headache
    D. Broadening of nasal bones.
41. Treatment of most of the nasal and paranasal malignancies consists of:
    A. Surgical excision
    B. Radiotherapy
    C. Chemotherapy
    D. All the above.
42. Which of the following is most frequently seen in the nose?
    A. Primary syphilis
    B. Secondary syphilis
    C. Tertiary syphilis
    D. Congenital syphilis.
43. Rhinosporiodosis is commonly seen in:
    A. Hilly areas
    B. Islands
    C. Tropical areas
    D. Throughout the world.
44. The most common etiological organism in the osteomyelitis of frontal bone is:
    A. *Pneumococcus*
    B. *Streptococcus*
    C. Anaerobic *streptococcus*
    D. *Staphylococcus aureus.*
45. Herniation of brain tissue with its dural coverings into the nasal cavity is called:
    A. Glioma
    B. Neurofibroma
    C. Encephalocele
    D. Olfactory neuroblastoma.
46. Unilateral nasal discharge suggests:
    A. Papilloma
    B. Nasal polyps
    C. Juvenile angiofibroma
    D. Foreign body.
47. Choanal polyps almost always originate in the:
    A. Posterior ethmoidal cell
    B. Nasopharynx
    C. Maxillary sinus
    D. Sphenoidal sinus.
48. Benign neoplasms of the nose and sinuses include all of th following, except:
    A. Dermoid
    B. Vestibular papilloma
    C. Juvenile angiofibroma
    D. Olfactory neuroblastoma.
49. Studer's syndrome is characterized by all of the following, except:
    A. Pain at root of nose and about the eye
    B. Pain beyond mastoid and in occiput
    C. Pain or itching of hard palate
    D. Myosis.
50. Cerebrospinal fluid rhinorrhea is characterized by all, except:
    A. Clear color
    B. Sediment formation after standing
    C. Containing glucose
    D. Being unilateral.
51. An uncorrected blow out fracture results in:
    A. Epiphora
    B. Exophthalmos
    C. Enophthalmos
    D. Cavernous sinus thrombosis.
52. Convulsion, unconsciousness and death following maxillary sinus irrigation suggests:

A. Meningitis
B. Air embolism
C. Septicemia
D. Maxillary artery thrombosis.

53. Mucocele of the frontal sinus:
A. Displaces the eye ball downwards and laterally
B. Produces proptosis and diplopia
C. Produces rarefying osteitis and erosion in the surrounding bone
D. All of the above.

54. Vidian neurectomy has been useful in treating:
A. Allergic rhinitis
B. Vasomotor rhinitis
C. Atrophic rhinitis
D. All of the above.

55. Injection of silicone may be useful in:
A. Treatment of atrophic rhinitis
B. Correction of small defects in the shape of nose
C. Both A and B
D. None of these.

56. The origin of osteomyelitis of the frontal bone:
A. In children is almost always the result of hematogenous spread
B. In adults is almost always the result of spread from an adjacent infection
C. Both A and B
D. None of these.

57. Cytologic examination of nasal secretions:
A. Suggests allergy when eosinophils are found
B. Rules out allergy when eosinophils are not found
C. Both A and B
D. None of these.

58. Headaches from sinusitis are:
A. Usually due to acute infection
B. Worse in the morning and usually improves by late afternoon
C. Aggravated by stooping or exertion
D. All of the above.

59. Rhinoscleroma is characterized by all, except:
A. Hard cartilage like nodules affecting upper respiratory tract membranes
B. Inflammation and ulceration of surrounding tissues
C. Presence of red shaped encapsulated bacilli
D. Response to streptomycin.

60. All of the following are related to cerebrospinal rhinorrhea, except:
A. Congenital defect of cribriform plate
B. Base of skull fracture
C. Retinoblastoma
D. Intranasal meningocele.

61. Which of the following is not a type of atopic allergy?
A. Bronchial asthma
B. Hay fever
C. Contact dermatitis
D. Eczema.

62. Which of the following tests are not related to allergic rhinitis?
A. Intracutaneous test
B. Scratch test
C. Patch test
D. Rast test.

63. All of the following lead to unilateral exophthalmos, except:
A. Tumors of the orbit
B. Malignant hypertension
C. Frontal sinus mucocele
D. Grave's disease.

64. Complications of sinus disease include:
A. Retrobulbar neuritis
B. Orbital cellulitis
C. Cavernous sinus thrombosis
D. All of the above.

65. Local defences of nose include:
A. Cilia
B. Film of mucous
C. Lysozymes
D. All of the above.

66. Prolonged use of vasoconstrictor nose drops results in:
A. Rhinitis sicca
B. Allergic rhinitis
C. Rhinitis medicamentosa
D. Mulberry turbinates.

67. The chief shortcoming of inferior meatal antrostomy has been:
A. Failure to eradicate sinus disease
B. Disruption of normal physiology
C. Inability to use procedure for bilateral disease
D. Closing of the window.

68. The most common etiological factor in hyperplastic rhinitis is:
A. Allergy
B. Chemical irritation
C. Septal deviation
D. Bacterial infection.

69. An endocrine dysfunction not infrequently found in vasomotor rhinitis patients is:
A. Hyperthyroidism
B. Hypothyroidism
C. Hyperparathyroidism
D. Diabetes mellitus.

70. In hereditary hemorrhagic telangiectasia:
    A. Bleeding time is prolonged
    B. Clotting time is prolonged
    C. Platelet count is increased
    D. All coagulation studies are normal.
71. An effective procedure for controlling epistaxis due to hereditary hemorrhagic telangiectasia is:
    A. Anterior ethmoid artery ligation
    B. Internal carotid ligation
    C. External carotid ligation
    D. Septal dermoplasty.
72. In severe epistaxis the pterygomaxillary fossa may be entered surgically in order to ligate the:
    A. Anterior ethmoid artery
    B. External carotid artery
    C. Posterior ethmoid artery
    D. Internal maxillary artery.
73. Regarding fibrous dysplasia all are true, except:
    A. Usually occurs before the age of 20 years
    B. Most often involves mandible
    C. Almost always appears radiologically translucent
    D. Is treated surgically.
74. The usual treatment of lethal midline granuloma is:
    A. Wide surgical removal
    B. Radiation therapy
    C. Antimetabolites
    D. Streptomycin.
75. Side effects of antihistamine include all, except:
    A. Hypertension
    B. Urinary retention
    C. Drowsiness
    D. Dryness of mouth.
76. Regarding ephedrine all are true, except:
    A. Is less potent than epinephrine
    B. Has a shorter duration of action than epinephrine
    C. Elevates blood pressure
    D. Produces bronchial muscle relaxation.
77. Conditions which respond significantly to antihistaminics include all, except:
    A. Common cold
    B. Hay fever
    C. Motion sickness
    D. Allergic dermatosis.
78. The usual nerve injured in maxillary fractures is:
    A. Anterior ethmoidal nerve
    B. Supraobital nerve
    C. Infraorbital nerve
    D. Sphenopalatine nerve.
79. Allergic contact dermatitis occurs most frequently in otolaryngology as:
    A. Vasomotor rhinitis
    B. Nasal polyposis
    C. Bronchial asthma
    D. External otitis.
80. A deflected nasal septum is corrected by:
    A. Straightening
    B. Inserting prosthesis
    C. Septoplasty
    D. Removal.
81. The clinical features of carcinoma of the maxillary antrum include all of the following, except:
    A. Entropion
    B. Proptosis
    C. Toothache
    D. Epiphora.
82. Regarding epistaxis which of the following is not true?
    A. If coming from the anterior part of the septum, the treatment is to pack the nostrils
    B. Sometimes requires arterial ligation
    C. May be a feature of hypertension
    D. Usually comes from little's area.
83. All of the following open into middle meatus, except:
    A. Nasolacrimal duct
    B. Anterior ethmoidal sinus
    C. Maxillary sinus
    D. Frontal sinus.
84. Features of fibroangioma of the nasopharynx include:
    A. It is highly destructive
    B. It is a benign tumor
    C. Never metastasizes
    D. All of the above.
85. All of the following are true about nasal polypi, except:
    A. Ethmoidal polypi are usually multiple
    B. Antrochoanal polyp is usually single
    C. They cause nasal obstruction
    D. They are sensitive to touch.
86. Which of the following is not true about rhinophyma?
    A. Nasal apex becomes bulbous in appearance
    B. Commoner in females
    C. It occurs due to hypertrophy of sebaceous glands at nasal apex
    D. The skin at nasal apex becomes coarse and pitted
    E. There is excessive secretion of sebaceous material at nasal tip.
87. All of the following features are of atrophic rhinitis, except:
    A. Commoner in males
    B. Fetor
    C. The patient is anosmic
    D. Nasal passages are roomy.
88. All of the following are true about chronic hypertrophic rhinitis, except:
    A. The main symptom is nasal obstruction

B. Hypertrophic posterior and inferior concha gives mulberry appearance on posterior rhinoscopy
C. The middle concha is usually affected
D. Sense of smell and taste may be impaired.

89. Cerebrospinal rhinorrhea may be caused by:
A. Leaking meningocele from anterior cranial fossa
B. Erosion of the cribriform plate of the ethmoid
C. Trans-sphenoidal hypophysectomy
D. All of the above.

90. Cysts of the maxillary sinus are usually of:
A. Nasal origin
B. Orbital origin
C. Dental origin
D. Auditory origin.

91. The olfactory nerves are about:
A. 5 filaments
B. 10 filaments
C. 15 filaments
D. 20 filaments.

92. Malignant tumors of the nose and sinuses:
A. Squamous cell carcinoma is the most common type
B. Retropharyngeal metastasis is common
C. Ameloblastoma is a rapidly growing, highly malignant tumor
D. Adenoid cystic carcinoma is associated with furniture workers.

93. Surgical treatment of allergic rhinitis:
A. Is preferable to long-term medication
B. Is indicated when nasal obstruction is due to polyps
C. Turbinectomy helps control excessive sneezing
D. In children, adenoidectomy is the first line of treatment.

94. Transitional cell papillomas (Ringertz tumors):
A. Most arise from the nasal septum
B. Malignant transformation is unknown
C. Radiotherapy is the treatment of choice
D. Complete removal is the treatment of choice.

95. All is true about Wegener's granulomatosis except:
A. Affects the nose, lungs and kidney
B. It is fatal without treatment
C. Steroids alone are favored to steroids with cytotoxic therapy.
D. The pathologic lesion is similar to polyarteritis nodosa.

96. Nasal lupus vulgaris:
A. Is a syphilitic skin infection
B. 'Apple jelly' nodules are seen histologically
C. Is a tuberculous skin infection
D. Tissue destruction can be reversed with drug treatment.

97. Septal hematomas:
A. May be due to blood dyscrasia
B. Unilateral nasal obstruction is the most common symptom
C. Usually resolve spontaneously
D. Treatment is conservative unless an abscess develops.

98. Bullet wounds in the head and neck region:
A. First principle of treatment is to safeguard the airway
B. First principle of treatment is to excise devitalized tissue
C. Primary closure is contraindicated
D. Fixation of fractures is not important.

99. Congenital choanal atresia:
A. Is most commonly membranous closure
B. Is most commonly bilateral
C. Occurs most commonly in males
D. Bilateral cases may be fatal.

100. Anosmia:
A. Causes no disturbance in the sense of taste
B. Can be assessed by simple objective methods
C. Is noticeable even if unilateral
D. May be due to a brain tumor.

101. Frontal sinus arterial supply is by:
A. Supraobital artery
B. Infraorbital artery
C. Facial artery
D. Greater palatine artery.

ANSWERS

1. A	14. B	27. D	40. B	53. D	66. D	79. D	92. A
2. A	15. D	28. D	41. D	54. B	67. D	80. C	93. B
3. B	16. B	29. A	42. D	55. A	68. A	81. A	94. D
4. B	17. B	30. C	43. C	56. A	69. B	82. A	95. B
5. D	18. D	31. B	44. D	57. A	70. D	83. A	96. B
6. D	19. D	32. B	45. C	58. D	71. D	84. D	97. B
7. C	20. D	33. D	46. D	59. B	72. D	85. D	98. A
8. D	21. D	34. A	47. C	60. C	73. B	86. B	99. A
9. D	22. D	35. A	48. D	61. C	74. C	87. A	100. D
10. A	23. C	36. B	49. B	62. B	75. B	88. C	101. A
11. C	24. A	37. D	50. B	63. D	76. B	89. D	
12. B	25. B	38. A	51. C	64. D	77. A	90. C	
13. A	26. D	39. C	52. B	65. C	78. C	91. D	

Section 3

Throat

Section Outlines

- Tracheostomy
- Disorders of Voice
- Tumors of the Larynx
- Block Dissection of the Neck
- Thyroid
- Bronchoscopy
- Esophagus
- Common Esophageal Diseases in ENT Practice
- Esophagoscopy
- Laser Surgery in ENT
- Principles of Radiotherapy
- Chemotherapy for Head and Neck Cancer
- Syndromes in Otorhinolaryngology
- Otolaryngologic Concerns in the Syndromal Child
- Head and Neck Cancer Staging
- Histopathology of Common Head and Neck Lesions
- Common ENT Instruments
- MCQs on Throat and Larynx

Chapter

41

Oral Cavity and Pharynx

Anatomy and Physiology of the Pharynx

The pharynx extends from the base of skull to the upper end of the esophagus at the level of the 6th cervical vertebra (**Fig. 41.1**). It is a fibromuscular structure consisting of the following layers from without inwards:

1. Outer layer of buccopharyngeal fascia
2. Muscular layer
3. Pharyngobasilar fascia
4. Mucosa.

The pharynx is divided into three parts: (i) nasopharynx, (ii) oropharynx, and (iii) laryngopharynx.

NASOPHARYNX

The part of pharynx which lies above the soft palate and behind the nasal cavity is called the nasopharynx.

Basisphenoid and basiocciput form the roof of the nasopharynx. The upper part of the posterior wall is formed by the anterior arch of the atlas. On the lateral, walls are the pharyngeal openings of the eustachian tubes about 1.25 cm behind the posterior end of the inferior turbinate. Above and behind, the tubal opening is a deep recess which is commonly a site for carcinoma and is called the *fossa of Rosenmuller.*

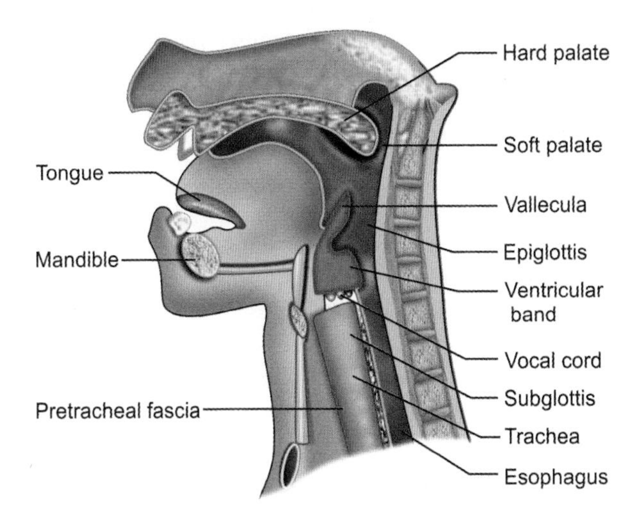

Fig. 41.1: Sagittal section through the upper air passages and esophagus

Nasopharyngeal Tonsil

It is a collection of lymphoid tissue under the mucosa of the nasopharynx situated at the junction of the roof and posterior wall of the nasopharynx. The collection disappears as the child starts growing. Hypertrophy of this lymphoid tissue is termed as adenoids. This lymphoid collection has no capsule. In the centre of the lymphoid mass is a depression called pharyngeal bursa. Thornwaldt's cysts, develop from the bursa.

OROPHARYNX

This is that part of the pharynx which extends from the level of the soft palate to the level of laryngeal inlet, below an imaginary horizontal line drawn at the level of the hyoid bone.

Anteriorly, the oropharynx opens in the buccal cavity at the oropharyngeal isthmus formed by the faucial pillars.

Tonsils

Tonsils are organized lymphoid structures situated between the faucial pillars. The tonsillar fossa is formed by the palatoglossal and palatopharyngeal folds and posterior part of the side of the tongue. A fold of mucous membrane, plica semilunaris connects the palatoglossal and palatopharyngeal folds superiorly. The *plica triangularis* is another fold of mucous membrane which connects the palatoglossal and palatopharyngeal folds at the lower pole of the tonsil.

The tonsil is covered by stratified squamous epithelium. The medial surface of the tonsil shows a number of crypts. An intratonsillar cleft is seen at the upper part of the tonsil and is a remnant of the second pharyngeal pouch.

The lateral surface of the tonsil is covered by a fibrous capsule attached loosely to the tonsillar bed.

Tonsillar bed: It is formed by loose areolar tissue, pharyngobasilar fascia, superior constrictor muscle and buccopharyngeal fascia. The internal carotid artery lies one inch lateral to the tonsil.

Blood supply of tonsil: Tonsillar branch of the facial artery is the main artery of supply. Branches of the following arteries also supply the tonsils:

i. Ascending pharyngeal artery
ii. Descending palatine artery
iii. Dorsalis linguae artery
iv. Ascending palatine branch of facial artery.

Veins: Veins emerge on the lateral surface and lower pole of the tonsil. Paratonsillar vein emerges on the lateral surface and pierces the superior constrictor muscle to end in the common facial vein and pharyngeal plexus of veins.

Lymphatic drainage: The efferent lymphatics emerge from the lateral aspect and end in the jugulodigastric group of deep cervical nodes. There are no afferent lymphatics.

Waldeyer's Ring

The lymphatic tissues of the pharynx and oral cavity are arranged in a ring-like manner around the oropharyngeal inlet (**Fig. 41.2**). The inner ring consists mainly of the nasopharyngeal tonsil, peritubal lymphoid tissues, faucial tonsil and lingual tonsil. The efferents from this ring drain to lymph nodes situated around the neck forming the outer ring. The lymphoid tissues have a protective function.

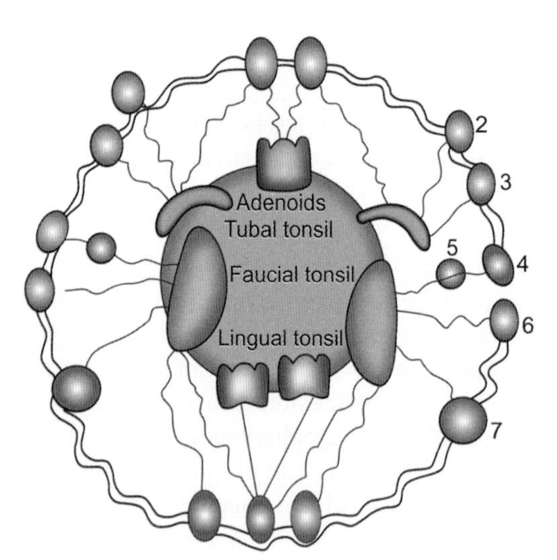

Fig. 41.2: Waldeyer's lymphatic ring and its connections

LARYNGOPHARYNX (HYPOPHARYNX)

This part of the pharynx lies behind the larynx and partly surrounds the larynx. Superiorly, it communicates with the oropharynx and starts at the level of the hyoid bone. Inferiorly, it extends up to the upper end of the esophagus at the lower border of the cricoid cartilage. It is divided into three parts: (i) pyriform sinus, (ii) postcricoid region, and (iii) posterior pharyngeal wall.

Pyriform Fossa

The pyriform fossa is a recess on each side of the larynx. It is bounded medially by the aryepiglottic fold, laterally by the thyrohyoid membrane in the upper part and medial surface of the thyroid cartilage in the lower part. Superiorly, the fossa is separated from the vallecula by the pharyngoepiglottic fold.

The fossa communicates below with the upper end of the esophagus.

Postcricoid Region

The postcricoid region is the lower part of the laryngopharynx and is formed by mucosa extending from the upper to lower border of the cricoid cartilage.

Posterior Pharyngeal Wall

This part of the hypopharynx extends from the level of the hyoid bone down up to the upper end of the esophagus. The rest of the mucosa is included into the lateral pharyngeal wall.

MUSCLES OF PHARYNX

Two layers of muscles form the pharyngeal wall. The circular layer is formed by the superior, middle and inferior constrictors which form the side and posterior wall of the pharynx. The longitudinal muscle layer is formed by the palatopharyngeus and stylopharyngeus muscles. The pharyngeal muscles help in deglutition. While the longitudinal muscles elevate the pharynx, the circular group help in propelling the bolus downwards.

NERVE SUPPLY

Pharynx is supplied through pharyngeal plexus which lies mainly on the middle constrictor muscle. This is formed by the pharyngeal branches of the vagus and glossopharyngeal nerves and sympathetic fibers around the vessels. The vagus supplies the motor fibers through its cranial accessory nerve. The glossopharyngeal is the main sensory nerve but supplies motor fibers to stylopharyngeus. The recurrent laryngeal nerve sends a branch to the inferior constrictor.

Soft Palate

It is a fibromuscular structure attached to the posterior edge of the hard palate by the palatine aponeurosis, which is formed by the expanded tendons of tensor palati muscles. Other muscles which take part in its formation are levator palati, palatoglossus, palatopharyngeus and musculus uvulae.

Laterally, the soft palate is attached to the pharynx. Posteriorly it is free.

NERVE SUPPLY

All the muscles of the soft palate except tensor palati are supplied by the cranial root of the accessory through the vagus. Tensor palati is supplied by the mandibular division of the trigeminal nerve.

The soft palate plays an important role in closure of the nasopharyngeal isthmus and, therefore, helps in deglutition and speech.

PASSAVANT'S RIDGE OR BAR

This is a rounded ridge which appears on the posterior pharyngeal wall during closure of the nasopharyngeal isthmus. The posterior free border of the soft palate comes in contact with this ridge to close the nasopharynx during deglutition. The ridge is raised by the contraction of upper fibers of the superior constrictor and the palatopharyngeus muscle.

Physiology of the Pharynx

The pharynx serves the following purposes:

1. It serves as an air and food passage.
2. Lymphoid aggregation in the nasopharynx and oropharyngeal isthmus have a protective role.
3. Pharyngeal muscles are important for deglutition.
4. The pharynx plays an important role in speech. It acts as a resonator of the voice. Besides, the pharynx is a site for various reflexes and is related to the opening of the eustachian tubes.

FUNCTIONS OF THE PHARYNGEAL LYMPHOID TISSUES

The exact functions of the subepithelial lymphoid tissues are not very clear. These probably play a defensive role. The strategic location of the faucial tonsils and nasopharyngeal lymphoid tissues suggests that these structures are concerned with sampling of air and food and thus constantly monitor the bacterial flora. Antibodies are formed against these microorganisms and thus help in the body's defence mechanism. Since, these lymphoid structures atrophy with the growth it appears that this defence mechanism is mainly active during childhood.

Deglutition

Deglutition is a process by which food passes from the oral cavity into the stomach through the esophagus. This process involves three stages:

First stage (voluntary): After the food is masticated and made into a bolus, the posterior part of the tongue propels the food into the oropharynx. The soft palate rises and closes the nasopharynx.

Second stage (pharyngeal stage): In this stage, food passes from the oropharynx into the esophagus. During this stage, the larynx is raised and laryngeal inlet gets closed to prevent food from going into the trachea. Retroversion of the epiglottis helps to close the approach to the laryngeal inlet. Breathing momentarily stops and the nasopharyngeal isthmus remains closed. The pharynx is elevated and the pharyngoesophageal junction opens to receive the bolus which is pushed down by contraction of the circular muscles of the pharynx.

Third stage (esophageal stage): This stage consists of passage of food down the esophagus. Once the cricopharynx opens, the food passes into the esophagus. It is carried down by peristaltic waves. The cardiac sphincter opens in response to the peristaltic waves and food thus enters the stomach.

In addition, deglutition also serves the following functions.

i. Disposal of dust and bacteria-laden mucus conveyed by ciliary action to the pharynx from nasal passages, sinuses, tympanic cavities, larynx and tracheobronchial tree.
ii. Opening of the pharyngeal ostia of pharyngotympanic tubes, to establish equalization of pressure on the outer and inner surfaces of the tympanic membranes.

The resting intrapharyngeal pressure is equal to the atmospheric pressure. During swallowing, there is a transitory rise of about 40 mm Hg pressure at the pharyngoesophageal junction. There occurs a region of raised pressure about 3 cm in length. During swallowing this pressure falls abruptly just before the pharyngeal peristaltic wave reaches this zone. This indicates a relaxation of the sphincter. Immediately after the bolus has passed, the sphincter contracts strongly with a rise of pressure to 50 to 100 mm Hg. This abrupt closure coincides with the arrival of the pharyngeal peristaltic wave and has the function of preventing reflux while peristalsis is occurring in the upper esophagus. When the bolus has passed further down the esophagus, the pressure in the pharyngoesophageal zone returns to normal, i.e. the sphincter returns to the normal state of tonic contraction.

SOUNDS DURING DEGLUTITION

Two sounds can be heard on auscultation over the esophagus during swallowing. They can be recorded electrically:

1. The first sound occurs immediately after the commencement of the act and is probably due to the fluids impinging on the posterior pharyngeal wall.
2. The second sound resembles a bubbling or trickling noise and occurs at a variable interval of 4 to 10 seconds after the first sound and persists for 2 to 3 seconds. It is heard

most clearly over the epigastrium. In recumbant subjects, the second sound is replaced by a few discrete squirting sounds, each of one second duration. When a solid bolus is swallowed, the second sound may be absent.

THIRST SENSATION

The sensation of thirst is composed of two components:

1. The first is a pharyngeal sensory element. This is due to dehydration causing decreased salivary secretion and drying of the pharyngeal mucosa with consequent stimulation of the special sensory receptors. Impulses from those receptors are conducted along fibers in the 9th and 10th nerves. This pharyngeal component can be abolished by stimulating salivary secretion or by local anesthesia of the pharyngeal mucous membrane.
2. The extrapharyngeal component or "thirst drive" is supposed to be the central component (not agreed by all). It seems to be related to intracellular osmolarity. Intravenous hypertonic saline or a high intake of salt with low water intake, causing intracellular dehydration and a rise in intracellular crystalloid osmotic pressure produces thirst. This osmotic effect acts on the osmoreceptor neurons in the hypothalamus.

Chapter 42

Common Symptoms of Oropharyngeal Diseases and the Method of Examination

Common Symptoms of Oropharyngeal Diseases

PAIN

Pain is a common symptom in the oropharyngeal area usually resulting from acute infections like tonsillitis, tonsillar abscess, trauma and sometimes due to carcinomas. Pain from the oropharyngeal diseases may be referred to the ear (referred otalgia).

Difficulty in Deglutition

Difficulty in deglutition may result from acute infections of the oral cavity.

Dysphagia means difficulty in swallowing. This can result from a variety of lesions in the oral cavity, pharynx and esophagus (**Fig. 42.1**). The lesions could be inflammatory, paralytic or neoplastic.

Odynophagia is painful deglutition caused by inflammatory lesions in the oropharynx or supraglottis. *Regurgitation* occurs in paralytic lesions of the soft palate when the ingested material regurgitates into the nose. Paralysis of the pharynx may lead to dysphagia as well as to aspiration into the trachea.

Difficulty in Respiration

Trauma, tumors and infections can lead to airway obstruction. Ludwig's angina, diphtheria and peritonsillar abscess may involve the larynx and result in dyspnea.

Difficulty in Speech

Palatal paralysis or sometimes adenoidectomy lead to improper closure of the nasopharyngeal isthmus with resulting hyper-nasality of voice called *rhinolalia aperta.*

Enlarged adenoids or nasopharyngeal tumors result in a closed nasal voice. This defect is called *rhinolalia clausa.*

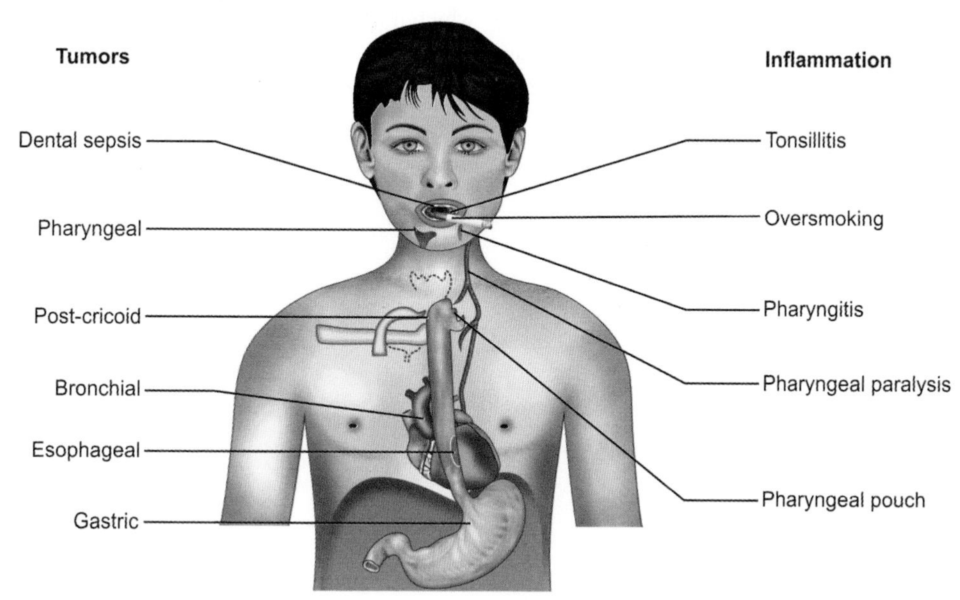

Fig. 42.1: Causes of dysphagia

Ulceration of Pharyngeal Mucosa

Ulceration of the pharynx may be manifestation of systemic diseases like leukemia, agranulocytosis or aplastic anemia.

Cervical Lymphadenopathy

Enlargement of the cervical nodes is commonly due to infective or neoplastic lesions of the oral cavity, pharynx, larynx and bronchi.

Method of Examination of the Oral Cavity and Pharynx

The clinical examination is done using a light source and head mirror in a systemic manner. The lips are examined first to note any color changes, ulcerations or tumor. The patient is asked to open the mouth and an inspection of the oral vestibule is done. A tongue depressor is used to retract the cheeks. The patient is asked to lift the tip of the tongue and orifices of the submandibular ducts and floor of mouth is seen.

Orodental hygiene is assessed and attention is given to the teeth as to the cause of pharyngeal disease. Movements of the tongue are noted for paralysis or neoplastic infiltration.

Faucial pillars and condition of the tonsils are noted. Pressure by the tongue depressor squeezes the debris from the tonsillar crypts in chronic tonsillitis. The color of the mucosa, ulcerations and membrane formation are looked for in the oropharyngeal and buccal mucosa.

The tongue depressor is used to depress the anterior two-thirds of the tongue for oropharyngeal examination. It should not be put on posterior-third of the tongue to avoid gagging. Surface of the hard and soft palate is noted for any clefts, ulcers or tumor. Movements of soft palate are observed by asking the patient to say *Ah*.

The postnasal discharge which indicates a nasal disease is seen trickling behind the soft palate. This may be the cause for many pharyngeal symptoms. The posterior pharyngeal wall is seen bulging in case of retropharyngeal abscess.

MIRROR EXAMINATION

A view of the nasopharynx by a postnasal mirror and that of the laryngopharynx by a laryngeal mirror is an important examination for diagnosing the pharyngeal diseases.

PALPATION

Finger palpation is necessary to examine the inside of the oral cavity and pharynx and should be routinely done. Bidigital examination of the submandibular salivary gland and its duct is done for calculus.

Palpation of the tongue (kept inside mouth) and that of the floor of the mouth is necessary for evaluating the extent of a tumor infiltration. Palpation of the tonsils and base of the tongue is necessary to diagnose certain infiltrative growths which may not show on the surface. An elongated styloid process may be felt on palpating through the tonsillar fossa. Palpation of the neck for lymph nodes forms an essential part of the examination.

INVESTIGATIONS

Hematological Tests

Like hemoglobin estimation total and differential counts are particularly required in ulcerations of the oral cavity and oropharyngeal mucosa. Serological tests are done to rule out syphilis.

Radiological Investigation

A plain X-ray of the neck (lateral view) provides clues for evaluating pharyngeal diseases. X-ray of the chest, lateral view of the nasopharynx, X-ray of the mandible are the other views which may prove useful.

CT scan of the neck, however, is the radiological investigation of choice for space occupying lesions.

Chapter

43

Common Diseases of the Buccal Cavity

Many lesions of the oral cavity are dealt by the dentists. Some of the common diseases of otolaryngologist interest are described here.

Stomatitis

Stomatitis is a general term for diffuse inflammation of the mouth. Inflammation of the oral mucosa can be caused by local and systemic diseases.

LOCAL CAUSES

Traumatic stomatitis: The trauma may be due to ill-fitting dentures, hot foods, corrosives, simple cut of the mouth, too vigorous use of a hard toothbrush, medicaments, fumes, smoke and radiotherapy.

Infective stomatitis: Inflammation of the oral cavity may result from viruses, bacteria or fungi.

1. Viral infections like herpes simplex or herpes zoster start as small painful vesicles which later ulcerate, involving the lip, buccal mucosa and palate.
2. Bacteria may produce inflammation like in acute ulcerative stomatitis (Vincent's angina), also known as trench mouth, with a characteristic fishy odor. Acute stomatitis can be caused by staphylococcal, streptococcal or gonococcal infections.
3. *Fungal stomatitis (moniliasis, thrush):* Stomatitis caused by *Candida albicans* is known as thrush or moniliasis.

The infection is common in debilitated patients, marasmic children and patients receiving broad-spectrum antibiotics. The lesions appear as white raised patches on the buccal mucosa, tongue and gingivae. These patches may coalesce to form a membrane which can be removed. Diagnosis can be confirmed by microscopical examination that show the fungal hyphae.

The disease is treated by local application of 1 percent gentian violet or a suspension of nystatin glycerine. The underlying debility needs attention.

Lichen planus: The mucous membrane lesions of this disease of unknown etiology appear as dull white or milky dots in a lace-like arrangement. The associated skin lesions help in diagnosis.

Other local causes are the following:

i. Aphthous ulcers
ii. Behcet's syndrome
iii. Pemphigus
iv. Stomatitis due to drugs
v. Excessive doses of bismuth, lead, iodides and mercury.

SYSTEMIC CAUSES

Deficiency of vitamins like the B-complex group and vitamin C also cause mucosal ulceration, particularly of the lips, angle of mouth and gingivae as in pernicious anemia, tropical sprue and malabsorption syndromes. Mucosal ulceration of the oral cavity and pharynx may be the presenting feature of agranulocytosis, leukemias, polycythemia and infectious mononucleosis.

RECURRENT ULCERATIVE STOMATITIS (APHTHOUS ULCERS)

Recurrent painful ulcerations of the oral mucosa is a common condition of unknown etiology. Various factors like viruses, endocrine disturbances, psychosomatic factors, habitual constipation and autoimmune reaction have been put forward as probable causative factors. The lesions, single or multiple, present as small superficial ulcers surrounded by erythema. These usually occur in the gingivobuccal groove, tongue or buccal mucosa and are very painful. There is no definite treatment but cauterization of the ulcers and local steroids in the form of hydrocortisone lozenges may help. Attention should be given to orodental hygiene and underlying nutritional deficiencies or constipation.

Behçet's Syndrome

This is a disease of unknown origin, characterized by ulcerations of the oral cavity, external genitalia and conjunctivitis.

Sometimes neurological manifestations like encephalitis and blindness may occur. Steroids may prove helpful in treating this disease.

PEMPHIGUS

Bullous lesions without erythema around them occur on the oral mucosa and the skin. The bullae rupture leaving a raw area. The cause is unknown. Treatment is by steroids.

IDIOPATHIC ORAL FIBROSIS (SUBMUCOUS FIBROSIS)

This consists of progressive fibrosis involving the oral mucosa and is accompanied by trismus.

Etiology

The exact etiology is not known but various predisposing factors are betel-nut, pan and tobacco chewing. Females are more affected than males and the disease is most common in the age group of 30 to 50 years.

Clinical Features

Various stages of the disease are the following:

1. *Prodromal stage:* In this stage, the patient complains of soreness and intolerance to spices and salts. The ulcers and blisters are not seen.
2. *Stage II:* In this stage, the patient has sense of stiffness inside the mouth and some difficulty in opening the mouth. There is pallor over the soft palate and fauces.
3. *Advanced stage:* The patient has marked trismus and difficulty in protrusion of the tongue. The incisor bite is reduced from the normal 4.5 cm to 2.5 cm. The mucosa of the oral cavity and oropharynx looks pale and rigid. The vestibule of mouth is obliterated and the patient cannot puff out the cheek. The anterior faucial pillars are markedly fibrosed with marked limitation of movement of the soft palate. The uvula looks like a rudimentary bud. It is not clear whether this should be regarded as precancerous condition or not.

Diagnosis

A history of betel chewing with the characteristic symptoms and signs suggest the diagnosis. The blood picture is of anemia and the ESR is raised.

Biopsy: It shows atrophy of the epithelial layers with increased mitotic activity of the basal layers. Subepithelial tissue shows increased thickening and hyalinized collagen and fibrous tissue and infiltration by lymphocytes and plasma cells.

Treatment

There is no satisfactory treatment. Various methods adopted are steroids (locally), sectioning of fibrotic bands and vitamin A administration. The anemia and hypochlorhydria are corrected.

TONGUE ULCERS

Various ulcers of the tongue are described in **Table 43.1**.

Table 43.1: Characteristics of various ulcer

Types of ulcer	Characteristic features
Simple	
1. Dyspeptic	Multiple, small, painful and on a red base.
2. Dental	Caused by irritation of a sharp tooth, has features of chronic simple ulcer. It has sloping edges, slight induration and heals on removal of the offending tooth.
Chronic nonspecific (e.g. following fissures)	Has the features of a chronic simple ulcer with slight induration.
Tuberculous	Usually associated with pulmonary tuberculosis, situated on the tip of the tongue, painful, undermined edges and thin pale granulation tissue on the floor.
Syphilitic	
1. Primary	Occurs on the lip, characteristic induration, enlargement of regional glands, scrapings of ulcer will show spirochete on dark ground illumination.
2. Secondary	Snail track ulcers and mucous patches.
3. Tertiary	Single gummatous ulcer on dorsum of tongue near midline with punched out appearance and wash lather base. No fixity of tongue. Rarely multiple gumma.
Herpetic	Multiple painful ulcers starting as vesicles.
Malignant	Usually at margin of anterior two-thirds (squamous epithelioma) not painful, local lesion may be an ulcer: (i) with raised everted edges with induration of base and surrounding area, (ii) a warty proliferation, (iii) a nodule in the tongue, or (iv) a fissure with restriction of free mobility. Regional lymph glands enlarged and hard.

ACQUIRED IMMUNODEFICIENCY SYNDROME

Acquired immunodeficiency syndrome (AIDS) was first recognized in 1981. The cause of the disease is the HIV virus. These patients have a specific impairment in the cell-mediated immunity. The disease is prevalent in homosexuals, intravenous drug users and those receiving repeated blood transfusion.

The common ENT manifestations of this disease include recurrent upper respiratory infection, oropharyngeal ulceration, mucocutaneous herpes simplex and Kaposi's sarcomas. Kaposi's sarcoma (KS) lesions are typically palpable but not exophytic, purple in color, discrete, initially painless and may involve any part of body.

Oral lesions including thrush, hairy leukoplakia and *aphthous* ulcers are particularly common in patients with untreated HIV infection.

Thrush due to *Candida* infection and oral hairy leukoplakia secondary to EBV infection are usually indicative of fairly advanced disease, i.e CD4 + T cell counts < 300/uz. Thrush appears as white cheesy exudates often on an erythematous mucosa in the posterior oropharynx. Most commonly seen in the soft palate, early lesions are seen along the gingival border. Diagnosis is by direct examination of the scrapings for pseudohyphal elements.

Oral hairy leukoplakia presents as white frond like lesions generally along lateral borders of the tongue or on adjacent buccal mucosa.

Treatment consists of topical podophyllin or systemic therapy with acyclovir.

Aphthous ulcers of posterior oropharynx are also seen with regularity in patients with HIV infection.

Topical anesthetics provide symptomatic relief of short duration.

Esophagitis secondary to *Candida*, CMV or HSV infections may present as odynophagia and retrosternal pain. Esophagus may also be the site of Kaposi's sarcoma and lymphoma.

Acute bronchitis and sinusitis are prevalent during all stages of HIV infection—severe cases occurring in patients with lower CD4 and T cell count. All sinuses can be involved although the maxillary sinus is the one most commonly infected. High incidence of sinusitis results from an increased frequency of infection with an encapsulated organism like *Haemophilus influenzae* and *Streptococcus pneumoniae*. In patients with low CD4 T cell counts, one may see mucormycotic infections of the sinuses. Mucormycosis of sinuses in patients with HIV infections may progress more slowly.

Management

Acquired immunodeficiency syndrome (AIDS) is a fatal disease. No definite treatment is available till date. Various antiviral drugs, amphotericin chemotherapy and modulation of the patient's immune system by various mechanism are under study.

Cysts of Mouth

Cysts of the oral cavity may be of developmental origin or may occur because of other lesions.

DEVELOPMENTAL CYSTS AND LINGUAL THYROID

Cysts may develop at the sites of embryonic fusion in the line of fusion of the two maxillae and from the tissues of the incisive canal (like nasopalatine cysts) or at the sites of fusion of the premaxilla with maxilla between the incisor and canine teeth.

Mucous Cysts

The orifice of a mucous gland may get blocked as a result of trauma or infection which leads to development of a mucous cyst. It is commonly seen on the lips and buccal mucosa.

RANULA

Retention cysts of the minor salivary glands or cystic degeneration of the sublingual salivary glands may lead to the development of a cystic swelling in the floor of mouth under the tongue called the *ranula* (**Fig. 43.1**). It presents as a grayish white, cystic swelling commonly seen in children. This swelling may sometimes burrow deep in the tissues of the floor of the mouth between muscles into the neck, when it is called a plunging *ranula.* Treatment is either complete excision or marsupialization of the cystic cavity.

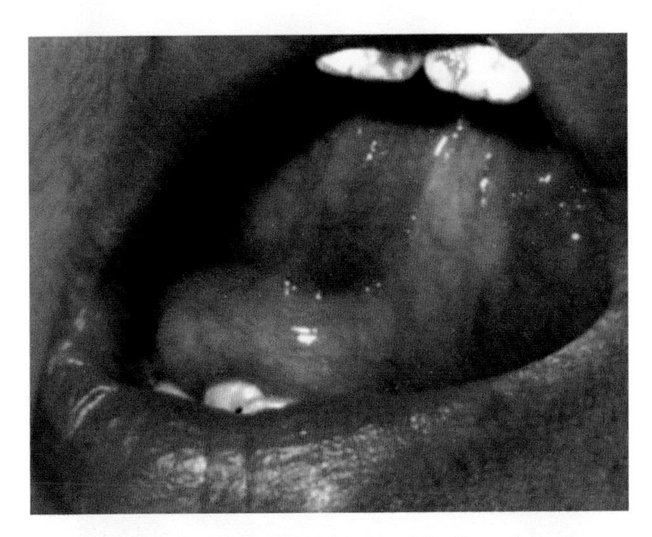

Fig. 43.1: Ranula on the right side of the floor of mouth

LINGUAL THYROID

It is an ectopic thyroid situated at the foramen cecum, at the junction of anterior two-thirds and posterior one-third of dorsum of the tongue. It may be only functioning thyroid tissue and may give rise to dysphagia, dyspnea, impairment of speech or hemorrhage (**Fig. 43.2**).

The tissue when operated upon can be transplanted in the form of slices at various sites in neck and in the submandibular salivary gland area.

Carcinoma of the Tongue

Squamous cell carcinoma is the most common cancer of the tongue. The etiology is uncertain but factors like chewing tobacco or betel nut, smoking, syphilis and poor orodental hygiene are thought to play a part. The disease affects males more frequently than females. The lesions present as a slough covered ulcerated mass with raised margins which bleed easily on touch. The surrounding areas are indurated and may involve the adjacent floor of the mouth. Lymph node metastasis is common, particularly from the posterior one-third, where the lesion is usually poorly differentiated and metastasis is bilateral.

TREATMENT OF CANCER OF THE ANTERIOR TWO-THIRDS

Lesions of size less than a centimeter can be either treated by implantation of radium needles or by surgical excision.

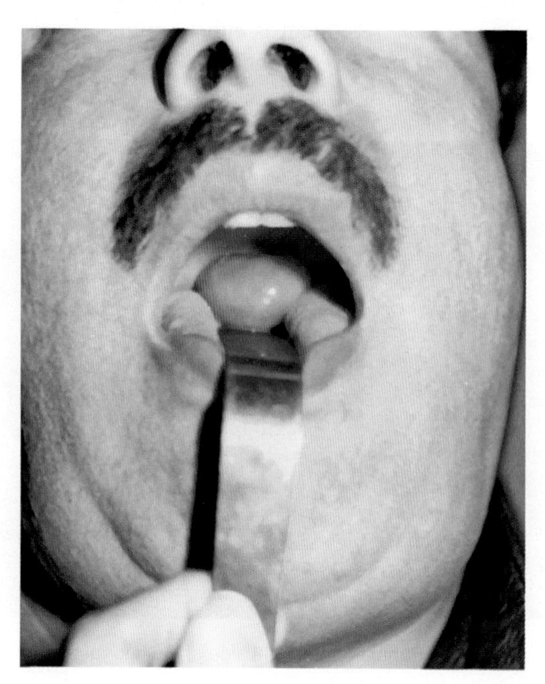

Fig. 43.2: Lingual thyroid

Larger lesions require hemiglossectomy. Growths involving the floor of the mouth and adjacent mandible are treated by removal of growth en bloc with the mandible and neck nodes (*Commando operation*).

Cancer of the posterior one-third is treated by external radiotherapy. If it does not respond to radiotherapy, surgical excision of the lesion with supraglottic or total laryngectomy is done. The latter is done to avoid aspiration.

Ludwig's Angina (Fig. 43.3)

This is an acute inflammatory condition producing cellulitis of the floor of the mouth, often caused by sepsis in the mouth. The patient is toxic and presents with swelling and edema of the floor of the mouth and brawny induration of the submandibular and submental region. There occurs difficulty in swallowing and breathing as the tongue is pushed up by the edematous tissues of the floor. The edema may spread to the larynx.

TREATMENT

Heavy doses of antibiotics, clindamycin with metronidazole are given. If the infection does not subside, it may require incision and drainage. Respiratory obstruction may need a tracheostomy.

Tumors of the Oral Cavity

Benign tumors commonly seen are:

PAPILLOMA

It may be solitary or multiple and may occur anywhere in oral cavity. The growth is seen as areas of multiple furfur like projections on the surface covered with keratinized epithelium;

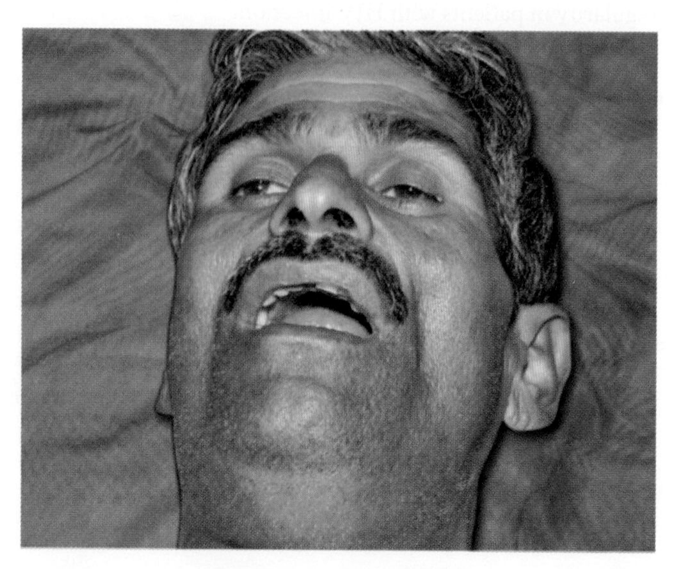

Fig. 43.3: Ludwig's angina

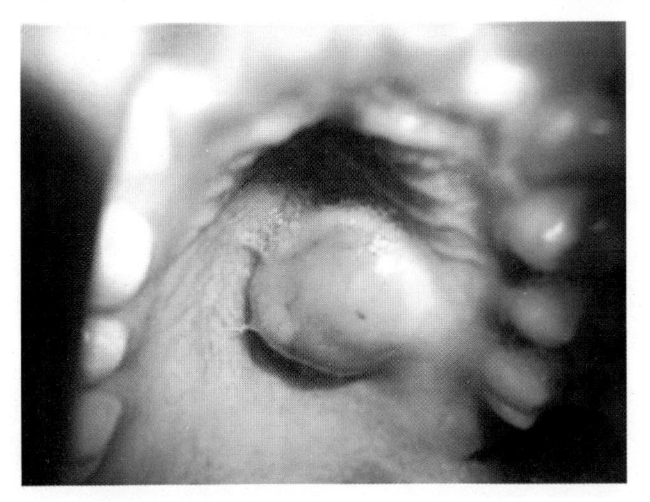

Fig. 43.4: Pleomorphic adenoma of the palate

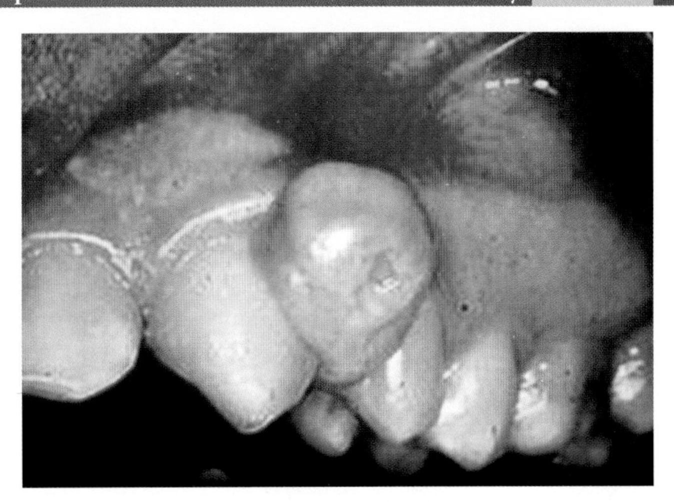

Fig. 43.6: Giant cell epulis

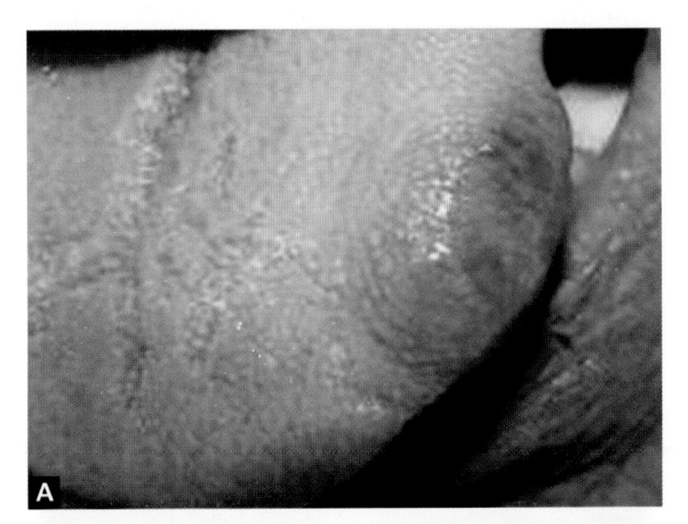

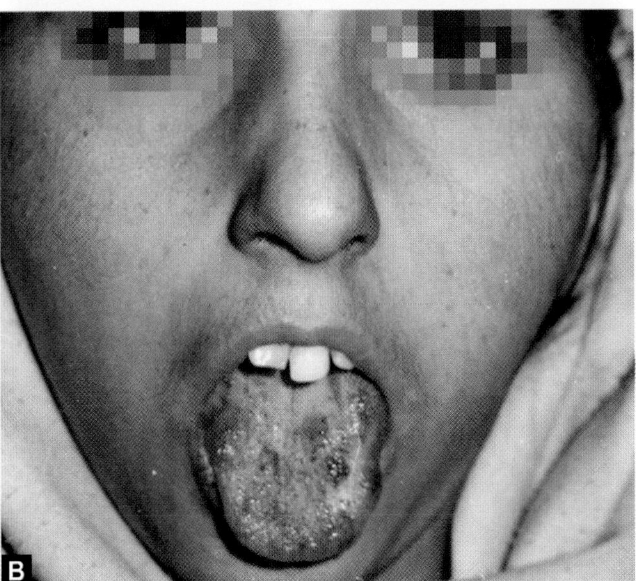

Figs 43.5A and B: Hemangiomas

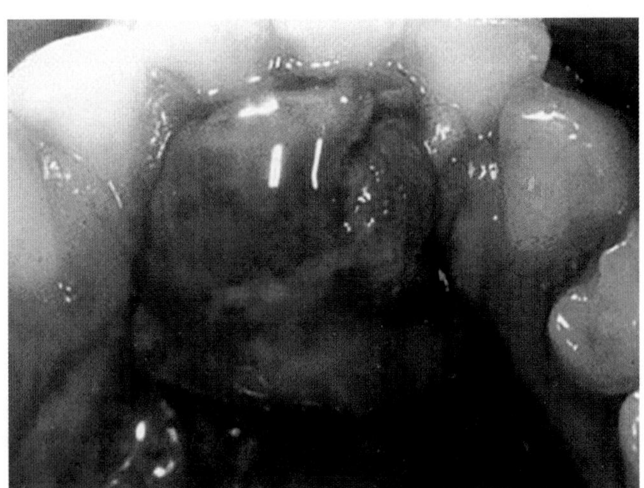

Fig. 43.7: Malignant epulis

papillomas or pleomorphic adenomas particularly on the palate (**Fig. 43.4**). Hemangiomas may sometimes occur on the oral mucosa or tongue (**Figs 43.5A and 43.5B**).

EPULIS

Epulis means a swelling on the gum.

Types of Epulis

Fibrous epulis: This presents as a sessile or pedunculated swelling on the gum between the teeth and may be few centimeters in diameter. Treatment is complete excision.

*Giant cell epulis (**Fig. 43.6**):* This tumor consists of multinucleated giant cells in a fibrous matrix with spindle cells. It is a vascular tumor and, therefore, bleeds easily. Surgical excision is the treatment of choice.

Malignant epulis: Squamous cell carcinoma may present as a swelling on the gum (**Fig. 43.7**). Biopsy confirms the diagnosis. Surgical excision along with its healthy margins is done. Alternatively, radiotherapy may be given.

Ameloblastoma (Adamantinoma) (Fig. 43.8)

This tumor arises frequently from the mandible. It is thought to arise from the remnants of epithelial *cells of Malassez* in the periodontal membrane. The tumor extends into the surrounding marrow spaces and causes expansion of the bone. It is a slowgrowing, histologically benign tumor but its recurrence is common. Radiologically the tumor gives a soap bubble appearance. Treatment is wide surgical excision to prevent recurrence.

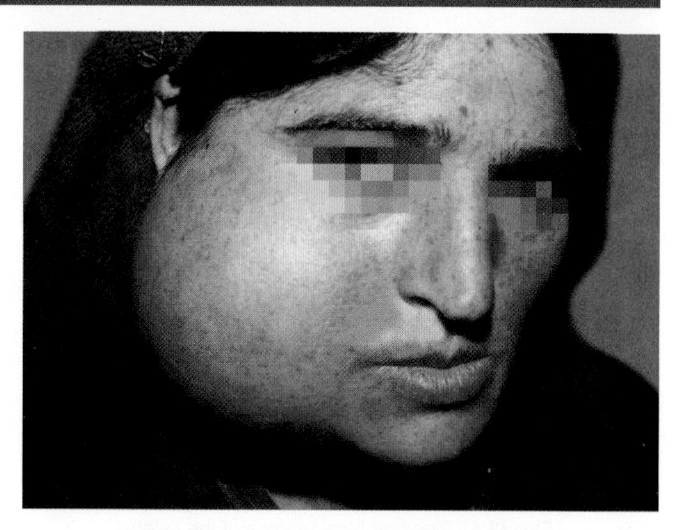

Fig. 43.8: Adamantinoma (right mandible)

Chapter 44

Evaluation and Management of the Patient with a Neck Mass

Neck masses are common clinical findings and can represent a variety of clinical diagnosis from the very simple ones to a very complex diagnosis. A systemic approach is essential to correctly distinguish the benign from the more sinister masses and the learning objective of this chapter is exactly that. By the end of this chapter, the student should have grasped the clinical anatomy of significance, the presentation and management of common benign and malignant masses in the neck in patients across all age groups (**Flow chart 44.1**).

Anatomical Considerations

TRIANGLES OF THE NECK

The thyroglossal cyst occurs as a dilated portion of the thyroglossal duct which extends from the foramen cecum at the base of the tongue to the isthmus of the thyroid gland. The tract passes through the hyoid bone or behind or in front of the body of hyoid (**Fig. 44.1**).

In 90 percent of the cases it is present in the midline, in 85 percent the cyst lies below the hyoid bone, in 8 percent above hyoid bone, in 5 percent low in the neck and in 1 to 2 percent at the base of the tongue.

Thyroglossal fistula develops from an infected cyst which has ruptured or from the incomplete removal of the sinus tract or cyst (**Figs 44.2A and B**).

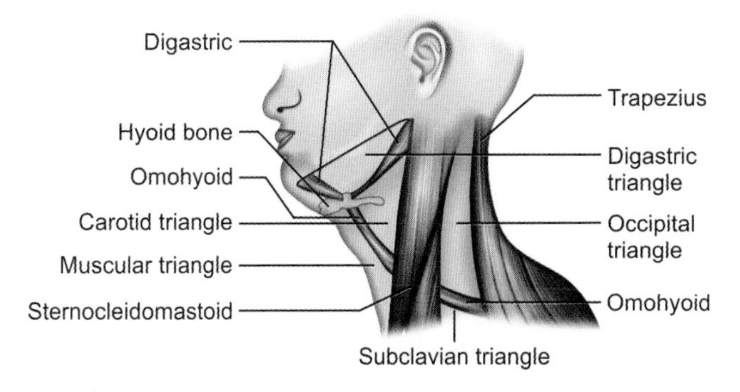

Fig. 44.1: Anatomy of neck

Treatment

Surgical excision of cyst along with the tract (Sistrunk's operation) is the treatment of choice.

Branchial Apparatus and its Abnormalities

At about 35 days of intrauterine life, 6 grooves appear on the side of the neck. These are the branchial clefts and intervening bars are the branchial arches. Each arch contains a central cartilage.

BRANCHIAL CYST

A cyst arising from the second branchial cleft is the most common, and usually occurs around 20 to 25 years (even up to 50) of age (**Figs 44.3A and B**).

The second arch branchial cyst is most commonly found at the junction of the upper two-thirds and the lower one-third of sternomastoid muscle, along its anterior border. The cyst is always lined by squamous epithelium.

The cyst fluid bears resemblance to tuberculous pus and under the microscope shows an abundance of cholesterol crystals.

Treatment

Treatment involves excision of the cyst.

BRANCHIAL FISTULA

A branchial fistula may be unilateral or bilateral and may represent a persistent second cleft. The external orifice of the fistula is nearly always found in the lower-third of the neck near the anterior border of sternomastoid.

Branchial fistulae which are clothed with muscle and are lined with columnar ciliated epithelium, discharge mucous and are often the seat of recurrent attacks of inflammation. When complete, the internal orifice of the fistula is commonly found in the anterior aspect of the posterior pillar of fauces, just behind the tonsil. As a rule, the track is blind and ends in the region of the lateral pharyngeal wall. It is frequently a

Flow chart 44.1: Relative frequency of specific neck masses within causative groups by age (years)

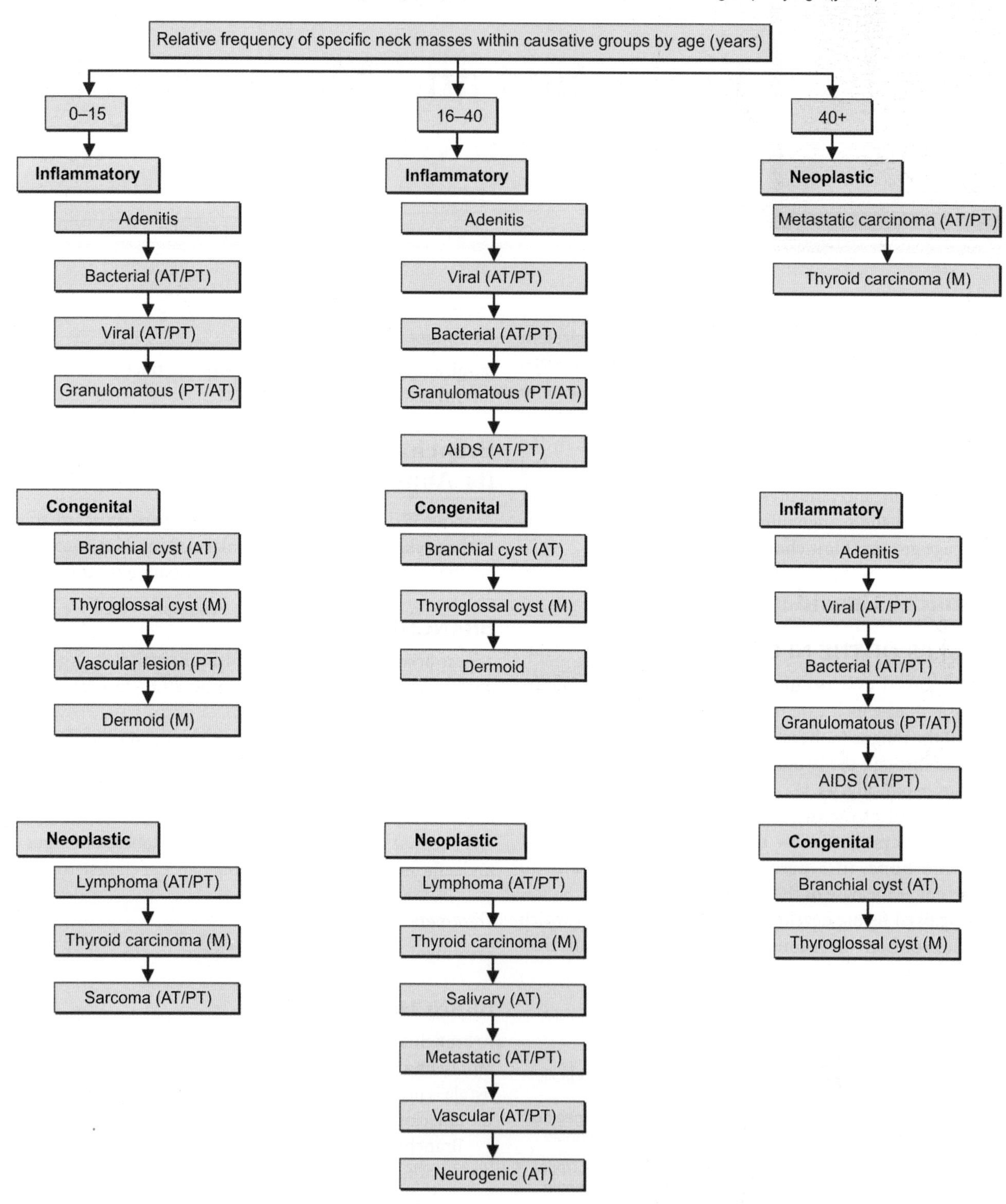

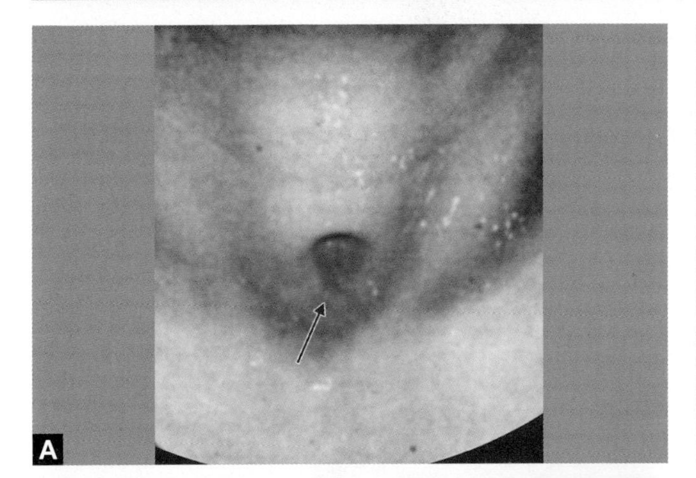

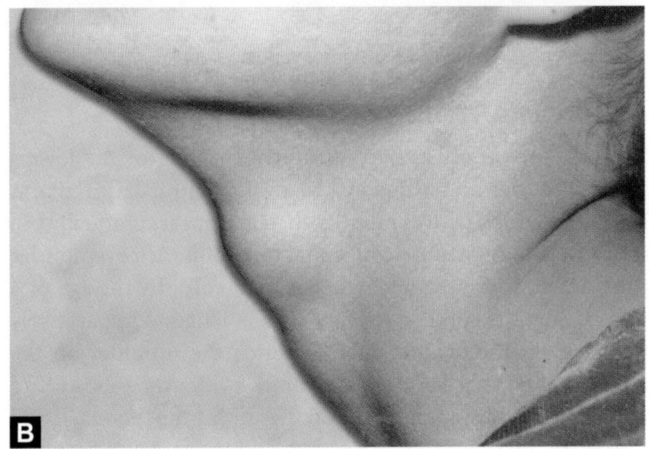

Figs 44.2A and B: (A) Thyroglossal fistula; (B) Thyroglossal cyst

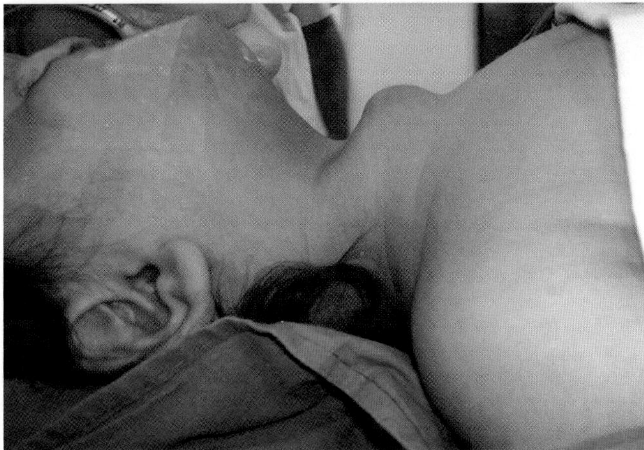

Fig. 44.3A: Branchial cyst (F)

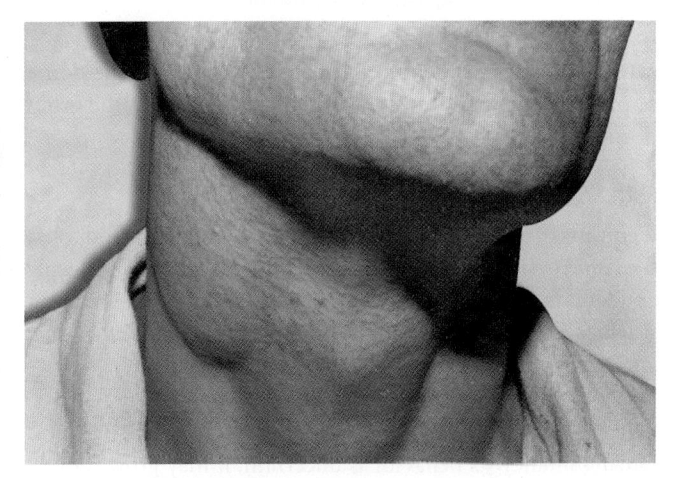

Fig. 44.3B: Branchial cyst (M)

congenital condition but can be acquired. The extent of fistula can be determined by radiography following the injection of a radiopaque medium.

Treatment

When causing troublesome symptoms, it should be removed by dissection. In a fistula without an internal opening, a purse-string suture is inserted subcutaneously round the external orifice 3 days before the operation. After a radiopaque medium has been injected, the suture is tied and a radiograph taken. Pent-up secretions distend the tract and can be followed more easily in depths of the wound.

Operation: A transverse incision is given and extended upwards as far as the limits of the wound permit. A second transverse incision is made at a higher level and the mobilized part of fistula is brought out of it till its termination, it usually passes through the fork of the common carotid and extends to the lateral pharyngeal wall.

Branchial cartilage and cervical auricle can be present at the site of external orifice of the branchial fistula.

CYSTIC HYGROMA

Etiology

At about the sixth week of intrauterine life, primitive lymph sacs develop in the mesoblasts. The principal pair is situated in the neck between the jugular and subclavian veins, and corresponds to the lymph hearts of the lower animals (**Fig. 44.4**). Sequestration of lymphatic tissue consequent upon failure of an important tributary of the primitive lymphatic system to link up with other lymphatic vessels or with the venous system accounts for the appearance of these swellings. Cystic hygroma, like sternomastoid tumor, is earliest to appear, usually during early infancy or may be present at birth.

Site

It occupies the lower-third of the neck and passes upwards towards the ear as it enlarges. Due to its many compartments and their intercommunications, the swelling is softly cystic and partially compressible but it is brilliantly translucent. It often

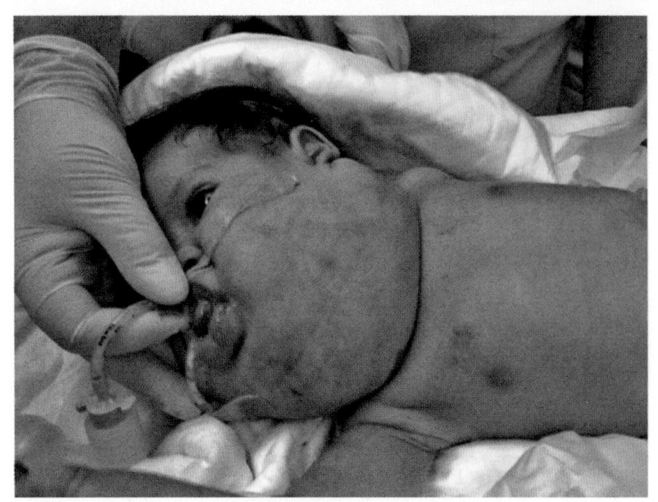

Fig. 44.4: Cystic hygroma

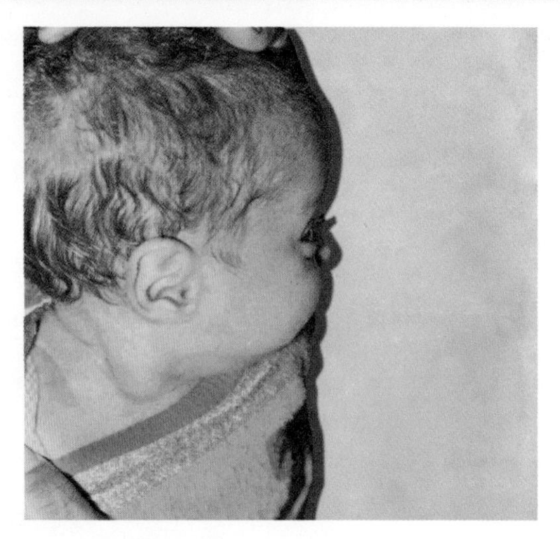

Fig. 44.5: Sternomastoid tumor

extends downwards behind the clavicle to lie upon the dome of pleura, sometimes into the axilla or may occur in the groin or mediastinum.

Pathology

It consists of an aggregation of cysts, like a mass of soap bubbles, the larger cysts are near the surface while smaller ones lie deeply and tend to infiltrate the muscle planes. Each cyst is lined by a single layer of endothelium, having the appearance of mosaic and is filled with clear lymph.

Clinical Course

During infancy its behavior is uncertain, it may grow rapidly and obstruct respiration and aspiration of the contents may be required. It may become the seat of inflammation from nasopharyngeal infection.

Treatment

Complete dissection of the cyst at an early age is the treatment of election. Later the cyst becomes more adherent and, therefore, its complete dissection becomes more difficult. If the cyst is removed incompletely, there is a danger of dehydration because of lymph leakage, unless the fluid balance is maintained. In all cases the wound must be drained for 48 hours.

SOLITARY LYMPH CYST

It is seen in adults but is otherwise akin to cystic hygroma. It is a single cyst filled with lymph and is usually found in the supraclavicular triangle.

Treatment

Treatment is excision.

STERNOMASTOID TUMOR

This usually occurs as hard, fusiform swelling of the lower-third of the sternomastoid at 1 to 2 weeks of birth. It remains stationary in size up to 3 months, then disappears gradually but if not treated may cause congenital torticollis. After 6 months, the affected muscle can be felt as a tight cord. By the age of 4 years, when the child's neck increases in length comparatively quicker and the head is down towards the shoulder on the affected side, the deformity becomes evident. Scoliosis and elevation of the scapula occur on the side of the lesions. If still untreated, facial asymmetry ensues and the face and cranium on the affected side fail to lengthen pari passu with the normal side (**Fig. 44.5**).

Pathology

The mass consists of white fibrous tissue. It can be regarded as Volkman's ischemia of the sternomastoid.

Theories of causation speculate ischemia resulting from malposition or sometimes fibroma as being the cause.

Treatment

1. *Manipulation:* It is done after the tumor disappears, by two persons, one holds the shoulders and other extends the neck towards the nonaffected side. This maneuver is repeated twice a day for years.
2. *von-Lackum's operation:* It is undertaken when the tumor is still present or soon afterwards. Through a transverse incision the swelling and muscle in the neighborhood is excised without injuring the eleventh nerve. No attempt is made to close the gap, but subcutaneous tissues are approximated accurately before closing the wound. No special after-treatment is required. The muscle regenerates.

Neck Masses

The likely sites of metastasis related to the site of primary tumor in head and neck based on Lindberg study are:

Level 1: Submental and submandibular groups—This consists of lymph nodes within the submental triangle and the submandibular group bounded by posterior belly of digastrics and body of mandible.

Level 2: Upper jugular group—This consists of lymph nodes located around upper-third of internal jugular vein and adjacent spinal accessory nerve extending from skull base down to level of carotid bifurcation where digastric muscle crosses the jugular vein. This part related to level of hyoid bone on CT scan. It contains junctional and sometimes jugulodiagastric nodes (**Fig. 44.6**).

Level 3: Middle jugular group—This consists of lymph nodes located around middle-third of internal jugular vein extending from carotid bifurcation superiorly down to upper part of cricoid cartilage (seen on CT) and represents the level where omohyoid muscle crosses the internal jugular vein. It usually contains the jugulo-omohyoid nodes and may contain jugulodiagastric node.

Level 4: Lower jugular group—This consists of lymph nodes located around middle-third of internal jugular vein extending from cricoid cartilage down to clavicle inferiorly. It may contain same jugulo-omohyoid node.

Level 5: Post-triangle group—These nodes are located along the lower half of spinal accessory nerve. The transverse cervical artery supraclavicular nodes are also included in this group. The posterior border is the anterior border of trapezius and anterior boundary is the posterior border of the sternomastoid muscle.

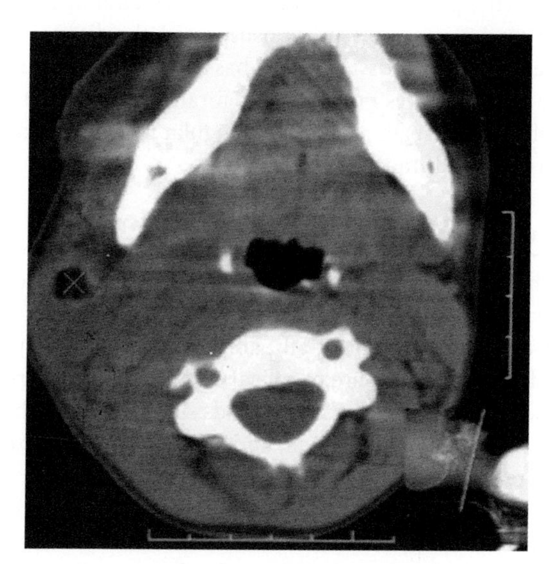

Fig. 44.6: Neck abscess (CT scan)

Level 6: Anterior compartment group (visceral group)—This consists of the lymph nodes surrounding the midline visceral structures of neck extending from hyoid bone superiorly to suprasternal notch inferiorly. The lateral border on each side is the medial border of sternomastoid muscle. It contains parathyroid, the paratracheal, perilaryngeal and prelaryngeal lymph nodes.

Level 7: Lymph nodes in upper anterior mediastinum

Management of Metastatic Cervical Nodes

Squamous cell carcinoma metastatic from stratified squamous epithelium of the upper aerodigestive tract is certainly the most common cell type and source of metastatic cervical nodes. Other sources of the same epidermoid cell cancer include the skin, esophagus, bronchi, and occasionally the uterine cervix. The most common site for squamous carcinoma is the larynx, but such cancers do not metastasize until they move off the true vocal cord into the lymphatic-rich mucosal beds. Lesions of the nasopharynx, lateral pharynx (tonsil), and hypopharynx (pyriform sinus and posterior-third of the tongue) metastasize earlier and more frequently than either oral or vocal cord lesions. When they are small, detection and performance of biopsies are more difficult. Sinus cancers are locally destructive but slow to metastasize to nodes.

Adenocarcinoma metastasis to cervical lymph nodes may originate in salivary glands, thyroid, or the gastrointestinal and genitourinary tracts. The source of enlargement of the supraclavicular nodes, especially those in the left medial supraclavicular position near the thoracic duct, is more likely to come from below the diaphragm. This is the classic Virchow's node.

Melanoma or lymphoma can metastasize to any node in the head and neck region. Melanoma, of course, usually arises in the skin but occasionally originates from mucous membrane. It is capable of skipping primary nodal drainage systems and appearing in a node some distance from the primary site (Lymphoma is more common and is usually manifest as a unilateral, large, soft node).

Diagnostic Work-up

There are endless tests that can be performed on a patient with a lump in the neck. The examinations and tests that are ordered should make sense and be based on the profile of the patient. The work-up should begin with the thorough history and then progress to the physical examination. After palpation and measurement of the mass, the extent of nodal disease in all patients should be staged according to the system proposed in the 1976 revision of the report of the American

Table 44.1: Staging of nodal disease

N1	Single clinically positive homolateral node <3 cm in diameter.
N2a	Single clinically positive homolateral node 3 to 6 cm in diameter.
N2b	Multiple clinically positive homolateral nodes not more than 6 cm in diameter.
N3a	Clinically positive homolateral node(s) >6 cm in diameter.
N3b	Bilateral clinically positive nodes.

Joint Committee on Cancer Staging and End Results Reporting (**Table 44.1**).

The physical examination must include more than the head and neck area to form a rational conclusion. Within this area, however examination should include inspection and palpation wherever possible of the salivary glands, thyroid, soft tissues of the neck, the lips, the mucous membranes of the cheek, the floor of the mouth, tongue, palate, alveolar ridge, soft palate, tonsils, nasopharynx, oropharynx, and hypopharynx including the base of the tongue and the pyriform sinus. In addition, indirect mirror laryngoscopy and nasopharyngoscopy should be done. If after inspection and palpation of these structures no suspicious mass is found, further studies are indicated. These studies are expensive and time-consuming and should be ordered only when the possible yield is realistic.

There are a variety of blood tests that, although not diagnostic, may provide a clue to the cause of the lymphadenopathy, especially when considered with other diagnostic criteria. These include complete blood count, mono tests, ASO titers, standard test for syphilis, T3 and T4 tests, carcinoembryonic antigen test, rheumatoid factor, and serum protein and serum calcium determinations.

The chest radiograph is absolutely critical. It should be of high quality with multiple views to discern a pulmonary primary. A barium swallow or cinefluoroscopic film of swallowing may be helpful in evaluating the esophagus prior to endoscopy. The radiograph cannot completely replace esophagoscopic examination. However, sinus X-rays are very important since there is no reasonable way of evaluating the sinuses by any other means except the Caldwell-Luc surgical approach for the maxillary sinuses.

Thyroid scans are helpful when the thyroid gland is bulky or the neck is obese. The scan is usually unable to detect a mass of less than 1 cm in diameter and most nodules over 1 cm in diameter can be palpated as easily as they can be scanned. Certainly there is no harm in ordering a thyroid scan in a nonpregnant individual, but it is of limited assistance.

OTHER BATTERY OF TESTS

1. *Nasopharyngoscopy:* Nasopharynx is one of the common sites of occult primary particularly from the area of fossa of Rosenmuller. Careful fibreoptic nasopharyngoscopic inspection is mandatory. If no gross tumor is seen, blind punch biopsies are advised.
2. *Laryngoscopy:* Careful fibreoptic examination of larynx and hypopharynx should be done. Hypopharynx and larynx constitute the common primary sites of squamous cell which metastatize to neck.
3. *Esophagoscopy/Bronchoscopy:* Tumors from upper end of esophagus and bronchi also metastasize to the neck, so careful esophagoscopy and bronchoscopy should be done.
4. CT scan/MRI of neck and chest.
5. Ultrasonograph/CT (Abdomen), if needed.
6. Bone scan, if needed.
7. Exploratory surgery.

Tumors of the Parapharyngeal Space

The tumors most commonly encountered in the parapharyngeal space include salivary gland neoplasms, neurogenic tumors, and metastatic deposits from primary carcinoma elsewhere in the body. The neurogenic tumors most commonly encountered include neurofibroma and paraganglioma. A vast array of other benign and malignant neoplasms may be rarely encountered. These lesions represent neoplastic degeneration of the tissues that exist in this potential space. There are reports of occasional patients with lipoma, rhabdomyoma, rhabdomyosarcoma, lymphoma, meningioma, and chondrosarcoma in the parapharyngeal space.

Metastatic involvement of the parapharyngeal lymphatics may be suspected in the patient with a known primary focus of carcinoma. The parapharyngeal space may be the first site of metastasis for patients with carcinoma of the nasopharynx, nasal cavity, palate, or maxillary sinus. In circumstances in which a primary neoplasm is unsuspected, the diagnosis may not be made until a tissue sample has been obtained. Paralysis of the cranial nerves in the jugular foramen as they enter the parapharyngeal space results in the jugular foramen syndrome or Vernet's syndrome.

Salivary Gland Tumors

Less than 5 percent of parotid tumors start in the deep portion of the parotid gland and extend into the parapharyngeal space. Nevertheless 50 percent of all parapharyngeal space tumors, excluding metastatsis, are of salivary gland origin. Neoplastic degeneration of minor salivary glands situated within the soft palate, lateral pharyngeal wall, and tonsilar pillars may result in a parapharyngeal space mass as well.

A presumptive diagnosis is often possible based upon physical examination and the characteristic radiographic findings. Pain is unusual. Bimanual palpation allows identification of a firm, relatively mobile mass. The preferred treatment for these tumors is surgical excision. Excisional biopsy is preferred. Incisional biopsy should be employed only for tumors considered inoperable. In circumstances in which histologic evaluation is considered necessary prior to excisional biopsy, fine needle aspiration is a useful too.

Neurogenic Tumors

PARAGANGLIOMAS

Paragangliomas are neoplasms that arise from the paraganglionic bodies of the autonomic nervous system. These microscopic composites are composed of granular cells that contain catecholamines. These cells are neuroectodermal in origin. The carotid paraganglioma of carotid body is sensitive to changes in pH, PO_2, and PCO_2.

Paragangliomas are well encapsulated brownish tumors with a firm consistency. Microscopic examination shows clusters of epithelial cells (Zellballen) in a highly vascular fibrous stroma. These lesions are histologically similar to the pheochromocytoma that may develop in adrenal medulla. In contrast to pheochromocytoma, however, cervical paragangliomas rarely secrete catecholamines. There have been isolated reports of secreting jugular, laryngeal, and carotid paragangliomas; however, routine preoperative screening for vasopressors in patients with solitary paragangliomas of the head and neck is not indicated unless the patient's clinical findings suggests the secretion of vasoactive substances. Fluctuating systemic hypertension, palpitations, and blushing would be an indication for further evaluation. Approximately 10 percent of patients with paragangliomas have a family history of the disease. Patients with familial paraganglioma may demonstrate multiple lesions. These patients are at a higher risk of having an associated pheochromocytoma and should undergo preoperative screening for vasoactive substances. Patients with familial paraganglioma should undergo angiography to rule out multiple clinically unrecognized lesions.

The paragangliomas are named according to their site of origin. Paragangliomas of jugular bulb are the glomus jugular paragangliomas. Technically, the glomus jugulare develops in the jugular bulb cephalad to the parapharyngeal space. Enlargement of the tumor may result in expansion along the great vessels into the parapharyngeal space. The site of origin may be difficult to demonstrate in large tumors. Paragangliomas originating in the parapharyngeal space at the site of the carotid body (between the internal and external artery) are called carotid paragnangliomas or chemodectomas, whereas a paraganglioma associated with the vagus nerve is called a vagal paraganglioma or a glomus intravagale.

Approximately 3 percent of all paragangliomas are associated with the vagus nerve. Metabolically active tumors secreting catecholamine have not been described. The vagal paraganglioma most commonly arises in association with one of the vagal ganglia. The jugular ganglion (superior) lies within the jugular fossa. One centimeter caudal to this lies the nodose ganglion. The tumors tend to be spindle-shaped and displace the carotid artery anteriorly.

The most common presenting symptom of a vagal paraganglioma is hoarseness and aspiration of fluids resulting from injury of the vagus nerve with subsequent motor and sensory deficits caused by injury to both the superior and recurrent laryngeal nerves. The finding of vocal cord paralysis in association with a mass along the course of vagus nerve is highly suggestive of vagal paraganglioma.

Tumors developing in the area of the jugular ganglion may be dumbbell in shape with an intracranial and extracranial component. It is important to identify this entity preoperatively so that adequate presurgical planning can be undertaken.

Neoplastic degeneration of the carotid body was termed *chemodectoma* by Mulligan in 1950. The term *carotid paraganglioma* better describes this neoplasm and its location. The most common presenting symptom of a carotid paraganglioma is a mass in the neck located at the bifurcation of the common carotid artery. Large lesions may produce pressure, dysphasia, cough, or hoarseness. Characteristically, the mass may be distinguished from cervical lymph node by virtue of the fact that is mobile in the lateral direction but cannot be move in a cephalocaudal direction. Carotid pulsations may be transmitted through the mass. Arteriographic evaluation demonstrates the findings of a vascular mass with early venous shunting in the bifurcation of the carotid artery. The diagnosis can be established preoperatively through CT scanning with enhancement or arteriography. Biopsy should not be undertaken prior to definitive operative removal.

The incidence of malignancy in paraganglioma is estimated to be less than 10 percent. Histologic evaluation may not adequately distinguish malignant from benign lesions. The findings of invasion of surrounding structures and metastases are indicators of malignancy.

Surgical management of paraganglioma is the treatment of choice. The indolent natural history of paraganglioma has led some authors to recommend no treatment for patients deemed too ill to tolerate surgical management or for elderly asymptomatic patients. Others have recommended radiation therapy.

Cole treated 22 patients with paraganglioma of the jugular foramen using radiation therapy. He reported that visible tumor typically remains unchanged for many years without progression of disease. Forty to fifty gray (Gy) was recommended. Patients treated with orthovoltage radiation therapy incurred a higher incidence of recurrence and severe complications. He subsequently recommended supervoltage radiation therapy.

The deferment of definitive surgical therapy has been associated with the development of pain and cranial nerve deficits, as uncontrolled tumors become larger. Current understanding of these lesions, skill in vascular reconstructive surgery, and the observation of progressive symptomatology in patients with paragangliomas suggest the advisability of surgical excision as the treatment of choice.

Other Neurogenic Tumors

Neurogenic tumors constitute 30 percent of primary tumors found in the parapharyngeal space. The vagus nerve is the one most often involved; however, these tumors may arise from any other nerves in the parapharyngeal space and, in some cases, it may not be possible to identify the nerve of origin.

EMBRYOLOGY OF THE PERIPHERAL NERVE

The neural tube gives rise to somatic motor axons and the preganglionic autonomic axons. All other peripheral axons, including postganglionic, sympathetic, and parasympathetic axons come from the neural crest. All peripheral axons are covered by Schwann cells. It is generally believed that Schwann cells are derived from the neural crest.

A number of terms are employed to describe lesions involving peripheral nerves, including *neurofibroma, neurinoma, nerilemmoma*, and *schwannoma*. The parent cell of all these lesions is, most likely, the Schwann cell. For practical purposes, only the terms *schwannoma* and *neurofibroma* are used in practice. Differences exist between neurofibroma and schwannoma, which have treatment implications.

SCHWANNOMA

The schwannoma is a solitary lesion that is almost never associated with von Recklinghausen's disease. Individual nerve fibers do not actually pass through the lesion but are draped over its surface. Therefore, it is possible to dissect the main trunk of the nerve away from the lesion during removal.

Pain and neurologic dysfunction are unusual. Unpleasant paresthesia with light palpations are characteristic. Malignancy rarely, or never, occurs.

The histologic pattern of a schwannoma demonstrates degenerative and cystic changes. A palisading array of nuclei around the central mass of cytoplasm is termed *Antoni type* A. When little distinctive pattern exists of stroma surrounding nerve fibers, the term *Antoni type* B is used. Occasionally, one type predominates over the other, but tumors are often composed of both patterns. The cells interwoven into palisades with fibrillary zones are termed *Verocay bodies*. Some schwannomas demonstrate hemorrhage and associated hemosiderin deposits. Pleomorphism with enlarged nuclei, irregular shapes, and occasional mitotic figures may be observed. These features do not imply malignancy. Schwannomas arising in cranial nerves in close proximity to a bony foramen may extend through the foramen, forming a dumbbell-shaped tumor. The schwannoma is uncommonly found in the lateral portion of the neck.

NEUROFIBROMA

The neurofibroma also arises from the schwann cell. Neurofibromas are often subcutaneous and may be multiple. The neurofibroma is not encapsulated. Nerve fibers are incorporated within the tumor and pass through it. This contrasts with the schwannoma. Cystic and degenerative changes are uncommon.

von Recklinghausen's disease is associated with a multiple neurofibroma. Sarcomatous transformation is reported in 6 to 16 percent of patients with von Recklinghausen's disease.

VON RECKLINGHAUSEN'S DISEASE

von Recklinghausen's disease is an autosomal dominant disorder observed in approximately 1/3000 births. In spite of this, only 50 percent of cases have a family history of the disease.

Characteristically, patients have light brown macules 1.5 cm or greater in diameter called *cafe' au lait* spots. Five or more *cafe' au lait* spots are considered diagnostic. Other neurologic abnormalities such as spina bifida and glioma may be observed.

Patients with von Recklinghausen's disease most commonly have cutaneous neurofibromas. However, the cranial nerves may be affected with the acoustic and optic nerves most commonly involved. Neurofibroma may arise on the cranial nerves in the parapharyngeal space.

MALIGNANT NEUROFIBROMA

Invasion of adjacent tissue or metastasis is an indication of malignancy. Malignant neurofibroma may occur sporadically however, it is more frequently found in patients with von Recklinghausen's disease. The clinical findings include sudden growth or recurrence after apparent complete removal of a benign neurofibroma. Malignant neurofibroma may be histologically indistinguishable from fibrosarcoma, except for its relationship to a nerve trunk. Electron microscopy demonstrates a basement membrane in malignant neurofibroma that is lacking in fibrosarcoma. Nevertheless, many pathologists will not make a diagnosis of malignant neurofibroma unless the patient has von Recklinghausen's disease.

Hemangioma (Fig. 44.7)

The most common head and neck neoplasms in children are hemangiomas. Although they are predominantly located on cutaneous surfaces, they may be found on mucosal surfaces as well. The scalp is the most frequently involved region, followed by the neck and face (**Fig. 44.7**). Girls are more frequently affected than the boys, and the tumors are more often solitary than multifocal (Batsakis, 1979).

Even though less than 33 percent of hemangiomas are present at birth, they are typically noted during the first

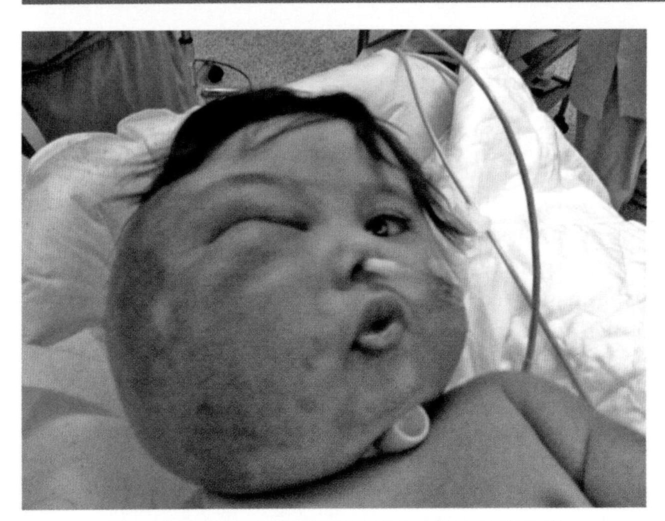

Fig. 44.7: Congenital hemangioma face and neck

month of life and progressively enlarge during the next year. In almost 90 percent of the cases, involution will occur and no therapy is necessary. Hemangiomas can be defined as benign, nonreactive processes in which there is an increase in the number of normal and abnormal appearing blood vessels. In addition, these malformations can be divided into active and inactive hemodynamic categories, which are determined by the presence of anteriovenous fistulas, vascular proliferation, and overall clinical behavior. Several different types have been described (Stal et al 1986).

The cutaneous birthmark (nevus flammeus) is an example of a capillary hemangioma that is located in the dermis. Capillary hemangiomas are composed of nests of capillary vascular channels that are lined by endothelial cells and surrounded by pericytes. In early lesions, the endothelial cells are quite plump, often obscuring the lumen of the capillaries. Thus, the lesion represents arrest in development of the mesenchymal primordial in the capillary network stage. When this occurs, the vascular nature of the lesion may not be readily apparent. The strawberry nevus is a subcutaneous mass that is actually a hypertropic type of capillary hemangioma. This growth is marked by a period of slow evolution, which is then followed by a rapid growth phase and, possibly, involution, most often beginning by 10 months of age (Stal et al 1986).

In contrast, cavernous hemangiomas are composed of tortuous, large vascular channels lined by endothelial cells. They are larger, more frequently involve deeper structures than the capillary hemangiomas, and are unlikely to regress spontaneously. Adventitial fibrosis is frequently present. Thrombosis may occur, with resultant dystrophic calcification and the development of phleboliths. Cavernous hemangiomas are found both in the skin and in the deeper tissues. If the lesions are not present at birth, involution is uncommon.

Arteriovenous hemangiomas frequently occur in the soft tissues of the neck and are referred to by some as arteriovenous malformations. In addition to many of the histologic features of a cavernous hemangioma, there is often times intimal thickening in veins. Additionally, serial sections of such lesions demonstrate diverse arteriovenous connections. Although the histopathologic findings are characteristic, equally important to that diagnosis is the clinical presence of a pulsatile mass with the physiologic manifestations of an arteriovenous shunt.

The radiographic evaluation of a cervical hemangioma is best done with a CT scan and angiography. The CT scan will demonstrate a deeply enhancing mass and graphically depict the soft tissue extent of the lesion. Angiographically, hemangiomas are well-circumscribed lobular masses that have a persistent dense tissue stain and are supplied by multiple slightly enlarged arteries. A proximal artery surrounds the lesion, and multiple smaller arteries enter the hemangioma at right angles. Arteriovenous shunting is usually not present. The angiographic appearance reflects the type of vessels that compose the hemangioma. Capillary venous malformations have dilatated, ectatic spaces that fill during the venous phase and demonstrate prolonged contrast pooling and more numerous vessels.

Hemangiomas that are located in the deep subcutaneous tissues, fascia, and muscles of the neck tend to be infiltrating and difficult to treat. Although the lesions do not undergo malignant degeneration or metastasize, local control is difficult and is frequently not achieved. The intramuscular hemangioma is an example of such an invasive lesion. It usually presents as a localized mass with a rubbery consistency and distinct margins. It is mobile and is not associated with a bruit, thrill, or pulsation. Cutaneous involvement may be present and there may be functional abnormality of the involved muscle. Patients often complain of pain secondary to compression.

The most common type of intramuscular hemangioma is capillary hemangioma. In the neck, the scalene, trapezius, and sternocleidomastoid muscles are frequently involved. This lesion is associated with a 30 percent recurrence rate following appropriate therapy because of its infiltrative nature. Cavernous intramuscular hemangiomas are the second most common type seen and they are associated with a 9 percent recurrence rate. Mixed types are uncommonly found and are associated with a 25 percent recurrence rate. Therapy for these intramuscular hemangiomas requires ligation of the feeding vessels and excision of the mass. As with lymphangiomas, the surgeon must remember that these are benign lesions and care must be taken to avoid injury to vital structures.

Because most congenital lesions involute spontaneously, conservative therapy is the rule for many hemangiomas. One must constantly reassure both the child and the parent that involution is expected. If the tumor shows unusually rapid growth, hemorrhage, or recurrent infection, biopsy is indicated, and definitive therapy must be initiated. This obviously must be individualized based on several factors, including patient age, site of lesion, size of lesion, depth of extension, and the general characteristics of the mass. Steroids are often a helpful adjunct to surgical excision, but radiotherapy and sclerosing agents, though often recommended in the past, are generally avoided. The steroids are felt to interrupt proliferation for several possible reasons, including blockage of estradiol receptors or interference with the release of heparin or angiogenic factors from mast cells.

Teratoma

Teratomas are developmental lesions that contain tissue elements derived from all three germinal layers. The cells found in the lesion may be in any stage of differentiation, and when cells are quite immature, malignancy is unusual, however, and the histologic changes most likely represent immaturity of the tissue.

Cervical teratomas generally present as a mass in the neck that is discovered at birth. It may be seen in stillborn children and rarely presents after the age of 1 year. An *in utero* diagnosis can be made on ultrasound when a cervical mass is demonstrated that is of mixed echogenicity and displaces the trachea posteriorly. Calcification may be present. There may be some confusion with cystic hygroma, but this mass typically presents as a multiloculated, noncalcified, cystic mass.

These lesions are encapsulated and are usually partially cystic, having a variegated appearance on cut section. Microscopically, the lesions are composed of a mixture of mature elements derived from ectoderm, mesoderm, and endoderm and of immature or embryonic tissue, including embryonic neuroectoderm. Consequently, most are classified as embryonal teratomas.

Cervical teratomas are sometimes referred to as teratomas of the thyroid gland. They cause symptoms secondary to pressure, and this frequently results in upper airway compression and obstruction, patients may present with stridor, cyanosis and possible apnea. In addition, there may be dysphagia secondary to esophageal compression. Plain neck radiographs reveal a soft tissue mass that contains speckled calcification in approximately 50 percent of cases; the trachea and the esophagus are displaced posteriorly, and there may be associated pulmonary atelectasis or collapse. On ultrasound, a teratoma is generally of mixed echogenicity and usually can be differentiated from a cystic hygroma, which appears as a multilocular cyst with possible mediastinal extension, or from a congenital goiter, which has a solid appearance.

Patients do not seem to have an increased incidence of other congenital anomalies, but maternal hydramnios has been incriminated as a predisposing factor. The differential diagnosis is broad and includes cystic hygromas, branchial cysts, cavernous hemangiomas, thyroglossal duct cysts, laryngoceles, goiters, desmoid tumors, and lipomas. Cystic hygromas are generally differentiated by their more cystic appearance and ill-defined margins. Branchial cysts, in contrast, are distinguished on the basis of their size, location, and fluctuance.

Once the diagnosis of a cervical teratoma is made, surgical excision is mandatory to prevent upper airway obstruction or pulmonary compromise. Without intervention, most patients die. Even in those patients who do survive long enough to undergo surgery, there is a mortality rate associated with the condition.

Chapter 45

Salivary Glands

General Epidemiology

- Eighty percent parotid, 80 percent benign, 80 percent pleomorphic
- *Submandibular gland:* 50 percent benign, 50 percent malignant
- Sublingual and minor glands (most common on hard palate): >80 percent malignant
- Children:
  - Five percent of all salivary tumors, but >50 percent are malignant
  - Most common benign tumor is pleomorphic
  - Most common malignant tumor is mucoepidermoid (some say adenoid cystic)
  - Most common parotid tumor overall is nonsalivary—the hemangioma.

Parotid Gland

ACUTE PAROTID GLAND INFECTIONS

Mumps

Mumps is caused by the mumps virus which spreads by droplet infection. It affects mainly children of school-going age and young adults. Most cases occur in spring. The incubation period is 18 days.

Clinical Features

Malaise, fever and pain in the angle of jaw is soon followed by a tender swelling of one or both parotid glands. The submandibular salivary glands may also be involved. The swelling subsides in a few days.

Complications

Orchitis, pancreatitis and encephalitis are the usual complications.

Treatment

Isolation, care of oral hygiene and symptomatic treatment is instituted. Difficulty in opening the mouth may need feeding through a straw. Steroids are given in cases where orchitis develops.

ACUTE PAROTITIS (FIG. 45.1A)

Infection reaches the parotid gland either from the mouth or through blood. In severe cases the causative organism is *Staphylococcus aureus.* The infection is often confined to one parotid gland.

Etiology

Acute parotitis may result from the following:

1. Postoperative.
2. As a complication of debilitating diseases like typhoid and cholera.
3. Secondary to obstruction of Stensen's duct. This may be due to parotid calculus and foreign bodies.
4. As a complication of septicemia.
5. Idiopathic.

Clinical Features

There is a painful swelling on the side of face. Signs of toxemia are usually present. Temperature is over 100°F. Pus can be expressed from the Stensen's duct.

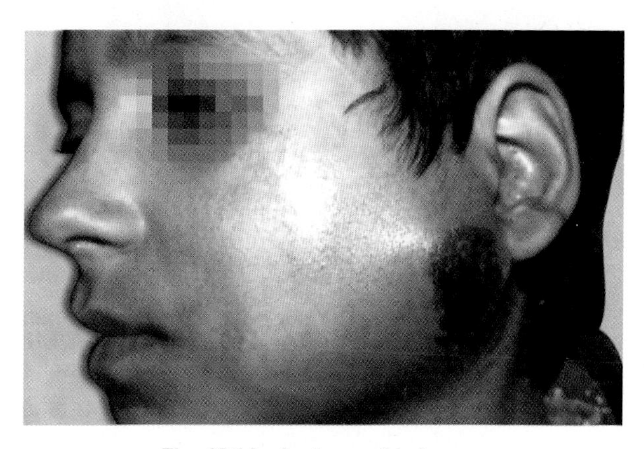

Fig. 45.1A: Acute parotid abscess

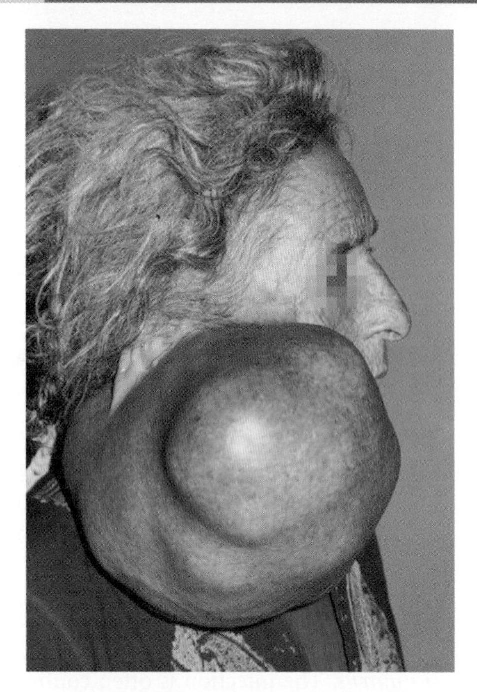

Fig. 45.1B: Pleomorphic adenoma

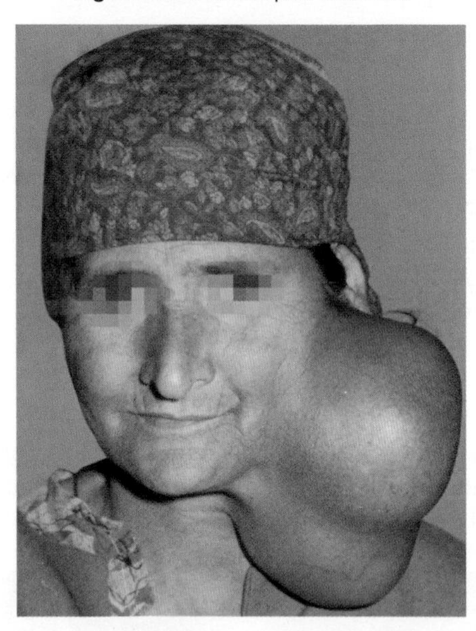

Fig. 45.1C: Parotid tumor

Treatment

Treatment involves cleaning the mouth correction of dehydration and administration of antibiotics.

In fulminating cases, decompression of the parotid salivary gland is done. An incision is made down to the capsule of the gland as used for parotidectomy. The skin is reflected anteriorly to expose the surface of the gland. The capsule is incised transversely. The skin is closed with interrupted sutures and drainage is provided at the lower end of the wound.

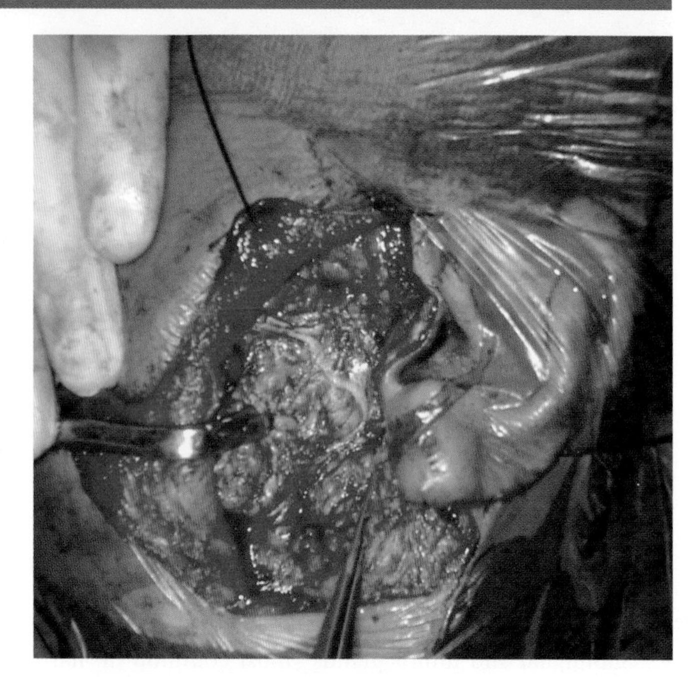

Fig. 45.1D: Superficial parotidectomy showing terminal branches of facial nerve

CHRONIC PAROTITIS

Chronic parotitis is more common than acute cases. The condition is frequently bilateral but may be unilateral. Purulent saliva can be expressed from the Stensen's duct if gentle pressure is exerted over the gland. A parotid calculus must be excluded by X-ray.

Sialography reveals sialectasis, calculus, or stenosis of the duct.

Treatment

Catheterizing the Stensen's duct with a fine ureteric catheter and injecting antiseptic fluid such as 1 percent mercurochrome or tetracycline are resorted to. These measures can be repeated if necessary. In long-standing cases, parotidectomy is done.

PAROTID CALCULUS

Parotid calculi are uncommon as compared to submandibular calculi. The patient complains of a painful swelling of gland occurring especially at meals.

Sialography demonstrates the parotid calculus.

Treatment

If a stone is found in the Stensen's duct, it can be removed by splitting the duct. If the calculus is deeply placed within the partoid tissue, the gland is exposed and calculus is removed through a transverse incision in the gland substance. If multiple stones are present superficial lobectomy should be done.

NEOPLASMS

Benign Disease

1. *Pleomorphic adenoma* ***(Figs 45.1B and C)****:*
   - Most common tumor overall, and most common for each type of salivary gland
   - Slow growing but can reach massive sizes
   - Also known as a mixed tumor, which describes the epithelial and mesenchymal components of tumor histology
     - Epithelial cells within mesenchymal (myxoid, chondroid, osteoid, fibroid) stroma
   - Incomplete encapsulation with multiple pseudopod extensions
     - These features account for high recurrence rate after enucleation, which is why adequate surgical therapy requires complete excision with margin of normal tissue.
2. *Warthin's tumor* ***(Fig. 45.2)****:* Comprises 10 percent of all parotid tumors. Also known as papillary cystadenoma lymphomatosum based on its histological appearance which usually is a double layer of papillary epithelium (with lymphoid stroma) projecting into cystic spaces, eosinophillic staining. Many mitochondria in cytoplasm [oncocytes—ground glass appearance] (hot on Tc-99m scan). Tends to occur more in elderly men, in region of parotid tail and can be bilateral in 5 percent of cases. They have a very slow growth rate, thus once FNA proven can be monitored in very elderly or non-surgical candidates.
3. *Oncocytoma:* Account for 1 percent of tumors, exclusive to parotid gland. Histologically have plump eosinophillic cells with indented nuclei, many mitochondria (appears hot on Tc99 scan). Can undergo malignant degeneration rarely, but if so have high rate of nodal metastases.
4. *Monomorphic adenoma:* Present as many subtypes, all of which are rare. Most common is basal cell adenoma.

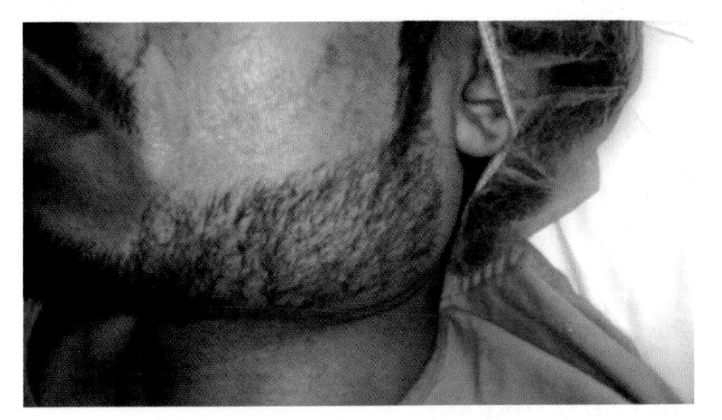

Fig. 45.2: Warthin's tumor left parotid

Malignant Disease

1. *Mucoepidermoid:* Is the most common malignancy overall, most common malignancy of parotid, with hard palate being next most common site. Generally classified as low (mostly mucous cells) or high (mostly epidermoid cells) grade, 30 percent cell proportion cut-off is used to classify them i.e. more than 30 percent mucous cells would mean the tumor is low grade and vice versa. High grade are disorganized tumors, may resemble squamous cell carcinomas, and require mucin/PAS stains to demonstrate mucinous cells and differentiate from them. They are also more aggressive with high propensity for metastases (50%). So even in the presence of N0 (no clinical or radiological evidence of neck nodes) neck need to have prophylactic block dissection. Most studies report a 20 to 50 percent 10-year survival.

   Low grade tumors have more mucoid cells with strands of epidermoid cells, have a more indolent course (nearly 95% 10-year survival reported).
2. *Adenoid cystic:* Is the most common malignancy of glands other than parotid. It can present with facial paralysis or facial pain and often infiltrates normal tissue. Histology appears as cylindric epithelial cystic formations within fibrous stroma. Typically have perineural invasion, and very difficult to assess extent clinically. Three basic histologic subtypes with worsening prognosis: tubular, cribriform, solid. Can present with very distant neural recurrence many years after surgery, thus needing long-term follow-up (30% 10 year survival reported).
3. *Acinic cell:* Thought to arise from serous cells (majority found in parotid gland). Is bilateral in 3 percent, often multicentric. PAS+ on staining, shows many mitochondria and appears hot on Tc-99m scan. Classified as a low grade malignancy, 80 percent of cases have a 10 year survival.
4. *Adenocarcinoma:* It is more common in minor salivary glands. Histologically resemble mucoepidermoids, but lack keratin. Although they can have low-grade phenotypes, generally tend to be aggressive and metastatic tumors (40–60% 10-year survival).
5. *Carcinoma ex-pleomorphic:* This aggressive tumor arises from a pleomorphic adenoma because the epithelial component of the pleomorphic has become malignant (a true malignant mixed from both tissue types is very rare). About 5 percent of pleomorphic adenomas undergo this change. Typically presents with a sudden increase in size from a previously stable mass. Histologically is similar to pleomorphics, but contains hemorrhage and necrosis. Poor long term prognosis (30% 10 year survival).
6. *Squamous cell carcinoma:* This occurs more commonly in submandibular gland and proper diagnosis requires exclusion of:

- Contiguous cutaneous primaries
- Metastases from cutaneous primaries
- High-grade mucoepidermoid.

  There is a high incidence of regional and distant mets, poor prognosis (50% 10 year survival).

7. *Undifferentiated:* Rare tumors, possible relation to Epstein-Barr virus has been suggested. These are very aggressive tumors with a poor prognosis (less than 50% 10 years survival).

ETIOLOGY

- In general poorly understood although smoking plays a factor in Warthin's tumors and irradiated parotid glands have higher tumor incidence after long latency period
- Occupational exposure to wood dust associated with increased incidence of minor salivary gland malignancies (adenoid cystic and adenocarcinoma), especially in sinonasal tract.

EVALUATION

Salivary gland masses generally present with a slow nonspecific enlargement

- Pain is unusual, carries worse prognosis as can be associated with neural invasion (studies have shown 50% decreased survival if pain present)
- Always examine oral cavity to see if tumor is bulging from parapharyngeal space
- Always examine CN VII (and all CNs in case of parapharyngeal space)
- Always examine scalp to assess for cutaneous primary.

Fine needle aspiration remains controversial:

- *Proponents say:* Aids in preoperative counseling, planning extent of resection and adjuvant therapy (or even if resection needed at all as in Warthin's)
- *Opponents say:* Makes no difference as lesion must come out anyways and adjuvant treatment can be planned later with no change in outcome.

Imaging is not often part of the general management, but certain indications exist. MRI is thought to be more useful overall as better for soft tissue and nerve imaging unless bone involvement (i.e. mandible, palate) is suspected in which case CT is complementary.

STAGING

Stage	Description
Tx	Tumor cannot be assessed
T0	No evidence of tumor
T1	<2 cm, no extraparenchymal extension
T2	2–4 cm, no extraparenchymal extension
T3	4–6 cm or extraparenchymal extension without CN VII involvement
T4	>6 cm, or invading CN VII or invading skull base

TREATMENT

Surgery is the treatment of choice and various surgical procedures are the following:

1. Extracapsular excision is done for very small superficial benign tumors.
2. Superficial parotidectomy with preservation of the facial nerve is done for most of the benign tumors when:
   i. Tumor has broken its confines, or
   ii. Tumor has recurred after local excision.

   As recurrence is very common following local excision only, superficial parotidectomy is now recommended as the treatment of choice even if the tumor is small in size.
3. Total parotidectomy (**Fig. 45.1D**) with or without block dissection of neck for malignant lesions of the parotid.

COMPLICATIONS OF PAROTIDECTOMY

1. *General complications of any surgery:* Infection, hematoma, seroma.
2. Anesthesia in distribution of great auricular nerve (very bothersome complaint)
3. Salivary fistula, skin flap necrosis, mild trismus, 1st bite syndrome (pain on initial mastication following parapharyngeal space surgery)
4. *Facial paralysis:* Temporary paresis is seen in 10 to 20 percent of cases and aim of any good surgeon should be to keep down the rate of permanent paresis to <1 percent.

FREY'S SYNDROME (AURICULOTEMPORAL NERVE SYNDROME)

This follows injury to fibers of the auriculotemporal nerve at the time of incision for relief of suppurative parotitis. In such cases on eating, the cheek becomes red, hot and painful followed by perspiration appearing upon it. There is also cutaneous hyperaesthesia in front and above the ear. This is due to the fact that when the nerve has been damaged, the axis cylinders conveying secretory impulses grow down the sheaths of cutaneous elements of the nerve. In this way the stimulus intended for saliva production causes cutaneous hyperaesthesia and sweating.

Treatment

- Nothing (most cases are asymptomatic)
- Topical antiperspirants
- Topical glycopyrrolate
- Atropine
- Jacobson's nerve neurectomy
- Insert flap between skin and nerve fibers.

MIKULICZ DISEASE

It comprises the following:

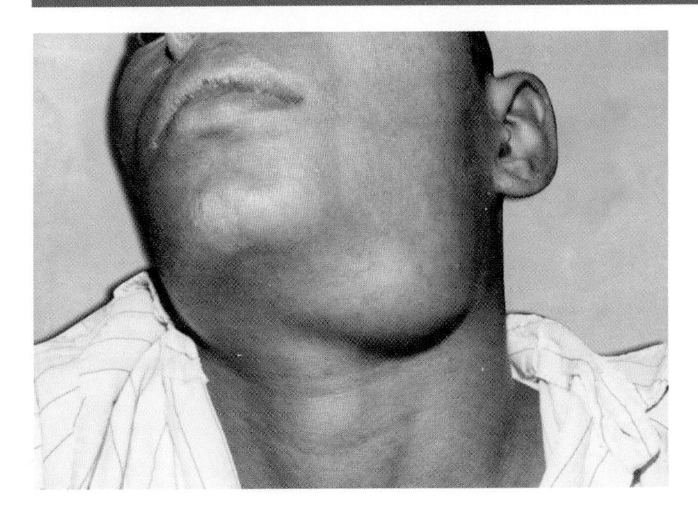

Fig. 45.3: Submandibular sialadenitis

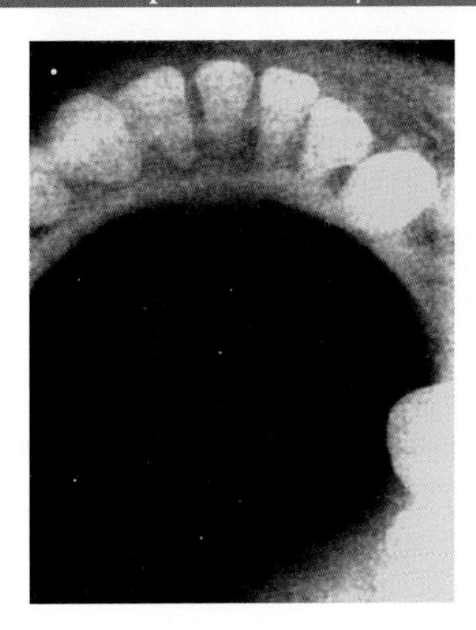

Fig. 45.4: Calculus in the left submandibular gland duct (X-ray floor of mouth)

i. Symmetrical enlargement of the salivary glands.
ii. Narrowing of the palpebral fissures due to enlargement of the lacrimal gland.
iii. Parchment like dryness of the mouth.

Submandibular Glands

The most common cause of the involvement of this gland is a foreign body in the duct or a stone.

CALCULUS

The most common site for salivary calculus is within the submandibular gland or its duct (Wharton's duct). It is fifty times more frequent here than in the parotid gland and its duct. This is because salivary secretions from the submandibular gland are more mucoid and are rich in calcium. These salivary calculi consist of phosphates of calcium and magnesium.

Clinical Features

Painful swelling of the gland (**Fig. 45.3**) before or during meals is characteristic of this condition. The patient should be given fruit juice to sip at the time of clinical examination. Little or no saliva pours out from the orifice of Wharton's duct on the affected side. A stone in the Wharton's duct can be detected by bidigital palpation.

Salivary colic sometimes occur at the commencement of a meal.

A calculus in the Wharton's duct or in the gland is seen in the lateral or occlusive view of the submandibular region (**Fig. 45.4**).

Treatment

1. Stones in the duct should be removed under local or general anesthesia. The tissues immediately behind the stone are grasped with tenaculum forceps, which steady the stone and elevate it. An incision is then made in the long axis of the duct and the stone slips out. The wound is left unsutured.
2. Stones in the gland necessitate removal of the gland.

Sialography

INDICATIONS

1. Differential diagnosis of swellings in the region of the salivary glands, e.g. sialectasis.
2. Obstruction of the duct due to stricture, calculus or foreign body.
3. Subacute and chronic infections, the degree of damage to the ducts and glands can be shown.
4. The extent of involvement of the gland by a neoplasm can be assessed.
5. To know the site of communication of the fistula with the duct which helps in planning treatment.

Chapter 46

Pharyngitis

Inflammation of the oropharynx can be classified into acute and chronic.

Acute Pharyngitis

Acute inflammation of the pharyngeal mucosa may be an accompanying feature of many local and systemic diseases. It may follow an attack of common cold and may be a feature of other infections like measles, chickenpox or influenza. Acute inflammatory lesions of the pharynx may develop after trauma by a foreign body or after instrumentation.

The patient's chief symptom is sore throat, associated with fever and other constitutional symptoms. Examination reveals diffuse congestion of the pharyngeal wall, uvula and adjacent faucial tissues. Depending upon the severity of infection, there may be edema of the lining mucosa and uvula and enlargement of the glands of the neck.

Treatment consists of bed rest, analgesics and antibiotics preferably penicillin or erythromycin.

Membranous Pharyngitis

Various diseases, local or systemic, are associated with membrane formation in the pharynx.

FAUCIAL DIPHTHERIA

The condition caused by *Corynebacterium diphtheriae* is associated with membrane formation on the faucial tonsils. The membrane is greyish white and extends to the uvula and soft palate. It cannot be easily removed and on removal leaves a raw bleeding surface (**Fig. 46.1**).

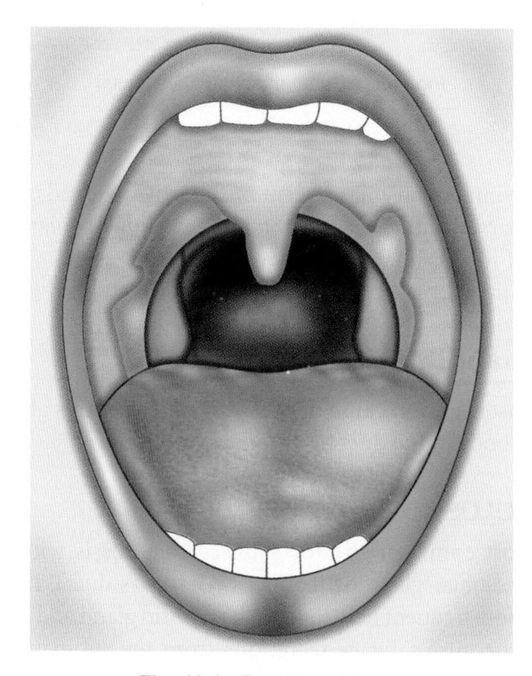

Fig. 46.1: Faucial diphtheria

There occurs marked toxemia associated with a fast pulse rate, disproportionate to the rise in temperature. Palatal and peripheral nerve paralysis and myocarditis are the complications that can occur up to the second or third week of infection.

VINCENT'S ANGINA

This condition is characterized by an ulcerative lesion on the tonsils, usually on one side. The lesions are covered by a slough, which may extend to the adjacent pharyngeal tissues and gums. Low grade fever and malaise are accompanying features. There occurs a characteristic fishy odor. Bacteriological studies reveal a fusiform bacillus and spirochete (*Spirochaeta denticola*). Treatment is by administering penicillin or erythromycin in addition to analgesics and mouthwashes.

AGRANULOCYTOSIS

This condition results because of sensitivity to drugs like chloramphenicol, sulphonamides, cytotoxic drugs and amidopyrine.

The patient presents with a history of sore throat, ulcerations in the buccopharyngeal mucosa and false membrane formation. Diagnosis is confirmed by the blood picture which shows marked reduction in neutrophils. Treatment is withdrawal of the drugs offending and prescription of heavy doses of penicillin, and of blood transfusion, if necessary.

LEUKEMIA

Acute lymphocytic leukemia may sometimes present as oropharyngeal ulcerations with membrane formation. Diagnosis is made from the blood picture.

INFECTIOUS MONONUCLEOSIS

It is viral disease which may sometimes be associated with oral lesions. The uvula may be swollen and there may occur inflammatory lesions in other parts of buccopharyngeal mucosa. The blood picture shows leukocytosis and relative increase in lymphocytes. The Paul-Bunnell test is positive.

MONILIASIS (THRUSH)

It is a fungal infection of the mouth due to *Candida albicans.* The lesions appear as white or grayish-white patches on the oropharyngeal mucosa surrounded by areas of slight redness. The membrane can be removed leaving a raw area. The condition is common in marasmic children. Treatment consists of local application of 1 percent gentian voilet or nystatin in glycerine, besides good nursing.

Chronic Pharyngitis

Chronic inflammation of the pharynx may be due to nonspecific or specific lesions.

CHRONIC NON-SPECIFIC PHARYNGITIS

Various etiological factors in the nose or oral cavity may produce secondary effects in the pharynx.

The infected discharge from the nose and paranasal sinuses as in rhinitis and sinusitis constantly irritates the pharyngeal mucosa, and often results in chronic inflammatory changes. Similarly, obstructive lesions in the nose like deflected septum, nasal polypi and adenoids lead to a habit of mouth-breathing, which is an important predisposing cause of pharyngitis.

Caries of the teeth and infected gums may also lead to pharyngeal infection. External conditions may play an important role in pharyngitis. People working in dusty atmosphere and smokers are the usual victims. Sometimes, pharyngitis may be a manifestation of dyspepsia or chronic suppurative lung diseases.

Clinical Features

The most constant symptom is discomfort in the throat with a foreign body sensation. Spasms of cough and tendency to clear the throat are common. Tiredness of voice and difficulty in swallowing may occur.

Diffuse congestion of the pharyngeal wall may be seen and prominent vessels are seen through the inflamed mucosa. This type of pharyngitis is called chronic catarrhal pharyngitis. Sometimes the chronic infection results in hypertrophy of lymph nodules on the pharyngeal wall presenting a granular picture, called chronic granular pharyngitis. This form of pharyngitis usually occurs in persons who use their voice excessively, particularly when the voice production is faulty like Clergymen (Clergymen's throat).

Treatment of Chronic Pharyngitis

It is rather difficult to reverse the chronic changes once, they have set in. However, the symptoms can be alleviated to a greater extent.

The primary etiological factor in the nose, nasopharynx or oral cavity should receive proper treatment. Such patients are usually in the habit of making frequent swallowing attempts in order to clear the throat. This should be forbidden as such attempts at clearing the throat or hawking only add to the misery. Cough suppressants like codeine phosphate linctus should be given to relieve the cough. Temporary relief may be achieved by local application of various soothing paints like Mandl's paint.

Alcohol, smoking, irritants and spicy foods should be avoided.

CHRONIC ATROPHIC PHARYNGITIS

The atrophic changes in the pharynx usually result as a direct extension of atrophic changes in the nose. The condition in its mild form is called *pharyngitis sicca.* It may also result from conditions which result in mouth-breathing. The main symptom is dryness of the throat which causes great discomfort. In later stages, the presence of crusts may cause a coughing and hawking sensation. Examination reveals a dry glazed appearance of the mucosa, sometimes covered with crusts.

Treatment

Local alkaline gargles or spraying help in the removal of crusts. Nasal condition should be properly attended to. Vitamin A may be useful. Smoking and irritant foods are avoided.

Keratosis Pharynges

It is a condition of unknown etiology which is characterized by whitish horny outgrowths on the faucial tonsils, base of the tongue and posterior pharyngeal wall. It results from hypertrophy and keratinization of the superficial epithelium. The lesions are hard and cannot be removed easily. There is no surrounding erythema and no constitutional symptoms except mild discomfort.

There is no specific treatment of this condition, it may subside within a few months. The patient needs only reassurance.

Specific Infections of the Pharynx (Fig. 46.2)

TUBERCULOSIS

Tuberculosis of the pharynx usually results as a secondary manifestation to advanced chronic pulmonary tuberculosis. Mucosal ulceration with undermined edges occurs in the oropharyngeal region. The chief complaint of the patient is pain with dysphagia. Treatment is by antitubercular drugs.

LUPUS VULGARIS

Lupus of the nose may extend posteriorly to involve the pharynx, soft palate and fauces. Tubercles appear on the pharyngeal mucosa which breakdown with subsequent cicatrization and scarring of the fauces and soft palate.

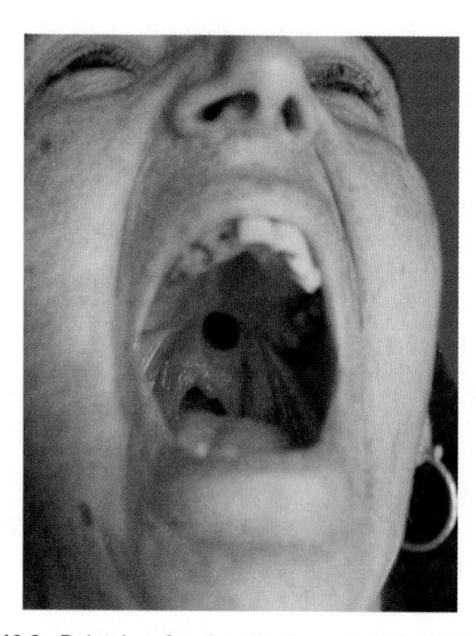

Fig. 46.2: Palatal perforation: Postgranulomatous infection

SYPHILIS

The pharynx is usually involved in the secondary stage of syphilis. It shows diffuse congestion and there occur mucous patches and snail-track ulcers with lymphadenitis. Spirochetes can be seen on smears from the mucous patches and ulcers.

In tertiary syphilis, the gumma may sometimes be a presenting feature on the fauces, palate and pharynx. The diagnosis is by biopsy and serological tests. Penicillin is the drug of choice for the treatment of syphilis.

Stenosis of the Pharynx

ETIOLOGY

Stenosis occurs due to scar tissue formation which may occur due to the following causes:

1. Infections
   a. Acute, e.g. scarlet fever or gangrenous tonsillitis
   b. Chronic, e.g. scleroma, syphilis, lupus
2. Operative measures
   a. For removal of neoplastic disease
   b. Removal of tonsils and adenoids
   c. Electric cauterization
3. Trauma
   a. Accidental wounds
   b. Corrosive poisonings.

Clinical Features

Difficulty in nasal breathing, altered voice (*rhinolalia clausa* or muffled speech) and dysphagia are the main symptoms.

Treatment

Treatment is dilatation with bougies or surgical division of the adhesions and Thiersch' graft may be undertaken.

Chapter

47

Tonsillitis

The palatine tonsils are subepithelial lymphoid collections situated inbetween the faucial pillars. These help in protecting the respiratory and alimentary tracts from bacterial invasion and are thus prone to frequent attacks of infection.

Acute Tonsillitis

Acute tonsillitis is mainly a disease of childhood but is also frequently seen in adults.

ETIOLOGY

It may occur as a primary infection of the tonsil itself or may secondarily occur as a result of infection of the upper respiratory tract usually following viral infections.

Common causative bacteria include hemolytic *Streptococcus, Staphylococcus, Haemophilus influenzae* and *Pneumococcus.*

Poor orodental hygiene, poor nutrition and congested surroundings are important predisposing factors for the disease.

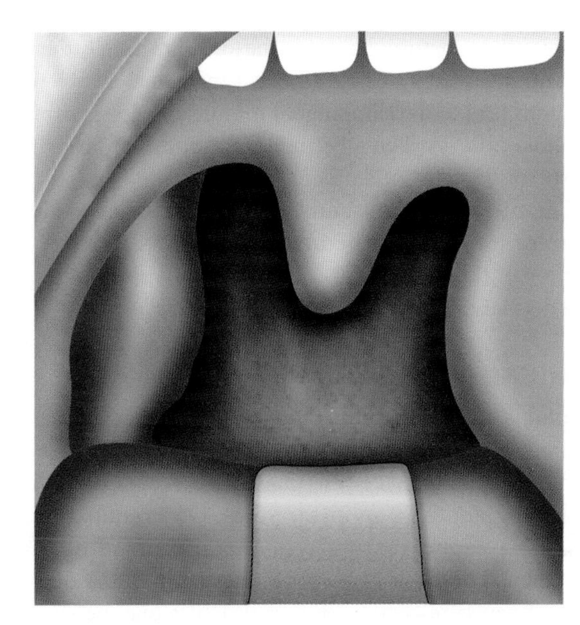

Fig. 47.1: Oropharynx showing follicular tonsillitis

PATHOLOGY

The process of inflammation originating within the tonsil is accompanied by hyperemia and edema with conversion of lymphoid follicles into small abscesses which discharge into crypts. When tonsils are inflamed as a result of generalized infection of the oropharyngeal mucosa, the condition is termed *catarrhal tonsillitis.*

When the inflammatory exudate collects in the tonsillar crypts, these present as multiple white spots on an inflammed tonsillar surface, giving rise to a clinical picture of follicular tonsillitis (**Fig. 47.1**). Sometimes exudation from crypts may coalesce to form a membrane over the surface of the tonsil, giving a clinical picture of *membranous tonsillitis.* When the whole tonsil is uniformly congested and swollen, it is called acute parenchymatous tonsillitis.

CLINICAL FEATURES

The patient presents with discomfort in the throat, difficulty in swallowing and generalized body symptoms like malaise, anorexia, fever and bodyache. On examination, the patient is febrile and has tachycardia. The tonsils appear swollen, congested with exudate in the crypts. There may occur edema of the uvula and soft palate.

The jugulodigastric (tonsillar) lymph nodes are enlarged and tender.

TREATMENT

General management of the patient includes bed rest, and giving plenty of fluids. Analgesics are given to relieve pain and fever. Antibiotics are prescribed according to the culture sensitivity report. However, penicillin is the drug of choice. Erythromycin and ampicillin may be needed for resistant cases.

COMPLICATIONS OF ACUTE TONSILLITIS

1. *Chronic tonsillitis:* Repeated attacks of acute tonsillitis result in chronic inflammatory changes in the tonsils.

2. *Peritonsillar abscess:* Spread of infection from the tonsil to the paratonsillar tissues results in development of abscess between the tonsillar capsule and the tonsil bed.
3. *Parapharyngeal abscess:* Infection from the tonsil or peritonsillar tissue may involve the parapharyngeal space with abscess formation.
4. *Acute otitis media:* Infection from the tonsil may extend to the eustachian tube and result in acute infection of the middle ear.
5. *Acute nephritis and rheumatic fever* are the other complications of streptococcal tonsillitis.

Chronic Tonsillitis

Chronic inflammatory changes in the tonsil are usually the result of recurrent acute infections treated inadequately. Recurrent infections lead to development of minute abscesses within the lymphoid follicles. These become walled off by fibrous tissue and surrounded by inflammatory cells.

The most common and the most important cause of recurrent infection of the tonsils is persistent or recurrent infection of the nose and paranasal sinuses. This leads to postnasal discharge which then infects the tonsils as well.

CLINICAL FEATURES

Symptoms include discomfort in the throat, recurrent attacks of sore throat, unpleasant taste (cacagus) and bad smell in the mouth (halitosis). Sometimes there occurs difficulty in swallowing and change in the voice. On examination, the tonsils may appear hypertrophic and protruding out of the pillars. These are diffusely congested, mouths of crypts appear open from which epithelial debris may be squeezed on pressure. The anterior pillars are hypermic. Sometimes the symptoms of sore throat and dysphagia are associated with small fibrotic tonsils (chronic fibrotic tonsillitis). Enlargement of the jugulodigastric lymph nodes is an important sign of tonsillar infection.

The diagnosis is based on the history of repeated attacks of sore throat or acute tonsillitis, associated with symptoms of dysphagia and discomfort. These symptoms if seen with enlarged tonsils, hyperaemic pillars and enlarged neck nodes, a diagnosis of chronic tonsillitis is well considered.

TREATMENT

As already mentioned, infections of the nose and paranasal sinuses forms the most important factor leading to chronic or recurrent infection of the tonsils. Treatment of these factors in the form of antibiotic cover, decongestants, mucolytics, mucokinetics and antihistaminics as well as surgical management like septoplasty for a deviated nasal septum, antral washouts, removal of nasal polypi if any, etc. might reduce or actually prevent any further infection of the tonsillar tissue.

If the above measures fail and the patient continues to have recurrent attacks of tonsillitis, surgical removal of the tonsils (tonsillectomy) might be needed.

COMPLICATIONS

These include, peritonsillar abscess, parapharyngeal abscess, intratonsillar abscess, tonsillar cyst, tonsillolith, rheumatic fever and acute nephritis.

Acute Lingual Tonsillitis

Lymphoid tissues of the base of the tongue are called lingual tonsils. Their inflammation is referred to as acute lingual tonsillitis. The causative factors are usually the same as for acute tonsillitis. Dysphagia is the main symptom. On examination, movements of the tongue are painful and the tongue base is tender on palpation. Mirror examination reveals the inflamed lingual tonsils.

TREATMENT

Antibiotics, usually penicillin or erythromycin are prescribed in association with analgesics.

The condition if untreated may lead to edema of the epiglottis and larynx or suppuration may occur (lingual quinsy).

Chronic Lingual Tonsillitis

Chronic inflammation of the lingual tonsils may be a problem after tonsillectomy when the lingual tonsils undergo compensatory hypertrophy.

The patient complains of discomfort in the throat, dysphagia and a thick plummy voice. Most patients respond to medical treatment of avoiding irritant foods, and application of local paints.

Sometimes diathermy or cryosurgery may be needed to reduce the size of the lingual tonsils.

Tonsillectomy

INDICATIONS OF TONSILLECTOMY

The tonsils get infected because of bad oral hygiene, unhygienic eating habits, constant postnasal discharge, mouth breathing and irritant eatables. Control of these, thus, can prevent infection. However, tonsillectomy may be indicated in certain cases.The indications of tonsillectomy can be classified as absolute and relative.

Absolute indications:

1. Hypertrophied tonsils causing obstructive symptoms like obstructive sleep apnea.

2. Suspicion of malignancy
3. More than one attack of peritonsillar abscess
4. Tonsillitis resulting in febrile convulsions
5. Persistent or recurrent tonsillar hemorrhage.

Relative indications:

1. Recurrent acute tonsillar infections either more than six per year or more than five per year for two consecutive years.
2. Cases with chronic enlargement of regional lymph nodes in association with sore throat.
3. Tonsillectomy is indicated when it is thought that tonsillar infection is producing secondary effects in other organs. Rheumatic fever and acute glomerulonephritis develop as an antigen antibody reaction to streptococcal infections. Though tonsillectomy does not help an established rheumatic heart disease or nephritis, recurrent attacks can be prevented by tonsillectomy. However, in such cases before undertaking tonsillectomy there should be no evidence of active throat infection.
4. Carriers of diphtheria and *Streptococcus haemolyticus* as proved by repeated throat swabs, who are a potential source of infection.
5. Eating or swallowing difficulties
6. Failure to thrive
7. Halitosis.

INDICATIONS FOR UNILATERAL TONSILLECTOMY

1. As excision biopsy of the tonsil to determine a possible malignancy.
2. As an approach to expose the glossopharyngeal nerve or enlarged styloid process in tonsillar bed, in stylalgia or idiopathic glossopharyngeal neuralgia.
3. Tonsillolith, tonsillar cyst, and impacted foreign body in the tonsil need tonsillectomy on the affected side.
4. In branchial fistula to remove the complete tract, one end of the tract being in posterior faucial pillar.

CONTRAINDICATIONS OF TONSILLECTOMY

1. Tonsillectomy should not be done during an epidemic of poliomyelitis as there is a high-risk of contracting bulbar poliomyelitis.
2. Blood dyscrasias like purpura, aplastic anemia, bleeding and coagulation defects.
3. Cases of uncontrolled systemic disease like diabetes.
4. Tonsillectomy should not be done during or immediately after an attack of infection or when the child has recently been exposed to infectious disease like measles.
5. Tonsillectomy is not done during menstruation or during pregnancy.

SELECTION OF TONSILLECTOMY CASES AND INVESTIGATIONS

In a case where an indication for tonsillectomy exists, it is necessary to look for any contraindication that may coexist.

Various investigations may be needed to avoid taking any unnecessary risk of anesthesia or operation. Blood examination is done to know the hemoglobin level and the state of coagulability (coagulation time) and capillary contraction (bleeding time). Urine analysis is another routine investigation to rule out any kidney damage or other metabolic disorders.

The instruments used for tonsillectomy are shown in **Figure 47.2**.

METHOD

Surgery is generally done under general anesthesia, but can be undertaken under local anesthesia also.

The dissection method is the procedure of choice for tonsillectomy. Guillotine tonsillectomy is not favored at present. Though this method is more quick in expert hands but it is not suitable for the cases with excessive fibrosis and does not provide an effective control for bleeding.

The dissection method allows complete removal of the tonsillar tissue under direct vision. Bleeding points are properly ligated. The following are the steps of the operation:

1. After the patient is put in Rose's position, a Davis Boyle's mouth gag is used to open the mouth and retract the tongue.

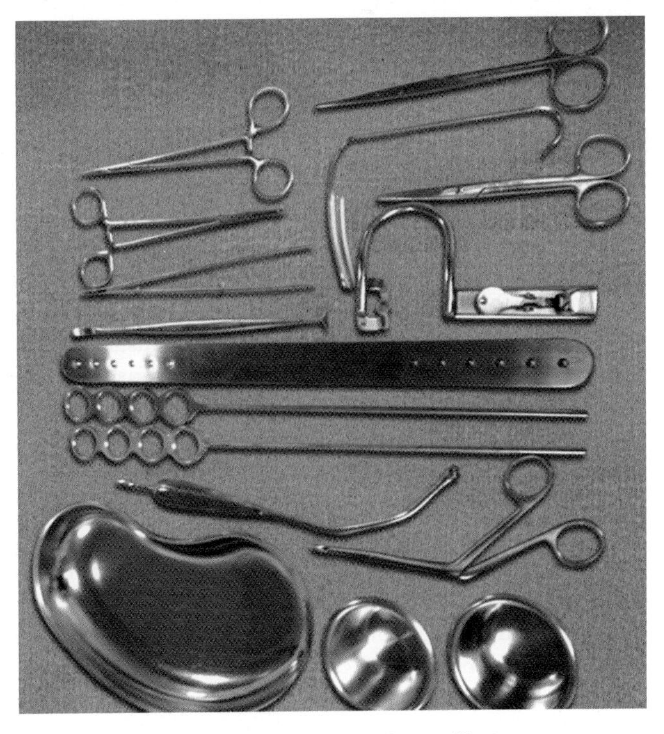

Fig. 47.2: Instruments used for tonsillectomy

The tonsil is grasped at the upper pole by a tonsil holding forceps and stretched medially.
2. The incision is made in the mucosa of the anterior pillar at the upper pole where it passes on to the tonsil.
3. With a blunt dissector or scissors, the upper pole of the tonsil is separated from the anterior and posterior pillars.
4. A blunt dissector or a blunt suction tip separates the tonsils with its capsule from the loose areolar tissue which binds it to the bed.
5. Dissection is continued to the lower pole.
6. Tonsillar snare is passed around the pedicle and is closed. It crushes and cuts through the pedicle and the tonsil gets separated.
7. The tonsillar fossa is packed for a few minutes to stop any oozing.
8. Prominent bleeding points are identified and ligated or cauterized and the procedure repeated on the other side.

POSTOPERATIVE CARE

Normal unaided respiration should be established before the patient leaves the operation theater. The patient is placed in tonsil position. This position allows free respiration and permits any blood and secretions, which may collect to run out of the nose and mouth.

A strict watch should be kept on the pulse and respiration of the patient. A rising pulse rate indicates hemorrhage. Cold drinks and soft diet are prescribed for the initial few days. Analgesics are given for pain. Antiseptic mouth washes help to keep the mouth clean.

Postoperative Complications

Hemorrhage: Besides the complications that may arise because of anesthesia, the main surgical problem is hemorrhage. It could be primary (during operation), reactionary (within the first 24 hours), or secondary (between fifth to tenth postoperative day) hemorrhage.

Excessive bleeding at the time of operation usually arises because of trauma to an aberrant vessel or paratonsillar vein.

Reactionary hemorrhage usually arises as a result of slipping of a ligature or because of the postoperative rise in blood pressure. If a clot has formed in the fossa, it is removed. This allows the muscular contraction and retraction of the blood vessel.

A gauze pack may also be held in the fossa for a few minutes to control the bleeding. However, if the bleeding does not stop, the patient is reanesthetized and the bleeding vessel is ligated. Sometimes, the tonsillar pillars may need to be stitched over a pack to control the bleeding.

Secondary hemorrhage is the result of infection. Bleeding is usually mild. Antibiotics, antiseptic mouth washes are given in addition to bed rest.

Surgical trauma: During tonsillectomy, trauma may occur to the pillars, soft palate, teeth or uvula.

Pulmonary complications: Pulmonary complications may result because of inhalation of blood or tonsillar tissue, with the result collapse, pneumonia or lung abscess may occur.

Peritonsillar Abscess (Quinsy, Paratonsillar Abscess)

Peritonsillar abscess is a complication of acute or chronic tonsillitis. The pathogenesis of peritonsillar abscess (**Fig. 47.3**) is described in the textbooks as being a direct communication and progression of acute exudative tonsillitis. Little study has been done on the true etiology and pathogenesis of peritonsillar abscess. A group of salivary glands (Weber's glands) proven to be located in the supratonsillar space have been shown to be implicated in its pathogenesis (**Fig. 47.4**). A review of peritonsillar abscess has been undertaken, and evidence has been presented to support the premise that the true cause for peritonsillar abscess is not necessarily an extension of an acute exudative tonsillitis, but an abscess formation of Weber's salivary glands in the supratonsillar fossa.

There occurs accumulation of pus between the tonsil capsule and tonsil bed. In most of the cases, pus collection occurs *anterosuperior* to tonsil but may sometimes occur laterally or posteriorly. A mixed bacterial flora of streptococci, staphylococci and pneumococci grows on culture of the pus.

CLINICAL FEATURES

The condition usually affects adolescents and is mostly unilateral. The patient complains of unilateral throat pain after

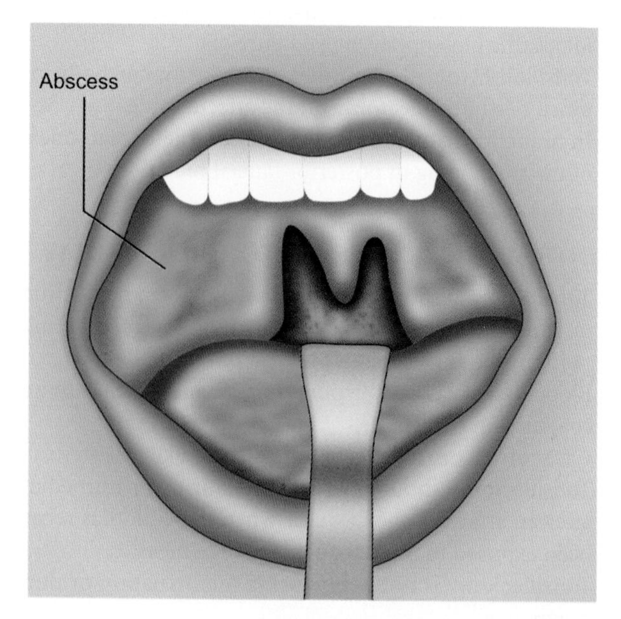

Fig. 47.3: Acute peritonsillar abscess

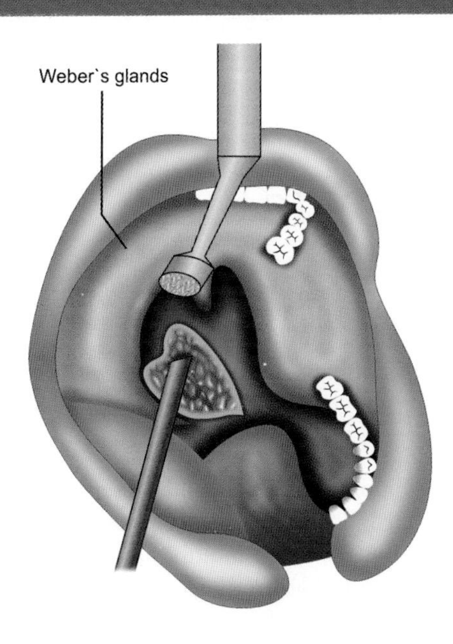

Fig. 47.4: Weber's gland in the supratonsillar space, resting on the superior pole of the tonsil (From Parkinson, RH: Tonsil and Allied Problems. Macmillan, New York, 1951)

a few days of sore throat. The pain gradually becomes severe and may radiate to the ear. Swallowing is markedly painful so the patient even allows the saliva to dribble out. The patient feels extremely ill.

Examination shows a toxic patient, with the head inclined towards the side of the abscess. There is trismus because of spasm of the pterygoid muscles. There is a unilateral swelling of the palate and pillars on the side of the abscess. The tonsil is displaced downwards and medially. The edematous uvula is pushed towards the opposite side with its tip usually pointing to the side of the lesion. Cervical lymph nodes on the affected side are enlarged and markedly tender.

TREATMENT

When pus is suspected, it should be drained. The following are the sites of drainage:

1. The most prominent part of the swelling should be selected and drainage done.
2. Alternatively, the intersection of an imaginary line drawn from the base of the uvula and another imaginary line drawn along the anterior faucial pillar is the site of drainage.
3. Sometimes the drainage is done through the supratonsillar crypt.

The peritonsillar abscess draining forceps is introduced and opened up to drain the abscess. The tip of a guarded sharp scalpel can be used to make an incision and the abscess drained by sinus forceps. Anesthesia is not needed as the pain is already intense and a sharp stab for the drainage does not add to it. Besides drainage, heavy doses of antibiotics, usually coamoxiclox or clindamycin are prescribed in addition to antiseptic mouth washes and analgesics.

Interval tonsillectomy: In view of the painful nature of this condition and the possible serious complications that may arise, tonsillectomy is advocated after 6 to 8 weeks, when the inflammation has subsided. Now, it is not thought to be necessary in all cases.

Abscess tonsillectomy (Quinsy tonsillectomy): This procedure of draining the peritonsillar abscess by removing the tonsil has been advocated by some surgeons. It is done on the assumption that since the tonsil forms the medial wall of the abscess, therefore, tonsillectomy would give drainage to the abscess as well as save the patient from interval tonsillectomy. However, this procedure is not favored as the abscess may rupture during anesthesia with consequent problems of aspiration. Besides as the tissues are acutely inflamed, there occurs severe bleeding and chances of systemic dissemination of infection are more.

COMPLICATIONS OF PERITONSILLAR ABSCESS

The abscess may rupture spontaneously and cause aspiration and asphyxia. Spread of infection to the parapharyngeal space can cause parapharyngeal abscess.

Thrombosis of the internal jugular vein or even a carotid artery rupture can occur because of extension of this abscess to the parapharyngeal space.

Extension of the inflammatory process from the peritonsillar space can lead to laryngeal edema with resultant asphyxia. Systemic infection with the development of septicemia and multiple abscesses may occur.

PERITONSILLITIS

It is a stage in the development of peritonsillar abscess before the pus formation. The clinical features are those of severe tonsillitis with trismus. The peritonsillar tissues are severely inflamed but there is no displacement of the tonsil. Heavy doses of antibiotics cure the condition and prevent abscess formation.

Chapter 48

Adenoids

Introduction

Hypertrophied nasopharyngeal tonsils (adenoids) are usually the seat of infection in children between 3 and 6 years of age. As the child grows, the size of the nasopharyngeal tonsils diminishes and they disappear by puberty.

Clinical Features

Hypertrophied nasopharyngeal tonsils may produce symptoms because of their size. The symptoms may be nasal or aural.

The common nasal symptoms include frequent attacks of cold, persistent nasal discharge, nasal obstruction and snoring.

The common aural symptoms include recurrent attacks of earache, deafness and ear discharge. The other important symptoms include headache possibly due to infected material in the nasopharynx and nocturnal cough because of postnasal discharge. Lack of appetite and mental dullness have also been attributed to adenoids.

Examination reveals mucoid or mucopurulent discharge in the nose.

Throat examination reveals postnasal discharge and in a cooperative child, posterior rhinoscopy shows enlarged mass of adenoids on the posterosuperior wall of the nasopharynx (**Fig. 48.1**).

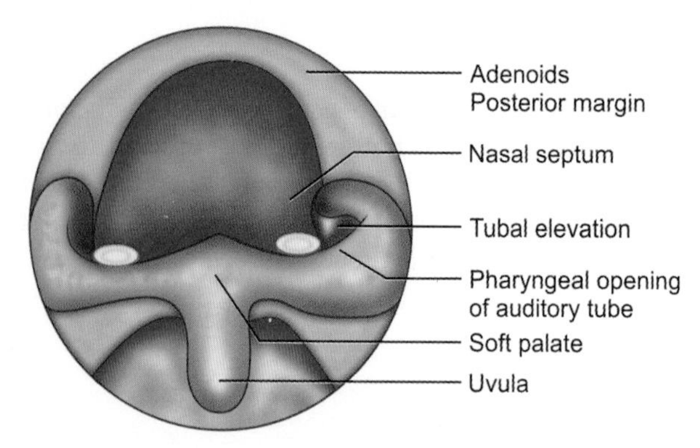

Fig. 48.1: Posterior rhinoscopic view of the nasopharynx showing adenoids

In a longstanding case, the child presents with a typical appearance called "adenoid facies" (**Fig. 48.2**). There is a dull look, pinched nostrils, open mouth, narrow maxillary arch, retracted upper lip and protruding teeth.

A lateral view X-ray of the nasopharynx may sometimes be done to show an adenoid mass.

Complications of Adenoids

These include recurrent attacks of otitis media, secretory otitis media, maxillary sinusitis and orthodontic disturbances. Besides, such patients are likely to encounter speech problems, like rhinolalia clausa (closed nose voice). Chronic infection may lead to the development of adenoid cysts.

Treatment

Conservative management includes decongestants (systemic and locally in the nose), systemic antibiotics to control the infection and antihistaminic preparations.

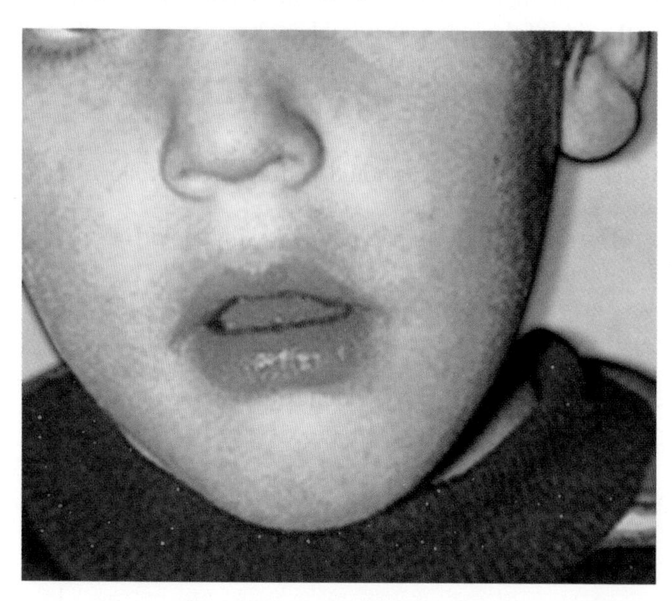

Fig. 48.2: Typical adenoid facies

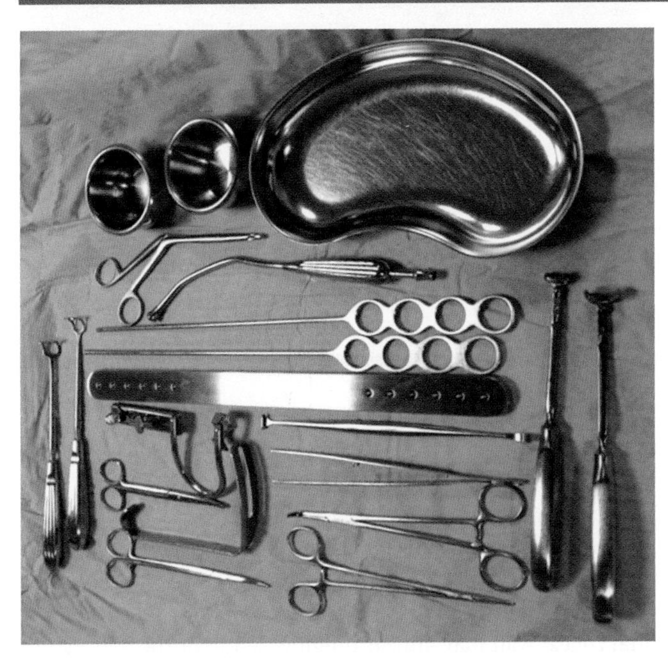

Fig. 48.3: Instruments used for adenoidectomy

Surgery: The operation of adenoidectomy is advocated if the size of adenoids is interfering with the nasal and eustachian tube function or causing difficulty in speech and feeding. Adenoidectomy may be needed if the adenoids are thought to be the cause of recurrent upper respiratory tract infection or recurrent otitis media.

Since the problem of adenoids and tonsils usually coexist, the operation of adenoidectomy is done in the same sitting as the tonsillectomy. The operation is performed under general anesthesia and oral intubation is preferred. St. Clair Thompson adenoid curette with a guard is the instrument more commonly used. **Figure 48.3** shows the instruments used for adenoidectomy.

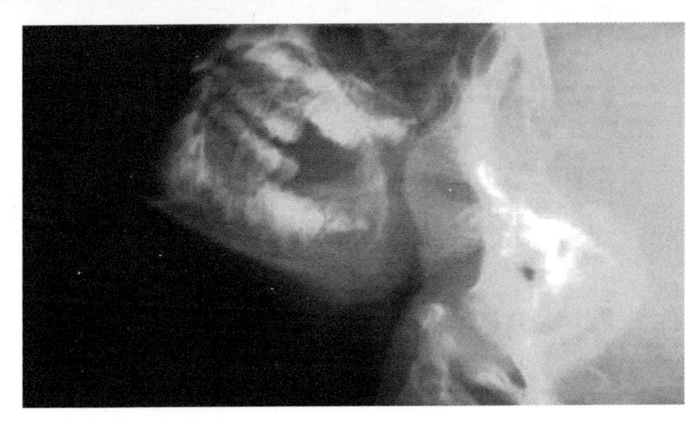

Fig. 48.4: Lateral neck X-ray showing hypertrophied adenoid

The adenoid curette is held in the right hand and passed behind the soft palate to the posterior end of the nasal septum. It is pressed against the roof of the nasopharynx to engage the adenoid mass. Then with a downward and forward sweeping movement, the adenoids are curetted out and are held up in the guard of the curette. A second stroke may be needed to clear the roof.

Adenoid mass from the lateral wall is displaced towards the center and curetted out. The postnasal cavity is packed for a few minutes to stop the bleeding. Postoperatively antibiotics and nasal decongestants are prescribed (**Fig. 48.4**).

The main complication of surgery is hemorrhage. Primary hemorrhage usually occurs due to leftover adenoid tags which may need further curettage. In case of severe bleeding the postnasal pack is kept for 24 to 48 hours. Secondary hemorrhage occurs due to infection and is treated by rest and antibiotics. Pulmonary complications like pneumonia, collapse or abscess may arise because of aspiration of blood or adenoid tissue tags.

Damage may occur to the eustachian tube openings and soft palate. Subluxation of the atlantoaxial joint, though a rare complication may result because of trauma, infection, decalcification of the vertebra or laxity of the anterior vertebral ligament.

Chapter 49

Pharyngeal Abscess

Besides the peritonsillar abscess, infection from a tonsil can travel to the retropharyngeal or parapharyngeal spaces and lead to development of an abscess.

Retropharyngeal Space

The retropharyngeal space is bounded anteriorly by the bucco-pharyngeal fascia and visceral fascia over the esophagus and posteriorly by the anterior layer of the deep fascia over the cervical vertebrae. Inferiorly this space communicates with mediastinum. The space contains lymph nodes of Ranvier's which drain the nasopharynx, part of oropharynx and the paranasal sinuses.

A retropharyngeal abscess develops because of infection in this space.

Parapharyngeal Space

It is a lateral pharyngeal space which extends from the base of skull above the level of the hyoid bone below.

It is bounded medially by the fascia over the pharynx and laterally by the fascia over the medial pterygoid muscle and the parotid glands. Posteriorly lies the carotid sheath with its contents. The space communicates with the retropharyngeal space and the submaxillary space and inferiorly with the mediastinum. It is divided into prestyloid and poststyloid portions by the styloid process.

Acute Retropharyngeal Abscess

ETIOLOGY

It is an uncommon condition, usually affecting children. It results from suppuration of the retropharyngeal lymph nodes secondary to infection in adenoids, sinuses or tonsils. The abscess may occur in adults after trauma by a foreign body or on endoscopy.

CLINICAL FEATURES

The patient complains of fever, malaise and difficulty in swallowing. The abscess in the late stages may present with respiratory difficulty.

The patient is ill, febrile and looks toxic. The posterior pharyngeal wall may appear bulging. X-ray of the soft tissues of the neck, shows a widened retropharyngeal space (**Fig. 49.1**). There is increased distance between the laryngotracheal air column and anterior border of the cervical vertebra.

TREATMENT

Systemic antibiotics are given. The abscess needs drainage. The patient is held supine on the table with the head end lowered to

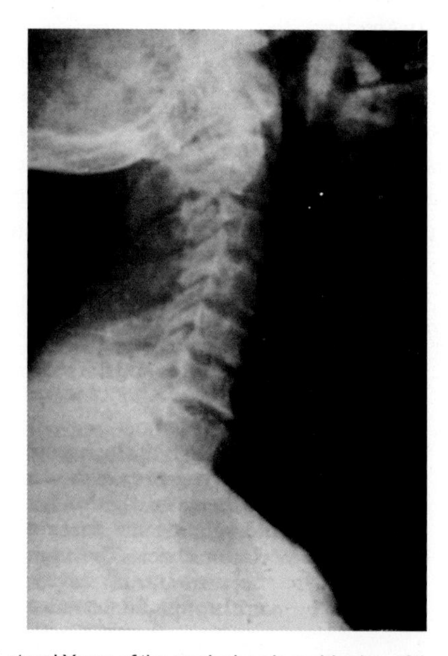

Fig. 49.1: Lateral X-ray of the neck showing widening of the prevertebral space in retropharyngeal abscess

prevent aspiration of pus into the larynx. An incision is given in the posterior pharyngeal wall and the pus sucked out.

Chronic Retropharyngeal Abscess

This occurs due to tuberculosis of the cervical spine. Radiography of the cervical spine shows destruction of the vertebra. Drainage is done through a neck incision in the posterior triangle.

Antitubercular treatment is given for the required period.

Parapharyngeal Abscess

The infection may travel to the parapharyngeal space from the tonsils, teeth or the other oropharyngeal or parotid lesions, as well as from the submandibular glands.

CLINICAL FEATURES

The patient looks ill, toxic and febrile and complains of difficulty in swallowing and may present with trismus.

The oropharyngeal examination may reveal a primary focus of infection. Examination of the neck shows a diffuse tender swelling below the angle of the mandible on the affected side.

TREATMENT

Antibiotics are given to control the infection. The abscess is drained through a lateral neck incision given anterior to the sternomastoid from the angle of the mandible to the hyoid bone.

Early drainage is done to prevent serious complications like thrombosis of major vessels and spread of infection to other spaces.

Chapter

50

Tumors of the Pharynx

Tumors of the Nasopharynx

Tumors of the nasopharynx can be benign or malignant. Benign tumors of the nasopharynx are rare. These are grouped as follows:

1. Juvenile angiofibroma
2. Hamartomas and dermoids
3. Craniopharyngiomas (from Rathke's pouch)
4. Lipoma, fibroma and neurofibroma.

Nasopharyngeal Angiofibroma

This is a benign but locally invasive lesion of the nasopharynx. It occurs almost exclusively in males between 10 and 25 years of age. The tumor tends to regress or stop growing after 25 years of age.

The etiology of the condition is unknown. Various factors which are thought to be causative agents include hormonal, traumatic and allergic factors. It is thought that the lesion arises from the ventral periosteum of the skull as a result of hormonal imbalance or persistence of embryonic tissue.

PATHOLOGY

The tumor consists of two main components, viz vascular and fibrous:

1. *Vascular component:* The great vascularity and abnormal structure of the vessel walls are striking. Blood vessels appear as multiple sinusoidal spaces lined by flattened endothelium and are devoid of the muscular wall. The blood spaces are variable in size.
2. *Fibrous stroma:* The stroma appears as loose connective tissue, highly cellular with some collagen fibers and fibroblasts.

SPREAD OF TUMOR

The tumor from its origin in the nasopharynx, fills the nasopharyngeal space and may spread anteriorly to the nasal cavities. It may extend to the pterygopalatine fossa and present in the orbit or cheek. The tumor can spread to the intracranial cavity by eroding its base or through its foramina.

CLINICAL FEATURES

Gradually increasing nasal obstruction and recurrent attacks of epistaxis are the common presenting symptoms.

Examination reveals a reddish vascular mass in the nasopharynx which may extend into the nasal cavities. There may be seen prominent blood vessel traversing over the tumor surface which bleeds easily and profusely on probing, therefore, probing or palpation of the nasopharynx should not be done.

INVESTIGATIONS

X-rays of the nasopharynx base of the skull and paranasal sinuses determine the extent of the tumor. External carotid angiography helps in its diagnosis (*tumor blush*), to determine the extent of tumors and to know the main blood supply.

The typical clinical features of this condition make preoperative biopsy unnecessary. Biopsy should be avoided due to risk of severe hemorrhage.

DIFFERENTIAL DIAGNOSIS

1. *Antrochoanal polyp:* It presents as a gray, pale polypoidal mass in the nasopharynx, unlike the firm, reddish, tumor mass with prominent vessels described above. Besides, there is no history of epistaxis.
2. *Nasopharyngeal carcinoma:* This lesion usually presents as a friable, proliferative or ulcerated mass with a high incidence of lymph node metastasis.

TREATMENT

These patients are usually anemic because of recurrent epistaxis, hence anemia should be corrected. Surgery is the treatment of choice. Through a transpalatal approach (Wilson's), the mucoperiosteum around the tumor mass is incised and with a strong periosteal elevator the tumor is separated from its bed. Lateral rhinotomy or Caldwell-Luc's procedures may be needed for tumors extending into the nose and antrum. To avoid profuse bleeding, it is important to go around the tumor mass and remove it *en masse*. Cryosurgery and diathermy have been helpful in reducing the bleeding during operation.

Hormonal therapy for the tumor is of doubtful value. Radiotherapy is used for the recurrent tumors and in patients unfit for surgery.

Prior external carotid artery ligation may be done with the hope of reducing hemorrhage. Recently external carotid artery embolization by gel foam has been tried as a temporary measure to reduce the bleeding during surgical removal.

MALIGNANT TUMORS OF NASOPHARYNX

Malignant tumors of the nasopharynx are more common than the benign ones of this region. Various types of malignant tumors of the nasopharynx are classified as follows:

- Squamous cell carcinoma, 90 to 95 percent are epithelial nasopharyngeal carcinomas
- Lymphoma, lymphosarcoma, osteosarcoma, myosarcoma
- Reticulum cell sarcoma
- Lymphoepithelioma
- Adenocarcinoma
- Chondrosarcoma
- Chordoma.

Etiological Factors in Carcinoma of the Nasopharynx

Highest incidence in southeast Asian geographic area, very rare elsewhere and shows HLA genetic predisposition. There is a dietary association with salt-preserved foods, notably fish and also a strong association with EBV in WHO III endemic subtypes. Males are more commonly affected and growths are more common in the relatively younger age group.

Histopathology: Three WHO subclassifications are described:

1. WHO I (keratinizing squamous carcinoma)
   - Accounts for higher proportion in nonendemic areas
   - Worse prognosis
2. WHO II (nonkeratinizing squamous carcinoma)
   - Least common
3. WHO III (undifferentiated)
   - Most common variant in endemic areas

Spread of Nasopharyngeal Growth

Direct involvement by the growth can cause destruction of the basisphenoid and basiocciput and spread can occur intracranially. The tumor may spread through the foramen lacerum in the roof near the lateral wall and involve the fifth and sixth cranial nerves.

Lateral spread can occur to the parapharyngeal space and cause paralysis of the last four cranial nerves including mandibular branch of the 5th nerve. The growth can spread anteriorly into the nasal cavities, ethmoids, orbits and downwards to the oropharynx.

Most cases of nasopharyngeal malignancy present with bilateral cervical node enlargement. Spread occurs usually to the upper deep cervical nodes but later the whole lymphatic chain of the neck may get involved.

Blood spread can lead to metastasis in the lungs and bones, particularly in the spine.

Clinical Features

Varied symptoms are characteristic of nasopharyngeal malignancy. The symptoms can be grouped as under:

1. *Nasal symptoms:* Nasal obstruction and epistaxis can occur.
2. *Aural symptoms:* Because of effects on the functioning of eustachian tube, the patient may present with conductive deafness because of serous otitis media or acute otitis media. So adults presenting with secretory otitis media need a fiberoptic scope examination of the nasopharynx to rule out nasopharyngeal mass.
3. *Neurological symptoms:* Malignant tumors of the nasopharynx are known to produce various neurological lesions particularly cranial nerve paralysis. Because of the intracranial and extracranial spread of tumor, multiple cranial nerve paralysis can occur. Nasopharyngeal malignancy is a common cause of the secondary trigeminal neuralgia, particularly in the distribution of maxillary division.

   Diplopia can occur because of involvement of 6th nerve or 3rd and 4th nerves, due to its spread along the foramen lacerum to cavernous sinus, where these nerves get involved.

   Paralysis of last four cranial nerves in the parapharyngeal space produces symptoms of pharyngeal and laryngeal paralysis.
4. *Nodal symptoms:* Most of the patients present with bilateral enlargement of neck nodes when first seen, even though the primary in nasopharynx is small or clinically not detectable (**Fig. 50.1**). The upper deep cervical glands are most commonly involved although all the lymphatic chain may get involved.

Diagnosis

Detailed examination of the nasopharynx is mandatory using a flexible nasopharyngoscope. Biopsy will tell about the histopathology and it may be necessary to take biopsy from nasopharynx, even if there is no obvious primary in a suspected case.

CT scan and MRI clinch the diagnosis. Metastatic work up in the form of CT Chest, abdomen and pelvis is recommended. Bone scan is also done to rule out any skeletal metastases.

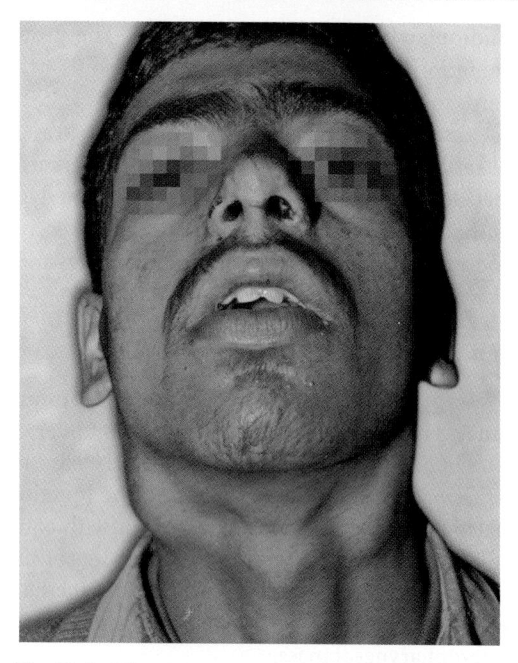

Fig. 50.1: Bilateral metastatic neck nodes in a case of nasopharyngeal carcinoma

STAGING

Most common system used is the American Joint Committee On Cancer (AJCC) system, but has prognostic shortcomings (places 80 percent of all patients into stage IV on presentation) (**Table 50.1**) and is being replaced by a different prognostic scoring system (that of Ho) based on risk factors.

Adverse risk factors in heme oxygenase system include:

- Increased number of symptoms
- Extension beyond nasopharynx
- Low neck adenopathy
- WHO I histology

AJCC staging is as follows:

Stage	Description
Tx	Tumor cannot be assessed
T0	No tumor
Tis	Carcinoma *in situ*
T1	Confined to nasopharynx
T2	Extends to oropharynx or nasal cavity (a or b = with/without parapharyngeal extension)
T3	Invading bone or sinuses
T4	Intracranial, orbital, or cranial nerve involvement

MANAGEMENT

Overall 5-year survival is 30 to 40 percent with a high-risk of local recurrence.

Table 50.1: Stage grouping

Stage 0	T1s	N0	M0
Stage I	T1	N0	M0
Stage IIA	T2a	N0	M0
Stage IIB	T1	N1	M0
	T2	N1	M0
	T2a	N1	M0
	T2b	N1	M0
Stage III	T1	N2	M0
	T2a	N2	M0
	T2b	N2	M0
	T3	N0	M0

Neoadjuvant chemoradiation: This is the main stay of the treatment of nasopharyngeal carcinomas. Currently low-risk patients with Stage I and II tumors receive radiotherapy only. High-risk patients receive cisplatinum (100 mg/m^2 over 6 hours on day 1 with standard hydration), mannitol and electrolyte replacement, and folinic acid (25 mg/m^2 every 6 hours for a total of six doses) as well as 5-fluorouracil (1000 mg/m^2 per day from day 2 for 5 days) as a continuous infusion. They receive three courses of chemotherapy every 21 days or on full blood count recovery, followed by irradiation. Patients not in complete remission after three courses of chemotherapy will receive concomitant cisplatinum (20 mg/m^2/day for 3 days with radiotherapy for two courses).

Surgery: It is limited to neck dissection to remove nodes not effectively treated with radiation. There are several small reports of primary skull-base surgical resection for T1 disease, T3-4 debulking or for local small recurrence.

EBV vaccination: It is postulated as primary preventative measure in high-risk populations, but no good trials or long-term data is available yet.

LYMPHOEPITHELIOMA

It is a special variety of epithelioma which arises in nasopharynx and oropharynx where there are subepithelial lymphoid tissue collections.

This type of tumor is characterized by its occurrence in young people, its early and widespread metastasis and sensitivity to radiotherapy.

Tumors of the Oropharynx

The common benign tumors from the oropharyngeal region include papilloma and pleomorphic adenoma.

PAPILLOMAS

Papillomas usually arise on the soft palate or the faucial pillars and form mobile warty growths. They are mostly asymptomatic. Treatment is surgical excision.

PLEOMORPHIC SALIVARY ADENOMA

Tumor may sometimes arise from the salivary glandular tissue distributed over the palate or faucial region.

It is a benign tumor with tendency to recur and a small proportion (5%) may undergo malignant change. Macroscopically, the tumor is firm, lobulated with a capsule surrounding it.

Microscopically it consists of epithelial cells in a hyaline stroma.

Treatment is surgical excision.

MALIGNANT NEOPLASMS OF THE OROPHARYNX

- Squamous cell carcinomas which account for >90 percent of lesions, with several variants
- Lymphomas (NHL) often found here in Waldeyer's ring nodes
- Minor salivary gland tumors
- Lymphoepithelioma
- Mucosal melanomas.

SQUAMOUS CELL CARCINOMA IN THE OROPHARYNGEAL REGION

It may arise from tonsils, palate or the posterior pharyngeal wall. The disease is common in men than in women. There is strong relationship of this disease with smoking and betel-nut chewing.

Symptoms usually occur late in the disease. Patients usually present with soreness or discomfort in throat and difficulty in swallowing. Excessive salivation and an earache may be presenting features. Examination reveals a proliferative or an ulcerative type of lesion in oropharynx. There is a high incidence of lymph node involvement, particularly the upper deep cervical groups of nodes are involved. High rates of nodes (50% overall) and second primaries (25% overall) are seen on presentation. All lesions larger than T1 are thought to have nodal metastases rate >25 percent

Diagnosis is confirmed by biopsy.

Staging

T1 — Tumor less than 2 cm in diameter.
T2 — Tumor 2 to 4 cm in diameter.
T3 — Tumor more than 4 cm.
T4—Massive tumor invading adjacent structures.

Treatment

A. Primary tumor (squamous cell carcinoma)

Surgery and radiation have equal efficacy for T1-2 lesions, such that one may be used to salvage the other. Deeply infiltrative lesions or those that involve significant tongue base are not well controlled by radiation, hence, are better treated initially with surgery + adjuvant therapy.

Indications for postoperative radiation are:
- Close or involved resection margins
- Perineural/perivascular invasion

B. Large lesions (T3-4) primary tumor (squamous cell carcinoma variant or nonsquamous cell carcinoma)
- Verrucous cancer requires wide local resection, no postoperative radiation
- Lymphoepitheliomas are exquisitely radiosensitive, hence, this is preferred primary therapy
- Minor salivary gland tumors
- Melanomas and sarcomas require wide local excisions neck dissection
- Lyphomas are treated with radiation and chemotherapy

Tumors of the Hypopharynx

This part of the pharynx lies posterior to the larynx and extends from the lower limit of the oropharynx up to the upper end of the esophagus. It includes two pyriform fossae, the postcricoid region and the lateral and posterior pharyngeal wall.

Benign tumors of this region are uncommon and present as smooth, slow-growing masses. The tumors of mesodermal origin are more common than papilloma or adenoma.

Malignant tumors of the laryngopharynx are common in India. The etiology is unknown. Plummer-Vinson syndrome and Bazex's syndrome (acrokeratosis paraneoplastica) paraneoplastic psoriatic changes of which 50 percent are associated with pharyngeal carcinoma are thought to be precancerous conditions. Betel-nut chewing and smoking may play a part in its causation.

Cancer of the laryngopharynx commonly affects the males of the elderly age group except cancer of the postcricoid region which is more common in females.

HISTOLOGY

Squamous cell carcinoma (moderately differentiated) is the most common type of cancer of this region. Adenocarcinoma, adenoid cystic carcinoma, and malignant lymphomas may also rarely occur.

Site and spread: Tumor usually seen in three subsites

1. Piriform sinus (2/3 of lesions)
   - Tumor spread laterally to thyroid cartilage and thyroid gland, medially to hemilarynx, cricoarytenoid joint, or cross over to other side
   - Seventy-five percent incidence of nodal spread on presentation.

2. Posterior pharyngeal wall (1/3 of lesions)
   - Invade prevertebral fascia, superior spread to tongue base, inferior spread to postcricoid region
   - Retropharyngeal mets to nodes of Rouviere in 40 percent on presentation.
3. Postcricoid (5% of lesions)
   - Circumferential spread along and into cricoid and cervical esophagus
   - Lowest metastases rate, and tend to spread to paratracheal nodes.

STAGING

Stage	Description
Tx	Tumor cannot be assessed
T0	No evidence of tumor
Tis	Carcinoma *in situ*
T1	Tumor limited to one subsite, <2 cm
T2	Tumors invades more than one subsite, <4 cm, no vocal cord fixation
T3	Tumor >4 cm or vocal cord fixation
T4	Invasion of adjacent structures (bone, tongue, skin of neck, etc...)

CLINICAL FEATURES

The patient usually presents in the late stages when the growth is well advanced. The early symptoms are vague and the patient may complain of discomfort in the throat or pain on swallowing.

Dysphagia is the main presenting symptom. It is usually complained of in the late stages and is progressive. The patient may present with a lymph node mass in the neck without any pharyngeal symptoms. Some patients present with pain in the ear (referred otalgia) or a muffled voice.

DIAGNOSIS

Flexible or indirect laryngoscopy usually reveals the growth in the laryngopharynx.

Pooling of saliva in the pyriform fossae is suggestive of an obstructive lesion and should arouse suspicion. Neck examination reveals lymph node involvement or the tumor mass. Laryngeal crepitus may be absent particularly in postcricoid malignancy. Imaging studies include Barium swallow which is good for detecting esophageal spread, but unable to accurately assess tumor thickness. CT is highly sensitive for tumor thickness, cartilaginous invasion, and involvement of nodes though it tends to overstage as cannot differentiate tumor from inflammatory edema. MRI has superior soft tissue resolution, and can differentiate edema from tumor on T2 weighed images.

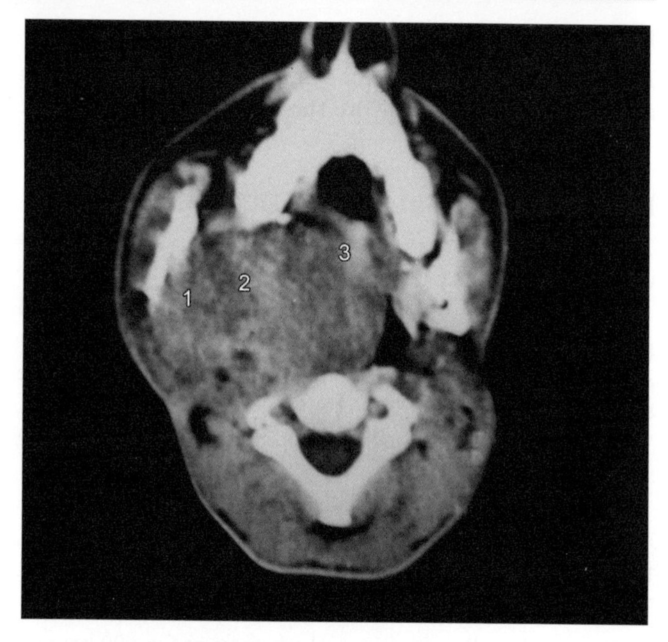

Fig. 50.2: Parapharyngeal tumor

Rigid hypopharyngoscopy and direct laryngoscopy are done to determine the site of growth, its extent and to take the biopsy. Biopsy is confirmatory **(Fig. 50.2)**.

TREATMENT

Generally combined modality therapy:

T1: Radiation alone (to primary and neck) with surgical salvage

- Some T1 lesions of piriform sinus are amenable to primary larynx-sparing surgery (lesions well away from apex of sinus)
- Some T1 lesions of posterior pharyngeal wall can be resected and reconstructed with split thickness skin grafts.

T3-4: Ablative surgery (laryngectomy with partial or total pharyngectomy) + postoperative radiation.

T2 lesions are controversial in terms of primary radiation vs surgery.

The role of inductive chemotherapy still is undefined +/– unproven, but goals include:

- Function preservation
- Increase disease-free survival or local control
- Sensitize tumors to radiation
- Make unresectable tumors resectable.

Neck dissection is generally reserved for bilateral II-IV neck nodes or bilateral neck radiation as indicated by primary therapy modality.

SURGICAL TECHNIQUES

Depending upon the extent of involvement the surgical procedures vary. There is hardly a tumor of the laryngopharynx which can be effectively treated by local excision. Laryngectomy is invariably needed in addition to removal of the growth in the laryngopharynx.

1. *Partial pharyngectomy with total laryngectomy:* This operation is done for the growth involving the pyriform fossa and larynx. The remaining mucosa is used to reconstruct the food channel.
2. *Total pharyngectomy with total laryngectomy:* This procedure is needed for the growth involving postcricoid, upper esophagus and lower part of the pyriform fossa, when no mucosa can be spared to construct the food channel. Second stage reconstructive surgery is done for restoration of continuity of the pharynx with the esophagus.
3. *Repair with skin:* Local skin flaps from the neck or a tubed flap from the upper part of the chest are mobilized and stitched to the pharyngeal end above and to the esophagus below.
4. *Repair with viscera:* Visceral transposition into the neck has been found useful for restoring continuity. The stomach, colon or intestines (free jejunal flap or gastric pull up) are mobilized and put between the pharynx and esophagus. Patients with advanced lesions and poor health may be given palliative radiotherapy and fed through gastrostomy.

Plummer-Vinson or Paterson-Brown-Kelly Syndrome

This condition is characterised by dysphagia, anemia, angular stomatitis and glossitis particularly affecting the women. The other associated features are achlorhydria, koilonychia and splenomegaly.

The anemia is of the hypochromic microcytic type and this condition is also called sideropenic dysphagia. There occurs thinning of the mucosa of the upper alimentary tract. Web formation may occur in the hypopharynx. Dysphagia is thought to be due to webs or muscular incoordination at the cricopharynx. Peripheral blood smear shows a picture of iron deficiency anemia. Serum iron level is reduced and iron binding capacity is increased.

Barium swallow may show web formation or narrowing.

TREATMENT

Follow-up is necessary as this condition is premalignant. There is a 10 to 15 percent risk of malignancy. Therapy with iron is helpful. Endoscopic dilatation of the postcricoid region may be required.

Chapter 51

Miscellaneous Conditions of the Throat

Globus Hystericus (Globus Pharynges)

It is a functional disorder in which the patient complains of a lump in the throat. There is no dysphagia. Examination reveals nothing significant in the throat. The patient often has a cancer phobia.

The patient needs to be reassured. Tranquilizers may be prescribed. If the symptoms persist, a barium study of the larynx or endoscopy may be done to rule out any hidden organic lesion.

Palatal and Pharyngeal Palsy

Paralysis of the soft palate (**Fig. 51.1**) and pharynx may occur in a variety of neurological disorders. The common causes are the following:

i. Diphtheritic neuritis
ii. Bulbar palsy
iii. Motor neuron disease
iv. Poliomyelitis
v. Encephalitis
vi. Vascular lesions in the brain
vii. Lesions at the jugular foramen.

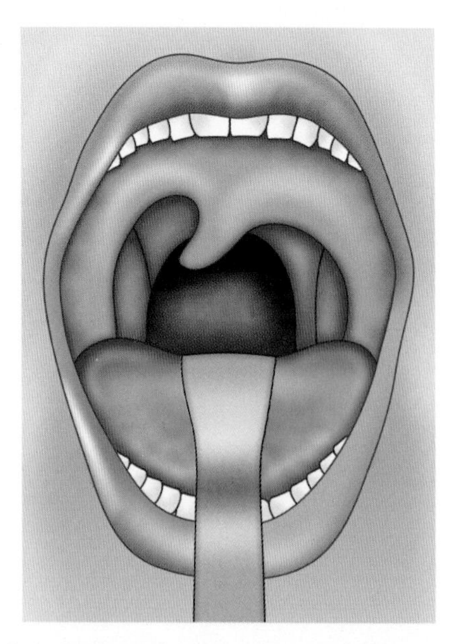

Fig. 51.1: Left sided soft palate palsy, uvula shifted to the right

Paralysis due to diphtheria usually occurs after the third week of the disease. A history of sore throat is forthcoming but sometimes, the patient may not have noticed any such symptom before.

The patient presents with a history of regurgitation of fluids through the nose and may notice a nasal twang of voice (*rhinolalia aperta*). The associated pharyngeal involvement leads to dysphagia and coughing on swallowing.

On examination, the palate on the corresponding side is immobile. If the patient is made to say "Ah" the palate is drawn towards the normal side.

TREATMENT

The treatment is directed towards the cause. In palatal palsy if diphtheria is suspected, then antidiphtheria serum is given. The patient is advised bedrest. A course of steroid therapy and neurotrophic vitamins may help. Regurgitation through the nose is prevented by asking the patient to pinch the nose during swallowing. If pharyngeal paralysis is associated then a Ryle's tube is used for feeding purposes. Oropharyngeal secretions need frequent suction. A tracheostomy using cuffed tube may be necessary to prevent pneumonia. Cricopharyngeal myotomy may help some patients in swallowing and prevents aspiration.

Pharyngeal Spasm

Spasms of the pharynx occurs in tetanus and rabies. The patient cannot swallow owing to lack of coordination of various movements during the process of deglutition and there occurs aspiration into the larynx. Attempts to swallow lead to spasms. Treatment is directed towards the cause. Tracheostomy may be needed to prevent aspiration pneumonia.

Pharyngeal Pouch

It is a pulsion diverticulum which occurs between lower cricopharyngeal and upper thyropharyngeal fibers of the inferior constrictor muscle of the pharynx. The area is known as *Killian's dehiscence.*

It is probably due to neuromuscular incoordination during swallowing which manifests as a failure of relaxation of the cricopharyngeal sphincter and its premature contraction before the bolus has passed down into the esophagus.

The patient presents with dysphagia and regurgitation. Patients with large pouches feel that they require a longer time to complete a meal as the food fills the pouch. Spill over from the pouch into the larynx may produce cough and aspiration.

Barium swallow is diagnostic of pouch formation.

TREATMENT

The pouch may be excised through a neck incision. Alternatively endoscopic division of the partition wall between pouch and esophagus is done by diathermy. Cricopharyngeal myotomy is successful in small pouches.

Trismus (Lock Jaw)

In general, this condition is regarded as the inability to open the mouth adequately. Under normal conditions in an adult, the mouth may open to a distance of 3.5 to 4 cm between the incisor teeth. The muscles which close the mouth are temporalis, masseter and medial pterygoids and muscles which open the mouth include mainly the lateral pterygoids, mylohyoid and infrahyoid muscles. The muscles of closure are more powerful than the muscles which open the mouth. It has been estimated that closing muscles exert a pressure of 100 to 300 pounds per square inch while the openers exert about 25 pounds per square inch. This relative weakness of the opening musculature is a primary factor in the patient's inability to open the mouth when some pathology involves the mandible and its surrounding tissues.

CAUSES

1. Muscle spasm as found in the following:
   a. Tetanus
   b. Arthritis of temporomandibular joint
   c. Acute parotitis
   d. Mumps
   e. Alveolar abscess
   f. Impacted wisdom tooth
   g. Hysteria.
2. Unreduced dislocation of the TM joint.
3. Contractures due to the following:
   a. Burns
   b. Lupus vulgaris

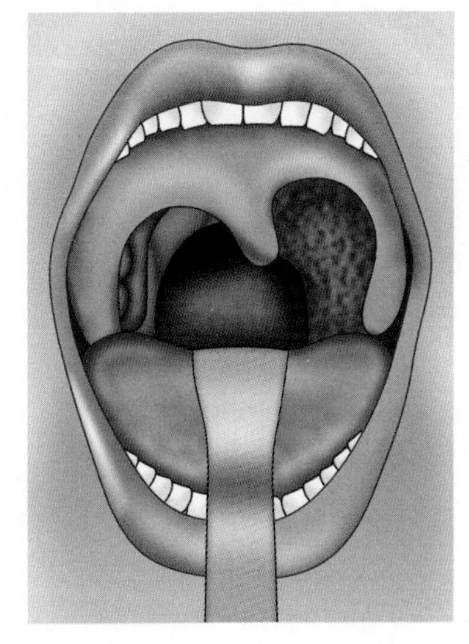

Fig. 51.2: Carcinoma of the left tonsillar fossa

   c. Cancrum oris
   d. Operated scars
   e. Application of radium
   f. Submucous fibrosis with adhesion bands.
4. Carcinoma of the cheek, tonsil (**Fig. 51.2**), maxilla, and parotid gland.
5. True ankylosis following arthritis of temporomandibular joint.

TREATMENT

Treatment is directed towards the cause. If due to true ankylosis, excision of condyle is the line of treatment. If due to false ankylosis due to external scarring, Esmaich's operation (removal of a wedge-shaped piece of bone with the narrow end towards the alveolus in the region of the angle of mandible forming a false joint at the site) is done.

Cleft Palate

Cleft palate (**Fig. 51.3**) can be of the following types:

1. Incomplete
   a. Bifid uvula
   b. Cleft of soft palate only
   c. Cleft of soft palate and part of hard palate.
2. Complete, involving both the soft and hard palate. It may be of the following types:
   a. Unipartite, when there is a cleft on one side of the premaxilla while the other side is fused with the alveolus.
   b. Bipartite, when there are cleft on either side of the premaxilla and cleft palate communicates with both the clefts.

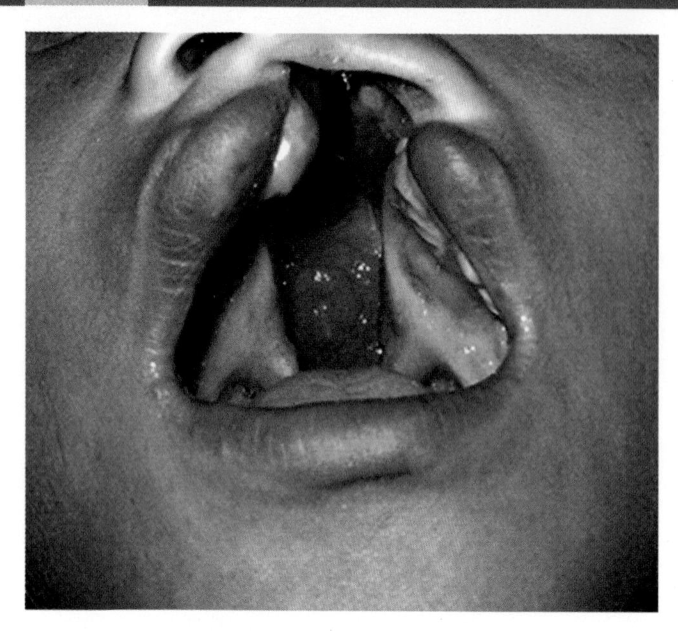

Fig. 51.3: Cleft palate and lip

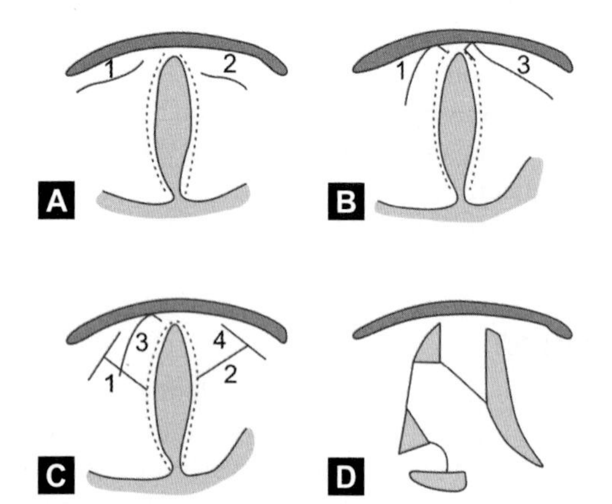

Figs 51.4A to D: Operations for cleft palate repair: (A) Two-flap method; (B) Three-flap method; (C) Four-flap method; (D) Cuthbert's operation

TREATMENT

Optimum peak for correction of the deformity is before the child begins to speak, i.e. about 18 months.

Various operative procedures followed are shown in **Figures 51.4A to D**.

Four-flap method: A release cut is made on either side at the periphery of the palate and an oblique cut from the point of junction of the soft and hard palate parts in the cleft reaching the releasing cut. The four flaps of mucoperiosteum thus shaped are raised from the bone. A "push back" of the flaps brings the edges together. The edges are paired, mucoperiosteal flaps are raised from the nasal septum and suture of these flaps closes the gap.

Elongated Styloid Process (Stylalgia)

The styloid process of the temporal bone is about 2.5 cm long in an adult. In 4 percent of the population the styloid process is grossly enlarged and may give rise to symptoms. The elongated styloid process can be felt through the pharynx in the tonsillar bed or posterior pillar and the process is in close relationship with the glossopharyngeal nerve.

CLINICAL FEATURES

Two types of symptoms may be present.

Classically, the patient complains of a dull or intermittent pain in the throat and ear on that side, especially after deglutition. Difficulty in swallowing and a foreign body sensation in the throat persist. On the other hand, the patient may present with the styloid process-carotid artery syndrome. An elongated styloid process may impinge against carotid arteries and cause disturbances in circulation as well as irritation of the nerve plexus around the vessels. The patient complains of parietal headache and pain along the distribution of the artery involved.

The diagnosis of an enlongated styloid process can be made by palpating for process through the tonsillar bed and by radiography, which shows an abnormally long process.

TREATMENT

Treatment of a symptomatic elongated styloid process is its surgical removal.

In transpharyngeal excision, tonsillectomy is done and the styloid process felt through the tonsillar fossa, where it is exposed by a dissecting forceps. The periosteum is elevated around the process and a portion of it is removed.

The enlarged styloid process can also be excised by an external approach. An incision is given along the anterior border of the sternomastoid from the tip of mastoid to the hyoid bone. The anterior border of the sternomastoid muscle is retracted, the process exposed by a deep dissection and a portion of it is removed.

Chapter 52

Development of Larynx and Tracheobronchial Tree

Development of Larynx and Tracheobronchial Tree

The larynx, trachea and lungs develop from the laryngotracheal groove which arises as a diverticulum posterior to the hypobranchial eminence from the foregut at about four weeks of embryonic life. As the groove deepens, its edges fuse and the groove gets separated from the developing esophagus.

The developing laryngotracheal tube gets elongated and becomes bilobed. Each lobe later becomes the primary bronchus and gives rise to the rest of the bronchial tree and lung tissues. The portion of the tube above the bifurcation becomes the trachea and its upper part forms the larynx.

Two swellings appear at the upper end of the fused ridges of the diverticulum and form arytenoids.

The epiglottis develops from the posterior part of the hypobranchial eminence and gets connected with arytenoids by aryepiglottic folds. The other laryngeal cartilages develop from the branchial mesoderm.

The thyroid cartilage develops from the fourth arch while the fifth and sixth arches form other cartilages.

Larynx

ANATOMY

Situated in front of the neck, the larynx lies opposite the third to sixth cervical vertebrae. The larynx has a cartilaginous framework supported by ligaments and muscles.

CARTILAGES OF THE LARYNX

The thyroid cartilage, epiglottis and cricoid cartilage are single while the arytenoids are paired cartilages. Besides, two small cartilages, (**Figs 52.1 and 52.2**) corniculate and cuneiform lie in each aryepiglottic fold.

Thyroid Cartilage

It is the largest cartilage and forms a prominence in the neck (*Adam's apple*). The two lateral laminae fuse together in midline in a V-shaped manner and its upper and lower ends are continued into horns called superior and inferior horns.

This cartilage is connected to the hyoid bone by the thyrohyoid membrane and to the cricoid cartilage by the cricothyroid membrane.

Epiglottis

This is a flattened leaf-like cartilage, attached to the angle between the thyroid laminae by the thyroepiglottic ligament. It projects upwards behind the hyoid bone and its superior margin is free.

Folds Extending from the Epiglottis

The aryepiglottic folds extend from its lateral margins to the arytenoid cartilage. The glossoepiglottic fold extends from the tongue to the lingual aspect of the epiglottis, creating two depressions on either side called valecullae. The pharyngoepiglottic folds the extend from the lateral margins of the epiglottis to the pharyngeal wall.

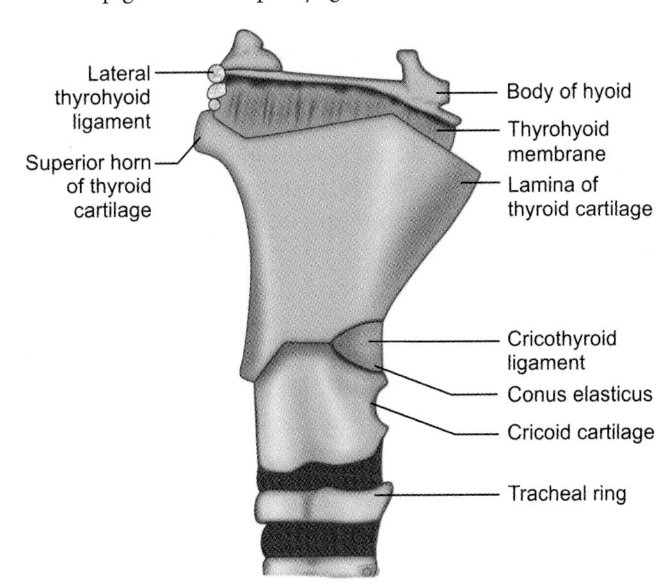

Fig. 52.1: Cartilages and ligaments of the larynx (lateral view)

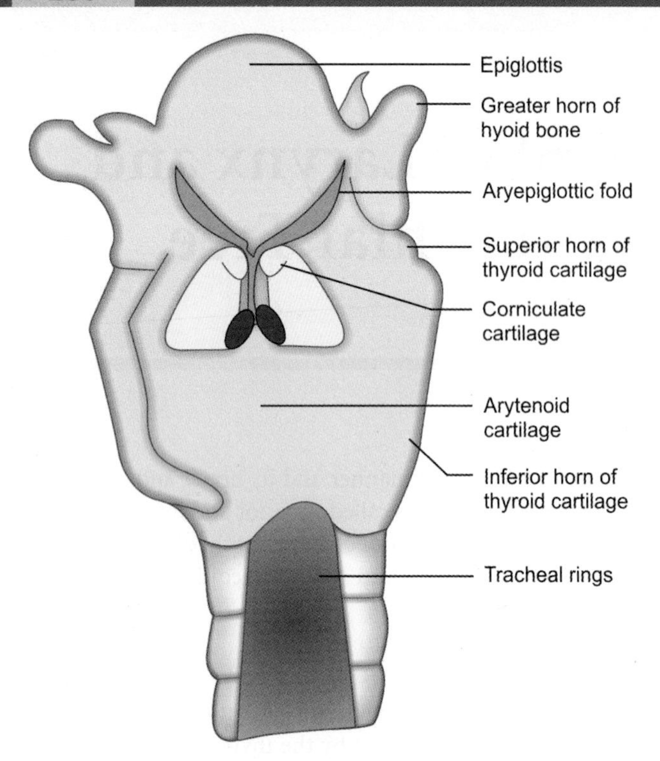

Fig. 52.2: Interior of the larynx

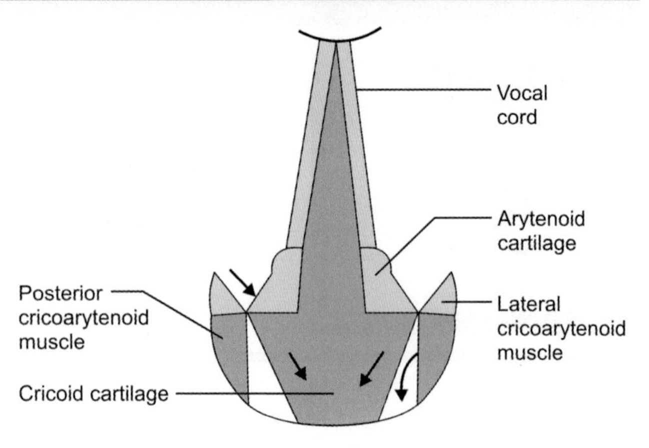

Fig. 52.3: Arytenoid cartilages

Pre-epiglottic space: This is a potential space in front of the epiglottis which contains lymphatic channels. It is bound in front by the thyroid cartilage, posteriorly by the epiglottis and above by the hypoepiglottic ligament. The space is important surgically as tumor cells may involve lymph vessels of this space and hence this space should be excised along with the growth area.

Paraepiglottic Space: Cricoid Cartilage

It is a ring cartilage which has a narrow anterior arch and a broad posterior lamina.

The anterior arch is connected with the inferior border of the thyroid cartilage by the cricothyroid membrane. The posterior lamina gives attachment to the muscles and articulates with the arytenoid cartilages at the cricoarytenoid joints.

Arytenoid Cartilages

These are pyramid-shaped cartilages situated on the cricoid lamina (**Fig. 52.3**). The base of the pyramid articulates with the cricoid facet to form the cricoarytenoid joints.

The anterior angle of the pyramid, known as vocal process, gives attachment to the vocal cord. The lateral process known as muscular process gives attachment to the muscles. The apex provides attachment to the aryepiglottic fold.

Corniculate Cartilage (Cartilage of Santorini)

This is situated at the apex of the arytenoid cartilages on either side in the mucous membrane of the aryepiglottic folds. It is conical in shape.

Cuneiform Cartilage (Cartilage of Wrisberg)

It is situated in each aryepiglottic fold just in front of the corniculate cartilage. It is club-shaped.

MUSCLES OF THE LARYNX

These are divided into two groups, extrinsic muscles and intrinsic muscles.

Extrinsic muscles: This group includes a various muscles which attach the larynx to other structures and includes the sternothyroid, thyrohyoid, sternohyoid, omohyoid, inferior constrictor and stylopharyngeus muscles. These muscles elevate and depress the larynx during deglutition.

Intrinsic group: The intrinsic muscles cause movements of the laryngeal cartilages and work during breathing and phonation.

The muscles are subgrouped according to their action and are named according to their attachments (**Figs 52.4A and B**).

1. *Adductors:* These include the lateral cricoarytenoid muscles, cricothyroids and the interarytenoid muscle. The lateral cricoarytenoid is the main adductor. It arises from upper border of the lateral part of the arch of cricoid and gets inserted into the muscular process of arytenoid.
2. *Abductor muscle:* The posterior cricoarytenoids are the sole abductors of the vocal cords. The muscles arise from the lower and medial surface of the posterior of cricoid lamina and are inserted into the posterior of the muscular process of arytenoid on the same side. When these muscles contract, they move the vocal cords apart causing widening of the glottis.

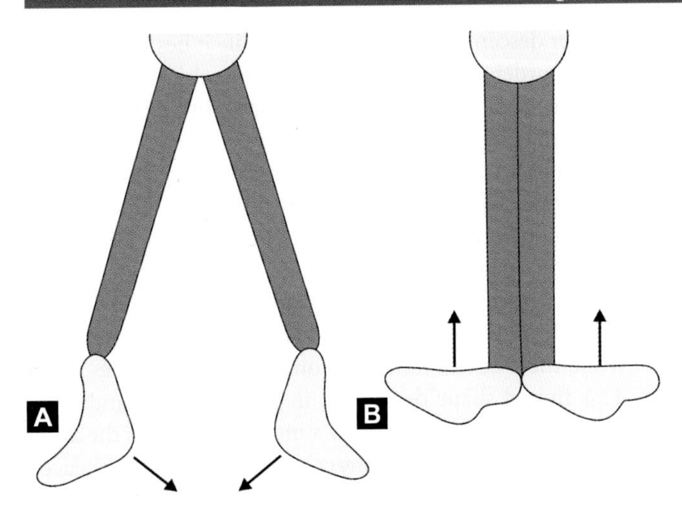

Figs 52.4A and B: Muscles of the larynx: (A) Abduction posterior cricoarytenoid; (B) Adduction lateral cricoarytenoid

3. *Tensors of vocal cords:* These include cricothyroid and thyroarytenoid muscles.

The thyroarytenoids arise on each side from the inner aspect near the angle of the thyroid cartilage and vocal ligament proceeding backwards to the arytenoid cartilage and its vocal process.

The transverse arytenoid muscle is a single muscle which extends from the posterior aspect of one arytenoid to the other and helps in closing the interarytenoid region.

Nerve Supply of Muscles

The cricothyroid muscle is supplied by the external laryngeal nerve which is a branch of the superior laryngeal nerve. Other intrinsic muscles are supplied by the recurrent laryngeal nerve.

INTERIOR OF THE LARYNX

The laryngeal inlet is bounded above and in front by the free margin of the epiglottis, laterally by the aryepiglottic folds, and posteriorly by the interarytenoid mucosa (**see Fig. 52.2**).

LARYNGEAL VESTIBULE

It lies between the inlet of larynx and the level of vestibular folds or false cords.

It is bounded above by margins of the laryngeal inlet, in front by the posterior aspect of the epiglottis, laterally by the inner aspect of the aryepiglottic fold, and posteriorly by the mucosa covering the anterior surface of the arytenoid cartilage.

SINUS OF THE LARYNX

It is a small recess, the opening of which lies between the vocal cord and the ventricular fold. It secretes mucus and thus lubricates the vocal cords.

SACCULE OF THE LARYNX

From the anterior part of the ventricle, a pouch called saccule of the larynx extends between the vestibular fold and inner aspect of the thyroid cartilage. Its dilatation is thought to be the cause of laryngocele.

VOCAL CORDS

These are fibroelastic bands which extend from the angle of the thyroid cartilage anteriorly to the vocal process of arytenoids posteriorly. These are formed by reflection of the mucosa over the vocal ligaments which are the free edges of the cricovocal membrane. The cords have stratified squamous epithelium with no submucous layer. These have a poor blood supply and are almost devoid of lymphatics.

The rima vestibuli and rima glottidis: The space between the two vestibular bands is called rima vestibuli while the space between the vocal cords is called rima glottidis. The average length of rima glottidis in an adult male is 23 mm and in an adult female is 16 mm.

BLOOD SUPPLY OF THE LARYNX

Larynx is supplied by the superior and inferior thyroid arteries. The superior thyroid artery is a branch of the external carotid artery while the inferior thyroid artery arises from the thyrocervical trunk of the subclavian artery.

LYMPHATIC DRAINAGE OF THE LARYNX

The part of the larynx above the vocal cords is drained by lymphatics which proceed upwards through the thyrohyoid membrane and end in upper deep cervical lymph nodes. The part of the larynx below the vocal cords is drained by lymphatics which end in the pretracheal, paratracheal and lower deep cervical nodes. The lymphatics may also end in lymphatics of the superior mediastinum.

The vocal cords themselves are practically devoid of lymphatics.

NERVE SUPPLY OF THE LARYNX

The superior laryngeal nerve is sensory to the laryngeal mucosa above the vocal cords. Besides it is motor to the cricothyroid muscle through its external laryngeal branch. Mucosa of the larynx below the vocal cords and all other intrinsic laryngeal muscles are supplied by the recurrent laryngeal nerves.

AVERAGE MEASUREMENTS OF ADULT LARYNX

Up to puberty the size of the larynx both in males and females is almost the same but thereafter in males it increases nearly

Table 52.1: Average measurement of adult larynx

	Males	Females
Length	44 mm	36 mm
Transverse diameter	43 mm	41 mm
Anterior diameter	36 mm	26 mm

twice in its anteroposterior diameter. The measurements are given in **Table 52.1**.

SURGICAL SUBDIVISIONS OF THE LARYNX

For clinicosurgical purposes, the larynx has been divided into three main regions:

i. Glottis
ii. Subglottis
iii. Supraglottis.

Glottis: It consists of the vocal cords, anterior commissure, and posterior commissure.

Anterior commissure is the area where the two vocal cords are attached to the angle of the thyroid laminae.

Posterior commissure is the area at the posterior end of the vocal cords, between the two arytenoids.

Subglottis: It is the area of the larynx which extends from 5 mm below the level of the vocal cords up to the lower border of the cricoid cartilage. The undersurface of the cords is excluded.

Supraglottis: It is the region of the larynx above the level of the vocal cords and includes the ventricles, vestibular bands and vestibule.

Comparison of infantile with the adult larynx:

1. *Size:* The difference in size is not only real, but also relative, for the lumen of infantile larynx and trachea is smaller in proportion to the body as a whole. The greatest "choke" is present in the subglottic region which predisposes to stridor. The normal subglottic diameter in infants is 6 mm, 5 mm is taken as reduced and 4 mm represents stenosis.
2. *Consistency of the tissues of the larynx:* In young children all the laryngeal tissues including the cartilaginous framework, musculature, and mucous and submucous tissues are softer than in adults.

   The cartilage is softer and more pliable and the mucosa loose and less fibrous.
3. *Position:* In the infant the larynx is placed high and it descends continually during development. In a fetus of 5 to 6 weeks the larynx is situated opposite the basiocciput but by the 4th month the lower border of the cricoid lies opposite the upper border of the 4th cervical vertebra. At seven months it lies about the middle of the 6th vertebra and it is still found in this position at full term. After birth further descent occurs until in adult life it lies opposite the lower border of the 6th cervical vertebra, while the top of the epiglottis lies opposite the lower border of the 3rd cervical vertebra.

   As a result of the higher position of the larynx in infants, the entry of the air current is straighter than in adults and the epiglottis less overhanging. In adult life the axes of the pharynx, larynx, and trachea meet at a more acute angle.
4. *Shape:* The upper end of the larynx and trachea is funnel-shaped in infants, the cricoid plate being tilted backwards while the tracheal lumen becomes smaller as it descends. This funnel shape disappears in older children and adult females while it reappears in a modified form in the adult male, the backward tilt of the cricoid cartilage being replaced by the forward tilt of the thyroid cartilage but the tracheal lumen no longer diminishes as in an infant.

Tracheobronchial Tree

ANATOMY

The trachea divides at the level of the upper border of the 5th thoracic vertebra into two main bronchi separated by a projection of the lowest ring of trachea called *carina.*

Right Main Bronchus

The right main bronchus is wider, shorter and more vertical than the left main bronchus.

It has the following ramifications:

1. *Right superior lobe bronchus:* It arises from the right principal bronchus and is divided into three segmental bronchi—apical, posterior, and anterior.
2. *Middle lobe bronchus:* It arises from the anterior aspect of the main bronchus, is directed forwards and downwards to be divided into two segmental bronchi, the lateral and medial.
3. *Right inferior lobe bronchus:* The inferior lobe bronchus gives the following segmental bronchi—apical, medial basal, anterior basal, lateral basal, and posterior basal.

Left Main Bronchus

The left main bronchus is longer, narrower and more horizontal. It divides into the following subdivisions:

1. Left superior lobe bronchus.
2. Left inferior lobe bronchus.

   The left superior lobe bronchus gives the following ramifications:

Lingular bronchus: It arises as its branch.

The superior lobe bronchus itself divides into the following

1. Apicoposterior, which divides into: (i) apical, and (ii) posterior segmental bronchi.

2. Anterior segmental bronchus.

The lingular bronchus which is a branch of the left superior lobe bronchus divides into: (i) superior lingular, and (ii) inferior lingular bronchi.

The left inferior lobe bronchus divides into the following segmental bronchi: (i) apical bronchus, (ii) anterior basal, (iii) lateral basal, and (iv) posterior basal.

There is no medial basal bronchus on the left side.

The successive divisions of the bronchial tree are termed principal bronchi, lobar bronchi, segmental bronchi, bronchioles and terminal bronchioles.

During inspiration the bronchial diameters increase. Absence of these movements on bronchoscopy denotes fixation of the bronchial wall by a neoplastic process. The advantage of this widening on inspiration is taken in removing a foreign body by forceps.

Chapter 53

Physiology of the Larynx

The larynx serves the following main functions:

1. *Respiratory passage:* It is a part of the upper respiratory tract and determines the resistance to air flow.
2. *Sphincteric action:* The larynx serves as a sphincter at the upper end of the respiratory tract and closure of this sphincteric mechanism helps in the following ways:
   a. Protective closing during swallowing, regurgitation and vomiting.
   b. Reflex protection against entry of foreign bodies.
   c. Closure of the sphincter helps in thoracic fixation and building of high intrathoracic pressure as required in straining, micturation, explosive coughing, etc. This sphincteric action is exerted at three different levels by the closure of the aryepiglottic fold, ventricular bands and vocal cords.
3. *Reflex action:* The larynx plays an important part in the cough reflex. It is a receptive field for reflexes.
4. *Phonation:* The larynx plays the main role in phonation and speech.

Phonation

Phonation involves the fundamental note produced by vibration of vocal cords.

The production of voice by the larynx involves the following mechanisms:

1. *Intratracheal high pressure column of air:* This is produced by contraction of the expiratory muscles in the thorax and the abdominal wall.
2. *Vibrating mechanism:* The vocal cords serve this function. The vocal cords are adducted and made tense by contraction of the laryngeal muscles and set into vibrations. The vibrating cords cut the expired column of air into a series of puffs, causing a series of compression and rarefaction waves of air. This constitutes the fundamental note. Various explanations have been given to explain the vibration of cords.
3. *Resonating mechanism:* The note produced at the larynx is feeble. This note is modified and enhanced by a resonating mechanism provided by the lung tissues, pharynx, oral cavity, nose and the paranasal sinuses. The resonating mechanism gives an individual quality to the voice.
4. *Function of larynx during deglutition:* The larynx moves up towards the base of the tongue and thus brings the pharyngo-esophageal junction nearer to the bolus. The epiglottis curls backwards and directs the food into the pyriform fossae. The sphincteric mechanism of the larynx comes into action and prevents the passage of food into the laryngotracheobronchial tree.

Chapter 54

Common Symptoms of Laryngeal Diseases

Symptoms due to involvement of the larynx include alteration or loss of its functions. Hence, the symptoms are referable to changes in voice, difficulty in breathing and incompetence of the laryngeal sphincters producing difficulty in swallowing.

Changes of Voice

Various changes in voice can be of the following types:

1. *Hoarseness of voice:* This phrase implies a rough, husky voice. Any disease which interferes with vibration of the vocal cords, approximation of the vocal cords or their movements produces a change in voice. A breathy voice occurs due to air leak as is seen in vocal cord paralysis.

   Loss of vocal range may occur in singers due to structural changes in cords like nodules, polyps and thickening.
2. *Puberphonia:* Crackling of voice or break in voice occurs at puberty in males as the larynx grows.
3. *Vocal asthenia:* Fatigue or weakness of the voice may occur particularly in weak elderly persons due to muscular weakness.
4. *Functional aphonia:* Complete loss of voice may occur in hysterical females. The patient can cough and vocal cords are seen to approximate on coughing.

Stridor and Dyspnea

Structural changes in the larynx may produce stridor and dyspnea. Stridor is noisy breathing produced by obstruction to air flow. It may occur during inspiration or on expiration depending upon the site of obstruction. An obstructive lesion in the larynx and trachea may produce dyspnea and cyanosis. Increased respiratory rate, indrawing of the larynx and trachea into the mediastinum, and recession of the intercostal spaces and supraclavicular fossae indicate a laryngeal or tracheal obstructive pathology.

Weak Cry

Diseases of the larynx in infancy produce distress and make the baby cry. Any lesion which prevents the approximation of the cords results in a weak cry.

Cough

Dry cough may be due to laryngeal involvement. Small neglected foreign bodies in the larynx and trachea, aspiration of fluids due to sphincteric incompetence, crusting in atrophic pharyngitis and laryngitis are the common factors in cough production.

Dysphagia and Odynophagia

Difficulty in swallowing (dysphagia) is not a common symptom in laryngeal diseases. Sometimes a vague feeling of a lump in the throat or difficulty in swallowing may occur in supraglottic tumors, particularly when involving the aryepiglottic folds. Acute epiglottitis and large supraglottic tumors produce dysphagia. Odynophagia (painful swallowing) may be a feature of laryngeal tuberculosis.

Chapter 55

Examination of the Larynx

Clinical examination of the larynx includes external palpation and indirect laryngoscopy. The complete examination may necessitate direct laryngoscopy, radiography and stroboscopy.

External Palpation

Examination of the neck is very important in laryngeal diseases. Laryngeal cartilages (thyroid and cricoid) are felt for thickening, tenderness and broadening.

The larynx remains stationary during quiet breathing but moves on deglutition and on deep breathing as during exercise and respiratory obstruction. It descends on deep inspiration and ascends on expiration.

When the larynx is moved laterally on the vertebral column, it produces a grating sensation which is normally elicited. In conditions like postcricoid malignancy or other retropharyngeal lesions this sign is absent as the larynx is pushed forwards and its movements over the vertebral column does not occur.

Examination of neck nodes: A detailed examination of the lymph nodes of the neck is done, particularly the nodes deep to the sternomastoids.

Indirect Laryngoscopy

This simple procedure provides the view of the interior of the larynx and is great clinical value. The following items are required:

1. A headmirror and a light source.
2. Laryngeal mirror (different sizes are available).
3. Tongue cloth (a piece of gauze for holding the tongue).
4. A spirit lamp or a hot water bowl for warming the mirror.

PROCEDURE

The patient and the examiner face each other. The procedure is explained to the patient to gain his cooperation and relaxation. The patient sits with his head upright and tilted slightly forward from the shoulders.

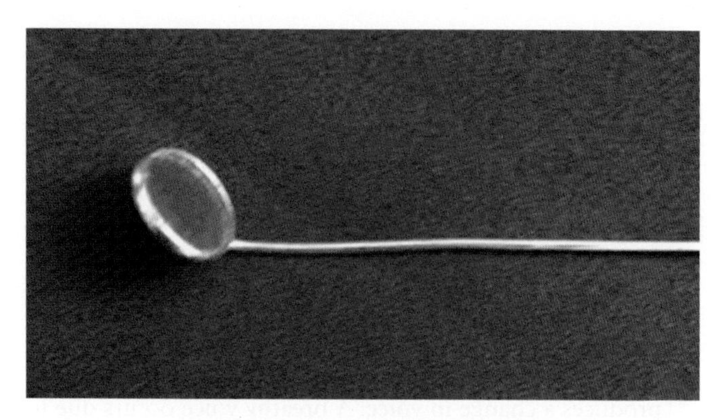

Fig. 55.1: Indirect laryngoscopy mirror

The light is focussed on the patient's lip. The mirror (**Fig. 55.1**) of proper size is warmed to prevent fogging of its surface. Its temperature is tested on the examiner's hand. The patient is asked to put out his tongue which is held by a gauze piece between the left thumb and middle finger. The left index finger retracts the upper lip of the patient. The warmed mirror is held in the right hand like a pen. It is passed through the angle of the mouth above the tongue with the mirror surface facing down. The mirror is carried backwards and placed at the base of the uvula with the face downwards. The patient is asked to breathe deeply. By tilting the mirror, various structures like the base of the tongue, endolarynx and hypopharynx are visualized. The larynx is also examined during phonation by asking the patient to say "E" so that the mobility of the cords is tested. All the structures are not visible in one view. The examiner has to tilt the mirror to visualize the various structures and then correlate the findings together.

Structures visible: The posterior part of the tongue, valleculae, and lingual aspect of the epiglottis and its margins are the structures seen first. By tilting the mirror, the laryngeal aspect of the epiglottis, arytenoids, aryepiglottic folds and false cords come into view. The false cords or vestibular bands

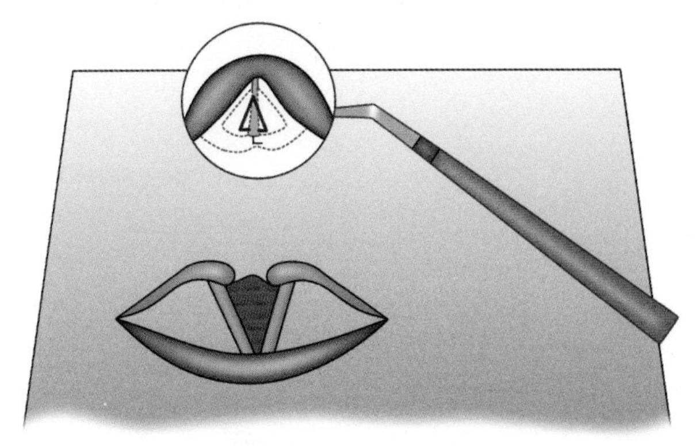

Fig. 55.2: Indirect laryngoscopic view

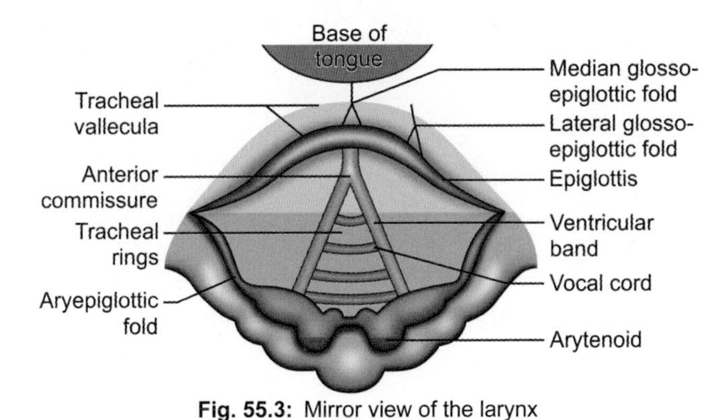

Fig. 55.3: Mirror view of the larynx

appear as dull red bands above the true vocal cords (**Figs 55.2 and 55.3**).

The vocal cords appear as whitish, flat, ribbon-like bands extending from the angle of the thyroid cartilage to the vocal processes of the arytenoids. Mobility of the vocal cords is tested on asking the patient to phonate "E".

Below the vocal cords, the walls of the subglottis are hidden from the view, only a few rings of trachea may be seen anteriorly.

By tilting the mirror, the pyriform fossae and a part of the posterior pharyngeal wall can be inspected.

DIFFICULTIES IN INDIRECT LARYNGOSCOPY

1. If the patient is not cooperative or is very sensitive, he may gag and thus makes the examination difficult. Local spraying with topical xylocaine helps in such cases.
2. In a short neck, the larynx is placed high up making laryngeal examination difficult.
3. The tongue may rise on phonation obscuring the view of the endolarynx.
4. Indirect laryngoscopy is difficult in children.

Blind areas of larynx: These are areas which are difficult to visualize and may conceal foreign bodies. These are the following:

1. Portion of the laryngeal aspect of epiglottis below its tubercle
2. Ventricle of the larynx
3. Anterior commissure
4. Subglottis.

USES OF INDIRECT LARYNGOSCOPY

1. It is useful in diagnosis and evaluation of laryngeal disease and forms a part of the routine ENT examination.
2. Sometimes, the procedure is used for taking a biopsy, for removal of small benign lesions, cauterization of ulcers, or for anesthetizing the larynx and trachea for direct laryngoscopy and bronchoscopy.

Direct Laryngoscopy

In this procedure, the larynx is directly examined with a rigid laryngoscope or fiberoptic laryngoscope.

INDICATIONS

1. *Diagnostic purposes*
   a. When a lesion in the larynx, as seen in indirect laryngoscopy, needs further evaluation to know its nature or extent, a direct view of the larynx is necessary.
   b. When indirect laryngoscopy is not possible as in children.
   c. If an elongated incurled epiglottis obscures the view of the endolarynx.
   d. To know about the pathological lesions in blind areas of the larynx.
2. *Therapeutic purposes*
   a. Direct laryngoscopy is done for intubation, for administering general anesthesia and to have a control on the airway.
   b. For removal of foreign bodies in the larynx, thickened secretions and crusts.
   c. For performing various operations like removal of cordal nodules, vocal polyps, cysts, taking a biopsy, etc.

CONTRAINDICATIONS FOR DIRECT LARYNGOSCOPY

1. In injuries and disease of the cervical spine, direct laryngoscopy is hazardous as the endoscopic procedure and the patient's movements might lead to spinal cord damage.
2. Trismus, long incisor teeth, and a short and thick neck make the procedure difficult.

ANESTHESIA FOR DIRECT LARYNGOSCOPY

The procedure can be done under general or local anesthesia.

Local anesthesia: After testing for xylocaine sensitivity, the oral cavity and pharynx are anesthetized by local spraying of 4 percent xylocaine. The larynx is sprayed with a laryngeal atomiser.

A piece of cotton soaked in xylocaine is placed in the pyriform fossa on each side by a curved laryngeal forceps. This pack is kept for a few minutes on each side to anesthetize the internal laryngeal nerve which lies under the mucosa of the pyriform fossa.

Local anesthesia is supplemented by sedation with pethidine or diazepam.

General anesthesia: General anesthesia is preferred. This provides proper relaxation and control over the airways, thus facilitating proper and detailed examination of the larynx.

A small endolaryngeal tube for anesthesia is desirable.

Various types of laryngoscopes are used for examining the larynx (**Figs 55.4A and B**).

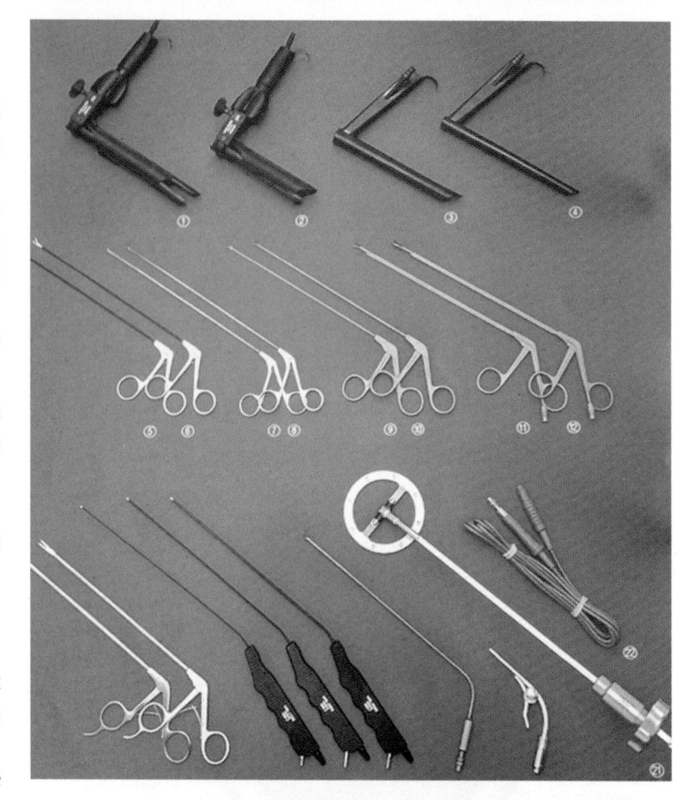

Fig. 55.4A: Instruments for direct laryngoscopy

INSTRUMENTS

The MacIntosh type of laryngoscope is a handy instrument needed for intubation and can provide a quick view of the larynx particularly in children.

Jackson's direct laryngoscope with a sliding blade is the common instrument used for examination and operative procedures.

The anterior commissure laryngoscope has a beveled end and is used particularly for viewing the anterior commissure and for operations on the vocal cords as it fixes the cords and thus allows proper excision of the cord lesions.

The anterior commissure laryngoscope is also helpful in examining ventricles and the subglottic area. The Negus type of endoscopes have a wide proximal end and a proximal light source.

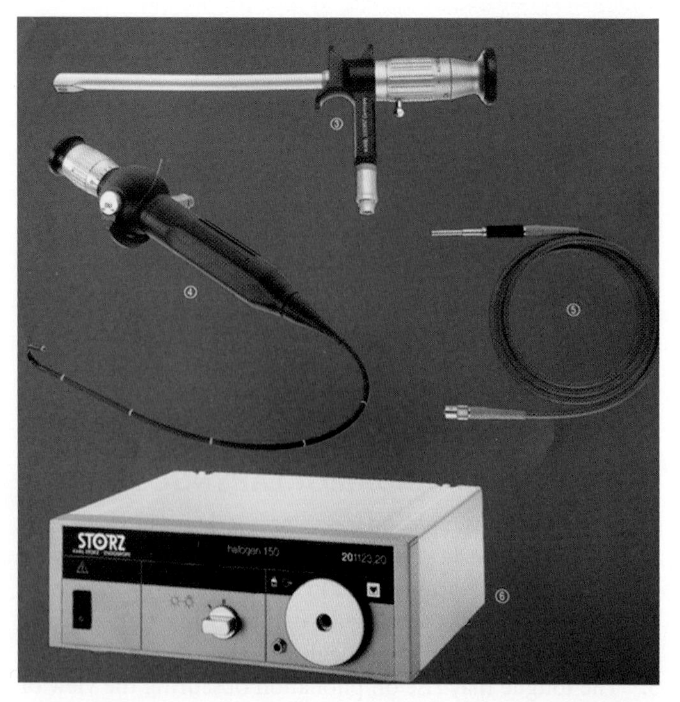

Fig. 55.4B: Instruments for telescopic and fiberoptic laryngoscopy

PROCEDURE

The patient lies supine on the operation table, his neck is flexed but the head is extended at the atlanto-occipital joint. This position brings the larynx in direct axis with the oral cavity and thus facilitates the introduction of the laryngoscope.

The laryngoscope is held in the right hand and passed from the right angle of the mouth. The teeth and lips are protected. The endoscope is passed into the oral cavity till the posterior part of the tongue is visualized. It is passed to the midline and the base of the tongue is elevated. This brings the epiglottis into view. The tip of the laryngoscope is guided behind the epiglottis and advanced, lifting the handle of the laryngoscope upwards. This brings the posterior part of the larynx into view. By proper manipulation, the anterior portion of the larynx is visualized. The chest support is fitted with the laryngoscope which keeps the instrument in position and allows both hands of the examiner to work. The operating microscope is placed in position, if needed.

During the endoscopic procedure, every effort is made to avoid pressure on the lip or teeth.

DIRECT LARYNGOSCOPY IN CHILDREN

Direct laryngoscopy is commonly required in infants and children having stridor and feeding difficulties. While examining such patients, it is necessary that the tip of the laryngoscope be placed anterior to the epiglottis, in the vallecula. In young children this brings the laryngeal inlet in line with the optical axis of the laryngoscope and allows a good view of the larynx. This is also important while looking for cord paralysis as in such a position the tip of the laryngoscope is not pressing on the aryepiglottic fold which might otherwise restrict the cord movements.

Stroboscopy

It is a method of laryngeal examination which facilitates the study of speech and analysis of voice production faults by observing the vibration of cords.

PRINCIPLE

Indirect laryngoscopy is done using an interrupted source of light. The frequency of flashes of interrupted light is adjusted to the frequency of note uttered on phonation in such a way that there remains a difference of 1 cycle/second between the frequency of the note and the light flashes. The cords appear vibrating, one excursion of vocal cord taking place each second.

Radiography of the Larynx

Radiology is of considerable help in the diagnosis and assessment of the laryngeal disorders such as the following:

1. Foreign bodies in the larynx.
2. Narrowing of the airway by edema or growth.
3. Surgical emphysema.
4. Fractures of the laryngeal cartilages.
5. Erosion of the laryngeal cartilage and assess the extent of disease in malignancy.
6. To note the degree and extent of laryngotracheal stenosis.
7. To note the position of the tracheostomy tube.

Usually the lateral view (X-ray of the soft tissues of neck) is helpful. CT of the larynx delineates the laryngotracheal air column and shows the valleculae, epiglottis, ventricle (space between true and false cord) and the subglottic region.

Fiberoptic Laryngoscopy

The laryngoscopy is done by a flexible fiberoptic instrument. The fiberscope is passed through the nose into the oropharynx and directed behind the epiglottis into the laryngeal lumen. Topical xylocaine is used for anesthesia. The instrument gives a

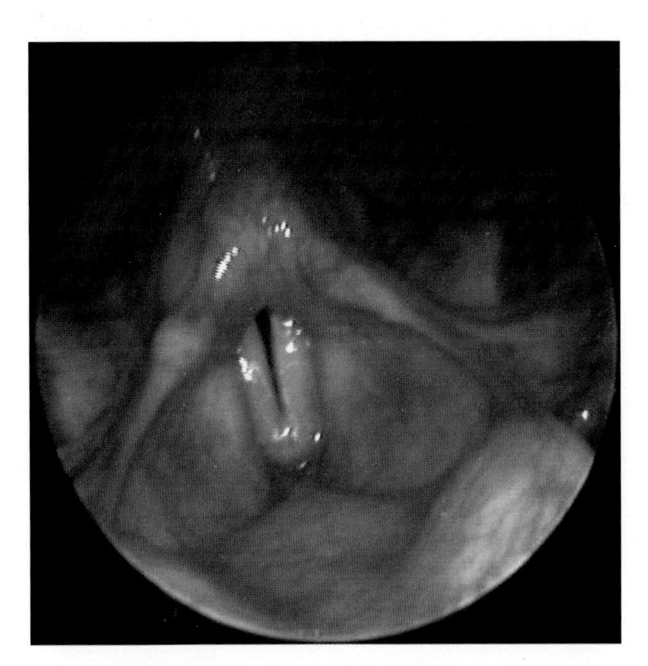

Fig. 55.5A: Normal larynx with adducted vocal cords

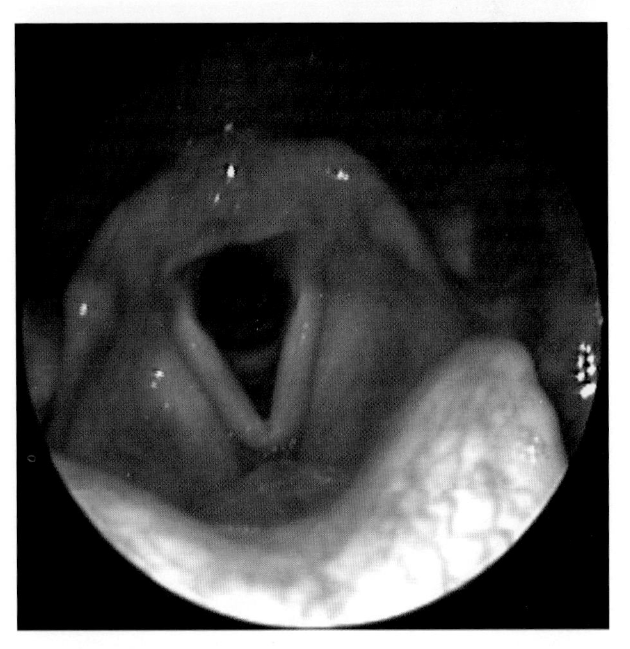

Fig. 55.5B: Normal larynx with abducted vocal cords

detailed and minute view and allows biopsy and photography. This instrument is particularly useful in conditions where direct laryngoscopy with a rigid endoscope is difficult.

Examination of the Larynx Under Microscope (Microlaryngoscopy)

The present day microsurgical techniques of the larynx are a credit to Kliensasser. A 400 mm objective lens is fitted to the operating microscope and the endolarynx visualized through a laryngoscope. This technique has revolutionized the treatment of various laryngeal conditions. It allows early detection of lesions and their accurate surgical removal. The surgeon can thus detect early malignancy as well as its extent and can take a biopsy from the properly selected area. Similarly, areas of leukoplakia are properly excised. Proper excision of the lesions like vocal nodules and vocal polyps under magnification prevents damage to the vocal cords and thus better functional results are obtained (**Figs 55.5A and B**).

Chapter

56

Stridor

The larynx may be divided into three compartments: supraglottic, glottic, and subglottic. Obstruction at each level produces characteristic physical findings that may be helpful in diagnosis. The supraglottis includes the epiglottis and false cords (vestibular folds). The glottis is bounded by the true cords. The subglottis extends below the true cords to the inferior edge of the cricoid cartilage.

Stridor is the hallmark of laryngeal obstruction.

Level of obstruction	Physical findings
Supraglottic	Stridor is inspiratory and characterised by a low-pitched flutter. Voice may be normal
Glottic	Stridor is inspiratory and expiratory and exhibits a phonatory quality. Dysphonia is present
Subglottic	Stridor is mainly expiratory. Voice may be normal. Brassy, barking cough is characteristic

Stridor is noisy breathing heard when there is obstruction to the free flow of air through the larynx or trachea. Stridor may be inspiratory or expiratory. When obstruction lies mainly in the larynx, stridor is inspiratory because a negative pressure develops below the site of obstruction and thus, laryngeal structures tend to collapse inwards narrowing the airway and causing a noisy breathing, while on expiration these structures are forced apart.

When the obstruction lies below the vocal cords, stridor is either heard both during inspiration and expiration or mainly during expiration depending upon the severity of obstruction. The timing of stridor with respiratory phase gives an idea about the site of obstruction. Similarly, if voice is hoarse, the lesion is likely at the level of cords. Stridor with a clear voice indicates that the obstruction is not at glottic level.

Stridor is produced by a number of conditions which cause narrowing of the larynx or trachea. It is mainly a problem of children, because the larynx is relatively small and laryngeal tissues are sensitive, lax, flabby and susceptible to edema and spasm.

Common Causes of Stridor

1. Laryngomalacia
2. Acute laryngotracheobronchitis and acute laryngitis
3. Diphtheretic laryngitis
4. Foreign bodies in the larynx and trachea
5. Laryngismus stridulous
6. Vocal cord paralysis
7. Multiple papillomas of larynx
8. Sometimes other rare conditions like laryngeal webs, bifid epiglottis and laryngeal cysts may be the etiological factors.

Congenital laryngeal stridor is not a diagnosis but a descriptive term for noisy breathing present from birth and could be caused by any condition which narrows the airway at birth.

LARYNGEAL STRIDOR IN INFANCY AND CHILDHOOD

Table 56.1 gives comparative information on the topic.

Laryngomalacia (Fig. 56.1)

It is a common cause of stridor in infancy. The condition manifests within a few weeks of birth and persists for 2 to 3 years. It is due to general flabbiness of the structures bounding the laryngeal aperture, particularly the flabbiness of the aryepiglottic folds. These get indrawn during inspiration thus producing narrowing and hence inspiratory stridor. While on expiration, the folds are forced apart, stridor is inconstant and is sometimes extremely marked. It tends to be worse with the child lying supine. Stridor gets more pronounced on crying and on exertion. Voice of the patient is normal.

Diagnosis is made on direct laryngoscopy, when indrawing of the aryepiglottic folds is evident and if the laryngoscope is passed between these folds, the stridor disappears.

Treatment

Stridor gradually decreases in severity and frequently disappears when the child is 2 to 3 years of age, as the flabbiness of folds disappears.

Table 56.1: Laryngeal stridor in infancy and childhood

		Congenital glottic stenosis	Congenital narrowing of laryngeal inlet	Laryngo-malacia	Intrinsic type laryngo-tetany and neonatal tetany	Reflex spasm	Spasm of inflammatory causation	Neoplastic
1.	Cause	Web	Incurved larynx	Softness of tissue, e.g. myasthenia gravis	Deficiency of calcium	FB adenoids whooping cough	Acute simple laryngitis, laryngotracheo-bronchitis, measles and diphtheria	Papilloma, cysts
2.	Age of onset	At or soon after bith	Soon after birth	Soon after birth	At birth to 2nd year	Variable	Variable	Usually before 2 years
3.	Onset of attacks	Not sudden	Not sudden	Not sudden	Sudden	Sudden	Sometimes sudden	Gradual
4.	General health	Not affected	Not affected	Usually weak	Weak	Adenoidal or temporary illness	Acute fever	Effects of obstruction
5.	Stridor by day	Inspiratory	Inspiratory	Inspiratory	During attacks mainly inspiratory	During attacks inspiratory or to and fro	Inspiratory or to and fro	Inspiratory or to and fro
6.	Stridor during sleep	Present	Diminished	Diminished	Attacks awake the patient	Only during attacks	Present, often worse	Present in severe cases
7.	Dyspnea	Variable	Variable	Variable	Severe during attacks	Severe during attacks	Often severe	Sometimes severe
8.	Cyanosis	Rare	Rare	Rare	Severe during attacks	Severe during attacks	Often severe	Sometimes severe
9.	Voice	Feeble	Clear	Clear	Clear	Nasal tone or hoarse	Hoarse	Hoarse
10.	Progress	Stridor improve but continues	Disappears in 2-3 years	Disappears in 2-3 years	Disappears in 8-9 years	Disappears after treatment	Dependent on response to treatment	Responds to treatment
11.	Danger	Fatal if severe	Slight	May be severe	During attacks	During attacks	Sometimes	Sometimes fatal
12.	Treatment	Laryngo-fissure cut and skin graft	No treatment	Better diet, oxygen, rarely tracheostomy	Fresh air stimulants artificial respiration treat debility	FB removal treatment of adenoids, worms	Oxygen treat the condition	Treat the cause

Reassurance is given to parents who are told to avoid rough handling of the child, to avoid sudden shocks to the child and to prevent exposure to changes in temperature. Tracheostomy is rarely needed.

Acute Laryngotracheobronchitis

It is a disease of infants and children and is rarely seen after the age of 7 or 8 years.

Etiology

The disease is considered to be caused by parainfluenza viruses. Bacteria like *Streptococcus, Pneumococcus, Staphylococcus* and *Haemophilus influenzae* are secondary invaders.

Pathology

The inflammatory process is diffuse in the larynx and tracheobronchial tree but the main area involved is the

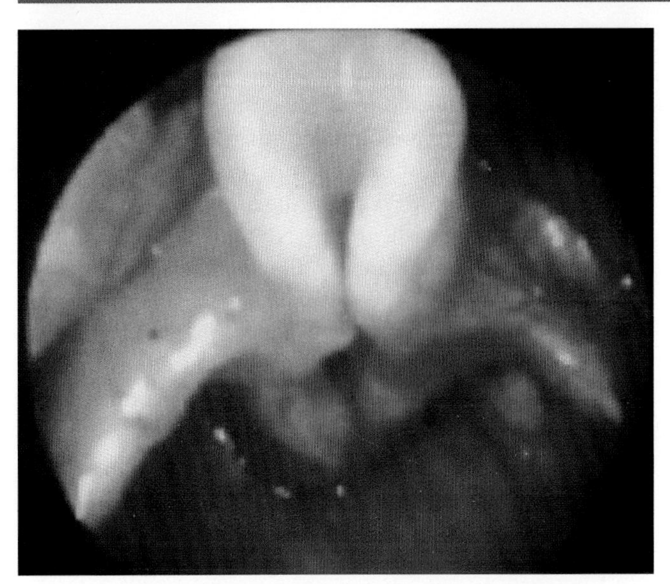

Fig. 56.1: Laryngomalacia (omega shaped epiglottis)

subglottic region of larynx. Inflammatory swelling of the mucosa occurs. The other characteristic feature is the production of tenacious, thick mucous which is difficult to remove. Edema, particularly in the subglottic region and the thick secretions cause severe difficulty in breathing and may lead to asphyxia.

Clinical Features

The disease usually start as a mild upper respiratory tract infection for a few days which is followed by symptoms and signs of severe respiratory obstruction. Dyspnea with recession of the intercostal supraclavicular and suprasternal spaces results. The child gets stridor and croupy cough. There is high fever, toxemia and restlessness. Examination of the chest usually does not reveal any marked abnormality. Direct laryngoscopy shows a congested larynx. Edema is the usual feature with semielliptical mounding of the subglottic tissues.

Treatment

Maintenance of the airway is of primary importance. Tracheostomy or endolaryngeal intubation may be needed in severe cases. Frequent suction of thick mucoid secretions is essential. Moist air should be provided to such patients. The room temperature should be kept about 91°F and humidity about 80 percent provided. This can be done by electrosonic nebulisers or by an oxygen tent erected over the bed and providing a boiling water kettle in the room.

Antibiotics like heavy doses of benzyl penicillin are given. These help to prevent complications by pathogenic organisms.

Corticosteroids help to reduce mucosal edema and effects of toxemia.

Acute Epiglottitis (Acute Obstructive Supraglottic Laryngitis)

It is a special form of laryngitis with definite clinical and pathological features. The disease is of bacterial origin and *Haemophilus influenzae* type B is the most common causative organism. The disease is rare and is seen usually in the age group of 3 to 6 years.

Pathology

There occurs marked swelling of the epiglottis which may extend to the supraglottic tissues. The main problem is marked respiratory obstruction that can occur within a few hours.

Clinical Features

The disease starts with a sore throat which quickly progresses to dysphagia and extreme difficulty in breathing. Because of the inflamed supraglottic tissues, the patient finds it very difficult to swallow. The voice may be muffled but is usually clear.

The degree of prostration and shock is most striking. The patient looks anxious and frightened because of choking. Examination of the throat shows marked swelling of the epiglottis and adjacent tissues.

X-ray soft tissue of the neck in the lateral view shows what is termed as the 'thumb sign; and this is due to the swollen epiglottis.

Treatment

Tracheostomy should be done to relieve respiratory difficulty. Antibiotics, usually ampicillin, are the drugs of choice. Steroids are helpful.

Acute epiglottitis in adults is still a rare condition, but takes a more dangerous course.

Diphtheria

The term diphtheria is derived from the Greek word diphtheria which means leather or membrane.

The disease affects children usually below the age of 5 to 6 years. The disease is still prevalent in underdeveloping countries including India.

Etiology

Corynebacterium diphtheriae also known as Kleb Loeffler's *Bacillus* is the causative organism. It is a gram-positive organism having a club-shaped appearance. Certain strains show a beaded appearance and grow in a "Chinese letter" fashion on culture.

There are three strains of this organism. These are classified as *gravis, intermedius,* and *mitis* depending upon the virulence of the strain.

Pathology

The faucial region is the most common site. From the faucial region, the disease can spread to the larynx although primary laryngeal or tracheobronchial diphtheria is known to occur. The infection produces hyperemia. Subsequently exudation occurs in the mucosa. The superficial layers of the epithelium get involved in a deposit of fibrin and leukocytes and thus there occurs formation of a membrane which can be removed with difficulty. The engorged capillaries also get trapped up in the membrane, hence, its removal leads to bleeding. The membrane is grayish white in appearance but may, sometimes, be brown or black due to hemorrhage in it. The underlying thrombophlebitis may sometimes produce necrosis of the mucosa leading to gangrenous diphtheria. The membrane is firmly attached over the areas lined by squamous epithelium and is loosely attached over ciliated columnar epithelium.

The *Bacillus* produces a powerful exotoxin which diffuses through lymphatics and blood vessels into the systemic circulation producing varying systemic effects of the disease. The degree of toxemia depends upon the causative strain of the *Bacillus* and the site of the infection. The cardiac and nervous tissues are more susceptible to toxemia. Myocarditis and neuritis are the usual complications produced.

Clinical Features

The disease is common in young children who have not received proper immunization.

The laryngeal lesions occur usually secondary to faucial diphtheria, however, the larynx may be primarily involved. The membrane forms over the cords and laryngeal vestibule and may spread over to the subglottis and trachea. The membrane is usually loosely attached to the ciliated columnar epithelium.

The main clinical feature is airway obstruction. The patient presents with stridor and dyspnea besides systemic toxemia. Direct laryngoscopy shows the membranous lesion of the larynx.

Patients with laryngeal diphtheria are detected early because of the respiratory difficulty which attracts the patient's and clinician's attention. Moreover, the membrane is loosely attached to the mucosa, hence, less of toxins are absorbed than in faucial disease where diagnosis is late and toxemia is severe.

Complications of Diphtheria

The main local complication is airway obstruction and asphyxia because of membrane formation and inflammatory edema. Toxemia produces certain systemic complications which may be cardiac and neurological.

1. *Cardiovascular complications:* These include acute peripheral circulatory failure, toxic myocarditis and varying degrees of heart block. In most cases, cardiac manifestations appear during the second week of the disease.
2. *Neurological complications:* Neuritis is the common manifestation. If frequently affects motor than sensory nerves. Paralysis of the soft palate is the most common complication which usually occurs during the third week of the disease. Other neurological complications that can arise include paralysis of the 3rd, 4th and 6th cranial nerves, and paralysis of the diaphragm.

Sometimes acute tubular damage of the kidneys may occur besides areas of toxic degeneration in the liver and spleen. Arthritis and septicemia are the other occasional complications of diphtheria.

Immunology

Schick test determines the susceptibility of a person to the infection. 0.1 ml containing 1/50 MLD of diphtheria toxin is injected subcutaneously. An area of erythema and induration of about 10 mm at about the 4th day indicates a positive test, i.e. a susceptible person while a negative test indicates that the person is immune. Immunity can be provided passively by injecting diphtheria antitoxin or by active immunization with diphtheria toxoid.

Treatment of Diphtheria

The main aim of treatment in such patients is restoration of the airway, if it is in danger, and neutralization of the circulating toxin.

Direct laryngoscopy may help to remove an obstructing membrane. If respiratory obstruction is impending, tracheostomy should be done.

To neutralize the circulating toxins, antidiphtheritic serum is given parenterally after a test dose. The dose varies according to the severity of infection. 10,000 IU to 50,000 IU are sufficient in mild to moderate cases. Heavy doses of benzyl penicillin or erythromycin are given. Systemic steroids help to reduce the toxemia and local inflammatory edema.

Other general measures include bedrest, adequate hydration and management of cardiac and neurological complications.

Chapter

57

Acute Laryngitis

Acute nonspecific laryngitis usually follows viral infections of the upper respiratory tract. Bacteria are the secondary invaders.

Predisposing Factors

Excessive vocal use, smoking, sinusitis and tonsillitis predispose to laryngitis. Similarly, irritant fumes, intubation and instrumental trauma are the other contributory factors.

Pathology

The mucosa of the larynx becomes congested and may become edematous. A fibrinous exudate may occur on the surface. Sometimes infection involves the perichondrium of the laryngeal cartilages producing perichondritis.

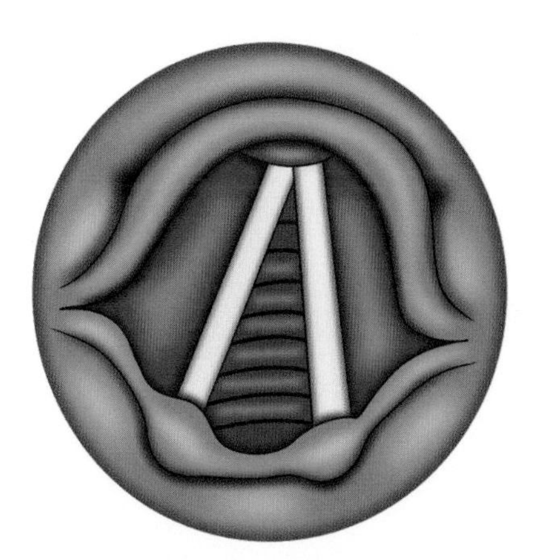

Fig. 57.1: Normal vocal cords

Clinical Features

The main complaint of the patient is the huskiness or hoarseness of voice and discomfort in throat particularly on swallowing. Dry irritating cough may be a troublesome feature of laryngitis. Dyspnea is present only in severe cases. Generalized features like fever, bodyache, and malaise are usually associated.

On examination the signs of upper respiratory tract infection are evident. Indirect laryngoscopy reveals a diffuse congestion of the laryngeal mucosa. The vocal cords look dull red and slightly edematous. Arytenoids, aryepiglottic folds and vestibular bands may show varying degrees of edema. Thick secretions appear on the surface of the laryngeal mucosa. The larynx in a normal person and in acute laryngitis is shown in **Figures 57.1** and **57.2**, respectively.

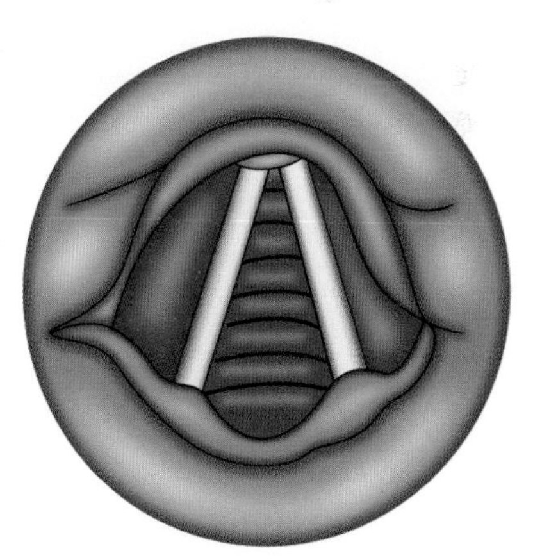

Fig. 57.2: Acute laryngitis

Treatment

Rest to the voice is important for speedy recovery. Steam inhalations are soothing to the inflamed mucosa and also provide humidification.

Analgesic and antipyretic drugs are given for relief of pain and control of fever. Antibiotics are prescribed for control of bacterial infection. In severe cases steroids may be needed.

Acute Laryngitis in Children

Acute nonspecific laryngitis in children usually follows exanthematous fevers and other bacterial infections of the upper respiratory tract. This disease follows a more severe course in children than in adults. It is so because the subglottic region of the larynx in infants is relatively smaller and the submucosal tissues of the larynx are very lax. Hence, the edema occurs readily causing obstruction of the airway.

CLINICAL FEATURES

The child usually presents with stridor, dyspnea and croupy cough, besides constitutional symptoms. The cry of the child becomes hoarse.

Diagnosis is made by direct laryngoscopy which reveals the acute inflammatory state of the larynx.

TREATMENT

Heavy doses of antibiotics, and steroids are prescribed for the control of disease. Signs of airway obstruction are looked for and endolaryngeal intubation or tracheostomy done to relieve the airway obstruction.

Chapter 58

Chronic Laryngitis

Chronic inflammation of the larynx may present as a diffuse lesion or produce localized effects in the larynx. A variety of factors are responsible.

1. *Chronic infection:* Chronic laryngitis may be produced by a chronic inflammatory focus in the tonsils, pharynx, teeth, gums or paranasal sinuses. The larynx is exposed to infected material from these sites and gradually develops features of chronic inflammation.
2. *Vocal abuse:* It is an important cause of chronic laryngitis. Teachers, salesmen, public speakers, etc. whose occupation demands a constant use of voice with strain and tension suffer more from this problem.
3. *Smoking:* Tobacco has harmful effects on the laryngeal mucosa. Inhalation of smoke produces edema and chronic inflammatory changes in the mucosa which eventually lead to hyperkeratosis and leukoplakia.
4. *Alcohol:* Alcohol produces chronic inflammatory changes in the pharyngeal mucosa and the nearby laryngeal mucosa gets involved. Moreover, alcohol drinking is often associated with smoking and vocal abuse.
5. *Irritant fumes:* Chronic irritation of the larynx may result from fumes inhaled in factories and is likely to produce chronic laryngitis.

Pathology

The histopathological examination shows mucosal thickening and infiltration with plasma cells and leukocytes. Capillaries appear engorged and the connective tissue elements are increased.

Clinical Features

The main presenting symptom of the patient is hoarseness of voice, i.e. change in the quality of voice. Tiredness of voice is also a frequent symptom. The patient may complain of some foreign body sensation in the throat and may frequently cough to clear his throat.

Examination reveals a red, hyperemic, and irregular laryngeal mucosa. It appears swollen and thickened. The mucosa is diffusely involved. The cords may appear granular and thickened.

Reinke's Edema

This condition is a bilateral polypoidal degeneration of the membranous vocal cords, producing smooth edematous swelling of the *Reinke's space* which is a subepithelial loose space on the membranous cords limited by the superior and inferior arcuate lines on the cords. Indirect laryngoscopy shows bilateral pale spindle-shaped swellings of the vocal cords.

The swelling results from the misuse of voice.

Treatment is microsurgical excision of the strips of mucosa from the membranous cords.

Vocal Nodules

Nodular thickening of the free edge of the vocal cords is a common disorder (**Fig. 58.1**). It involves females more than males.

ETIOLOGY

These lesions are common in people who use their voice excessively, such as teachers, hawkers, singers and preachers. These are common in people with a hyperkinetic personality, who are vociferous and of aggressive nature.

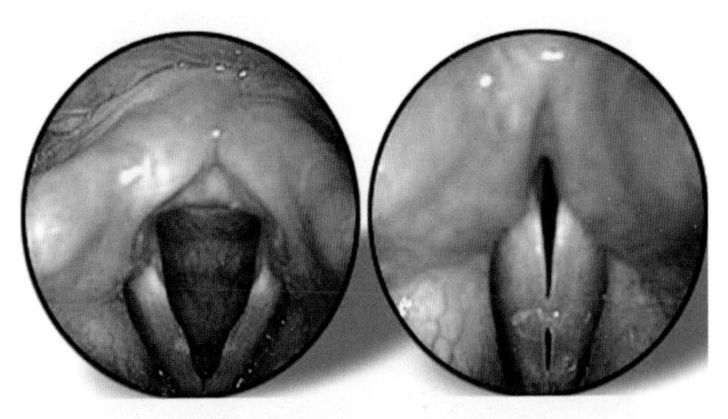

Fig. 58.1: Vocal nodules: abducted cords (left) and adducted cord view (right).

PATHOLOGY

The nodules are usually bilateral, symmetrical occurring at the junction of anterior and middle one-third. It is at this junction that maximum work load occurs on the cords. The nodules develop as hyperplastic thickening of the epithelium because of vocal abuse. Focal hemorrhage occurs in the subepithelial tissue which gets organized and results in nodule formation. The nodules rarely exceed 1 to 5 mm in size.

CLINICAL FEATURES

The patient complains of hoarseness of voice as the cords do not approximate completely. The voice tires easily. Constant efforts to improve the voice may strain the muscles and the patient may complain of pain in the neck. Indirect laryngoscopy reveals the nodules on the cords.

TREATMENT

In the initial stages, voice rest may help the patient. This might mean a vocal rest for several weeks and the patient should be advised to stop hemming and hawking. He should be trained to use the voice properly. Smoking should be stopped and attention given to any septic focus in the tonsils, nose, sinuses and teeth. When these measures do not help, microsurgical excision should be undertaken. The nodule is excised close to its base. Postoperative voice rest and speech therapy are a must.

Vocal Cord Polyp

Polypoid lesions of the cords are more common in males than in females. The etiology is obscure but there is usually a history of vocal abuse (**Fig. 58.2**).

Theories of etiology include inflammatory irritation and localized vascular disease but these have not been substantiated.

PATHOLOGY

Localized vascular engorgement and microhemorrhages occur, followed by edema (**Fig. 58.3**). The stroma is scanty, relatively acellular and distended with mucoid exudate. The epithelium is

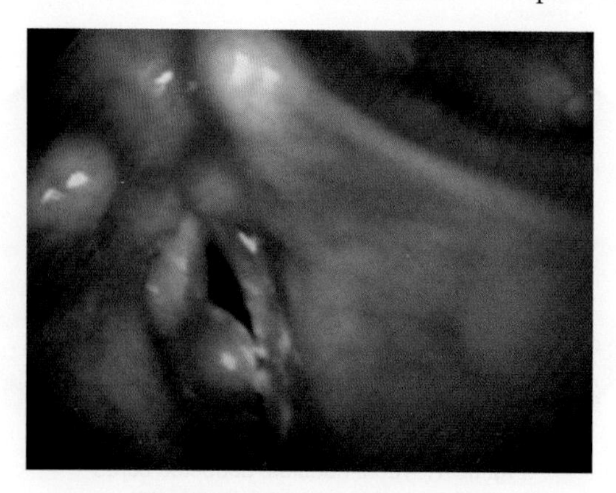

Fig. 58.2: Right vocal cord cyst

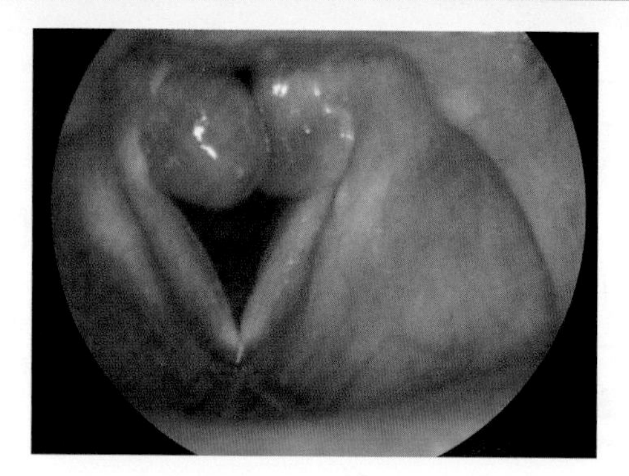

Fig. 58.3: Vocal cord polyps

normal. Histology may differentiate the polyp into three types: *gelatinous, transitional* and *telangiectatic.*

CLINICAL FEATURES

The main symptom is hoarseness of long duration. A large polyp may result in choking spells. Laryngoscopy reveals translucent sessile or pedunculated lesion arising from the vocal cord usually near the anterior commissure and sometimes it arises from both the cords.

The polyp may hang down into the subglottic region and become visible only on coughing or phonation.

TREATMENT

Treatment is microsurgical excision. The polyp should be properly grasped, pulled medially and carefully trimmed off by the scissors without causing damage to the cords.

Contact Ulcer

It is a form of localized lesion characterized by epithelial thickening on the vocal processes of the arytenoid cartilage. There is no true ulceration so the better term for this condition is contact pachydermia. The condition results from the misuse of voice. It results from the faulty production of voice rather than from its excessive use (**Fig. 58.4**).

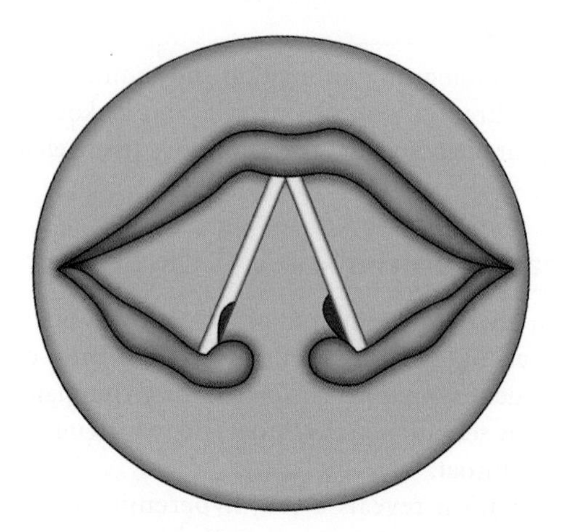

Fig. 58.4: Contact ulcer

The lesions appear on the vocal processes. The thickened hyperplastic epithelium gets heaped up around a crater, at the floor of which lies the vocal process. On indirect laryngoscopy, the heaped edge of one side may appear fitting in a crater on the opposite cord giving an appearance of an ulcer. The condition responds to voice rest and proper speech therapy. Surgery is required if conservative treatment fails. Microsurgical excision of the hyperplastic epithelium is done. Postoperatively, vocal rest and speech therapy are a must for the surgical treatment to succeed.

Hyperkeratosis and Leukoplakia

Sometimes circumscribed epithelial hyperplasia and keratinization occur in chronic laryngitis. Hyperkeratosis is a thickening of superficial layers of the epithelium. The area may appear as having warty or grayish papillomatous appearance. Leukoplakia appears as a white patch usually on the cords and may look like a small prominent patch or a nodular plaque.

The lesions may be single or multiple. In hyperkeratosis histologically there is thickening of the stratum corneum with little or no inflammatory reaction in the underlying tissues. Hyperkeratosis and leukoplakia lead to premalignant dysplasia. The cellular atypia is evident. Treatment of these lesions is microsurgical excision.

Atrophic Laryngitis

Atrophy of the laryngeal mucosa occurs usually in association with atrophic rhinitis and atrophic pharyngitis. The atrophic process involves the mucosa, the glands disappear and there occurs crusting of the mucosal surface.

The patient's main complaint is dryness of throat, irritant cough and blood-stained thick mucoid secretion. The voice becomes hoarse.

Voice rest is important. Attention is given to the nasal, sinus and pharyngeal diseases, besides prescribing local lubricating preparations.

Tuberculosis of the Larynx

Tuberculosis of the larynx occurs almost always secondary to pulmonary tuberculosis. The spread of infection is usually direct through the infected sputum. The infection may reach to the larynx through lymphatics and rarely through the blood stream. The disease commonly occurs between 20 and 40 years of age.

PATHOLOGY

Tubercle formation is the characteristic lesion. The tubercle bacilli invade the mucosa and are surrounded by polymorphs, macrophages and mononuclear cells. The macrophages destroy the bacilli and form epitheloid cells, which coalesce to form gaint cells. Coagulative necrosis occurs in the center of tubercle and caseation results.

The initial stage is infiltration which is followed by the proliferative stage when tumor like masses appear. Thereafter the ulcerative stage occurs and the tubercles breakdown and small superficial ulcers, with undermined margins appears. Finally healing by fibrosis may occur which is called the stage of cicatrization.

SITES OF INVOLVEMENT

The posterior part of the larynx is the most common site of involvement. The posterior commissure has a folded mucosa which forms the crevices where the tubercle bacilli get lodged easily.

Laryngeal ventricles, false cords and arytenoids are commonly involved. Subepithelial infiltration by the tubercular granulation tissue produces swelling of the aryepiglottic folds and epiglottis leading to *turban-shaped epiglottis.* Ulcers with mouse-nibbled appearance may appear on the false and true cords.

CLINICAL FEATURES

The history is suggestive of pulmonary tuberculosis. Weakness of the voice is a typical feature. The patient complains of odynophagia (painful deglutition), which is more for solids than for semisolids, as the semisolids form a coating over the ulcers having exposed nerve endings. The pain may radiate to the ears.

Examination of the chest reveals features of pulmonary tuberculosis. Laryngoscopy shows interarytenoid thickening or heaping of the mucosa. Arytenoids may appear edematous and the epiglottis may appear turban-shaped. Superficial ulcerations may be visible on the ventricular bands or vocal cords. Mucosa of the laryngeal ventricle may show a prolapse.

Adduction weakness of the vocal cords is considered an early sign of tuberculosis. A positive sputum and X-ray of the chest are suggestive of tuberculosis and make biopsy unnecessary, which, however, should be done in doubtful cases.

TREATMENT

Treatment is voice rest and proper antitubercular chemotherapy.

Laryngeal Lupus

Lupus vulgaris is an indolent form of tuberculosis. It is a rare disease which affects females more than males. It involves a slow destructive process. Laryngeal lupus is always secondary to lupus vulgaris of the nose. The nasal lesions itself may be active or may have healed. The epiglottis, aryepiglottic folds and arytenoids are the most treatment common sites involved. The disease may cause destruction of the epiglottis. Superficial ulceration, areas of cicatrization and characteristic pallor of the surrounding mucosa are typical features.

The disease runs a painless course and it is often the active or healed nasal lesions which attract the attention during examination. Antitubercular treatment should be given if the lesions are active.

Chapter 59

Laryngeal Trauma

Trauma to the larynx and trachea may be caused by external injury like vehicular accidents, blows, suicidal cut throat attempts, endoscopic procedures, intubation or tracheostomy.

Pathology

The degree of damage depends upon the nature and severity of the injury. Displacement or fracture of the laryngotracheal cartilages may occur with or without mucosal tear of the larynx and pharynx.

Lateral blows may fracture the thyroid cartilage in the midline with tearing of the vocal cords. Supraglottic fracture of the thyroid cartilage with displacement of the epiglottis may occur and occasionally there may occur total separation of the larynx from the trachea.

Clinical Features

Hoarseness of voice, difficulty in breathing, stridor and pain on swallowing may be the presenting symptoms.

Swelling of the soft tissues of the neck, subcutaneous emphysema and tenderness of the laryngeal tissues may be present on external examination. Laryngoscopy may show mucosal ecchymosis, laceration, edema and distortion of the endolaryngeal contours. X-rays of the soft tissues of the neck and cervical spine are helpful. Tomograms provide a detailed view of the injured tissue.

Treatment

Tracheostomy may be needed for restoration of the airway. Exploration of the larynx may be required for restoration of the normal anatomy. The displaced and fractured cartilages are repositioned and wired together to avoid subsequent stenosis. Mucosal lacerations are stitched and antibiotics given to prevent infection.

Laryngeal Stenosis

Laryngeal stenosis may occur because of congenital webs, atresia, inadequately treated laryngotracheal injuries, high tracheostomy or as a sequelae to injury by intubation.

The presenting features include hoarseness of voice and difficulty in breathing.

MANAGEMENT

A proper assessment of the degree of stenosis is made on clinical and radiological examination. CT of the neck is needed for proper evaluation. Small webs and stenotic bands are released on direct laryngoscopy.

A severe degree of stenosis requires laryngofissure. The stenotic area is released or excised. Mucosal or skin grafts may be needed to cover the raw area over an endolaryngeal stent. The stent is put in position for 3 to 4 weeks, after which it is removed.

Chapter 60

Laryngocele

A laryngocele is an air filled sac produced in the larynx due to dilatation of the laryngeal saccule which is vestigial in human beings. The dilatation may occur congenitally or due to raised intrathoracic pressure as occurs in persons engaged in playing wind pipe instruments or weight lifting.

Types

Internal laryngocele: The dilatation remains confined to the larynx. This produces a cystic swelling under the vestibular bands and aryepiglottic folds (**Fig. 60.1**).

External laryngocele: The dilated air sac may project through the thyrohyoid membrane into the neck, producing a compressible cystic swelling in the region of the thyroid cartilage. Sometimes a combination of the internal and external varieties occurs.

Symptoms

Majority of the cases are asymptomatic. The internal laryngocele produces hoarseness of voice and may produce dyspnea due to pressure changes. The external laryngocele presents as a cystic swelling in the neck.

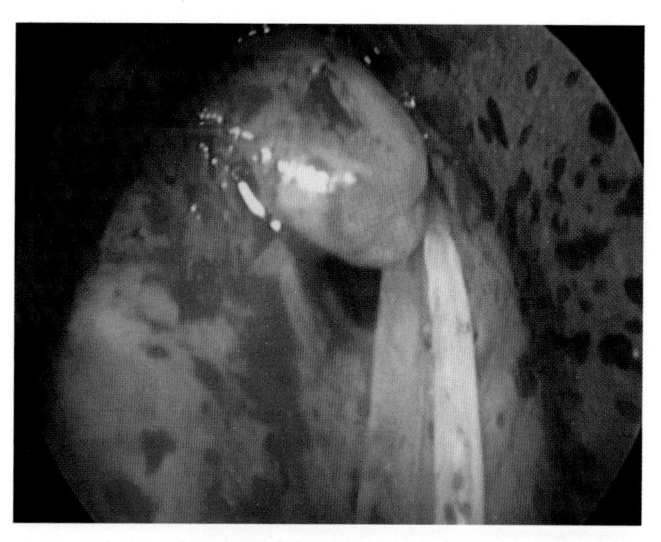

Fig. 60.1 Internal laryngocele

Diagnosis is done by clinical examination. The swelling increases in size on performing the Valsalva's maneuver.

X-ray of the neck, anteroposterior view, shows an air filled sac which becomes prominent on the Valsalva's maneuver. If symptoms are troublesome, the sac is excised.

Chapter 61

Edema of the Larynx

Edema of the larynx is not a disease as such but is a manifestation of various conditions affecting the larynx or the body as a whole (**Fig. 61.1**).

Etiology

1. *Inflammatory*
   a. Acute laryngitis, laryngotracheobronchitis, epiglottitis, diphtheria, acute perichondritis or abscess of the larynx.
      Inflammatory lesions like peritonsillar abscess, retropharyngeal abscess and Ludwig's angina may spread to larynx leading to laryngeal edema.
   b. Chronic inflammatory lesions like tuberculosis, syphilis and leprosy.
2. *Traumatic*
   a. Foreign bodies in larynx
   b. Trauma to the larynx by external injuries, endoscopy, and intubation
   c. Inhalation of irritant fumes
   d. Swallowing of corrosives
   e. Postoperative as after the operations on the larynx itself, pharynx, tongue and floor of the mouth.
3. *Neoplastic:* Neoplastic diseases of the larynx when associated with ulceration and infection are associated with edema.
4. *Angioneurotic edema:* Edema may develop in larynx due to allergy.
5. *Systemic diseases:* Laryngeal edema may be the manifestation of prolonged heart failure, renal failure and myxedema.

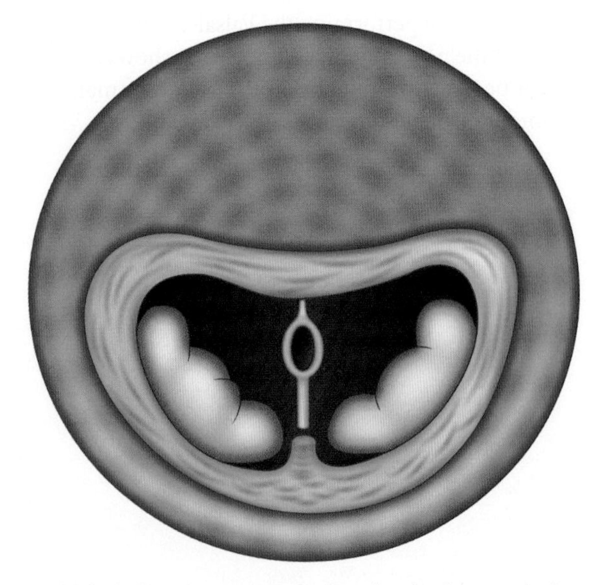

Fig. 61.1: Indirect laryngoscopic view showing laryngeal edema

Angioneurotic Edema (Quincke's Edema)

Allergic edema due to antigen-antibody reaction may involve the larynx. This may be due to sensitivity to some foods, drugs including antibiotics, insect bite, parenteral sera or because of worm infestation. Some cases remain idiopathic.

Generalized urticaria with sudden respiratory difficulty may occur because of edema of the larynx affecting the supraglottic and subglottic tissues.

Immediate attention should be given to the maintenance of the airway. This may need tracheostomy or intubation. Injection of 0.5 ml adrenaline 1:1000 is given subcutaneously. Parenteral steroids are started and repeated at periodic intervals. Antihistaminic drugs are prescribed and the offending drug or food withdrawn.

PATHOLOGY

The edema may occur as a result of irritation, allergy or inflammation. There occurs distension of the submucosal tissues with tissue fluid, lymph and inflammatory exudate. Swelling of the laryngeal tissues seen in tuberculosis and myxedema is called *pseudoedema.* In tuberculosis the swelling is caused by inflammatory infiltration with accumulation of cells. In myxedema, the swelling of the tissues is caused by myxomatous changes.

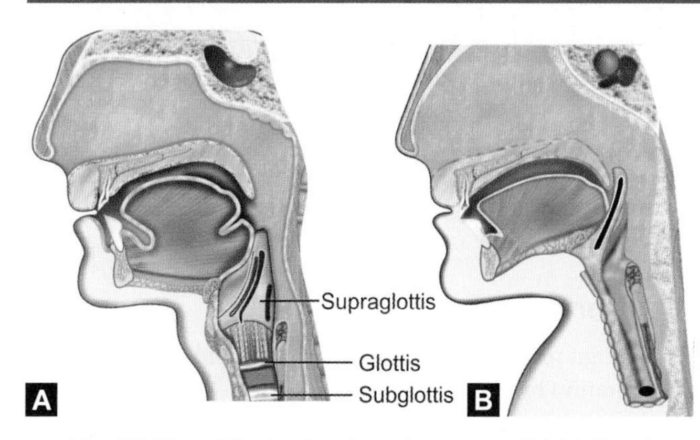

Figs 61.2A and B: Adult and newborn larynx. (A) Adult and (B) Newborn

Airway Obstruction in Children and Adults

The human newborn is an obligate nasal breather by virtue of the intranarial position of its larynx (**Figs 61.2A and B**). Approximation of the epiglottis with the soft palate provides a continuous, uninterrupted airway from the nose to the bronchi. This configuration, similar in all mammals, is peculiarly lost in humans four to six months after birth. The structural change provides the potential for oral respiration at an early age as the larynx descends in the neck with postnatal maturation. Therefore, if untreated, nasal obstruction in the newborn period could and often does prove fatal, whereas in adulthood, nasal obstruction may be regarded as a mere annoyance.

Differentiation of upper from lower airway obstruction is crucial. Stridor, supraclavicular, sternal, and intercostal retraction with cyanosis are consistent with upper-airway obstruction. On the other hand, lower-respiratory obstruction often produces asymmetry of chest expansion with wheezing on auscultation. Dullness to percussion, decreased breath sounds, or presence of rales support obstructive atelectasis. Hyperresonance suggests obstructive emphysema. Rarely is lower-airway obstruction by itself an immediate threat to life; upper-airway blockage represents a true emergency.

Obstruction at the laryngeal level produced by congenital laryngeal deformities and infection are common to childhood development. Neoplastic obstruction of the laryngeal aperture and vocal cord paralysis are often diseases of adulthood.

CAUSES OF OBSTRUCTION IN THE NEWBORN

Choanal Atresia

Choanal atresia, if bilateral, produces marked retraction and cyanosis in the newborn. However, if the infant is made to cry, airway obstruction is relieved and the color improves. Diagnosis is made by the passage of nasal catheters. Emergency treatment consists of establishing an oral airway followed by transnasal surgical repair. Tracheostomy is to be avoided.

Laryngomalacia

It comprises 75 percent of all laryngeal problems in infancy. Stridor consisting of a low-pitched inspiratory flutter is produced by an abnormally floppy epiglottis. Voice and cry are clear and strong. Aspiration is usually not a problem. Stridor is often exaggerated in a supine position and relieved in the prone. Diagnosis is made on direct laryngoscopy, which reveals an omega-shaped epiglottis. Gentle displacement to expose the glottic aperture will relieve stridor immediately. Symptoms ordinarily subside within months as the laryngeal framework enlarges and stiffens with growth.

Subglottic Stenosis (Fig. 61.3)

It comprises the second largest group of newborn laryngeal abnormalities. Obstruction results from:

i. Congenital hypoplasia of the cricoid cartilage, resulting in inspiratory and expiratory stridor. The luminal diameter of the subglottis measures 6 to 8 mm in the normal newborn. A subglottic diameter of 4 mm or less is regarded as abnormal. Diagnosis may be made radiologically or endoscopically. Treatment consists of tracheostomy and serial dilatations of the larynx.
ii. *Acquired subglottic stenosis* may be a result of direct trauma or high tracheostomy, but is most commonly found after a period of prolonged intubation, either during the neonatal period or following cardiac surgery. Premature neonates with a variety of metabolic and respiratory problems may often require prolonged endotracheal intubation with or without assisted

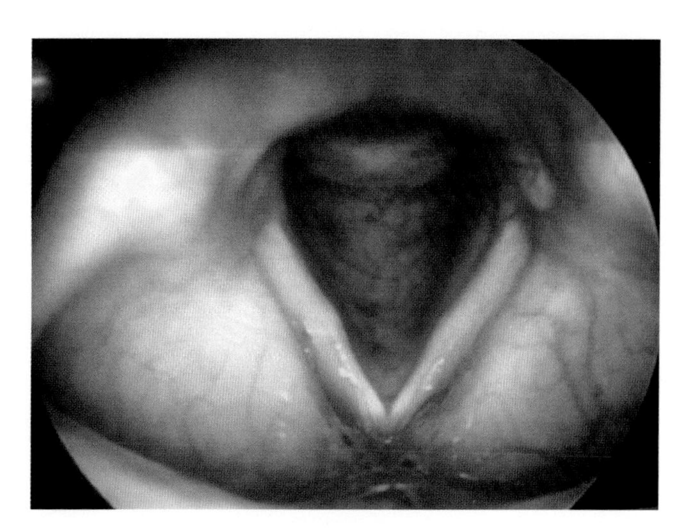

Fig. 61.3: Subglottic stenosis

ventilation and if the intubation has to be repeated frequently, the risk of subglottic mucosal damage and subglottic stenosis is increased. The incidence of this complication can be reduced drastically by careful fixing of tube, avoidance of infection and regular physiotherapy.

Children with severe acquired subglottic stenosis will require tracheostomy and this should be done between the fifth and sixth tracheal rings to avoid interference if surgical repair is required.

Laryngeal Webs

Laryngeal webs arise due to arrest of laryngeal development at about the tenth week of fetal life. Approximately 75 percent are located at the glottic level, the remaining 25 percent at the supraglottic. Because most webs occur at the glottis, symptoms include inspiratory and expiratory stridor. The patient's voice may be hoarse or he may be totally aphonic. Thin webs may respond to serial laryngoscopic dilatation, whereas thicker webs require tracheostomy and insertion of a laryngeal keel until cordal re-epithelialization occurs.

Laryngeal Spasms

Spasms of the larynx or choking may occur due to number of lesions.

ETIOLOGY

1. Foreign materials in the larynx (solids and liquids)
2. Irritation by instrumentation
3. Anaphylactoid reactions
4. Irritant fumes
5. Laryngismus stridulus (calcium deficiency)
6. Tetanus, rabies.

Urgent steps are taken to establish the airway by intubation or tracheostomy. Treatment is directed towards the underlying cause.

Chapter 62

Foreign Body in the Larynx and Tracheobronchial Tree

Foreign body in the larynx and tracheobronchial tree is one of the most important causes of stridor and dyspnea in infancy and childhood. There may or may not be a history of inhaling a foreign body. Sudden occurrence of dyspnea in a previously healthy child raises suspicion. Effects of the foreign body vary according to its size, nature and location in the larynx and tracheobronchial tree.

Small and smooth metallic foreign bodies such as pins allow uninterrupted passage of air, while a larger foreign body may cause a total occlusion of the airway.

The nature of the foreign body is also important. Vegetable foreign bodies like peas and beans produce severe pneumonitis and are also difficult to remove. The effects on the patient and his respiratory system depend also on the location of the foreign body in the respiratory tract. If the foreign body gets arrested in the larynx, it obstructs both the phases of respiration and rapidly produces laryngeal edema. In the trachea, if the foreign body is large, there is an equal danger of total respiratory obstruction.

Foreign Bodies in the Larynx

A foreign body lodged in the larynx obstructs inspiration as well as expiration and produces change in the voice. There may occur complete asphyxia which is further aggravated by the glottic edema.

Foreign Bodies in the Trachea

The main symptom is dyspnea with stridor. The changing position of the foreign body in the trachea may give rise to signs like an audible slap and a palpatory thud. Depending upon the obstruction one can hear an asthamatic type of wheeze in such cases.

Foreign Bodies in the Bronchus

Foreign bodies usually get arrested in the right main bronchus because it is wide and is more in line with the trachea than the left main bronchus.

The immediate effect of the foreign body in the bronchus is respiratory obstruction which could be partial or complete.

PARTIAL OBSTRUCTION

If the foreign body is smaller than the size of the bronchus, initially it allows the passage of air in both directions with little interference, like a bypass valve. A foreign body which is just of the size of the bronchus allows the flow of air only on inspiration and blocks the expiratory phase. It thus acts as a check valve. This sort of action depends upon the expansion of the bronchus on inspiration and its contraction on expiration. Such foreign bodies will produce obstructive emphysema with overdistension of the affected lobe and respiratory embarrassment.

TOTAL OBSTRUCTION

If the blockage of the bronchus is complete, either by the foreign body itself or by mucosal edema, a stop valve type obstruction results. There occurs no passage of air even on inspiration, so the air in the distal portion of the lung soon gets absorbed leading to collapse of a segment or lobe of the lung. Sometimes the foreign body may get arrested at the bifurcation producing a complete obstruction of one bronchus but only a partial obstruction in the other. Then the blocked segment of the lungs shows collapse while the partially obstructed one becomes emphysematous.

Patients in whom the foreign bodies are neglected may develop bronchiectasis, lung abscess and empyema in the long run.

Clinical Features

The clinical features of a case of foreign body in the larynx and tracheobronchial tree vary from mild symptoms to asphyxia. These depend upon the site of lodgement of the foreign body and the resultant pathological changes. The history may or may not be suggestive. A sudden episode of choking, coughing and dyspnea are important features.

Such patients present with dyspnea, cough and wheezing. If the effect produced is partial obstruction, then there are signs of obstructive emphysema with the trachea and mediastinum shifted away from the distended hyper-resonant lobe. In patients with complete bronchial obstruction there are signs of collapse with shifting of the mediastinum to the affected side.

Investigations

X-rays of the chest are of great help. These reveal the nature and position of the foreign body (if radiopaque) as well as the effects produced in the lung, like collapse or obstructive emphysema (**Fig. 62.1**).

Bronchoscopy may be done as diagnostic investigation and as a therapeutic procedure in cases where X-rays are not helpful but the history is suggestive.

Treatment

Foreign bodies in the larynx and the subglottic region are removed by direct laryngoscopy. Tracheostomy may be required initially to overcome the respiratory obstruction. The foreign body is then removed by direct laryngoscopy. Foreign bodies in the trachea and bronchi are removed by bronchoscopy. Impacted foreign bodies in the bronchus may require thoracotomy.

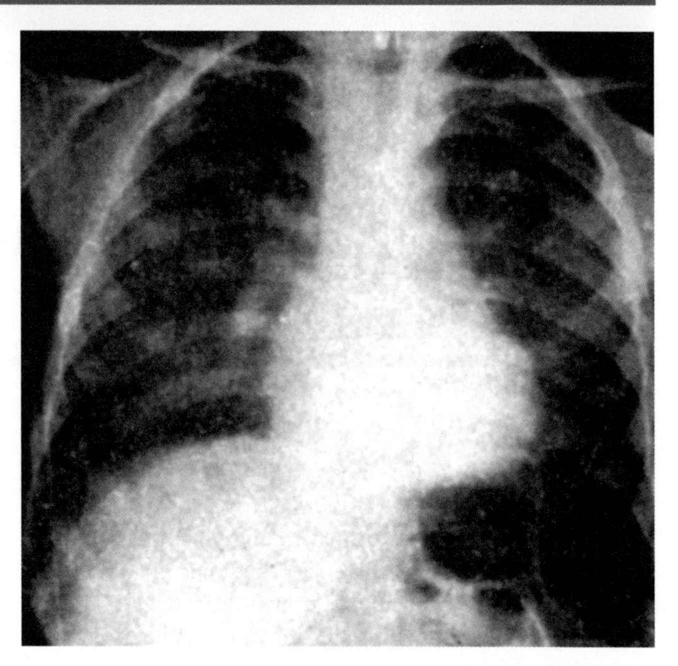

Fig. 62.1: X-ray of the chest showing a safety pin (foreign body) in the trachea

Chapter

63

Laryngeal Paralysis

The larynx is supplied by the vagus. The superior laryngeal nerve is sensory to the larynx but supplies motor fibers to the cricothyroid muscle through its external laryngeal branch. The recurrent laryngeal nerve is sensory to the larynx below the level of the cords and also supplies motor fibers to all laryngeal muscles except the cricothyroid.

These nerves can get involved in a variety of lesions in the brain, at the base of the skull, in the neck and in the chest. The right recurrent laryngeal nerve leaves the vagus at the level of the subclavian artery and then loops around it to ascend up in the tracheoesophageal groove to supply the larynx. The left recurrent laryngeal nerve has a longer course. It hooks around the ligamentum arteriosum and then ascends back into the neck to supply the larynx. **Figures 63.1A to C** show the position of vocal cords during respiration and phonation.

Etiology of Laryngeal Paralysis

Laryngeal paralysis can be caused by a variety of lesions. The sites of paralysis can be supranuclear or infranuclear. The former gives rise to a spastic type of paralysis and because larynx has bilateral representation in the cortex, only a widespread lesion of the cortex causes such paralysis (**Figs 63.2A to C**).

Infranuclear paralysis is common and can be due to following causes:

1. *Intracranial causes*
   a. Acute bulbar palsy
   b. Motor neuron disease
   c. Vascular lesions
   d. Tumors.
2. *Lesions at the base of skull*
   a. Nasopharyngeal tumors
   b. Fractures of the base of the skull
   c. Secondary deposits in the lymph nodes at the base of the skull.

   The laryngeal paralysis due to these causes is usually complete (superior laryngeal and recurrent laryngeal nerve paralysis) and may be associated with other cranial nerve paralysis (described later).
3. *Causes in the neck*
   a. Thyroid diseases, usually malignant
   b. Thyroid surgery
   c. Trauma to the neck
   d. Tumors and trauma to the esophagus and trachea in the neck
   e. Secondaries in the neck nodes.

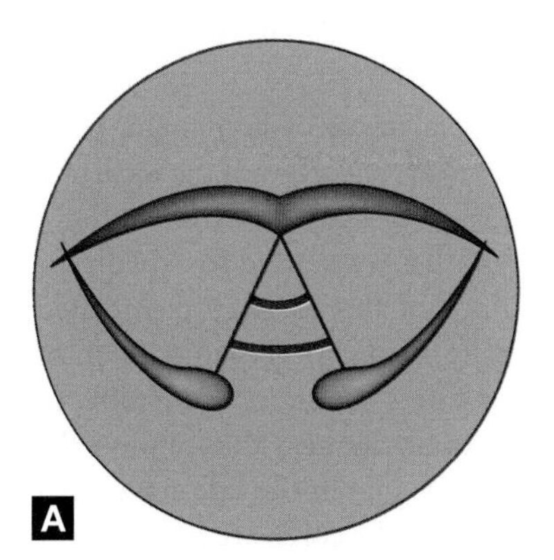

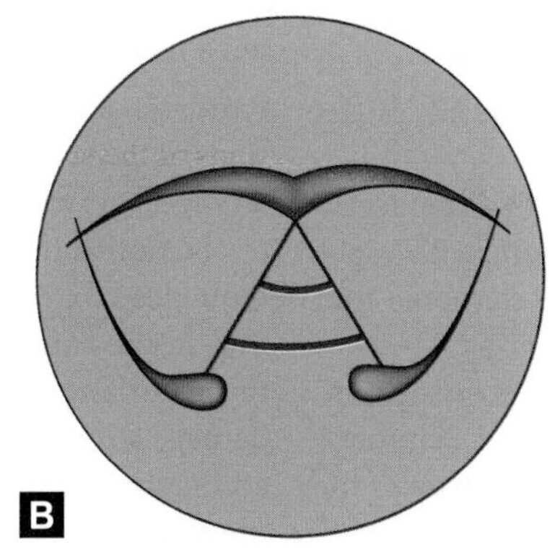

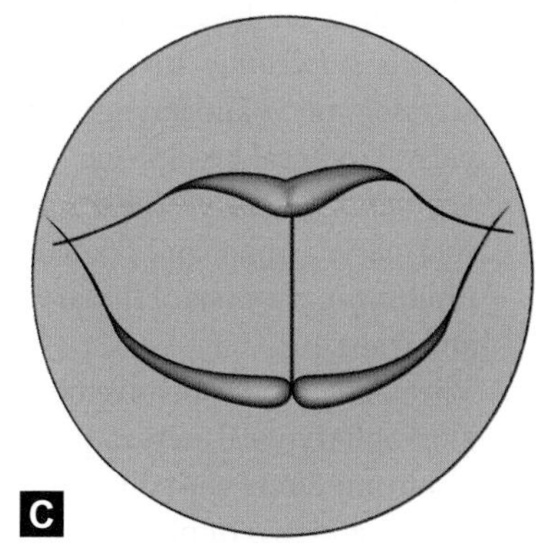

Figs 63.1A to C: Various positions of vocal cords. (A) Quiet respiration; (B) Deep inspiration; (C) Phonation

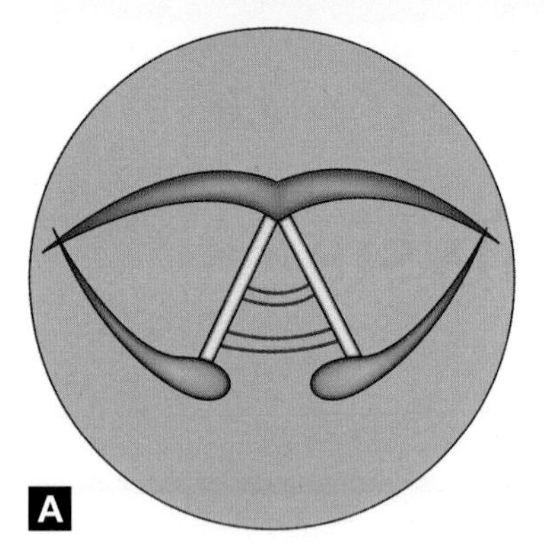

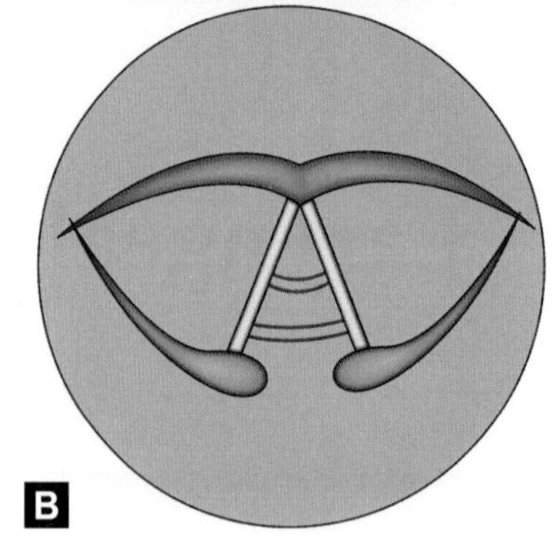

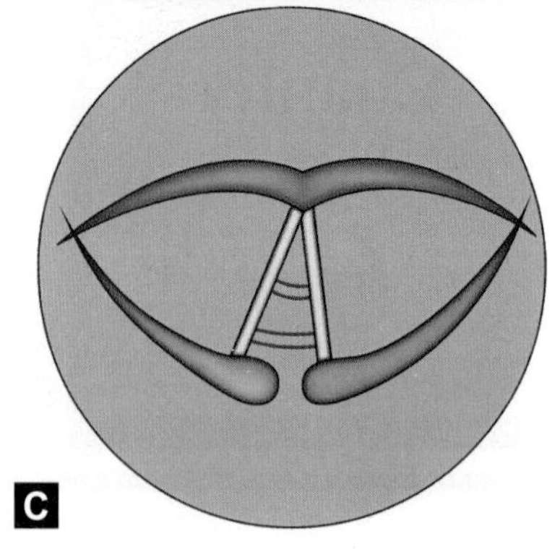

Figs 63.2A to C: Positions of paralyzed vocal cords. (A) Unilateral abductor paralysis; (B) Bilateral abductor paralysis; (C) Unilateral paralysis with compensation by unparalyzed cord

4. *Causes in the chest*
   a. Bronchogenic carcinoma with secondaries in the mediastinal nodes
   b. Esophageal malignancy
   c. Apical tuberculosis
   d. Aortic aneurysm.
5. *Miscellaneous causes:* Neuritis due to alcohol, diphtheria, lead poisoning, avitaminosis, diabetes, polyarteritis nodosa and sarcoidosis.
6. *Idiopathic:* Almost one-third of the cases of laryngeal paralysis are idiopathic. However, such a diagnosis is only made after proper investigations when all other known causes have been ruled out.

Laryngeal Paralysis in Association with other Cranial Nerve Dysfunction

Paralysis of the recurrent laryngeal nerve and superior laryngeal nerve may occur in association with paralysis of the other cranial nerve as a result of lesions at the base of skull or in the neck.

1. *Involvement of the hypoglossal and recurrent laryngeal nerve:* This may occur in the neck producing paralysis of the tongue and larynx on the same side known as *tapia syndrome.*
2. *Avellis-syndrome:* Involvement of the cranial root of accessory nerve and laryngeal nerves on the same side causes palatolaryngeal hemiplegia.
3. *Schimdt's syndrome:* There is involvement of the accessory nerve (spinal and cranial divisions) along with vagus resulting in paralysis of the larynx, soft palate, sternomastoid and trapezius.
4. *Vernet's syndrome:* Involvement of the vagus, accessory and glossopharyngeal nerves produces features of Schimdt's syndrome along with diminution of taste at the base of the tongue and loss of pharyngeal sensation.
5. *Hughlings-Jackson syndrome:* Involvement of the tenth, eleventh and twelfth cranial nerves produces homolateral associated paralysis of the larynx, soft palate, tongue and muscles of the neck (sternomastoid, trapezius).
6. *Collet-Sicard syndrome (Villaret's syndrome):* Involvement of the last four cranial nerves and the cervical symphathetic trunk in the region of the jugular foramen produces symptoms and signs of their paralysis.
7. *Klinkert syndrome:* Involvement of the recurrent laryngeal nerve and phrenic nerve, usually at the root of the neck or mediastinum produces this syndrome.
8. *Ortner's syndrome:* Paralysis of the recurrent laryngeal nerve may occur as a result of cardiomegaly particularly because of the dilated left atrium in mitral stenosis.

Paralysis of the superior laryngeal nerve: Involvement of this nerve produces sensory paralysis of the same side of the larynx. Laryngeal anesthesia and paresthesia occur on the side of lesion. Sometimes neuralgia is the presenting feature. Because of laryngeal anesthesia, there occur choking spells, particularly on drinking fluids. The patient also has some vocal weakness because of paralysis of the cricothyroid muscle.

Indirect examination reveals an oblique glottis and deviation of the posterior commissure to the side of paralysis. There may be a level difference of the cords as the affected cord lacks tension, because of cricothyroid paralysis.

Paralysis of the recurrent laryngeal nerve: The changing positions of the vocal cords as seen on laryngoscopy in the recurrent laryngeal nerve paralysis have been the subject of controversy.

Semon and Rosenback hypothesis was used to explain the sequence of paralytic conditions of the vocal cord. It stated that in the course of a gradually advancing organic lesion of the recurrent nerve, abductor fibers are more vulnerable to damage so the vocal cords approximate near the midline, the adduction is still possible and it is only in the late stages that the adductor fibers get involved and the cords are paralyzed in the intermediate position (cadaveric position), and the reverse happens during recovery.

Many diverse views have been proposed to explain the vulnerability of the abductors in laryngeal paralysis. However, neither separate grouping of the abductor and adductor fibers has been demonstrated in the nerve trunk, nor has any other explanation been found valid to explain the cord position on this hypothesis.

The opposition to this hypothesis came from *Wagner and Grossman*. They postulated that median or paramedian position of the paralyzed vocal cord in recurrent laryngeal nerve paralysis is due to intact function of the circothyroid muscle, which is innervated by the superior laryngeal nerve.

The intermediate position (cadaveric position) of the vocal cord is because of combined paralysis of the recurrent laryngeal nerve and the superior laryngeal nerve, as now the cricothyroid muscle also gets paralyzed.

It is now an accepted theory and so the laryngologist must consider mainly two positions, viz paramedian and intermediate. The apparent small variations in these two positions are due to compensation by the normal cord across the midline or atrophy and scarring of the paralyzed vocal cord.

MANAGEMENT OF LARYNGEAL PARALYSIS

The treatment in laryngeal paralysis is directed towards the causative lesion and to the effects of the paralysis.

Many cases of *unilateral vocal cord paralysis* do not require any active treatment as there are adequate compensatory movements by the normal cord, thus producing good voice.

Glottic rehabilitation with Teflon injection: For the return of voice, cough and laughter, the injection of Teflon glycerine mixture into the vocal cord is a procedure that can be used. The method has its most particular application in cases where there is a lateral lying paralyzed vocal cord. It is also useful in building up functioning scars after cordectomy and may help to correct cord deformities.

Teflon $(C_2 Fu)_n$ is a product of the research of the Manhattan project of Atomic Energy Commission. It is one of the most nonreactive substances known. For this reason it has been used as a graft for artery replacement. Animal studies have shown minimum tissue response. Left in tissues for a long time, it has not been found to be carcinogenic. Particles between 50 to 100 microns in diameter, mixed with glycerine as a vehicle to form air, are used to make an injectable paste. Teflon is not digested, absorbed or extruded as a foreign body. Since the average granule size is larger than the diameter of the lymphatic drainage channels, it remains where it has been placed. The glycerine vehicle is soon absorbed.

The following instruments are used:

1. Laryngoscope
2. Long needle to traverse the laryngoscope
3. Laryngoscope holder
4. Screw type syringe.

Local anesthesia is used and the patient is asked to attempt phonation.

Involvement of both the recurrent laryngeal nerves causes paralysis of both vocal cords in the paramedian position. Tracheostomy is needed to relieve respiratory distress. If recovery does not occur by 6 months to 1 year, the following options are considered:

1. The patient remains with permanent tracheostomy. He can be fitted with a speaking valve tracheostomy tube for speech. This tube has a valve which closes during expiration and allows the air column through the cords during phonation.
2. Alternatively, the patient is considered for surgery. Surgical procedures (cordectomy and cordopexy) are aimed at widening the glottis.

These procedures allow normal airway through the larynx but suffer from the disadvantage of poor voice.

Cordopexy: The procedure is termed *Woodman's operation.* The larynx is exposed laterally, the arytenoid is removed and the posterior end of the vocal cord is attached to the inferior cornu of thyroid cartilage, thus widening the glottis.

Cricoarytenoid Joint Arthritis

Arthritis of the cricoarytenoid joint causes fixation of the vocal cords. The patient gives a history of pain in the throat and odynophagia may be present. The fixed cord does not fall in a particular position as in laryngeal paralysis. Passive mobility test by a probe helps to differentiate this condition from paralysis. The joint mobility is impaired in arthritis.

Fixed and Paralyzed Cord

Fixation is due to infiltration of malignancy, adhesions and scarring of the vocal cord.

The important clinical signs to differentiate between the two conditions are given in **Table 63.1**.

Table 63.1: Differentiating points between paralyzed and a fixed vocal cord

	Paralyzed cord	Fixed cord
1.	There is bowing of the cord and it appears toneless.	The cord is straight and looks shortened.
2.	There is medial deviation of the arytenoid cartilage on the affected side.	The position of the arytenoid depends on the condition causing fixation.
3.	Vocal cord shows a flicker on phonation.	No flicker is seen.
4.	On probe test the paralyzed cord shows vibrations.	No vibrations are seen.

Chapter

64

Tracheostomy

Anatomical Relations of Trachea

Before considering the operative procedure, some important anatomical relations are reviewed.

Anteriorly, the trachea is covered by skin, superficial and deep fascia, sternohyoid and sternothyroid muscles. The isthmus of the thyroid gland lies deep to the strap muscles and covers the trachea from the second to the fourth ring. Below the isthmus lies the inferior thyroid vein.

On each side of the trachea are thyroid lobes enclosed in the pretracheal fascia, carotid sheath and other greater vessels and nerves of the neck. Posteriorly, the trachea lies on the esophagus and the recurrent laryngeal nerves ascend on each side between the trachea and the esophagus. The instruments used for tracheostomy are shown in **Figure 64.1**.

TRACHEOSTOMY

This is a procedure wherein an opening is made in the anterior tracheal wall which is brought to skin by inserting a tube.

Indications for Tracheostomy

1. Tracheostomy may be needed to relieve respiratory obstruction which may be due to the following:

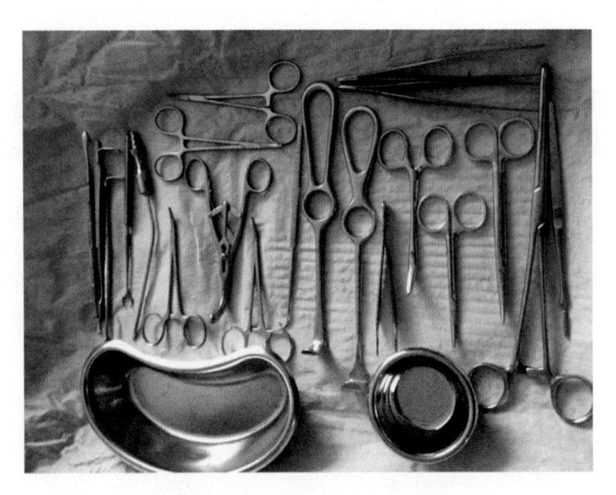

Fig. 64.1: Tracheostomy set

   a. Inflammatory diseases of the upper respiratory tract like acute laryngotracheobronchitis, laryngeal diphtheria and acute epiglottitis.
   b. Impacted foreign bodies in the larynx or trachea.
   c. Trauma such as laryngeal injury, maxillary and mandibular fractures, inhalation of irritant fumes or corrosive poisoning causing laryngeal edema.
   d. Angioneurotic edema.
   e. Tumors and cysts of the larynx and laryngopharynx.
   f. Bilateral vocal cord paralysis.
2. Tracheostomy may be needed to prevent aspiration of fluids, pus or blood from the trachea. Diseases like bulbar paralysis leads to pharyngeal paralysis and incompetence of the laryngeal sphincteric mechanism which leads to overspill of oral secretions into the larynx. Hence, tracheostomy is required to separate the lower respiratory tract from the pharynx.
3. Tracheostomy is indicated in certain diseases which lead to retention of secretions in the lower respiratory tract. Inadequate clearance of secretions from the tracheobronchial tree produces hypoxia and hypercapnia, further, these secretions serve as an ideal culture medium for bacteria. These conditions include bronchiectasis, lung abscess, chronic bronchitis, etc. Tracheostomy may be needed in various conditions like head injury and diabetic coma for proper suction of secretions in the lower respiratory tract.
4. Tracheostomy is indicated in certain conditions leading to respiratory insufficiency. Tracheostomy with a cuffed tracheostomy tube enables intermittent positive pressure respiration. The diseases which cause respiratory insufficiency are poliomyelitis, polyneuritis, chest injuries (flail chest), etc.
5. Muscular spasms and recurrent laryngeal nerve spasm as in tetanus necessitate a tracheostomy.

Types of Tracheostomy

The urgency with which a tracheostomy may be done is used to classify this operation.

1. *Emergency tracheostomy:* This type of operation is done when the laryngeal obstruction is acute and demanding an urgent relief. Under such circumstances, the patient's head and neck are extended and the trachea palpated. An incision is given with a knife deep in the midline and trachea opened for restoring respiration through tracheostomy (**Fig. 64.2**).
2. *Elective tracheostomy:* This is a planned operation. The patient and surgeon are both prepared. Proper instruments and anesthesia are arranged. The incision given is shown in **Figure 64.3**. It may be: (i) prophylactic, or (ii) therapeutic.

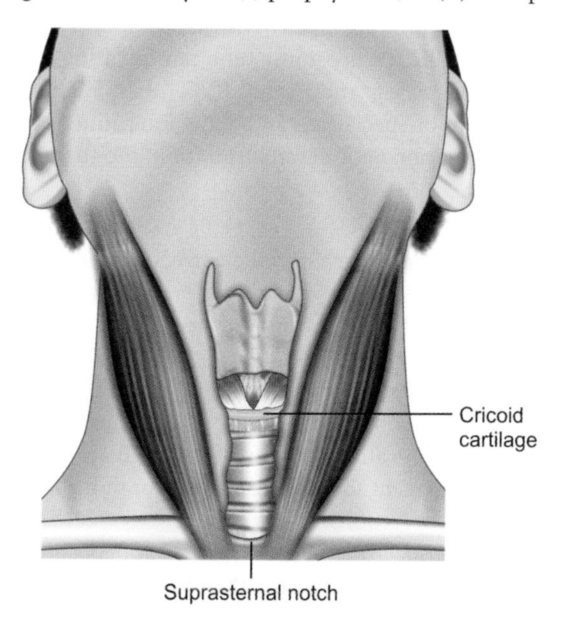

Fig. 64.2: Tracheostomy incisions—vertical incision for beginners and in emergency

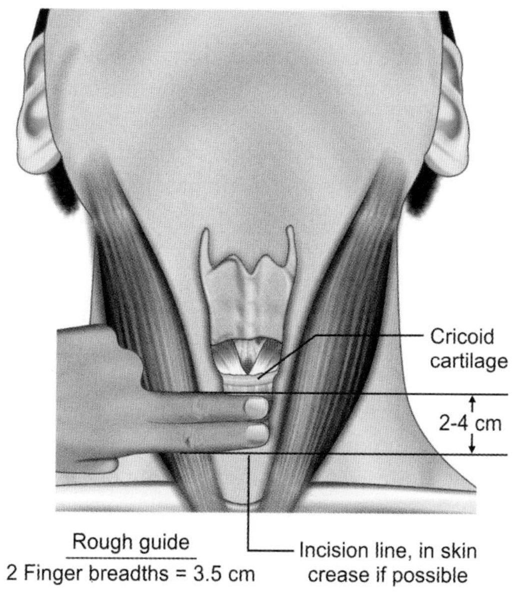

Fig. 64.3: Tracheostomy incisions—horizontal incisions in elective operation

3. *Permanent tracheostomy:* This may be required for patients with bilateral abductor paralysis, laryngeal stenosis, laryngectomy or laryngopharyngectomy, lower tracheal stump is brought, to surface and stitched to the skin.

Operative Technique (Figs 64.4 and 64.5)

A vertical incision is given in the suprasternal space extending down from the cricoid cartilage through the skin, subcutaneous fat and deep cervical fascia. The infrahyoid muscles are exposed and separated in the midline to expose the thyroid isthmus and trachea.

The thyroid isthmus is either retracted or cut to expose the tracheal rings. An assistant pulls the soft tissues and muscles laterally with retractors. The cricoid cartilage is hooked up to stabilize the trachea.

An opening is made in the tracheal wall, usually at the level of the 3rd or 4th ring and the tracheostomy tube is placed in position and secured by tapes around the neck.

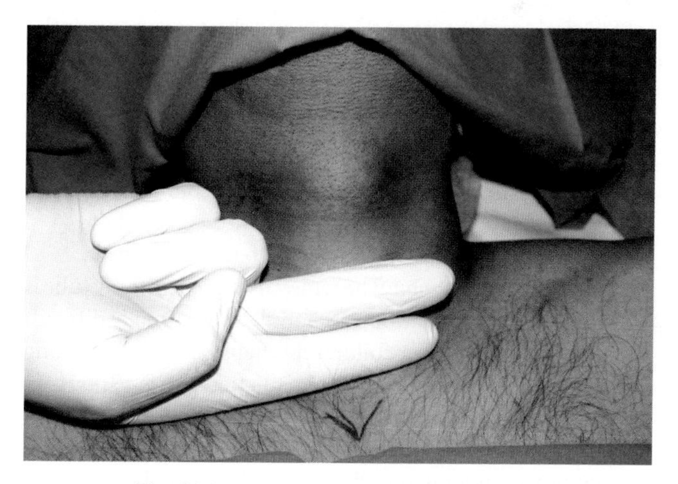

Fig. 64.4: Marking incision for tracheostomy

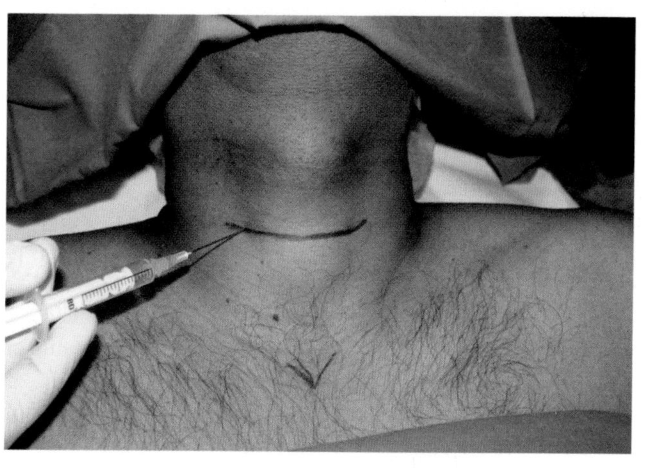

Fig. 64.5: Infiltration of tracheostomy incision

A tracheostomy is called high when the tracheal opening is made above the thyroid isthmus, i.e. through the first ring. There are chances of damage to the cricoid cartilage and subsequent subglottic stenosis.

A low tracheostomy means, making the tracheal opening below the thyroid isthmus. Care of such tracheostomy becomes difficult. Midtracheostomy is the ideal procedure where the opening is made behind the isthmus on the 3rd ring.

Complications of Tracheostomy

Various complications may arise during or after the operation. Complications that can arise during surgery include hemorrhage mainly due to trauma to the thyroid veins. Trauma during surgery may be to thyroid gland, esophagus, recurrent laryngeal nerve, great vessels of the neck or the domes of the pleura.

Sudden decrease in PCO_2 in the blood and correction of hypoxia may lead to apnea.

Postoperative Complications

1. Surgical emphysema of the neck and chest may occur as the air may leak into the cervical tissues.
2. *Displacement of tube:* Improper opening in the trachea, improper size and securing of the tube may lead to displacement of the tube with the formation of a false passage.
3. A high tracheostomy may damage the cricoid cartilage with resultant subglottic stenosis.
4. Damage to tracheal rings can lead to tracheomalacia.
5. *Difficult decannulation:* The removal of tracheostomy tube is known as decannulation. Decannulation is usually difficult in infants and young children perhaps because the young child has no airway reserve. It is better to use expiratory valve to begin with, thus restoring physiological expiratory thrust and stimulating the reflex for vocal cord abduction. Once this is tolerated well the cannula should be gradually blocked and reduced in size.
   Factors causing difficult decannulation are the following:
   i. Persistence of the condition that originally necessitated the tracheostomy
   ii. Granulation around stoma
   iii. Edema of the tracheal mucosa
   iv. Inability to tolerate upper airway resistance on decannulation
   v. Emotional dependence on tracheostomy
   vi. Subglottic stenosis
   vii. Tracheomalacia
   viii. Incoordination of the laryngeal opening reflex
   ix. Impaired development of the larynx as a result of long-standing tracheostomy.
6. *Pulmonary infection:* Lack of proper defence mechanism of the upper air passages and improper care of the tracheostomy may lead to pulmonary infection.
7. *Tracheal stenosis*
8. Fatal hemorrhage might occur due to erosion of a great vessel (innominate artery) by the tube end.

Types of Tracheostomy Tubes

A tracheostomy tube may be metallic or nonmetallic.

A metallic tracheostomy tube has an inner and an outer tube. The inner tube is longer than the outer one so that secretions and crusts form in it can be removed and the tube reinserted after cleaning without difficulty. However, they do not have a cuff and cannot produce an airtight seal.

A nonmetallic tracheostomy tube can be of the cuffed or noncuffed variety, e.g. rubber and PVC tubes. Silastic cuffed PVC tubes are of special use and allow intermittent positive pressure respiration and prevent aspiration into the trachea.

Care of Tracheostomy

1. Proper attention is given to the correct positioning of the tracheostomy tube by selecting a proper-sized tube and securing it with tapes around the neck.
2. *Removal of secretions:* In addition to the original pathology, the tube itself irritates the mucosa and thus produces copious secretions. The removal of secretions is done by using a sterile catheter for suction. Instillation of a few drops of 5 percent sodium bicarbonate or saline may cause thinning of secretions.
3. *Cleaning of tracheostomy tube:* Secretions deposited on the tube, dry up and form crusts thereby causing difficulty in breathing. The inner tracheostomy tube is periodically removed and cleaned, so is the outer tube, if necessary.
4. The tracheostomy wound is properly dressed to avoid infection.
5. If a cuffed tube has been used, the cuff should be periodically deflated to prevent necrosis of the mucosa and tracheal stenosis.
6. *Humidification and prevention of crusting:* The tracheostomy bypasses the upper air passages. Therefore, the function of air conditioning done by the nose is prevented which produces crusting in the trachea. To overcome this difficulty, a piece of moist gauze is put over the outer opening of the tube so that air takes up the moisture. A boiling water kettle in the room provides humidified air for such patients. Better techniques are available for humidifying the inspired air and include a condenser humidifier, ultrasonic humidifier, etc.
7. A tracheostomised patient cannot shout or call for help. So a call bell or nurse should be available and set of tracheostomy instruments should always be kept ready at bedside.

Other procedures for immediate airway establishment: When airway obstruction is so marked as to allow no time to do an orderly tracheostomy following measures can be taken:

1. *Endotracheal intubation:* This is the most quick method using a direct laryngoscope, laryngeal inlet is visualized and an endotracheal tube of correct size is inserted between the vocal cords, which makes patient to breath freely. No anesthesia is needed, but it is a temporary procedure. After intubation, if need is there a planned tracheostomy can be performed.
2. *Cricothyrotomy or laryngotomy:* Here, patient is made to lie on table with head and neck extended to identify lower border of thyroid cartilage and cricoid ring. The skin over here is incised vertically and then circothyroid membrane is cut with a transverse incision, which is kept open with a small tracheostomy tube or handle of small knife by turning it at right angle. This again is a temporary procedure.

Chapter 65

Disorders of Voice

The common disorders of voice encountered in ENT practice are the following:

Functional Aphonia

It is a hysterical manifestation occurring commonly in young females. Emotional crisis is the usual precipitating factor. The patient complains of sudden loss of voice though she is able to whisper, cough and cry normally. Laryngeal examination reveals normal vocal cords which are mobile but do not completely adduct on phonation. However, the cords meet in the midline on coughing.

Reassurance and persuasion will help in re-establishing the voice. Psychiatric advice may be needed. Tranquillizers are given.

Dysphonia Plicae Ventricularis (Ventricular Band Voice)

The voice in this disorder is produced by the apposition of the ventricular bands instead of the vocal cords. The voice produced is rough, harsh and unpleasant. This is regarded as a functional vocal disorder which may develop to compensate for the vocal disorder of the true cords.

Examination shows thickened ventricular bands which meet on phonation, obscuring the view of the true cords.

The condition can be helped by voice rest and speech therapy. Any organic lesion of the true cords should be ruled out.

Myasthenia of the Larynx (Phonasthenia)

Weakness of the phonatory muscles of the larynx may occur due to prolonged misuse and abuse of voice in singers and other such professionals. The thyroarytenoid and interarytenoid muscles are usually affected.

Examination shows hyperemic cords. The vocal cords do not completely approximate but leave an eliptical area in between due to weakness of the thyroarytenoid muscles.

The treatment is vocal rest, and vocal hygiene.

Mogiphonia

It is a psychoneurotic disorder in which phonic spasm occurs in professional voice users when they appear in public. Initially the voice is normal but soon the vocal cords get adducted and the person cannot speak. The treatment is vocal rest, speech therapy and the treatment of the underlying psychoneurotic problem.

Puberphonia (Mutational False to Voice)

In boys, the larynx matures at puberty as the vocal cords lengthen and voice changes from high pitch to lower pitch—normally. In emotionally immature and psychologically disturbed boys, this normal changes does not occur leading to persistence of childhood high-pitched voice. Treatment is to train the boy to produce low-pitched voice by Lustzmann's pressure test—where thyroid prominence is pressed backwards or downwards—which relaxes the overstretched cords producing lowpitched voice.

Other disorders of voice though not related to larynx are:

RHINOLALIA OPERTA OR APERTA OR HYPERNASALITY

It is due to defective closure of oropharynx from nasopharynx or abnormal communication between the oral and nasal cavities, e.g. in velopharyngeal insufficiency, cleft palate, short soft palate, wide nasopharynx, paralysis of soft palate, oronasal fistula, postadenoidectomy, habitual or familial speech pattern, etc.

RHINOLALIA CLAUSA OR HYPONASALITY

When there is absence of nasal resonance for words like syringe which normally resonate in the nasal cavity—the dull voice or "potato in mouth" voice is produced. The cause is in the nose or nasopharynx, e.g. catarrh or common cold, allergic rhinitis, polypi or growth in the nose, adenoid hypertrophy, nasopharyngeal growth and habitual or familial speech pattern.

STAMMERING OR STUTTERING

Though some children have normally dysfluency of speech between two to four years of age but children feeling psychologically insecure, or overattention of parents, imitating some stutters, may make this behavior pattern fixed. In early stage at grade I, the fluency of speech is affected and there may be hesitation to start the speech or repetition or prolongations or blocks in the flow of speech. Later stage in grade II child develops secondary mannerisms such as facial grimacing, eye blinking and abnormal movements of head, legs or arms. Stuttering is cured by speech therapy and psychotherapy, encouraging the child to speak normally without fear and tension. The parents and the teachers should be given proper education as not to overact to child's dysfluency in early stages of speech development.

Chapter

66

Tumors of the Larynx

The tumors of larynx can be benign or malignant.

Benign Tumors of the Larynx

The following are the benign tumors of the larynx:

1. Papillomas
   a. Solitary papilloma
   b. Multiple papillomas
2. Hemangioma
3. Fibroma
4. Chondroma

SOLITARY PAPILLOMA

Papilloma of the larynx is the most common benign lesion in the larynx. A solitary papilloma is common in adults, particularly in males. These usually arise from the edge of the vocal cord in the anterior part and may be pedunculated.

Indirect laryngoscopy shows a pink warty growth of varying size in the anterior commissure.

The main presenting symptom is hoarseness of voice.

Treatment

Direct laryngoscopy and excision of the papilloma is done, preferably using a microscope. The excised tissue is sent for histopathological examination as it is a premalignant condition.

MULTIPLE PAPILLOMAS OF THE LARYNX

The multiple papillomatosis of the larynx is a disease of children. The lesions subside at puberty. The etiology of this condition is not definitely known but it appears that it is of viral origin. The disease may occur in early childhood with a definite tendency for the papillomas to disappear at puberty.

Multiple papillomatous tumors appear on the vocal cords, false cords and other areas of the larynx and present with multiple problems. Not only do these tumors interfere with laryngeal function thereby causing hoarseness of voice and respiratory difficulty but because of their multiplicity, the tumors are difficult to excise. Besides, these papillomas have a tendency to recur and may spread to other areas of the larynx, trachea and bronchi causing a very frustrating situation for the laryngologist.

Treatment

Various medical modalities of therapy like antibiotics, steroids, hormones and vaccines have proved of no use. Repeated surgical excision is the treatment of choice. Microsurgical excision of the papillomas is done at repeated sessions to avoid damage and subsequent scarring. Instruments used are shown in **Figure 66.1.** Cryosurgery and laser are also used.

PRECANCEROUS CONDITIONS OF THE LARYNX

Precancerous lesions are those conditions which are not histologically malignant but for which there is satisfactory proof that cancer occurs in them with higher incidence than the corresponding normal tissues. Chronic inflammatory conditions of the larynx like chronic laryngitis give rise to lesions which may develop into malignancy. It is in such situations that hyperkeratosis, leukoplakia, carcinoma *in situ* and eventually

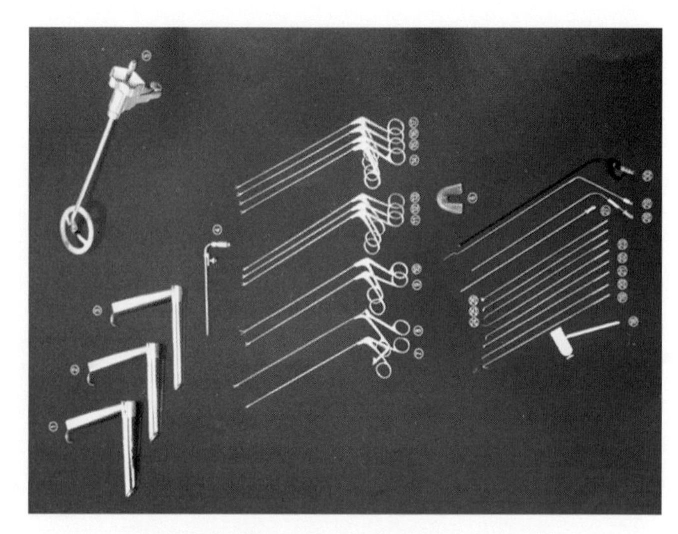

Fig. 66.1: Microsurgical laryngeal instruments

invasive carcinoma appears. Papilloma of the larynx in adults occasionally becomes malignant. Similarly, radiation burns of the larynx are sometimes known to proceed to cancer.

Malignant Tumors of the Larynx

CLASSIFICATION

Isambert (1876) and Krishaber (1879) separated tumors into two main groups:

i. Intrinsic
ii. Extrinsic

Thomson and Colledge (1930) divided them into four subdivisions.

i. Intrinsic
ii. Subglottic
iii. Extrinsic
iv. Mixed

From the pathological and therapeutic point of views, Lederman's classification of laryngeal tumors is as follows (**Figs 66.2 and 66.3**):

1. Supraglottis (**Table 66.1**)—includes the following sites:
   a. Marginal zone
      i. Posterior surface of the suprahyoid epiglottis including tip
      ii. Aryepiglottic folds
      iii. Arytenoids
   b. Supraglottis, excluding epilarynx
      i. Infrahyoid epiglottis
      ii. Ventricular bands
      iii. Ventricular cavity
2. Glottis
   a. Vocal cords
   b. Anterior commissure
   c. Posterior commissure

Table 66.1: Supraglottis

T	Primary tumor
TIS	Carcinoma *in situ*
T1	Tumor confined to the region with normal mobility
T1a	Tumor confined to one site of the region
T1b	Tumor from one site of the region extending to another site of the same region
T2	Tumor with extension to the adjacent region without fixation
T3	Tumor confined to the larynx with fixation and/or extension to involve postcricoid area, medial wall of pyriform sinus or pre-epiglottic space
T4	Tumor with direct extension beyond the larynx
Glottis	
TIS	Carcinoma *in situ*
T1	Tumor confined to vocal cord(s) with normal mobility
T2	Supra or subglottic extension of tumor with normal or impaired cord mobility
T3	Tumor confined to the larynx with cord fixation
T4	Massive tumor with thyroid cartilage destruction and/or extension beyond the confines of the larynx
Subglottis	
TIS	Carcinoma *in situ*
T1	Tumor confined to the subglottic region
T2	Tumor extension to vocal cords with normal or impaired cord mobility
T3	Tumor confined to the larynx with cord fixation
T4	Massive tumor with cartilage destruction extension beyond the confines of larynx into the soft tissues of the neck, or both
Regional lymph nodes	
NO	No evidence of lymph node involvement
N1	Movable homolateral regional nodes
N2	Movable contralateral or bilateral regional lymph nodes
N3	Fixed regional lymph nodes
M	Metastases
MO	No distant metastasis
M1	Evidence of distant metastasis

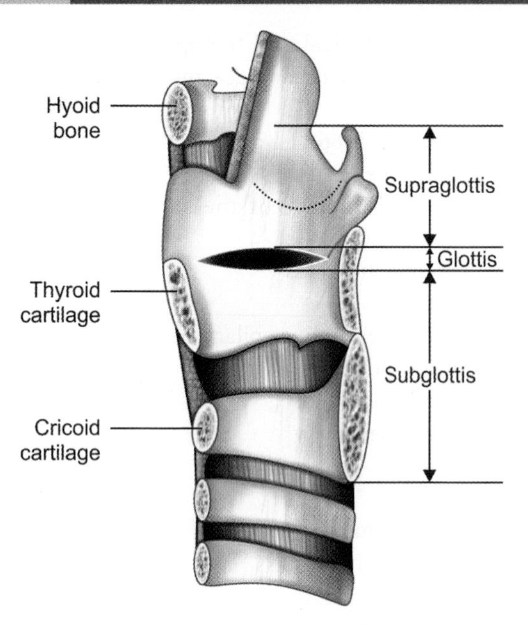

Fig. 66.2: Divisions of the larynx

3. Subglottis

The TNM classification is the universal method of classification at present.

Staging of Carcinoma Larynx

Stage I: T1 NO MO
Stage II: T2 NO MO/ TO-T2 N1 MO
Stage III: T3 NO-2 MO
T1, T2, T3, NI, MO/TO-3N2 MO
Stage IV: T4 NO-1 MO; Any T N2, N3, MO
Any T, any N, MI

Squamous cell carcinoma is the most common type of laryngeal cancer. Sarcomas are very rare.

Etiology

The exact etiology is not clear but carcinoma is relatively common in Indians. Chronic irritation by smoking, alcohol and chewing of betel nut and tobacco may be contributory factors, prolonged vocal strain plays a significant role.

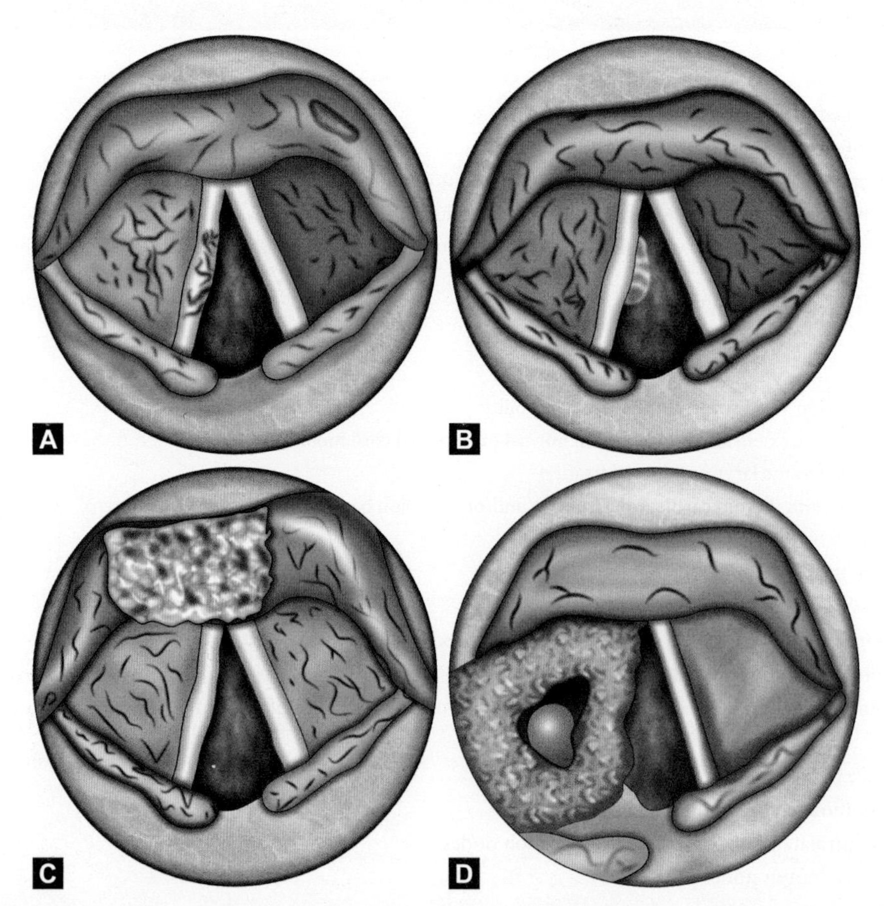

Figs 66.3A to D: Malignancy of larynx (Indirect laryngoscopy view): (A) Growth confined to right vocal cord; (B) Growth involving the free margin of right vocal and subglottis; (C) Growth involving anterior commissure, and anterior portion of vestibular folds, and epiglottis; (D) Growth right laryngopharynx

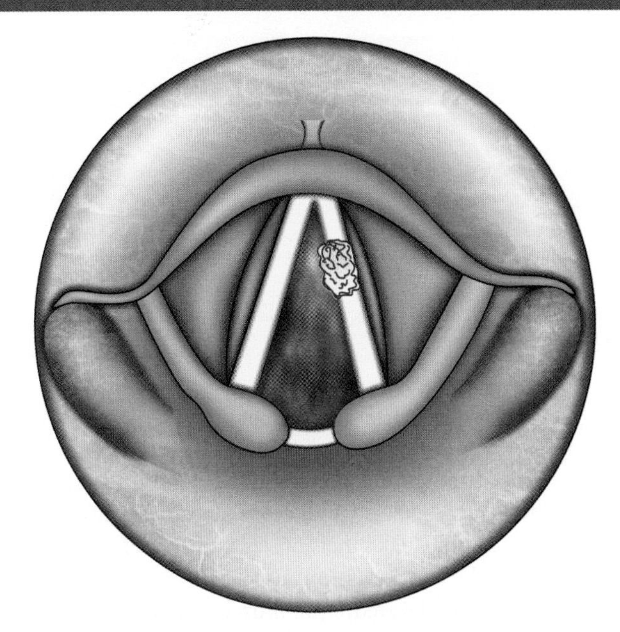

Fig. 66.4: Tumor confined to one vocal cord

Glottic cancer: It is the most common type of laryngeal neoplasm in adults. It usually arises from the free margin of the upper surface of true vocal cord in its anterior two-third (**Fig. 66.4**). The spread occurs locally along the cord to the anterior commissure and may involve the other cord. Lymph node involvement is a very rare phenomenon in glottic cancer as the vocal cords are practically devoid of lymphatics. Prognosis is excellent if the tumor is treated early.

Subglottic cancer: The subglottic region is usually involved by the downward extension of cordal growth and it is very rare that a primary starts in the subglottis itself. Subglottic cancer is difficult to diagnose, hence present very late and spread occurs to pretracheal, paratracheal and mediastinal lymph nodes making radical cure very difficult. The prognosis is bad.

Supraglottic cancer: Commonly epiglottis is the site of tumor in this region. Laryngeal ventricle and false cords are rare sites. The tumors present in the late stages. Epiglottic tumors send metastasis to both sides of the neck. Marginal zone tumors include tumors of the tip of the epiglottis and aryepiglottic folds. These carry a poor prognosis because these tumors are detected in advanced stages and gain an early access to the lymph nodes.

The spread of laryngeal cancer may occur directly to the adjacent tissues or through lymphatics to the regional lymph nodes. Rarely, spread may occur through the blood, usually to the lungs, liver and bones.

Clinical Features

The disease commonly affects elderly males. Progressive continuous hoarseness of voice is the main early symptom particularly in glottic cancer. The other symptoms include a feeling of discomfort in the throat, irritable cough particularly in supraglottic growths and hemoptysis and many times the patient presents with features of respiratory obstruction like dyspnea or stridor, dysphagia and swelling in the neck in advanced cases.

The growth may be seen on indirect laryngoscopy or fiberoptic laryngoscopy as raised nodular, papilliferous or an ulcerative lesion, with or without fixation of the cords and involvement of neck nodes.

Radiological examination includes, soft tissue X-ray and CT scan of the neck which shows extension of the lesion and involvement of cartilages, etc.

X-ray of the chest rules out the presence of secondaries and other associated pathology. CT is helpful to determine the extension of the tumor and to rule out any micronodal metastasis.

Direct laryngoscopy and biopsy determine the extent and nature of the lesion.

Treatment of Laryngeal Cancer

Ninety five percent of patients with laryngeal carcinomas are treatable. Currently two principal modalities of curative treatment are used in treating laryngeal cancer, viz. surgery and radiotherapy. The choice of treatment depends on the extent, site and histology of the tumor, presence or absence of the neck nodes and distant metastasis.

Each modality has its advantages and disadvantages. Radiotherapy preserves the larynx, so the patient retains the voice as well as the normal air passage. Surgery is the sure way of removing the disease as against radiotherapy, particularly in large growths.

Glottic growths: Tumors limited to the cords can be treated by surgery or radiotherapy. The results of both methods of treatment are the same. These types of cancers carry a better prognosis as they present early and metastasis is late.

Radiotherapy is the treatment of choice for cordal cancer because laryngeal functions are preserved with equal chances of cure.

Subglottic cancer: Surgery followed by radiotherapy is the treatment of choice. Total laryngectomy with or without neck dissection of lymph nodes is performed. Since, there is a chance of the disease having spread to the mediastinum, hence, postoperative radiotherapy is given to the neck fields and superior mediastinum.

Supraglottic cancer: Growths limited to the supraglottic region are either treated by *supraglottic laryngectomy* or by radiotherapy. Surgery, if planned, may or may not be associated with neck dissection of the lymph nodes.

Transglottic growth: Those growths which extend through the glottis to the other regions are usually dealt with by total laryngectomy. Neck dissection is done if the nodes are palpable.

Chemotherapy may play an adjuvant role in addition to radiotherapy and may be of some help in inoperable cases.

Partial CO_2 Laser Cordectomy

Partial CO_2 laser cordectomy is an excellent option for the treatment of TI squamous cell carcinomas involving one vocal fold when the following criteria are met: (i) adequate endoscopic exposure of the entire lesion and (ii) absence of *anterior commissure*, vocal process, ventricular or subglottic involvement. Using these criteria cure rates are equivalent to those reported with radiation therapy.

Total Cordectomy

Total cordectomy is another form of surgical therapy for early glottic cancer. It includes the entire vocal fold from the vocal process of the arytenoid to the anterior commissure, with the depth of resection down to the thyroid perichondrium. No thyroid cartilage is removed in this procedure. Cordectomy can be performed either endoscopically or through a laryngofissure. The indications for this procedure can be extended to T2 carcinoma of the glottis.

Hemilaryngectomy

A vertical hermilaryngectomy removes half of the larynx, including the ipsilateral thyroid ala, arytenoid, true vocal fold, and often the false vocal fold. Frequently, a neoglottis is constructed with strap muscle or a local mucosal flap to compensate for the resected tissue.

Extended Partial Laryngectomies

Various types of extended partial laryngectomies have been designed as alternative to the standard total laryngectomy when oncologically safe. Their presumed advantage lies in improved speech without the need for a prosthesis.

TOTAL LARYNGECTOMY

The patient should be meticulously assessed before operation. He should be made to understand what sort of life he will have after laryngectomy as he is going to lose his voice and will have a permanent tracheostomy.

Procedure

1. There should be no focus of infection in the nose, paranasal sinuses or in the oral cavity.
2. General condition of the patient should be fairly good.
3. Preliminary tracheostomy is done before undertaking laryngectomy.

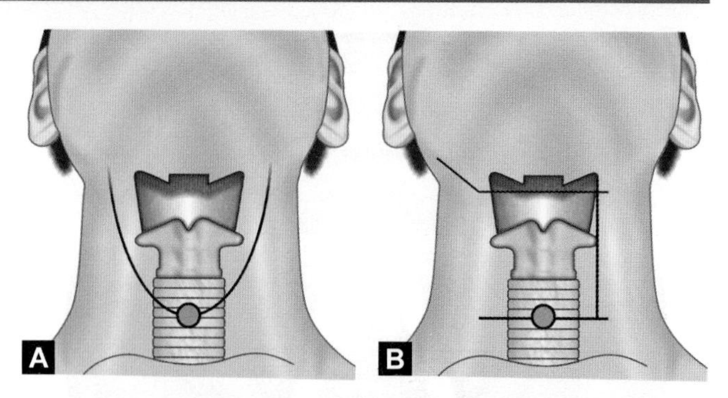

Figs 66.5A and B: (A) Sorenson's; (B) Gluck's incision for total laryngectomy

4. The procedure should preferably be done under general anesthesia, can be done under local anesthesia also.
5. Sorenson's and Gluck's incisions as shown in **Figures 66.5A and B**, are the usual incisions used.
6. The skin flap is elevated, strap muscles cut, larynx exposed, suprahyoid attachments cut, thyroid isthmus transected in the middle exposing the trachea, pyriform mucosa elevated from the inner aspect of thyroid laminae and then the larynx is removed either from above downwards or from below upwards.
7. The pharynx is closed in layers after passing the Ryle's tube.
8. Trachea is connected with the skin creating a permanent tracheostomy.
9. The skin is closed after keeping the corrugated rubber drains.

Postoperative Care

1. Care of the tracheostomy tube with proper suction is important.
2. Vital signs, viz. pulse, BP and respiration must be monitored.
3. The patient should be encouraged to sit and to cough, so as to prevent pulmonary complications.
4. He should be put on heavy antibiotics and IV fluids.
5. Daily dressings should be done to keep the wound healthy. Stitches should be removed on the seventh to the tenth day.

COMPLICATIONS

The following are the complications of laryngectomy:

1. Cardiac arrest
2. Hemorrhage
3. Pulmonary embolism
4. Pulmonary complications like bronchopneumonia, and atelectasis, etc.
5. Pharyngocutaneous fistula.

After laryngectomy the patient can be trained to speak by esophageal speech, use of electronic larynx or by surgical procedures aimed at constructing the "neoglottis".

Organ Preservation Therapy

In this study, laryngeal preservation was attained in 64 percent of the patients who received induction chemotherapy followed by radiation therapy. To date, the quality of the speech in these organ preservation protocol patients has been evaluated adequately.

Alaryngeal Communication

There are three major methods of communication used by patients after undergoing a total laryngectomy: artificial larynx, esophageal speech, and TE speech. They all possess various advantages and disadvantages, and it is clear that the optimal method of alaryngeal speech has yet to be developed.

Voice rehabilitation after total laryngectomy: It is important to make patient to converse to make his day-to-day life purposeful. Following methods are being used and tried:

a. *Esophageal speech*: Patient is taught to swallow air which is held in upper esophagus and then slowly ejected from esophagus to pharynx. These patients when trained can speak about 8 to 10 words by reswallowing air, voice is loud but rough.
b. *Artificial larynx:* In patients who cannot learn esophageal speech following devices are used to make them speak.
   i. *Electrolarynx*: It is a small transistorized, battery operated device having a vibrating disk which is held against the soft tissue of neck and a low pitched sound is produced in the hypopharynx which is further modified into speech by the tongue, teeth, palate and lips.
   ii. *Transoral pneumatic device*: Another type of artificial larynx is a transoral device. Here, vibrations produced in a rubber diaphragm are carried by a plastic tube into the back of oral cavity where sound is converted into speech by modulators. This is a pneumatic type of device and uses expired air from the tracheostome to vibrate the diaphragm.
   iii. *Tracheo/Esophageal speech:* Here, attempt is made to carry air from trachea to esophagus or hypopharynx by the creation of a skin lined fistula or putting an artificial prosthesis. The vibrating column of air entering the pharynx is then modulated into speech. This technique has the disadvantage of food entering the trachea. These days prostheses are being used to shunt air from trachea to esophagus. They have inbuilt valves which work only in one direction, thus preventing problems of aspiration.

Phonosurgery

Phonosurgery is undertaken in order to restore or retain the function of phonation.

There are multiple procedures designed to improve the voice (phonation) in different conditions which affect the proper voice production (phonation).

These procedures may be:

i. Microlaryngeal procedures for excision of benign or malignant disease.
ii. Vocal cord injection for augmentation and medialization.
iii. Laryngeal framework surgery which is further classified into four types of surgical procedures based on functional alteration of vocal cords:
   a. Medial displacement
   b. Lateral displacement
   c. Shortening or relaxation
   d. Elongation or tensioning procedures.
iv. Laryngeal reinnervation procedures, and
v. Reconstructive and rehabilitative procedures after tumor resection.

The microlaryngeal procedures have already been discussed.

PATIENT EVALUATION AND SELECTION

Degree of impairment may be determined by:

i. Subjective criteria based on the patient's symptoms, e.g. breathiness, aspiration or exertional intolerance.
ii. Objective criteria obtained through various tests like:
   a. Mean or maximum phonation time.
   b. Spectrographic analysis, measurement of fundamental frequency.
   c. Measurement of phonatory airflow, e.g. directly by pneumotachography or indirectly by using hot wire anemometry.
iii. *Videostroboscopy* is the most useful objective test, for preoperative and postoperative evaluation of patients with unilateral vocal cord impairment.
iv. Electromyography is a valuable test for evaluating the integrity of laryngeal innervation in the presence of vocal cord motion impairment.

VOCAL CORD AUGMENTATION OR MEDIALIZATION

Transoral Injection

Transoral injection may be performed in selected patients. Topical 4 percent lidocaine solution is applied to the pharyngeal mucosa. With the patient holding the tongue forward, allowing indirect visualization, the injection is performed using a curved laryngeal needle. Right and left needles are available so that the bevel is directed away from the midline to minimise the possibility of an intramucosal injection.

Laryngoscopic Injection

Ideally, the procedure is performed under local anesthesia to monitor the changes in vocal quality during injection. When local anesthesia is inadequate, the injection may be performed under general anesthesia with jet ventilation using the Sanders device, avoiding the use of an endotracheal tube. Superior laryngeal nerve blocks with lidocaine should be avoided, as they will alter vocal cord tension due to cricothyroid muscle paralysis and adversely affect voice quality.

First cord is lateralized exposing the ventricle, the laryngeal needle is inserted lateral to the vocal cord 2 mm deep.

Teflon or Gelfoam paste is injected at single click interval. It is must to wait after each click as there is continued extension of material for several seconds. A second injection is made lateral to vocal cord at the junction of anterior and middle thirds. After injection a spatula is used to massage the vocal cord to distribute the material more evenly. The laryngoscope is relaxed and patient asked to phonate. There are some complications of vocal cord injections like:

i. Excessive and incorrect placement of injected material.
ii. Inspiration with obstruction.
iii. Phonation with vocal cord overlap.
iv. Teflon granuloma.

Percutaneous medialization by injection should be considered in patient with short life expectancy and aspiration or severe dysphonia.

Vocal Cord Medialization by Injection

The use of injectable material for vocal cord medialization remains a standard procedure for laryngeal rehabilitation. In the absence of arytenoid ankylosis and when adequate residual vocal cord structure remains to allow needle placement for augmentation, medialization of a paralyzed vocal cord by injection using Gelfoam or Teflon. Recently transoral and percutaneous approaches have added a new. In selected patients, medialization can be accomplished quickly and effectively in the office setting. These procedures are relatively simple and yield immediate results with little discomfort to the patient.

When vocal cord paralysis has been found to be permanent, Teflon may be used to medialize the vocal cord. If recovery of vocal cord function is likely, Teflon is contraindicated and alternative methods must be considered. Gelfoam may be used as a temporizing measure in this setting. The use of Gelfoam injection as a trial before Teflon injection should be discouraged, as this will result in redundant surgical procedures. Percutaneous injections may be performed without sedation using local anesthesia alone. Flexible fiberoptic laryngoscope is required to visualize position and adequacy of injection, given their advantage and ease of performance, percutaneous injections are becoming the airway management is a potential problem, injection in a controlled setting during direct laryngoscopy should be considered.

A distinction should also be made between vocal cord medialization and intrachordal injection. With injection for medialization, the material is injected lateral to the vocal muscle leaving the mucosa overlying the vocal cord unaltered.

MEDIALIZATION THYROPLASTY

It has been introduced in 1915 by Payr:

1. It is performed with local anesthesia with minimal or no discomfort to the patient.
2. Patient positioning is more anatomic, allowing better assessment of voice during the procedure.
3. It is potentially reversible, and
4. Because the prosthesis is placed lateral to the inner perichondrium of the thyroid lamina, structural integrity of the vocal cord is preserved, allowing medialisation in the presence of a mobile vocal cord.

Disadvantages include the following:

1. The patient is subjected to an open procedure,
2. The procedure is technically more difficult, and
3. Intubation for surgery subsequent to medialization may result in displacement of the prosthesis or mucosal erosion secondary to endotracheal tube pressure.

Medialization thyroplasty is currently applicable for management of vocal cord paralysis, vocal cord bowing resulting from aging or cricothyroid joint fixation, sulcus vocalis, and soft tissue defects resulting from excision of pathologic tissue. Treatment for paralytic dysphonia is indicated when the likelihood of recovery is negligible.

When recovery is anticipated, medialization thyroplasty may be considered for management of aspiration or severe dysphonia as an alterative to repeated injections with Gelfoam. Generally, dysphonia by itself should be managed conservatively if recovery is anticipated.

TECHNIQUE

Medialization is performed through a window in the thyroid lamina at the level of the vocal cord. The inner perichondrium should remain intact. Factors that affect outcome include size and shape of the implant, position of the implant, maintaining proper position of the implant, and limiting the duration of the surgical procedure.

With the patient in the supine position and prepared for a sterile procedure, a paramedian horizontal incision is outlined over the middle aspect of the thyroid lamina. Local anesthesia is administered subcutaneously and in four quadrants over the ipsilateral lamina. A 5 to 6 cm incision is made through the platysma. Superior and inferior flaps are elevated in the subplatysmal plane exposing the thyroid notch and inferior border of the thyroid cartilage. The strap muscles are split in the midline and retracted laterally off the thyroid lamina, leaving the outer perichondrium intact. A single large skin hook is implanted in the anterosuperior aspect of the contralateral ala and retracted laterally, providing exposure of the ipsilateral lamina. The perichondrium is scored with electrocautery applied to a window template placed 8 mm posterior to the ventral midline with the superior edge at the level of the vocal cord. The outer perichondrium is incised and elevated off the window. Cartilage and osteoid material are removed precisely from the rectangle. Where ossification has occurred, the window may be drilled out or removed with a Kerrison punch. Regardless, care must be taken to preserve the inner perichondrium, which is now elevated in circumferential fashion off the thyroid lamina using a # 4 penfield elevator. One of four sizing prosthesis templates (3 to 6 mm) is inserted through the window and rotated 90 degree with the bevel directed inferiorly. All retractors are removed and the patient asked to phonate while moving the template through all four quadrants of the window to determine the optimal position. Smaller or larger templates may be selected as needed. Once the appropriate size and position have been determined, the retractors are replaced and the implant is inserted and secured with the corresponding shim.

If the window is fashioned correctly, the shim will fit securely preventing migration of the implant. The wound is then litigated with antibiotic solution. A one-fourth penrose drain is placed deep to the strap muscles and brought out through the incision. Strap muscles and platysma are approximated with 4-0 chronic suture and skin is closed with a running 4-0 nylon suture. A dry fluff compression dressing is applied for 24 hours, at which time the penrose is removed. Decadron is given preoperatively to minimize edema and prophylactic.

It is better to use the largest prosthesis possible while maintaining quality of voice. Overmedialization is supported by Isshiki et al (1989), who found deterioration in voice quality overtime as intraoperative edema resolved in the postoperative period. Where early medialization is performed, muscle atrophy may also result in voice deterioration postoperatively. Minimizing operative time is critical in obtaining optimal results. Fabricating implants before the procedure and rapid determination of size and position will facilitate the procedure.

Complication associated with type I thyroplasty include:

i. Penetration of the endolaryngeal mucosa, wound injection.
ii. Chondritis
iii. Implant migration or extrusion, and
iv. *Airway obstruction:* Airway compromise is a potential problem require in patient observation for a minimum of 24 hours.

MANAGEMENT OF BILATERAL VOCAL CORD MOVEMENT IMPAIRMENT WITH AIRWAY OBSTRUCTION

The least invasive of the lateralizing procedures involves endoscopic surgery. An arytenoidectomy may be performed through the laryngoscope. Lateralization of the vocal cord by suture placement is an alternative procedure. The laser has been suggested as a method for excising a portion of the vocal cord. Although this method has proved successful in removing the anterior two-thirds of the vocal cord, the posterior third represented by the arytenoid is more difficult to remove successfully with the CO_2 laser.

ELEVATE PITCH

Lengthening the vocal cord and elevating vocal pitch may be achieved by advancing the anterior commissure or by cricothyroid approximation lengthening procedures have been advocated for vocal cord bowing resulting from aging or trauma, postsurgical defects, androphonia, and gender transformation. An alternative approach to elevate pitch is to decrease vocal cord mass, thereby increasing the frequency of vibratory cycle. Decreased vocal cord mass may be achieved by removing tissue with the CO_2 laser or by mechanically inactivating the vocal muscle. Other techniques designed to decrease mass, including vocal cord stripping, laser vaporization, and steroid injection, are less well controlled and may potentially result in deterioration of vocal quality.

LENGTHENING PROCEDURES

Expansion of the thyroid ala. Alar expansion to elevate pitch was first described by Isshiki et al (1977, 1983). Unilateral alar expansion is performed by the junction of the anterior and middle one-third of the thyroid ala. A silastic strip implant is secured between the edges. Greater pitch elevation may be achieved with bilateral alar expansion, and if indicated, simultaneous medialization may be performed.

ANTERIOR COMMISSURE ADVANCEMENT: LEJEUNE PROCEDURE

Advancement of the anterior commissure was first described by Lejeune et al (1983) using an inferiorly based cartilaginous flap. Tucker (1985) modified this procedure using a superiorly based flap that allows greater advancement of the anterior commissure. A silastic or tantalum shim is used to maintain position of the flap. Anterior commissure advancement may also be combined with a medialization procedure by developing a pocket between the inner perichondrium and thyroid lamina via the anterior cartilage incisions.

The anterior flap technique is simpler in design and results in a more direct pull on the vocal cord than alar expansion.

CRICOTHYROID APPROXIMATION

Surgical approximation of the cricoid and thyroid cartilage to simulate contraction of the cricothyroid muscle was first described by Isshiki et al (1974). Four nonabsorbable mattress sutures are placed, first through the cricoid cartilage and then through the thyroid cartilage. Sutures should be placed anteriorly, 3 to 4 mm off midline, parallel to the rectus division of the cricothyroid muscle. Silastic or cartilage bolsters are used to distribute pressure over the thyroid lamina as the sutures are gradually tightened, alternating right and left while an assistant approximates the cricoid and thyroid cartilages. Maximum closure should be obtained, as some relaxation generally occurs postoperatively.

REINNERVATION PROCEDURES

The details of the reinnervation surgical technique are described by Tucker (1977). In the absence of ankylosis determined by direct laryngoscopy or history, and when spontaneous recovery is not anticipated, reinnervation may be attempted under local or general anesthesia, horizontal incision is made at the lower half of the thyroid lamina extending from the anterior midline posteriorly to the sternocleidomastoid muscle. The jugular vein and omohyoid muscle are exposed while the ansa hypoglossus and nerve branches to the anterior belly of the omohyoid muscle are identified. The nerve is carefully dissected to the muscle insertion site. The nerve typically several millimeters between muscle fibers before reaching the motor end plate region. Two stay sutures are placed adjacent to the insertion site and a block of muscle is removed, 2 to 3 mm per side. A posterior-based perichondrial flap is elevated and an inferior window created below the level of the vocal cord. It is possible to use the same window created for the type I thyroplasty; however, the inner perichondrium must be opened and the thyroarytenoid muscle incised superficially. The muscle pedicle is sutured in place using the previously placed stay sutures.

RECONSTRUCTION AND REHABILITATIVE PROCEDURES AFTER LARYNGECTOMY

Since most of the patients who have a total laryngectomy are elderly their motivation to attend speech therapy classes and practice esophagus speech is very low, hence neoglottis operations are performed for them initially a fistula used to be made between trachea and esophagus. Later different tubes were made in the form of tunnels from the base of tongue to the trachea or between the trachea and esophagus. The aim was to allow air to go up but to prevent fluid coming down other external devices like electric larynx were used to produce speech.

In the process of neoglottis formation Blom-Singer valve and Panje valve gave some promising results.

OPERATIVE PROCEDURE

A preliminary low tracheostomy is performed since a good length of supratracheostomal trachea is required for constructing the neoepiglottis from its posterior wall. A routine total or Kitamuras supracricoid laryngectomy (1970) with or without radical neck dissection is carried out leaving a long trachea above the tracheostome.

The trachea is separated from the esophagus by blunt and sharp dissections for about 4 cm taking care not to perforate through the posterior membranous wall of trachea. In that case neoepiglottis cannot be constructed. The trachea is retracted anteriorly and a tongue-shaped flap of the full thickness of the posterior tracheal wall is raised basing superiorly about 1.5 cm inferior to the upper cut margin of the trachea. This is the future neoepiglottis. The base is about 1.5 cm and height of the flap is 1.5 cm. The inferior margin is rounded. An endotracheal tube is fenestrated passed through the cricopharyngeal ring into the esophagus with the fenestra looking forward. A transverse incision of 1.5 cm is made on the fenestra through the anterior wall of the base of the neoepiglottis. The tube protects the posterior esophageal wall from possible injury by the knife. Two anchoring silk stitches are applied to the anterior esophageal wall, just lateral to the ends of the transverse incision. Another anchoring stitch is applied to the lower end of the neoepiglottis in order to facilitate its introduction into the esophagus through the transverse cut. A small cartilage bar (1 cm long and 2–3 mm thick) is cut out from the uninvolved thyroid ala and is placed transversely on the anterior esophageal wall just below the transverse cut. The esophageal mucosa is everted and brought down over the bar and stitched to the raw anterior esophageal wall with 4-0 vicryl, thus completely submerging the bar. The semirigid lower margin of the transverse cut with its mucosa-lined cartilage bar is meant to work as the vocal cord. A long artery forceps is introduced through the cricopharyngeal sphincter into the esophagus and the tip is shown at the transverse cut. The anchoring thread of the neoepiglottis is introduced through the transverse cut and is caught by the artery forceps placed in the esophagus while the assistant gently pulls the esophageal anchoring silks superiorly, laterally and anteriorly to stabilize the anterior esophageal wall in order to facilitate the introduction of the neoepiglottis into the esophageal lumen. The forceps in the esophagus is pushed downwards thus taking along with it the neoepiglottis through the transverse cut into the esophagus. While doing this maneuver, the trachea is pushed backwards and held in apposition with the anterior esophagus and thus the tracheal fenestra, resulting from raising the neoepiglottis, is closed by the anterior esophageal wall. The adjacent tracheal and esophageal walls are stitched to each other with 2-0 vicryl in order to prevent relative movements between the trachea and esophagus. The anchoring stitches and the forceps are removed. A rectangular silastic sheet (5 cm by 1.5 cm) is introduced through the neoglottis, situated between the mucosal surface of the neoepiglottis and the mucosa lined inferior margin of the transverse cut, into the esophagus from the tracheal aspect and left *in situ* for 3 weeks and anchored by a silk stitch to its tracheal end and brought out through the tracheostome and secured to the skin of the neck with an adhesive tape. After 3 weeks the sheet is removed by pulling on the thread. This is meant to prevent possible adhesions and stenosis of the neoglottis. Two wedges are removed from the lateral upper cut margin of the trachea is closed 2-0 vicryl stitches. So, the tracheal lumen ends in a cul-de-sac at its upper end. The pharynx and the skin wounds are closed in the usual way after inserting a nasogastric feeding tube and Redevac drainage. The patient is put on antibiotics and metronidazole for 2 weeks. Oral feeds are started on the tenth day after test feed. The silastic sheet is removed after three weeks. A fenestrated plastic or metal tracheostomy tube, preferably with a speaking valve, is inserted and the patient is asked to phonate closing the tracheostomy tube with his finger (if it is an ordinary tube) and he does it immediately. The phonetic steam, being bstructed by the upper end of the cul-de-sac, passes through the neoglottis into the oesophagus and upwards through the pharynx and the oral cavity for articulation. He is advised to talk, talk and talk which would keep the neoglottis patent.

Chapter 67

Block Dissection of the Neck

Many carcinomas of the head and neck sooner or later metastasize to the lymph nodes of the neck which form a barrier that prevents further spread of the disease for many months. The standard operation for dealing with metastatic glands in the neck is that of radical neck dissection described by Crile in 1906. In this operation, the different groups of deep cervical lymph nodes, internal jugular vein, sternocleidomastoid muscle, submandibular gland, tail of the parotid and the accessory nerve are removed en bloc with the primary tumor, if possible. Hence, the operation is also called block dissection of the neck. The block neck dissection is elective when no palpably enlarged lymph nodes are present, definitive or therapeutic when enlarged lymph nodes are present, and functional when the sternocleidomastoid muscle and internal jugular vein are preserved.

American Academic Committee for head and neck surgery and oncology has adopted the following classification for various neck dissections:

1. Radical neck dissection
2. Modified radical neck dissection
3. Selective neck dissection
4. Extended radical neck dissection.

Radical Neck Dissection

It consists of removal of all lymph node groups (level I-V) and all three nonlymphatic structures (spinal accessory nerve, sternocleidomastoid muscle and internal jugular vein).

Modified Radical Dissection

It consists of removal of all lymph node groups with preservation of one or more nonlymphatic structures. In type 1, the spinal accessory nerve is preserved. In type II, the spinal accessory and the IJV are preserved and in type III, all the three structures are preserved and this is known as functional neck dissection.

Selective Neck Dissection

It consists of preservation of one or more lymph node groups and all three nonlymphatic structures. The dissections are named according to the lymph node group removed.

Extended Radical Neck Dissection

It consists of removal of all the structures resected in radical neck dissection and one or more additional lymph node groups (levels VI orVII)or nonlymphatic structures. Neck dissection may be extended to remove paratracheal, pretracheal and retropharyngeal nodes and other nonlymphatic structures like hypoglossal nerve, levator scapulae muscles or carotid artery.

INDICATIONS

Block dissection of the neck is indicated in the following:

1. When the tumor has extended to lymph nodes of the neck.
2. In a patient of head and neck cancer with no apparent involvement of the neck nodes but who is unlikely to return for follow-up and has a tumor with a known high incidence of neck node metastasis.
3. When there is reasonable expectation of controlling the primary tumor.

CONTRAINDICATIONS

1. A mass in the subclavian triangle.
2. A large fixed mass.
3. Primary lesion which cannot be removed and controlled.
4. Distant uncontrollable metastasis.
5. Poor general condition of the patient.

INCISION

Various incisions used for block dissection of the neck are shown in **Figures 67.1A to G**. The structures that are preserved after a radical neck dissection are shown in **Figure 67.2**.

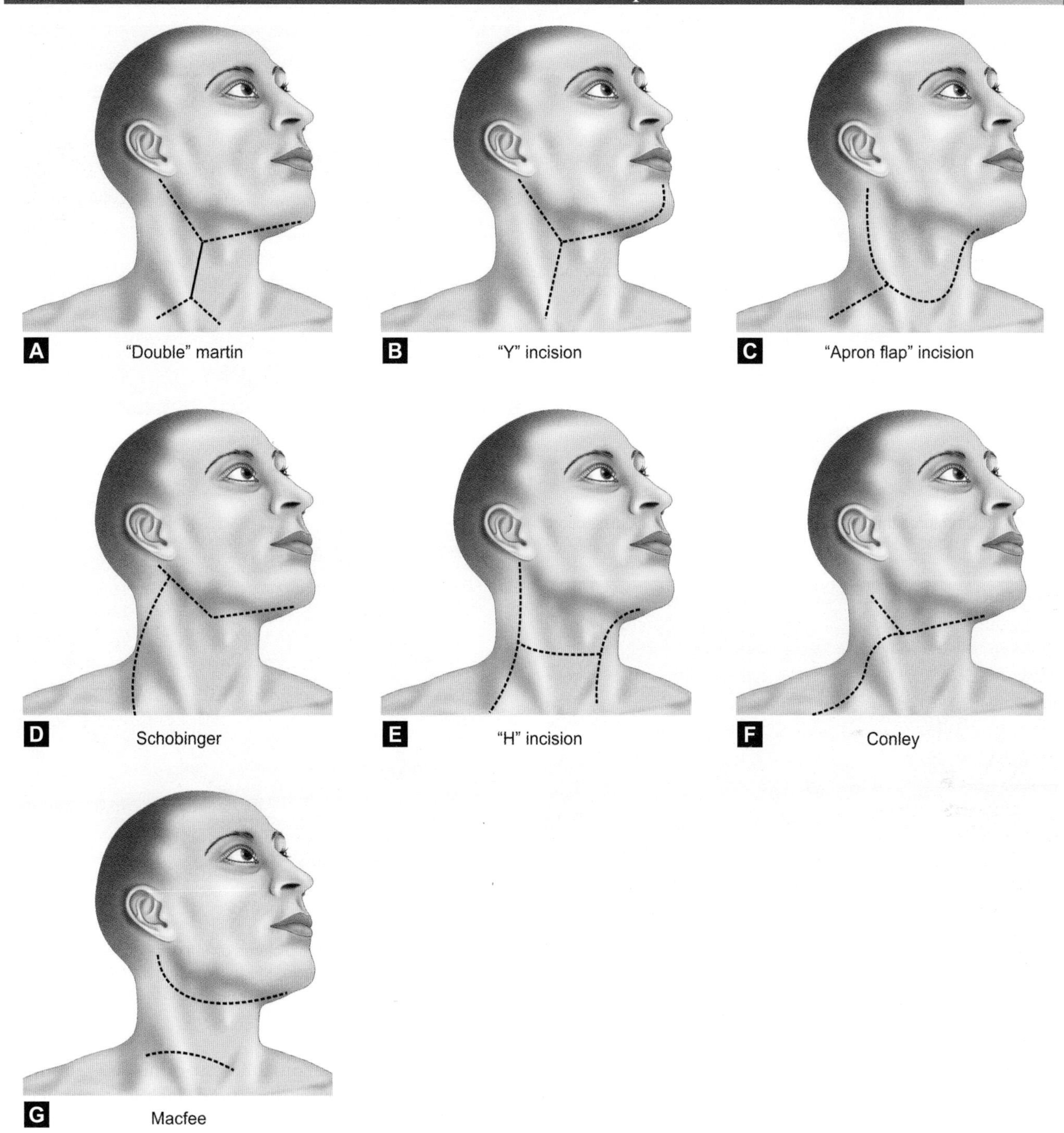

Figs 67.1A to G: Various incisions used for block dissection of neck

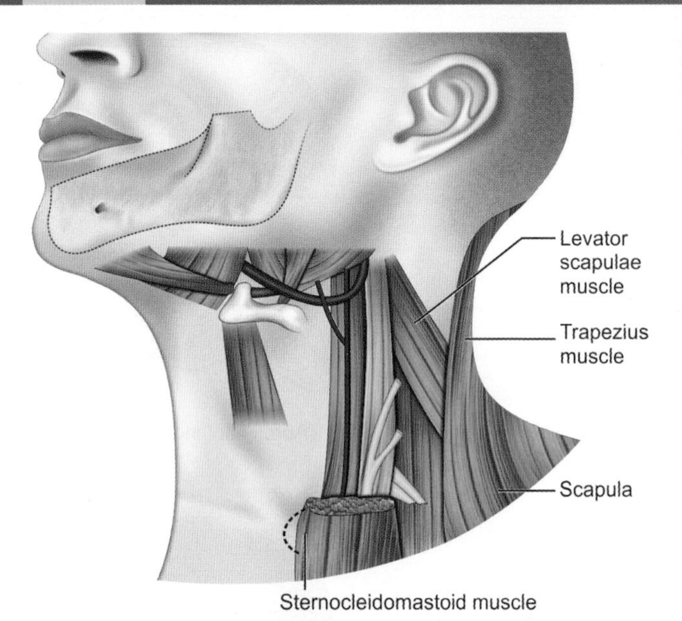

Fig. 67.2: Structures that are preserved after radical neck dissection

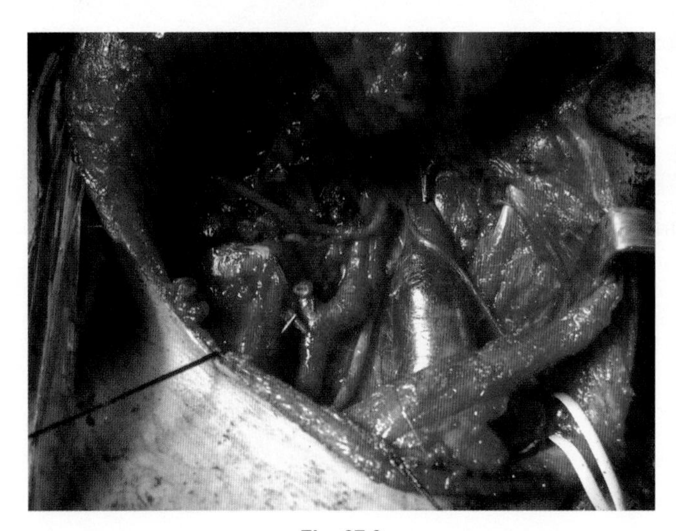

Fig. 67.3

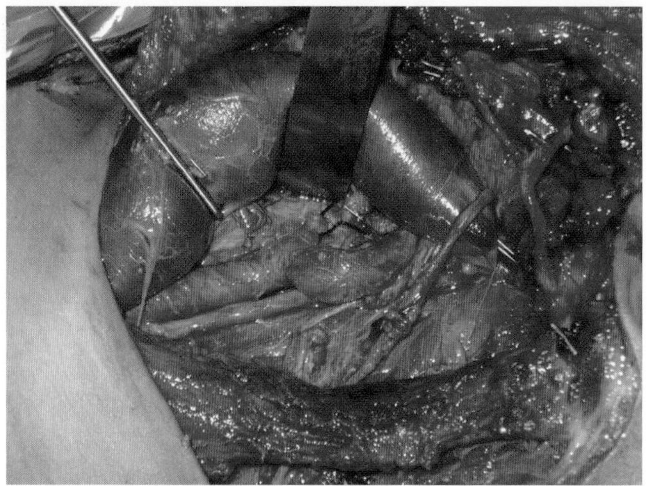

Fig. 67.4

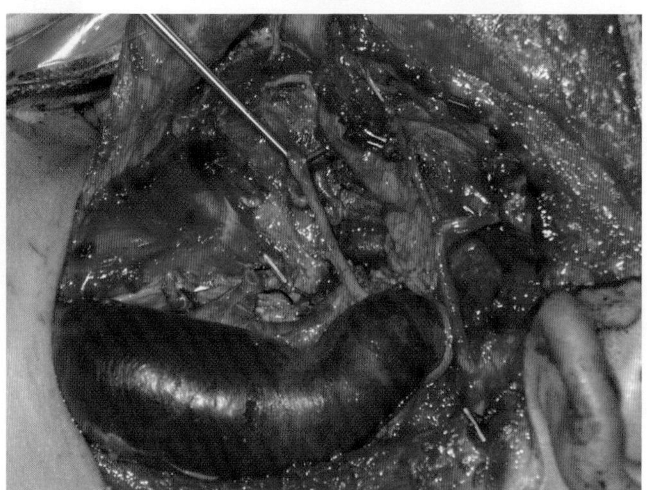

Fig. 67.5

Figs 67.3 to 5: Intraoperative pictures of left neck dissection showing the sternocleidomastoid muscle, the external jugular vein, the carotid artery and its bifurcation, the accessory nerve and the hypoglossal nerve

COMPLICATIONS

1. *Hemorrhage:* From the upper or lower end of the internal jugular vein, subclavian vein or carotid artery can be a serious problem during the operation, while subcutaneous hematomas may form in the postoperative period.
2. *Airway problems*: Kinking of the endotracheal tube, pneumothorax or postoperative laryngeal edema in cases of bilateral neck dissection may be the cause of respiratory embarrassment.
3. Air embolism
4. *Nerve damage*: The spinal accessory nerve is routinely sacrificed in radical neck dissection. This leads to postoperative shoulder drop and pain in that region. The nerves which may be damaged during dissection are the superior laryngeal nerve, vagus, facial, lingual, hypoglossal and phrenic nerves, brachial plexus and cervical sympathetics.
5. A chylous fistula may form due to thoracic duct injury.
6. Wound infection and gangrene of the skin flap are the other complications that can occur.

Chapter 68

Thyroid

The thyroid gland mainly develops from the median bud of the pharynx (thyroglossal duct) which passes from the foramen cecum at the base of the tongue to the isthmus of the thyroid gland. A lateral bud from the fourth pharyngeal pouch of each side amalgamates with it and completes the corresponding lateral lobe.

Enlargement of Thyroid Gland

ETIOLOGY

1. Nontoxic (simple)
   a. Physiological
      i. Puberty
      ii. Pregnancy
      iii. Menopause
   b. Nodular colloid
      i. Multiple endemic
      ii. Solitary sporadic
      iii. Adenoma
2. Toxic
   a. Primary
   b. Secondary to nodular
3. Struma lymphomatosa (Hashimoto's disease)
4. Lymphadenoid
5. Inflammatory.
6. Malignant disease
   a. Carcinoma
   b. Reticulosarcoma
   c. Secondary neoplasms

Nodular Goiter

It can be sporadic or endemic.

ETIOLOGY

1. Iodine deficiency
2. *Goitrogens:* If the iodine intake level falls to a critical level, the addition of one of the goitrogens can cause thyroid enlargement, e.g. calcium excess, fluoride excess, and water pollution.

PATHOLOGY

Endemic goiter passes through a stage of diffuse epithelial hyperplasia followed by involution and the formation of a colloid goiter. Recurring cycles of hyperplasia and involution continue and unequal responses by different portions of the gland result in gross nodularity. The nodules though circumscribed by delicate capsule, are difficult or impossible to enucleate. Later most of the nodules form cysts filled with brown, green or black watery fluid or jelly-like material. Cholesterol crystals are present and in some cases fibrous tissue overgrows and later on calcification occurs.

CLINICAL FEATURES

In severe endemic areas, by the age of 6 years, about 20 percent boys and 30 percent girls present a visible and palpable smooth, soft enlargement of the thyroid gland (**Fig. 68.1**). It may regress or disappear in some while in others it becomes multinodular by 30 years of age.

COMPLICATIONS

1. Pressure upon the trachea—dyspnea, tracheal shift
2. Secondary thyrotoxicosis—iodine basedown
3. Malignancy—in 8 percent cases.

TREATMENT

Partial thyroidectomy is the treatment of choice.

Retrosternal Goiter

This is mostly acquired though a few cases are congenital in origin. It is of the following varieties:

1. *Substernal:* There is a prolongation of a cervical goiter downwards behind the sternum.

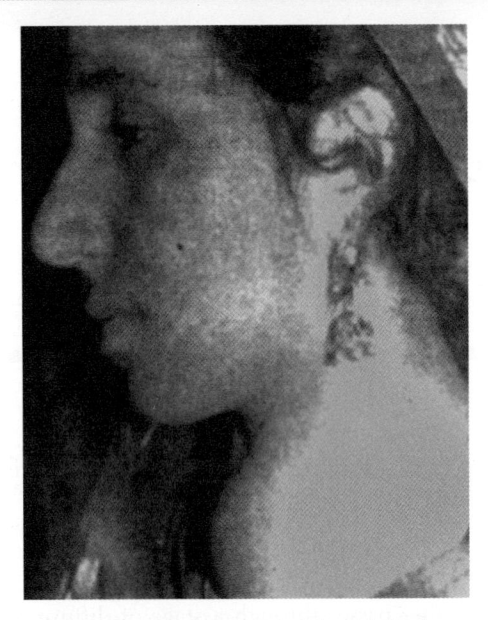
Fig. 68.1: Enlargement of thyroid gland

2. *Intrathoracic:* The whole thyroid is situated within the thorax between the great veins and resting upon the aorta.
3. *Plunging goiter:* The thyroid is wholly intrathoracic but from time to time it is forced into the neck by raised intrathoracic pressure due to coughing.

Hashimoto's Thyroiditis

It occurs mostly in women at menopause. The glands feels like Indian rubber and may be tender.

TREATMENT

Dessicated thyroid, 3 doses (200 mgm) daily causes regression or L-thyroxine is used.

Thyroid Neoplasms

Thyroid cancer is uncommon and the most common way for it to present is as a solitary thyroid nodule. Thyroid nodules are more common in women and increase in frequency with age. The female to male ratio for malignant tumors of thyroid gland is about 2.5:1. Fine needle aspiration cytology is an important investigation for many of these patients and further evaluation and subsequent treatment usually involves assessment by head and neck surgeon, a clinical oncologist and an endocrinologist.

HISTOPATHOLOGICAL TYPES OF THYROID TUMOR

Solitary non-functioning nodules of the thyroid gland are either cystic or solid, and the latter are either benign adenomas or cancers. From 10 to 20 percent of non-functioning solid nodules will prove to be malignant. The thyroid may less commonly be involved by direct spread of cancers from adjacent organs or very rarely through hematogenous spread from a distant malignant lesion.

Benign enlargement of the thyroid gland is common. Colloid and adenomatous goiters, characterized by multiple nodules of varying size and consistency, are the types most often encountered. Microscopically, they contain nodules of various sizes with flattened follicular epithelium.

The adenoma is the most common benign thyroid neoplasm. This usually presents as a solitary thyroid nodule or as a dominant nodule in a multinodular goiter (**Fig. 68.2**). Adenomas are most common in middle-aged females, are not pre-malignant and rarely become toxic, but may function and become autonomous. These are capsulated and the microscopic patterns include follicular, microfollicular, hurthle cell and embryonal. Teratomas have been reported in infants.

Malignant tumors of the thyroid gland can originate from any of the cellular components of the gland, follicular and parafollicular cells, lymphoid cells and stromal cells. The vast majority, however arise from follicular cells, and other types are rare. Follicular cell neoplasms can be classified into three major categories: papillary, follicular and anaplastic. The only known neoplasm of parafollicular cell origin is the medullary carcinoma. Malignant lymphomas are uncommon, usually arising from a lymphocytic thyroiditis and sarcomas are very rare. Only a few cases of squamous cell carcinoma of the thyroid have been described. Much more common is direct spread by continuity and contiguity from carcinomas of either the larynx or postcricoid region.

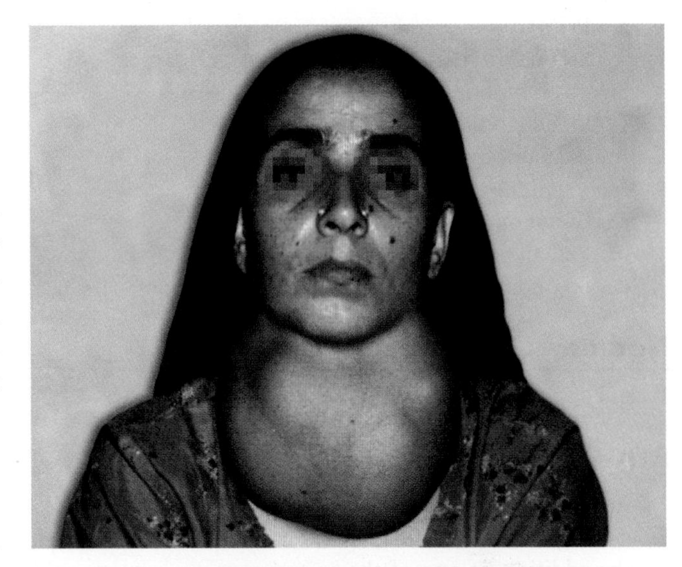
Fig. 68.2: Huge multinodular goiter

NEOPLASMS

Three types of thyroid neoplasms are common:
1. Papillary carcinoma
2. Follicular carcinoma
3. Medullary carcinoma.

Papillary Carcinoma

This is the most common malignant tumor of thyroid, accounting for 80 percent of all thyroid tumors. The tumor may present as a solitary thyroid nodule, but the rest of the gland may also contain microscopic nodules. Female to male ratio is 3:1, and 10 percent of patients have had prior neck irradiation.

Characteristic histology features includes papillary architecture, nuclear grooving, cytoplasmic inclusions, "Orphan-Annie" nuclei and Psammoma bodies (stippled calcific concretions thought to be remnants of colloid follicles). Papillary carcinoma has various common subtypes, but behavior is mostly the same in all patients under age 45:

a. Follicular variant (mostly follicular as opposed to papillary) = 10 percent
b. Tall call (3:1 height:width in >30% of specimen) = 4 percent of lesions (more aggressive variant in older patients)
c. Others include sclerosing, oxyphillic, and clear cell types.

Spreads by regional lymphatics, though the incidence of lymphatic spread is high but this is of minimal significance in the overall survival rates.

Follicular Carcinoma

Accounts for 10 percent of all thyroid cancers. The female to male ratio = 3:1. Is more prevalent in areas of endemic goiter or I-deficiency, as tumor does not concentrate I well. Capsular/vascular invasion is required for differentiation from adenoma. Fifty percent show microinvasion, 50 percent show marked invasion. The nodal spread is less than papillary Ca. (<20%). Insular variant of this tumor is more aggressive in behavior and an important variant is the Hurthle cell tumor.

Medullary Carcinoma

Originate from parafollicular calcitonin-producing C-cells [embryological remnant of the ultimobranchial body (4th branchial pouch)]. Account for 5 percent of thyroid cancers. Cellular characteristics include: nests of small polygonal cells, amyloid, dense calcifications, and neurosecretory granules. Produce calcitonin and CEA, and both are useful as recurrence markers. Lymph node metastases occur in 50 to 80 percent of cases. Four subtypes:

i. Sporadic lesions, these form 75 percent of the lesions and 30 percent of these are bilateral. They have the best prognosis.
ii. Familial (25%), 100 percent have bilateral multiple foci. Following subtypes are described:
   - Isolated familial (best prognosis of familial subtypes)
   - MEN IIA [comprise of medullary thyroid CA, pheochromocytoma (50%), hyperparathyroidism (25%)]
   - MEN IIB [Medullary thyroid CA, pheochromocytoma (50%), mucosal ganglioneuromas, Marfanoid habitus]

All families should be screened and there is no minimum age for performing a prophylactic thyroidectomy (mets can occur as early as age 1) or neck dissection (for MEN IIB families). Five-year survival is 50 to 80 percent, lower if nodes present during the surgery.

ANAPLASTIC CARCINOMA

One percent of all thyroid malignancies. Highly aggressive undifferentiated tumor, with average survival postdiagnosis of <6 months. Generally affects elderly patients. Cellular characteristics: giant and spindle cells, haphazard and heterogeneous. Thought to represent transformation of prior stable well-differentiated tumor, so any long-standing goiter which undergoes rapid change should be evaluated aggressively. In most cases surgery (beyond tracheostomy) will offer no benefit, although there is some suggestion that various trials of chemoradiations are potentially of survival benefit.

AJCC staging for thyroid neoplasms

T	N	M
T0: No primary	N0: No nodes	M0: No mets
T1: Tumor <1 cm	N1a: Ipsilateral nodes	M1: Distant mets
T2: Tumor 1–4 cm	N1b: Any other nodes	
T3: Tumor >4 cm		
T4: Tumor extracapsular		
	Age <45	Age >45
Stage I	Any T, N, M0	T1, N0, M0
Stage II	M1	T2-3, N0, M0
Stage III		T4 or N1
Stage IV		M1

Medullary

Stage I	T1, N0, M0
Stage II	T2, T3, T4, N0, M0
Stage III	Any T, N1, M0
Stage IV	Any T, any N, M1

MANAGEMENT

Imaging is vital and includes:

Ultrasound

- Differentiates solid from cystic in 80 percent of cases, but prognostic significance for malignancy is dubious (20% solid, 10% cystic)

- Very useful for size determination, needle aspiration and contralateral lobe evaluation.

CT

- Used in cases of massive or substernal lesions, to evaluate lymphadenopathy, and examine for signs of malignancy (i.e. carotid encasement, invasion of trachea or esophagus)
- Calcifications suggestive of papillary (speculated) or medullary (dense)

Fine needle aspiration can be reported as benign, malignant, suspicious or inconclusive and carries 90 to 95 percent sensitivity/specificity when conclusive.

Treatment

Thyroid neoplasms are treated by surgery (thyroidectomy) supplemented by radio-iodine (I^{131}) and external radiotherapy depending upon the stage of disease. The patient is put on thyroid hormone replacement therapy after surgery.

Treatment Policy

PAPILLARY ADENOCARCINOMA

A patient with papillary adenocarcinoma with a large mass in one lobe of the thyroid associated with metastatic lymph nodes in the neck requires a total thyroidectomy and neck dissection. Treatment strategy for differentiated (papillary and follicular) thyroid cancer in high-risk patients including all males and females over 45 years is total thyroidectomy. High-risk tumors including the papillary and follicular carcinomas greater than 1 cm in size are also treated with total thyroidectomy, as are the tumors associated with significant multifocality, local or distant spread. Patients under 16 years with a diagnosis of differentiated thyroid cancer should be regarded as high-risk, and are usually best treated aggressively. The intermediate group of thyroid malignancy of the differentiated type may either be treated by Hemi or by total thyroidectomy and if recurrence occurs following the conservative surgery further treatment (completion thyroidectomy) is likely to be curative. The intermediate group of patients consists of a low-risk patient (female under 45 years) with high-risk tumor or a high-risk patient with low-risk tumor (including papillary carcinoma of less than 1 cm in size). Low-risk patient with a low-risk tumor is treated with hemi thyroidectomy. Tumors of the isthmus can be treated by an isthmusectomy and a 1 cm margin.

FOLLICULAR ADENOCARCINOMA

The management of follicular adenocarcinoma is very similar to that of papillary tumors. The main stay of treatment is surgery. The neck and mediastinum are managed as for papillary carcinoma. Subsequently ablation of any thyroid remnants is performed, followed in 3 months by screening for residual disease in the neck or distant metastasis. Hurthle cell cancers should be managed as follicular cancers.

MEDULLARY CARCINOMA

The principal treatment advised for the patient with medullary carcinoma is total thyroidectomy and removal of any enlarged lymph node masses. Palpable disease requires modified radical or radical neck dissection. The operation is extended into superior mediastinum if necessary. As these tumors arise from parafollicular cells, it is not surprising that they do not concentrate radio-iodine. Postoperative radio therapy is indicated if there is any suggestion of macroscopic residual disease in the neck and/ or multiple large nodal metastasis with extracapsular extension.

THYROID LYMPHOMA

Although no surgery other than biopsy is usually considered to be necessary for lymphoma at other sites, surgical removal of bulky disease has been shown to improve both local control and survival in patients with thyroid lymphoma. Thyroidectomy is, therefore, sometimes indicated (but not usually feasible), so that radiotherapy remains the principal treatment for this condition. Patients with high grade histology and more advanced disease should, in addition, receive appropriate chemotherapy, if permitted by their general condition.

ANAPLASTIC TUMORS

A biopsy is mandatory to confirm that a patient suspected to have an anaplastic carcinoma does not have lymphoma which may be curable. Sometimes isthmus may need to be divided and tracheostomy performed if there is airway obstruction. Regression may be achieved by radical radiotherapy and chemotherapy, but early recurrence is the rule, leading almost inevitably to death within 6 to 12 months.

Chapter

69

Bronchoscopy

The endoscopic examination of the bronchi is necessary for various diagnostic and therapeutic purposes.

Indications

Bronchoscopic procedure may be needed for the following:

1. Examination of the bronchial tree in patients, who present with abnormalities like unexplained lung shadows on X-ray, hemoptysis, collapse of the lung, slowly resolving pneumonia.
2. For biopsy of an endobronchial growth.
3. For removing foreign bodies from the bronchus.
4. For bronchial aspiration in cases of lung abscess and aspiration pneumonia.

The examination is carried by a rigid metallic tube which has arrangements for lighting and aspiration. The bronchoscope has side holes to allow respiration to take place through the bronchi which are not occupied by the bronchoscope.

The bronchoscopes are of various sizes designed to fit the bronchi at various ages as the bronchi do not allow over distension. Bronchoscopic telescopes are available and allow a more detailed magnified view of the subglottis, trachea and bronchi. Forceps of various shapes are available for endobronchial manipulation. The instruments used for bronchoscopy and esophagoscopy are shown in **Figure 69.1**.

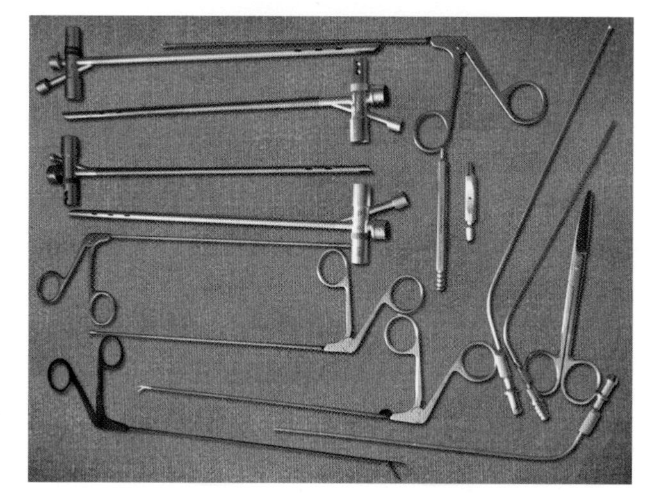

Fig. 69.1: Bronchoscopy set

Contraindications for Bronchoscopy

1. Diseases of the cervical spine, where it may be impossible to pass a rigid metallic tube.
2. Vascular tumors like aneurysms of aorta.
3. Fulminating suppurative pneumonitis or morbid condition of the patient.

PROCEDURE

Bronchoscopy can be done under local or general anesthesia. The patient lies in supine position with the neck slightly elevated and the head extened at the atlanto-occipital joint. This brings the buccal cavity, pharynx and larynx in a straight line, thus allowing easy passage of the bronchoscope (Boyce's position).

The bronchoscope help in the right hand is passed in the right side of angle of the mouth to the posterior-third of the tongue, which is raised to visualize the epiglottis. The epiglottis is lifted on the beak of the bronchoscope and the tube is gradually advanced to the glottis. The tip of the bronchoscope is held in the long axis of the glottis to allow easy passage of the bronchoscope into the trachea.

The trachea is properly examined and the bronchoscope advanced to the carina which divides the trachea into right and left main bronchi. The carina appears as a sharp vertical spur. Any broadening or thickening of the carina is pathological.

The tip of the bronchoscope is directed towards the bronchus under examination while the patient's head is directed to the opposite side.

The right main bronchus is more vertical and shorter than the left main bronchus. On right bronchial examination, the orifices of the upper lobe, middle lobe, lower lobe bronchi are identified and a detailed examination with the help of the telescope which are retrograde, straight and right angled.

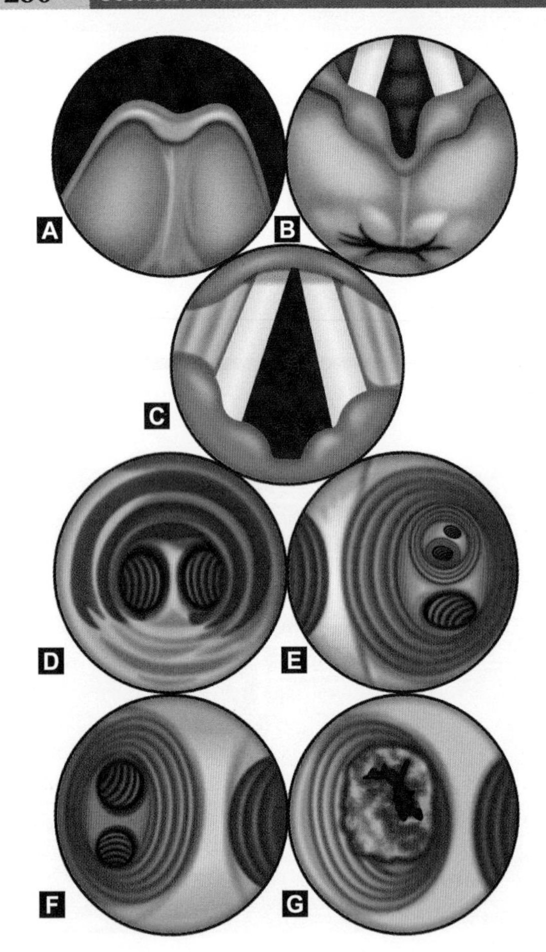

Figs 69.2A to G: Different structures which come in view on bronchoscopic procedure, as one proceeds, are as under: (A) Valleculae and lingual surface of epiglottis; (B) Posterior commissure, arytenoids and posterior 1/3rd of vocal cords; (C) Full view of glottic aperture and vocal cords; (D) Carina and openings of two main bronchi; (E) Right main bronchus and openings of upper, middle and lower lobe bronchi; (F) Left main bronchus and openings of upper and lower lobe bronchi; (G) Growth seen in left main bronchus

Examination of the left main bronchus is similarly done and its subdivisional bronchi viewed (**Figs 69.2A to G**)

The pathological lesions are examined and if necessary biopsy taken and suction done. Aspirations may be sent for bacteriological and cytological examination.

COMPLICATIONS OF BRONCHOSCOPY

1. *Laryngeal edema:* Instrumentation of the larynx may induce edematous swelling, particularly of the subglottic region.
2. Hemorrhage may occur during bronchoscopy following biopsy particularly of a vascular tumor.

FIBEROPTIC BRONCHOSCOPY

This method is simple and quick. It enables the inspection and biopsy of all segmental and subsegmental bronchi.

Types of Bronchoscopes

1. Chevaliar-Jackson type
2. Negus type
3. MC Gibbon type (1942) emergency bronchoscope
4. Fiberoptic with microphotography bronchoscopes.

The various sizes of the bronchoscopes available are shown in **Table 69.1**.

Table 69.1: Various sizes of the bronchoscopes

	Internal diameter (mm)	Circum-ference (mm)	Length (cm)
1. For suckling	4.1 × 3.2	15	15
2. For infants	5.4 × 4.1	19.5	25
3. For adolescents	8 × 6.7	26	30
4. For children	7 × 5.7	29	40
5. For adults	10 × 8.7	35	40

Chapter

70

Esophagus

Surgical Anatomy

Esophagus is a fibromuscular tube about 25 cm long extending from the cricopharyngeal sphincter to the cardia of the stomach. In an adult 4 cm of this tube lies below the diaphragm. The musculature of the upper one-third is striated and that of the lower two-thirds is smooth. It is lined by squamous epithelium and the portion below the level of the diaphragm is lined by gastric type of mucosa (without oxyntic or peptic cells).

At birth the greatest diameter of the empty esophagus is 5 mm, at one year of life it is 9 mm, at five years of life it is 15 mm, and it is 20 mm in adult. After distention it increases about 30 mm.

There are three physiological constrictions in the esophagus at the level of 15, 25, 40 cm from the upper incisor tooth (**Fig. 70.1**). They are the sites of anatomical narrowing where difficulties may be experienced in the passage of instruments and where foreign bodies may be arrested. They are also the sites of predilection for benign strictures and for carcinoma of the esophagus.

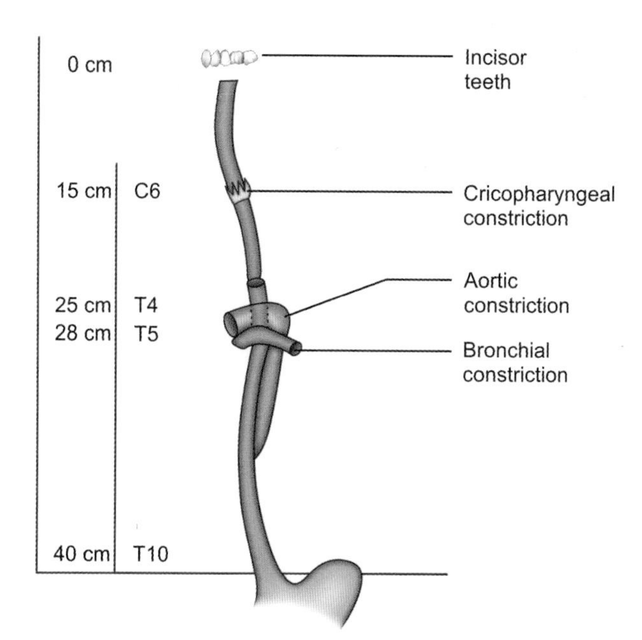

Fig. 70.1: Various constrictions of esophagus

NERVE SUPPLY

The parasympathetic nerve supply is mediated by the vagus through the extrinsic and intrinsic nerve plexuses. The intrinsic plexus has no Meissner's network which is present elsewhere throughout the alimentary canal, and Auerbach's plexus is present in the lower two-thirds only. Sympathetic supply is by nerves surrounding the vessels which supply the esophagus.

Investigations for an Esophageal Disease

The following investigations are undertaken in an esophageal disorder:

i. Radiography
ii. Endoscopy
iii. Esophageal pressure study.

RADIOLOGICAL INVESTIGATION

1. *X-rays of the chest and neck (AP and lateral view)* are helpful to diagnose conditions like foreign bodies in the esophagus and esophageal rupture with complications.
2. *Barium screening:* It is a common investigation required for an esophageal disease.

   During screening, the passage of a mouthful of barium from mouth to the stomach is followed and the following points are noted.

a. Physiological constrictions.
b. Pathological dilatations, constrictions, webs, filling defects or holdups and the exact site of the constriction, stricture or holdup.
c. The type and amplitude of peristaltic waves and competence of the esophagogastric sphincter.
d. Any diversion of normal flow.

A radiolucent foreign body in the esophageal lumen may be demonstrated on screening by giving the patient a piece of cotton impregnated barium to swallow, which gets arrested at the site of the foreign body.

Cine-radiography: Image intensification with cine-radiography is an improvement over the barium swallow examination. It is particularly helpful in abnormal patterns of deglutition such as cricopharyngeal spasm.

BARIUM MEAL X-RAY OF THE ESOPHAGUS

X-ray films taken during barium screening are helpful in determination of the site of holdup and to note the extent of the obstructing lesions like tumor or stricture. Spillage of barium into the lungs suggests a tracheoesophageal fistula.

The mucosal irregularity and diverticulum are demonstrated. Extraluminal pressure on the esophagus by an enlarged atrium, aorta or a mediastinal tumor may be evident as an area of compression and displacement.

ESOPHAGEAL PRESSURE STUDY

Manometric pressure studies of the esophagus have been done and found useful in neuromuscular disorders affecting peristalsis.

Chapter 71

Common Esophageal Diseases in ENT Practice

Congenital Abnormalities of the Esophagus

Congenital lesions that may affect the esophagus include atresia, congenital stenosis and tracheoesophageal fistula.

Congenital esophageal atresia with tracheoesophageal fistula is the more common abnormality encountered. An infant presents with excessive salivation, cyanosis and the inability to swallow. The diagnosis is confirmed by passing a lubricated rubber catheter which gets held up in the blind esophageal pouch. The atresia is shown on X-ray if 1 to 2 ml of iodized oil is passed through the catheter.

MANAGEMENT

The patient is prepared for surgery and through transpleural route, the two esophageal segments are defined, fistula closed and anastomosis between the two segments is established.

Injuries to the Esophagus

The ENT surgeon may come across esophageal injuries in the following situations. *External trauma* of the neck may result from cut throats or during tracheostomy.

ACCIDENTAL PERFORATIONS OF THE ESOPHAGUS

Perforations of the esophagus from within its lumen result from penetration by pointed foreign bodies like metallic pins, pointed dentures, fish or meat bones. Perforation may also result on esophagoscopy during removal of foreign bodies, dilatation of strictures or on taking a biopsy specimen. Forcible passage of the esophagoscope, particularly at the level of the anatomical constrictions can also lead to instrumental trauma to the esophagus.

Clinical Features of Esophageal Perforations

The patient complains of severe pain in the neck, chest or epigastrium depending upon the site of perforation. The general condition of the patient deteriorates. Surgical emphysema may be noticeable in the neck. A fall in blood pressure and increase in pulse rate may occur.

X-ray examination of the chest may show pneumothorax or air in mediastinum.

Treatment

When the diagnosis is made, nothing should be given orally. A Ryle's tube is passed. Systemic antibiotics are given in massive doses.

Indications for surgery: Surgical exposure is needed in the following:

i. Progressive surgical emphysema.
ii. Evidence of pleural effusion.
iii. Worsening of the patient's general condition.
iv. Formation of a mediastinal abscess.

CORROSIVE INJURY OF THE ESOPHAGUS

Corrosive poisoning may be accidental or suicidal and is caused by swallowing acids or alkalies. It results in severe burns with consequent local edema and disturbances of acid-base balance.

It is, however, the late changes that are of importance surgically. The degree and extent of these changes are proportionate to the amount and concentration of the corrosive fluid swallowed. In addition, the presence or absence of vomiting or regurgitation of the ingested material is of considerable significance, thereby causing second exposure chemical trauma.

Pathology of Stricture Formation

Initially cellular death takes place. This area is surrounded by an intense zone of inflammation. Necrotic tissue sloughs out during the first week, leaving behind an ulcerated surface. The level of tissue necrosis depends upon the nature of the corrosive ingested. Alkalis cause liquefication necrosis and therefore a deeper level of tissue injury and are thus associated more with perforations of the esophagus. Acids on the other hand cause coagulative necrosis and as such although the burns are severe tend to be confined to the superficial muscular coats of the esophagus. Repair follows by the formation of granulation tissue. It is important to note that the granulation tissue does not function like damaged muscle tissue. Instead, healing occurs by dense scar tissue which forms the stricture. Strictures due to corrosive burns are usually single although these may be multiple. "Skip areas", virtually free of involvement, are noted in multiple strictures. These are explained on the basis of spasm and peristalsis.

Clinical Features

There is a history of swallowing of a corrosive liquid. There occurs intense pain and difficulty in swallowing. The acute symptoms subside within 2 to 3 weeks followed by apparent improvement. However, within a few weeks the patient presents with dysphagia and regurgitation. Barium meal X-ray reveals the character of the stricture, its severity, location, extent and whether it is single or multiple. Typically a corrosive stricture is single, involving a large segment of the esophagus.

Treatment of Corrosive Burns of Esophagus

Immediate attention is given to the general condition like maintenance of fluid and electrolyte balance and preservation of adequate airway. Systemic antibiotics are given to control the infection.

Prevention of Stricture Formation

As soon as the patient's general condition allows, a Ryle's tube is passed down the gullet. It not only maintains the lumen during the healing stage but also helps in feeding the patient.

Steroid therapy is started within two or three days of the illness. This helps to minimize the fibrosis and thus prevents stricture formation.

Benign Strictures of the Esophagus

Besides corrosive burns of the esophagus, other important causes of the esophageal strictures include trauma by foreign body or instruments, reflux esophagitis, systemic infections like scarlet fever and collagen diseases.

Barium X-ray confirms the diagnosis. Esophagoscopy reveals the stricture area. At the stricture site the mucosa is pale and there is lack of elasticity of the esophagus.

COMPLICATIONS ASSOCIATED WITH STRICTURE ESOPHAGUS

1. Nutritional deficiences consequent to long-standing dysphagia.
2. Foreign body impaction.
3. Increased chances of instrumental perforation because of less elasticity.
4. Pulmonary complications because of frequent regurgitation and aspiration of food material.
5. Malignancy may develop at the stricture site.

TREATMENT OF ESOPHAGEAL STRICTURE

Bougies of increasing size are passed down the lumen to dilate it. The procedure needs frequent repetition. If bouginage fails, external operation is required wherein the stenosed area is removed and anastomosis done.

HIATUS HERNIA AND GASTROESOPHAGEAL REFLUX

This is yet another condition where there is failure of the lower esophageal mechanism. The outcome is the regurgitation of the gastric contents into the esophagus. The hernia may initiate due to either a laxity at the hiatus or an increase in the intra-abdominal pressure. However, once established the resultant reflux causes progressive esophageal fibrosis resulting in the shortening of the esophagus. Laparoscopic hiatus hernia repair with fundoplication offers a feasible alternative to open surgery.

Esophagiectasia (Cardiospasm)

It is a disease of unknown etiology affecting men more frequently than women, usually between the age group of 30 and 60 years.

PATHOLOGY

The main pathological change noticed is degeneration of the ganglion cells in the Auerbach's nerve plexus particularly in the lower part of the esophagus. No coordinated peristalsis occurs in the esophagus and the lower esophageal sphincter fails to relax in response to swallowing. Thus, there is retention of food in the esophagus and distension of its lumen. The mucosa gets ulcerated.

CLINICAL FEATURES

There is long-standing history of epigastric discomfort which progresses to dysphagia, more for liquids than solids as the solid food can pass down the sphincter because of its weight. Dysphagia may be marked by temporary remissions unlike in carcinoma. Regurgitation is another troublesome symptom. Swallowed foods and liquids associated with mucous usually foul smelling, are regurgitated.

DIAGNOSIS

Barium X-ray shows a spindle-shaped narrowing of the cardiac end through which little or no barium passes down. However, the narrowing is smooth and regular unlike in carcinoma. The esophagus is shown as a fusiform dilated organ and no regular peristalsis is seen.

On esophagoscopy, after the retained food material is cleaned, the dilated esophageal lumen becomes evident. The mucosa is hyperemic and at places ulcerated.

COMPLICATIONS

These include nutritional deficiencies and pulmonary complications because of frequent regurgitation. The chances of developing esophageal malignancy are around 20 percent.

TREATMENT

Conservative management includes administration of antispasmodic drugs. Repeated dilatation may help. Diagnosis is confirmed using esophageal manometry. Laparoscopic cardiomyotomy has shown results comparable to open cardiomyotomy minus the attendant problems. Performing a fundoplication simultaneously also takes care of the attendant reflux. The hospital stay is shortened, the patient mobilises early and the overall period for recovery is much decreased. The successful outcome depends on observing the surgical principles for cardiomyotomy at all times. These include an incision at least 6 cm long with 1 cm extending onto the cardia.

Surgical treatment is by *Heller's operation*. In this operation, the obstruction at the lower end is relieved by cutting through the muscular layer of the esophagus. Through the left-sided thoracotomy, the lower part of esophagus is exposed. An anterior longitudinal incision is made in the muscular wall of the esophagus at the cardioesophageal junction down to the mucosa but not through the mucous membrane.

Foreign Bodies in the Upper Food Passages

Foreign bodies in the upper food passages is a common emergency in ENT practice. Any object which is retained in the pharynx or esophagus is a foreign body.

FOREIGN BODIES IN PHARYNX

Small fish or meat bones are the commonly encountered foreign bodies in the pharynx. These may get lodged in the tonsils, valecullae, base of tongue and the pyriform fossae.

Diagnosis

The history is suggestive. The patient complains of pain and discomfort in the throat. Proper examination of the throat should be done and a detailed mirror examination usually reveals the site of lodgement of the foreign body. Ulceration gives a further clue. X-ray of the soft tissues of the neck may sometimes be required to detect an otherwise invisible foreign body.

Once the foreign body has been located it is removed with an appropriate forceps.

FOREIGN BODIES IN THE ESOPHAGUS

A variety of objects may be retained in the esophagus as foreign bodies. Coins and meat bones are the most common objects followed by metal hooks, artificial dentures and meat lumps.

Etiology

Children are usually in the habit of swallowing anything they can get hold of. Similarly, foreign body lodgement is common in the elderly because of improper mastication and week propulsive movements of the gullet.

Loose fitting artificial dentures may be swallowed during mastication or sleep. Certain esophageal conditions like benign strictures or malignancy and sites of anatomical narrowing of the esophagus may arrest a foreign body.

Clinical Features

The patient, if an adult, usually gives a history of having swallowed a foreign body. If the foreign body is arrested in the upper part of the esophagus, the patient is very often able to localize the pain and site of the lodgement of the foreign body. If the foreign body is lower down, localization is vague. Dysphagia is another important symptom of foreign body in the esophagus and should raise the suspicion, particularly in children.

A detailed examination of the pharyngeal wall, tonsils, valecullae and pyriform fossae should be carried out.

Plain films of the neck and chest are taken. Ideally both the anteroposterior and lateral views are taken to know the exact location and disposition of the foreign body (**Figs 71.1 to 71.3**).

Foreign bodies in the esophagus, particularly flat objects like coins lie in the coronal plane in contrast to laryngeal or tracheal foreign bodies which lie in the sagittal plane.

If the foreign body is not visualized, screening of the chest and abdomen is done to note whether it has passed down.

In case of nonopaque foreign bodies, a little barium sulfate is given and its passage down the esophagus is observed. Barium may be held up or the flow of barium may be split at the site of the foreign body. Sometimes a little cotton soaked in barium paste or a gelatin capsule filled with barium is swallowed and its arrest in the esophagus on the foreign body noted. However, if the clinician is still in doubt, esophagoscopy should be done to be sure regarding the presence or absence of the foreign body.

Complications

Complications of foreign body in esophagus include the following:

1. Impaction of foreign body
2. Esophagitis
3. Periesophagitis
4. Perforation
5. Paraesophageal abscess.

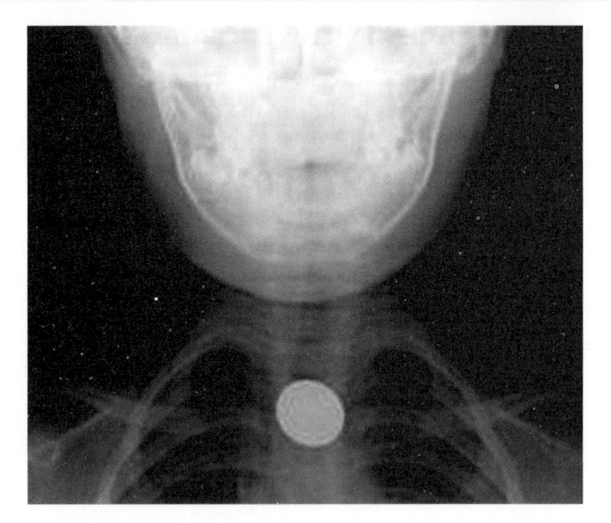

Fig. 71.1: Foreign body (coin) in the upper esophagus

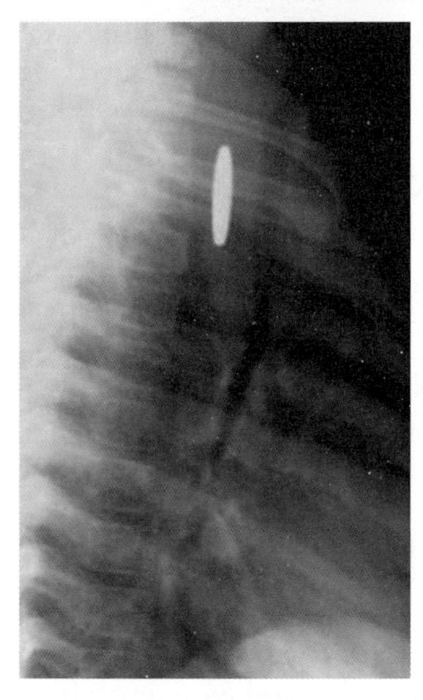

Fig. 71.3: Lateral X-ray film showing foreign body in esophagus

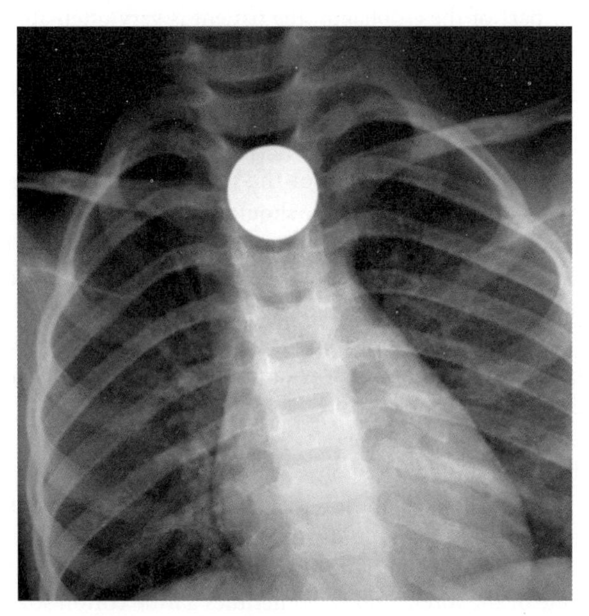

Fig. 71.2: Foreign body in the esophagus

Treatment

Foreign bodies in the esophagus should always be removed. It is not good to wait and allow the foreign body to pass down as it may get arrested leading to fatal complications. Though foreign body removal is an emergency, the surgeon must have a knowledge of the location and disposition of the foreign body so that he selects the proper endoscopic instruments and orients himself to the situation.

Esophagoscopy for removal of the foreign body can be done under local and general anesthesia. If the size of the foreign body is bigger than the diameter of the esophagoscope, then after having caught the foreign body, all three articles, the foreign body, forceps and esophagoscope are removed as a single unit.

With all long foreign bodies, the aim is to search the proximal end. In case of pins and needles, their point must be searched for.

The mortality which may follow the failure to remove a foreign body does not justify the violent method of its removal and no harm should be done, if one cannot remove the foreign body.

Dentures in the esophagus present many problems. They often have sharp edges and associated metallic hooks which cause their impaction. Hence, such cases should be properly studied before attempting haphazard removal. They may require division by a sheer before they can be removed.

Indications of removal by external route include an impacted foreign body and periesophageal abscess associated with a foreign body.

In the cervical esophagus, foreign bodies can be removed by left lateral esophagotomy while lower down, thoracotomy is needed to expose the esophagus and remove the foreign body.

Neoplasms of the Esophagus

Benign neoplasms of the esophagus are very rare. These include leiomyomas, fibromas, papillomas and hemangiomas.

MALIGNANT TUMORS OF THE ESOPHAGUS

The malignant lesions of the esophagus occur more frequently in males than in females. This neoplastic disease is commonly found in regions where rice is the staple diet as in Kashmir and Assam. The exact etiology of the disease is not known. Bad oral hygiene, smoking, spicy and hot foods and large quantities of hot salt tea have been found as the usual irritating factors. Long-standing esophagitis, fibrous stricture, esophagectasia, Plummer-Vinson syndrome and pharyngeal diverticulum are the predisposing conditions.

Histology

Squamous cell carcinoma (well-differentiated) is the most common type of tumor. Adenocarcinomas may occur at the lower end of the esophagus. Mesodermal tumors like fibrosarcoma, leiomyosarcoma and rhabdomyosarcoma are very rarely seen.

Site of Lesion

Carcinoma develops most frequently in the middle-third of the esophagus followed by lower-third and the upper-third.

Spread of the Tumor

The tumor, usually of the ulcerative type, may infiltrate the esophageal wall and spread submucosally to encircle the lumen. Spread by submucosal lymphatics may produce satellite lesions at some distance from the original lesion.

Spread beyond the esophagus involves the trachea, bronchi and recurrent laryngeal nerves. Lymphatic spread involves the mediastinal lymph nodes in the root of neck or nodes in abdomen (celiac group). Blood-borne metastasis occurs commonly to the lungs and liver.

Symptoms of Carcinoma Esophagus

The patient commonly presents with rapidly progressing dysphagia. The dysphagia which is initially for solids occurs later for liquids also. The patient may present with absolute dysphagia and dehydration. A history of anorexia and weight loss is common. The patient may present with an impacted foreign body.

Diagnosis

A history of progressive dysphagia is important and should raise suspicion of this disease. Barium screening of the esophagus is frequently suggestive. A holdup and irregularity of the lumen may be noted. Barium meal X-ray of the esophagus may show a typical rat-tail deformity (**Figs 71.4 and 71.5**).

Esophagoscopy (**Fig. 71.6**) allows proper visualization of the obstructing lesion.

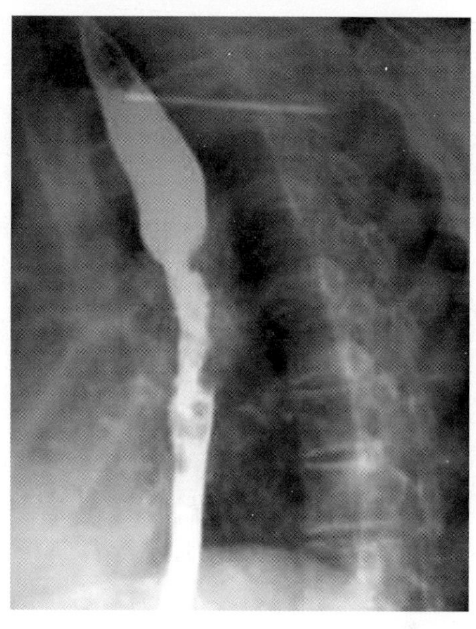

Fig. 71.4: Barium X-ray of the esophagus showing irregular narrowing with dilatation above (malignancy)

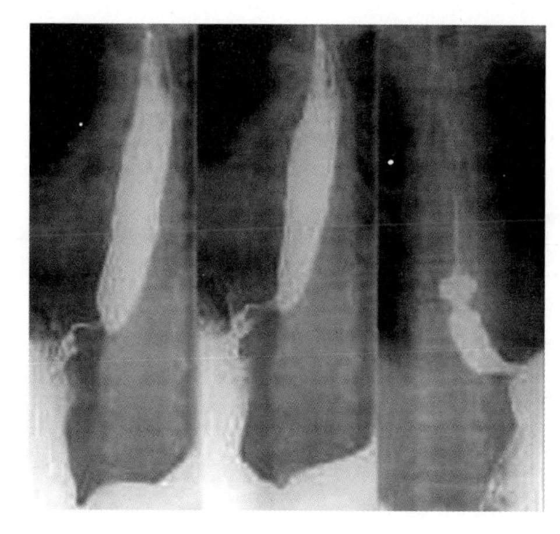

Fig. 71.5: Barium X-ray of the esophagus (rat-tail deformity due to malignancy)

Proliferative or ulcerative lesions and areas of mucosal irregularity are looked for an endoscopy. The extent or spread, its site and distance from the upper incisor teeth is noted. Mobility of the esophagus seen on inspiration, may be absent. Biopsy from the suspected lesion is confirmatory.

Treatment

The prognosis of esophageal cancer at present is poor. Majority of the cases are inoperable. The symptoms present late, and,

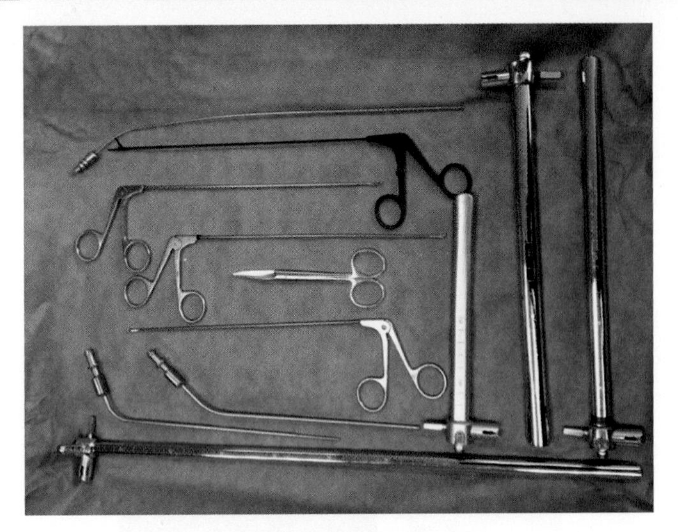

Fig. 71.6: Esophagoscopy set

many times only palliative radiotherapy is given to relieve them. If the growth lies below the level of the thoracic inlet, endoluminal plastic tubes may be inserted through the growth area to maintain patency. Soutter's or Mousseu-Barbin tubes may be used for providing nutrition. Feeding gastrostomy may be only choice in very advanced lesions.

Surgery: Esophagogastrectomy for growths involving the lower end of the esophagus offers better chances of survival provided the patient presents early.

Involvement of the bronchial tree and recurrent laryngeal nerve indicate an inoperable growth.

Chapter 72

Esophagoscopy

Introduction

Endoscopic inspection of the esophagus is known as esophagoscopy. The procedure may be needed for diagnostic or therapeutic purposes.

INDICATIONS

1. *Diagnostic*
   a. Foreign body in the esophagus
   b. Stricture of the esophagus
   c. Growth in the esophagus
   d. Esophageal varices
   e. Tracheoesophageal fistula.
2. *Therapeutic*
   a. Removal of foreign bodies
   b. Bouginage to dilate stricture or spasm
   c. Sclerotherapy of esophageal varices
   d. Endoscopic excision of pharyngeal pouch.

CONTRAINDICATIONS TO ESOPHAGOSCOPY

1. Aneurysm of aorta
2. Severe spinal deformities or cervical spondylosis
3. Mediastinal growth
4. Trismus.

TECHNIQUE

The procedure can be done under local or general anesthesia. The patient is kept in *Boyce's position* with the neck flexed and the head extended at the atlanto-occipital joint. A piece of gauze protects the teeth on the upper jaw and retracts the upper lip.

The esophagoscope is held by the right hand and guided forwards gently by the left thumb so that it is passed through the oral cavity on the right side of the tongue, pharynx and along the right pyriform fossa till the cricopharynx is visualized. After a little pause, the cricopharyngeal sphincter relaxes and the esophagoscope is passed down again with very gentle movement taking care of the anatomical curves of the esophagus, and visualizing the lumen for any abnormality like narrowing, bulging, varices, stricture or growth. The direction of the tip of the esophagoscope should be towards the left anterosuperior iliac spine because in the lower-third, the esophagus is directed forwards and curves towards the left to join the cardiac end of the stomach.

COMPLICATIONS OF ESOPHAGOSCOPY

Esophageal perforation usually results if the esophagoscope is passed forcibly or an attempt to remove the foreign body is made without exactly knowing its position and nature.

FIBEROPTIC ESOPHAGOSCOPY

The flexible fiberoptic esophagoscope is more frequently used these days for diagnostic purposes. It is flexible; hence there are no contraindications or dangers that are associated with the rigid metallic esophagoscope. It allows proper inspection and biopsy from a representative area of the lesion. However, the rigid esophagoscope is still useful for removing foreign bodies, for dilatation of strictures and occasionally for injection of esophageal varices.

The metallic esophagoscopes are available in various sizes. Commonly in adults 16 mm (Internal diameter) × 45 cm (length) and in children 6 mm × 35 cm esophagoscopes are used.

TYPES OF ESOPHAGOSCOPES

1. Burning, Kahler, Haslinger's (proximal light type)
2. Chevalier Jackson (distal light type)
3. Negus (oblique light type)
4. Fiberoptic esophagoscope.

The sizes available of the esophagoscopes are shown in **Table 72.1**.

Table 72.1: Esophagoscopes of various sizes

		Internal diameter	Circumference	Length
1.	For children	10 × 8 mm	35 mm	35 mm
	Chevalier Jackson	7 mm	35 mm	35 mm
2.	For middle of esophagus	15.6 mm 13.6 mm	55 mm	35 cm
3.	Adult size full lumen	17.6 × 15.6 mm	60 mm	45 mm

Chapter

73

Laser Surgery in ENT

Introduction

Laser, by definition, means *light amplification by stimulated emission of radiation.* The history of laser begins with the Father of Modern Physics, Einstein who first discussed stimulated emission. In 1960, the first laser was built by the Hughes Aircraft Company. In 1965, the first CO_2 laser was developed. ENT was one of the first specialties to use the laser.

Various materials used for this purpose include carbon dioxide, "Nd:YAG", "Ruby", "Argon", KTP 532, helium, neon.

Principles of Laser Surgery

Normally, an atom is having an equal number of electrons and protons orbiting the nucleus at a fixed distance so is in stable form. If energy is given, the electrons change their orbits away from the nucleus, making atom excited but this state does not last long as atom releases the absorbed energy quickly which is called spontaneous emission. If these excited atoms are struck by photons, the decay of atom is accelerated releasing stimulated emission. Lasers have an optical resonating chamber, two mirrors (one partially transmissive), and a space between the mirrors filled with active medium and when external energy excites the medium, spontaneous emission occurs in all directions. Only those photons in perpendicular to the mirrors are reflected back into the medium causing stimulated emission of radiation. This generates more photons in the same axis with same energy and wavelength and a steady state is achieved when the amount of radiation leaving the optical cavity is balanced with the pumping rate of excited atoms. There are some essential elements to a laser:

A. Monochromatic, which means: (1) can target blood vessels and allows for the selective photothermolysis of vascular lesions and (2) specific wavelength changes the depth of penetration of a tissue by the laser light, the amount of hemostasis achieved, and influences the zone of thermal necrosis.

B. Coherence which means not only is the light emitted in the same direction, it is also emitted in phase with all the other light. Not very clinically applicable/useful.

C. Collimated means white light is emitted in all directions. If the lens is placed close to the object to collect light, than the image is large. If you pull the lens away to get a small image, then the image is very dark.

Laser produces a pencil beam of parallel light. Easy to focus down to a small spot, and does not matter how far the lens is placed from the laser, it is easy to collect all the laser beams with the lens.

D. High Power density reflects the ability to focus the laser beam to a small point allowing the use of laser for ablation. This crucial aspect of laser, the ability to focus light to a minimum spot size and have the highest energy density to allow for tissue ablation is made use of in the medical application of lasers. The clinical application of these beams also depend on their wavelength and absorptive power of the tissues on which used.

Function of laser beams can be to:

i. Vaporize
ii. Cut or
iii. Coagulate the tissues.

Carbon dioxide laser is the one commonly used. It has a wavelength of 10.6 m in the infra-red region. Its effect on tissue is, therefore, purely thermal and produces no ionization. At this wavelength, the energy is completely absorbed. Tissue destruction is in part proportional to its water content.

The laser beam can be used to vaporize predetermined volume of tissue in a precisely controlled fashion by using an appropriate amount of energy. A foot-switch controlled interval timer operates the shutter for the beam to strike the target area for an appropriate period. For precise microsurgery, a power setting of 15 watts is commonly combined with a time exposure of 1/15 sec, for gross dissection 15 to 25 watts of power may be used quasi-continuously in the manual mode, bypassing the timer, using the foot switch to start and stop the dissection. In contrast to pulsed lasers, the continuous wave CO_2, laser has comparatively little shock effects, so that it has minimal tendency to scatter in soft tissue.

In the ENT region, laser has been successfully used for:

i. Nose, e.g. papillomas, rhinophyma, telangiectasis, nasal polypi, choanal atresia, turbinectomy. It is very beneficial in patients with bleeding dyscrasias and coagulopathies.
ii. Oral cavity, e.g. multiple areas of leukoplakia, erythroplakia, small superficial cancers, debulking of large recurrent or inoperable tumors. Advantages are transoral approach, precision surgery, hemostasis and less postoperative edema and pain.
iii. Oropharynx, e.g. tonsillar and pharyngeal tumors. Laser tonsillectomy is done in cases of coagulopathies or hypertension.
iv. Larynx, e.g. papilloma larynx, laryngeal web, subglottic stenosis, capillary hemangioma. In adults, it has been used for vocal nodule, leukoplakia of cord, papilloma, polypoid degeneration of cord, endoscopic laser arytenoidectomy, malignant T1 lesions of the vocal cord.
v. Trachea and bronchi, e.g. recurrent papillomatosis, tracheal stenosis, granulation tissues and bronchial adenoma, debulking of obstructive malignant lesions of trachea and bronchi.
vi. Plastic surgery, e.g. benign and malignant tumors of skin, vaporization of nevi and tattoos.
vii. Neuro-otology, e.g. removal of acoustic neuromas, stapedectomy.

Advantages of Laser Use in Laryngeal Cancer Surgery

1. No tracheostomy needed
2. Shorter operating time
3. Decreased incidence of pharyngo-cutaneous fistula
4. No neck incisions
5. Resumption of swallowing is quicker following laser surgery (**Figs 73.1A to C**).

Indications of Endoscopic Laser Laryngeal surgery: This includes tumors of size—T1/T2 suprahyoid epiglottis and

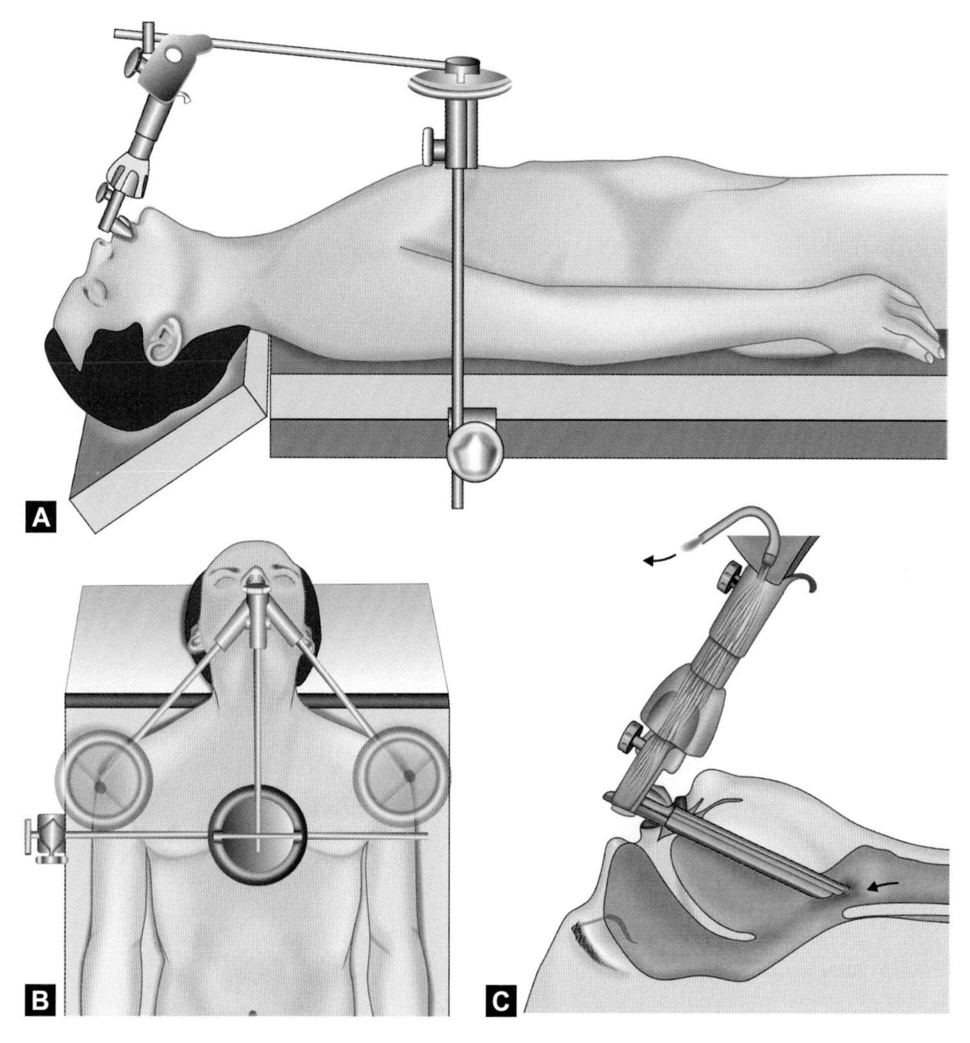

Figs 73.1A to C: Positioning of the patient during laryngeal surgery by laser

growths limited to aryepiglottic fold, vestibular fold and tumors with minimal pre-epiglottic space involvement.

PRECAUTION IN THE USE OF LASER

a. *Education of staff:* The surgeon, anesthesiologist, nursing and operation theater personnel should be educated in laser safety.
b. *Protection of eyes:* Protective eye glasses specific for the wavelength of laser being used should be worn by the personnel to prevent accidental burns to the cornea or retina.

   Patient's eyes should also be protected by a double layer of saline-moistened eyepads.
c. *Protection of other exposed areas*: All exposed skin and mucous membranes of the patient not in surgical field should be protected by saline-soaked towels, pads or sponges which are kept wet by moistening them periodically. Teeth should also be protected.
d. *Evacuation of smoke:* Two separate suctions, one for the blood and the other for smoke and steam, which is produced by vaporization of tissues, should be used.
e. *Anesthetic gases and equipment:* Only non-inflammable gases like halothane or enflurane should be used. When using CO_2 laser, red rubber or silicone tube should be wrapped by reflective metallic foil. Cuff should be inflated with methylene/blue colored saline and protected with saline-soaked cottonades.

   The safest tube to use with Nd:YAG laser is colorless or white polyvinyl or silicone endotracheal tube that does not have any black or dark lettering or a lead lines marking along the side. Negligence in these precautions can cause endotracheal tube fires.

Management of Airway Fire

- Douse fire with saline
- Stop all anesthetic gases including O_2
- Remove endotracheal tube
- Supported ventilation
- Rigid bronchoscopy to assess airway damage
- Remove eschar
- Give antibiotics and steroids
- Maintain high humidity

Repeat bronchoscopy 3 to 5 days postincident.

Chapter

74 Principles of Radiotherapy

Human cells as many other organic cells are created to perform certain biological functions. These functions are controlled by the genetic makeup of the cell. There are hundreds of thousands of chemical reactions which will result in a change of either the physical function or the chemical function. The disturbance of chemical reactions is either due to an abnormality in the cellular genetic code or path physiological factors which affect those reactions. The cellular growth and physiology are the functions of the cellular genetic code, hence, if there are abnormal genetic code, the growth may be affected and cancer may occur.

In order to reverse the abnormal and uncontrolled "cancer" growth, one has to either correct the abnormality of the genetic code or eliminate the abnormal cell. The effort of correcting the abnormality in the genetic code has not been very successful as there are two aspects to be considered:

First: An effective method to identify the genetic abnormality. There are thousands of research studies exploring this aspect with limited success. The abnormality in the genetic coding is not always limited to one cell, which makes it very difficult and not all cancer cases or even cells in the given tumor exhibit the same genetic abnormality.

Second: Even if the abnormality is identified, a successful methodology to correct the problem must be identified.

Virology has proven the ability of viruses to duplicate using human cells. Genetic material studies use viruses as a vehicle to enter an abnormal cell and replace the abnormal cellular genetic material with the normal cell they carry.

The other way to eliminate cancer is to eliminate the abnormal cell. The cellular kill can be achieved by either physical or chemical ways. Chemotherapy acts in different cellular levels in order to kill the cell. Radiotherapy kills the cell by either direct DNA damage or indirect DNA damage. More detail about direct and indirect radiation damage will be presented below.

One might wonder why these chemical and physical methods selectivity kill the abnormal cells and leave the normal cells. The answer is simple, both chemical and physical results will kill the normal and abnormal cells. However, because the normal cell has a good DNA repair mechanism, it will correct the damage quickly while the abnormal cell will not be able to correct the damage since its repair mechanism is not normal. Further details of these mechanisms will be presented below.

Radiobiology

Radiation causes cellular damage by energy transfer from the radiation to the cell. The larger the energy transfer the more extensive the damage. The energy transfer can be measured by linear energy transfer (LET). Different types of radiation have different LET.

The effect of radiation depends on:

1. *Type of radiation:* High LET (Heavy charged particle) cause more damage than low LET.
2. *Type of organism:* There are different radiation sensitivity between different organisms and different animals, while dogs and pigs are considered to be sensitive; turtles are resistant, as well as bacteria and viruses are very resistant.
3. *Type of cells:* In the human not all cells are equally sensitive to radiation. Lymphocytes are very sensitive and nerve cells are more resistant.
4. *The cell cycles phase:* Radiation sensitivity also depends on the phase of the cell cycle; the most sensitive phase is G2-M phase (**Fig. 74.1**).

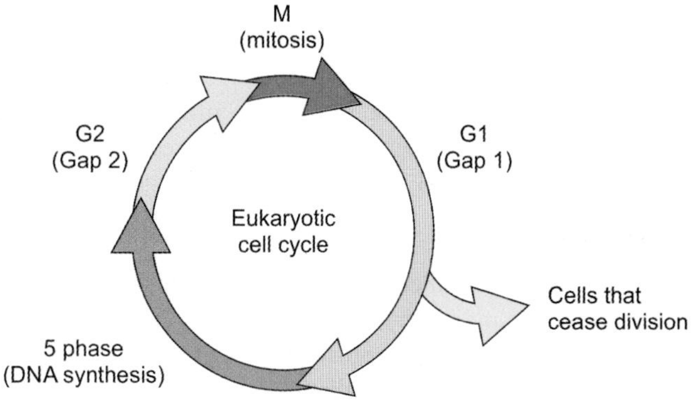

Fig. 74.1: Cell cycle

5. *Radio enhancer or radio protector:* Certain chemicals may enhance radiation damage, e.g. oxygen; chemotherapy or some may protect against radiation damage.

The radiation damage occurs either through direct cellular damage or indirect cellular damage.

a. *Direct damage:* The energy transfer to the cellular DNA causes DNA break which lead to death. This type of damage happens less than 20 percent in conventional radiation treatment however, with high LET (charge particles) this damage if predominant.
b. *Indirect damage:* The radiation interacts with the cellular water to form free radical. The free radical causes DNA damage. This type of interaction is predominant (80 and 0 in conventional radiation treatment.

If the radiation causes the damage, why does it kill the tumor cells while preserving the normal cells? The damage occurs in both the normal and the abnormal cells but the normal cells have a fast and active repair mechanism which fixes the damages while the abnormal cells have a defective repair mechanism. When the radiation dose is administered, the cell's active repair mechanism is initiated; however, if the radiation dose is high the damage will occur in spite of the repair mechanism. The better the repair mechanism, the more resistant the cell is to the radiation. In order to utilize the differences in repair mechanism between normal cells and tumor cells "radiation fractionation" was established. By administering the radiation in multiple fractions you allow normal cells to repair the damage while tumor cells are killed. The gain of maximum tumor cell kills while reducing the radiation complication is the ideal goal of the therapy. While it is true that if you maximize tumor control you will introduce a certain percentage of normal tissue damage, fractionation, radio sensitizers, and radio protectors are employed to achieve a good therapeutic ratio.

The normal cells as we indicated earlier are different; some cells are fast growing with active reproduction and others are slow with slow reproduction. Damage to fast growing, early responding cells will cause early radiation reactions like mucositis, and dermatitis, while damage to late responding tissue will cause late reaction, e.g. blindness, fibrosis.

In head and neck cancer an important factor to be considered is tissue oxygenation. The hypoxia will reduce the charge of cell kill and reduce the likelihood of tumor control. Many studies have shown a correlation between anemia and a reduced number of tumors controlled due to hypoxemia (low oxygen).

BASIC PHYSICS

Radiation can be classified into two main categories:

1. Nonionizing radiation (cannot ionize matter)
2. Ionizing radiation (ionize matter): Ionizing radiation is the type used in therapeutic radiation and can be divided into (**Flow chart 74.1**):

Flow chart 74.1: Classification of radiation

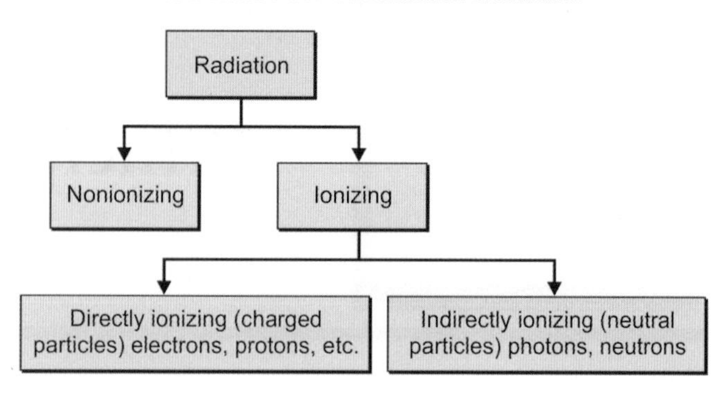

a. Direct ionizing radiation
b. Indirect ionizing radiation

Radiation can be found in nature as isotopes which can be used in different industries, as well as, sources of therapeutic radiation; examples of natural isotopes—cesium, iridium and iodine.

Radiation can also be produced by machines as a linear accelerator. The use of radiation as a mode of treatment for cancer depends on.

1. Energy of radiation
2. Distort of radiation.

The radiation interaction with tissue depends on the energy of radiation. Low energy radiation can be used for diagnostic purposes, however, high energy radiation can be used for cancer treatment. When radiation is delivered from a distance, i.e. from a machine we call it teletherapy and when radiation is inserted or placed close to the area we need to treat it is called brachytherapy.

TREATMENT PLANNING

In order to achieve a good balance between higher tumor cell kill with less tissue damage one how has to be meticulous in measuring the radiation doses to both normal and abnormal tissue. The radiation is measured by gray and each type of tissue has a radiation tolerance which should not be exceeded. Before radiation is delivered, physicists and dosimeterists use sophisticated computer programs to show the radiation delivered to the different tissue. Radiation oncologists work closely with the physicist to choose the type of radiation, how the radiation is delivered and the appropriate doses.

CLINICAL RADIOTHERAPY

Radiotherapy is used for cancer treatment in one of three (3) ways:

1. As neoadjuvant:
   Which means radiation is given before the definite

treatment. This type is not commonly used in treatment in head and neck cancer.
2. Sole treatment: Radiation can be used alone as a sole treatment as in early stage larynx cancer and chemotherapy in nasopharyngeal cancer and laryngeal and hypopharyngeal cancer.
3. Adjuvant treatment: This means radiation is used as a supplement to the definite treatment. Radiation is used in most advanced head and neck cancer after surgery.

Radiation also has an important role in palliation either to alleviate symptoms or reduce progression.

PROCESS OF RADIATION TREATMENT

Before offering radiation treatment to patients one has to complete certain processes.

Phase one—Diagnosis and staging: Every patient has to complete a diagnostic work-up which is aimed at:
1. Confirming pathological diagnosis.
2. Evaluating local extension of the disease.
3. Assessing regional mode involvement.
4. Excluding distant metastasis.

Phase two—Treatment decision: After completion of diagnostic work-up, the patient's condition is discussed in tumor board and mode of treatment is decided.

Phase three—Immobilization: Before starting radiation a planning fixation device is done in order to ensure fixation of head and neck region during treatment.

There are many fixation devices but "Aquaplast" is the most commonly used.

Phase four—Planning: The patient will undergo CT Scanning and in some cases MR Scanning for planning purposes. The images are transferred to the planning program. The radiation oncologist marks the tumor, potential area at risk and critical structure. Physicist starts planning to ensure maximum radiation dose to tumor area and minimum dose to critical structure.

Phase five—Treatment: After completion of the plan and carefully checking the plan, the patient undergoes a daily treatment. Port films which are X-ray films produced by the treatment machine are checked by the radiation oncologists to ensure that there is no deviation position between the plan and treatment.

Patient is seen weekly by physician to evaluate radiation side effects.

RADIATION COMPLICATION

As we indicated earlier radiation affects both normal and abnormal cells. The radiation side affects occur as a result of normal tissue damage. The damage to fast growing cells such as mucosa cells and skin lead to an early reaction or acute side effects, while the damage to slow growing cells such as connection tissue lead to late or chronic side effects. To measure the grading of side effects there are many scales, however, the "RTOG" scale is the most commonly used.

RTOG RADIATION SIDE EFFECTS SCORING SYSTEM

Guidelines

- The acute morbidity criteria are used to score/grade toxicity from radiation therapy. The criteria are relevant from day 1 of the commencement of therapy, through day 90. Thereafter, EORTC/RTOG criteria of late effects are to be utilized (**Tables 74.1 and 74.2**).
- The evaluation must attempt to discriminate between disease and treatment related signs and symptoms.
- An accurate baseline evolution prior to commencement of therapy is necessary (**Fig. 74.2**).

  The toxic reactions are graded from 1-5 and any toxicity which causes death is grade 5.

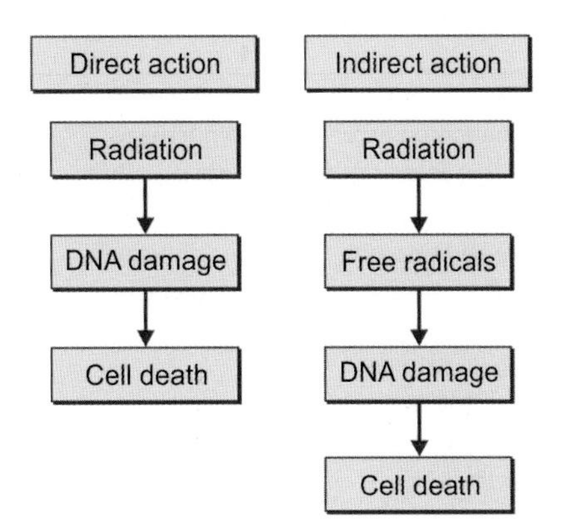

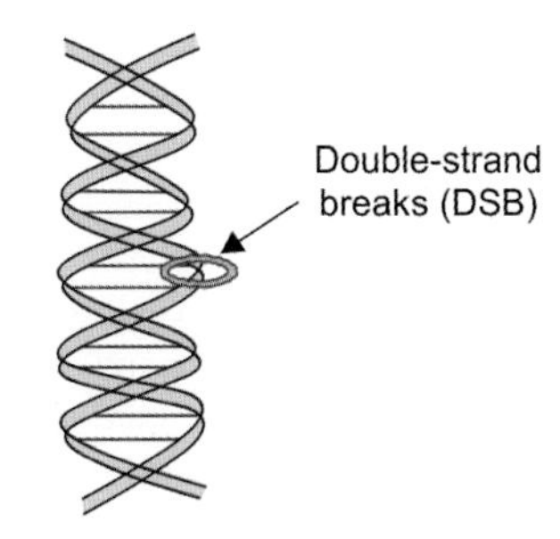

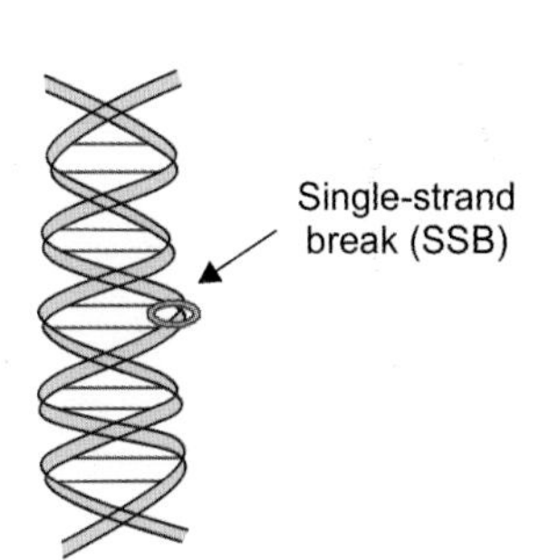

Fig. 74.2: Radiation effects on cells

Table 74.1: RTOG/EORTC late radiation therapy morbidity scoring scheme

Organ tissue	Grade 0	Grade 1	Grade 2	Grade 3	Grade 4	Grade 5
Skin	None	Slight atrophy, pigmentation, change some hair loss	Patch atrophy, moderate Telangiectasia total hair loss	Marked atrophy, gross telangiectasia	Ulceration	Death directly related to radiation late effects
Mucous membrane	None	Slight atrophy and dryness	Moderate atrophy and telangiectasia Little mucous	Marked atrophy with complete dryness Severe telangiectasia	Ulceration	
Eye	None	Asymptomatic cataract Minor corneal ulceration or keratitis	Symptomatic cataract Moderate corneal ulceration Minor retinopathy or glaucoma	Severe keratitis Severe retinopathy or detachment Server glaucoma	Panopthalmitis/ blindness	
Esophagus	None	Mild fibrosis Slight difficulty in swallowing solids No pain in swallowing	Unable to take solid food normally swallowing Semi-solid food dilation may be indicated	Severe fibrosis able to swallow only liquids may have pain on swallowing Dilatation required	Necrosis/ perforation Fistula	
Subcutaneous tissue	None	Slight indurations (fibrosis) and loss of subcutaneous fat	Moderate fibrosis but asymptomatic slight field contracture <10% linear reduction	Severe indurations and loss of subcutaneous tissue field contracture	Necrosis	
Salivary glands	None	Severe dryness of mouth Good response on stimulation	Moderate dryness of mouth Poor response on stimulation	Complete dryness of mouth No response on stimulation	Fibrosis	
Larynx	None	Hoarseness Slight arytenoids edema chondritis	Moderate arytenoids edema chondritis	Severe edema Severe chondritis	Necrosis	

Table 74.2: Acute radiation therapy morbidity scoring scheme

Organ tissue	0	1	2	3	4
Skin	No change over baseline	Follicular, faint or dull erythema/ epilation/ dry desquamation/ decreased sweating	Tender or bright erythema, patchy moist Desquamation/moderate edema	Confluent, moist desquamation other than skin folds, pitting edema	Ulceration, hemorrhage, necrosis
Eye	No change	Mild conjunctivitis with or without scleral injection increase tearing	Moderate conjunctivitis with or without keratitis requiring steroids and/ or antibiotics/dry eye requiring artificial tears/ iritis with photophobia	Severe keratitis with corneal ulceration/ objective decrease in visual acuity or in visual/fields/ acute glaucoma/ Panopthalmitis	Loss of vision (unilateral or bilateral)

Contd...

Contd...

Organ tissue	0	1	2	3	4
Salivary glands	No change over baseline	Mild mouth dryness/ slightly thickened saliva/may have slightly altered taste such as metallic taste/these changes not reflected in alteration in baseline feeding behavior such as increased use of liquids with meals	Moderate to complete dryness/thick sticky saliva/ markedly altered taste of mouth	—	Acute salivary gland necrosis
Larynx	No change over baseline	Mild or intermittent hoarseness/cough not requiring antitussive/ erythema of mucosa	Persistent hoarseness but able to vocalize/refereed ear pain, sore throat, patchy fibrinous exudates or mild arytenoids edema not requiring narcotic/ cough requiring antitussive	Whispered speech, throat pain or refereed ear pain requiring narcotic confluent fibrinous exudates, marked arytenoids edema	Marked dyspnea, stridor or hemoptysis with tracheotomy or intubation necessary
Mucous membrane	No change over baseline	Injection/may experience mild pain not requiring analgesics	Patchy mucositis which may produce an inflammatory serosanguinous discharge/ may experience moderate pain requiring analgesia	Confluent fibrinous mucositis/may include severe pain requiring narcosis	Ulceration hemorrhage, necrosis
Ear	No change over baseline	Mild external otitis with erythema, pruritis, secondary to dry desquamation not requiring medication. Audiogram unchanged from baseline	Moderate external otitis requiring topical medication/serious otitis media/hypoacusis on testing only	Severe external otitis with discharge moist desquamation/ symptomatic hypoacusis/ tinnitus/ not drug related	Deafness
Pharynx and esophagus	No change over baseline	Mild dysphagia or odynophagia/ may require topical anesthetic or non narcotic analgesics/may require soft diet	Mild dysphagia or odynophagia/ may require narcotic analgesics/ may require puree or liquid diet	Severe dysphagia or odynophagia with dehydration or weight loss (<15% from pre-treatment baseline) requiring N-G feeding tube. IV fluids or hyper alimentation	Complete obstruction ulceration/ perforation fistula

PATIENT CARE DURING RADIOTHERAPY

As patient shows certain reactions during and after radiotherapy special care is to be taken for:

i. *Nutrition*—if patient can swallow nicely, his diet should be supplemented by more proteins, vitamins, iron and minerals. If facing difficulty in swallowing, nasogastric tube feeding should be done. If blood counts fall, substitute blood or platelet transfusion should be given.
ii. *Oral hygiene*—dental check-up is must and due care to be given for proper oral cleaning and care for candidiasis, thrush or ulcers, e.g. stomatitis and glossitis treated by local application of nystatin or clotrimazole. No spices, smoking, alcohol or irritants to be taken.
iii. Skin reaction is often seen during radiotherapy though with megavoltage therapy reaction is very less. However, patient should take following precautions for irradiate skin, e.g. skin to be kept dry, no soap or water washing to be done, avoiding exposure to sunlight or heat and wet shaving, or plaster dressing or irritants. Topical application of antibiotic or antiallergic ointments may be used and the area covered with soft silk.

Chapter 75

Chemotherapy for Head and Neck Cancer

Chemotherapy as a treatment option in the management of head and neck cancer is useful in the setting of micrometastases or in the regional control of massive disease. Generally chemotherapy is more effective if used as combination with other agents. Chemotherapeutic agents decrease effect of cell resistance and increase kill rates at various points in cell cycle. The various drugs which are approved for the therapy generally are studied via clinical trials, which are undertaken in 3 phases:

Phase I: To assess safety, dosage, side effects

Phase II: Assess therapeutic activity at defined doses

Phase III: Compare new therapy to existing therapies with similar actions or efficacies.

Roles in Management of Head and Neck Cancer

A. For unresectable/unradiatable or metastatic disease, most studies give a figure of overall palliative response of 3 to 6 months with chemo alone in 33 percent of patients.
B. For unresectable advanced disease, chemotherapy offers improved survival with concurrent chemoradiation although higher combined rate of adverse effects are seen with this therapy.
C. For resectable advanced disease (neoadjuvant therapy), many studies have pointed out the advantage of this therapy in the presence of limited disease, e.g. 40 to 60 percent laryngeal organ preservation with concurrent chemo-rads has been reported to have 8 to 12 percent survival advantage.
D. Curative in select cases of nasopharyngeal Ca.

Chemo Agents Commonly Used

METHOTREXATE

- Binds to and inhibits dihydrofolate reductase → inhibits DNA synthesis
- *Side effects:* Myelosuppression, mucositis, N/V, hepatic fibrosis.

CISPLATIN

- DNA cross-linking agent
- Overall survival trend improval as compared with methotrexate
- *Side effects:* Nephrotoxicity, ototoxicity, neurotoxicity, myelosuppression
- Carboplatin (an analog) has ↓ nephro/ototoxicity, but slightly less anticancer action than cisplatin
- Major side-effect is myelosuppression.

5-FLUOROURACIL

- Blocks conversion of uracil to thymidine, thus inhibits DNA synthesis
- Adds to effect of cisplatin, but toxicity increased
- *Side effects:* Myelosuppression, mucositis, cardiac.

TAXANES (PACLITAXIL, GEMCITABINE)

- Block microtubule synthesis thus prevent mitosis
- Very active against head and neck cancer
- Undergoing Phase III trials.

RETINOIDS

- Recall field cancerization theory of Slaughter (clonal proliferation of CA cells along contiguous mucosa)
- Therefore, if some dysplastic cells are sensitive to a prophylactic agent, all should be postulated role in chemoprophylaxis of cancer, but literature sparse and toxicity high so not generally used yet.

PHOTODYNAMIC THERAPY

- Systemic photosensitizer which is preferentially incorporated into tumor cells
- Illumination (local/endoscopic) activates compound and kills cells.

Chapter 76

Syndromes in Otorhinolaryngology

Syndrome in ENT

ALBRIGHT'S SYNDROME

Symptoms and Signs

- It is an asymmetric disease of bones of face (osteitis fibrosa cystica) with melanotic pigmentation of skin
- Sexual precocity.

Treatment

- Facial asymmetry can be corrected by surgical procedure.

ALBRICH'S SYNDROME

Symptoms and Signs

- Chronic eczema
- CSOM
- Anemia
- Thrombocytic purpura.

Etiology

- Transmitted as sex linked recessive disorder.

ALPORT'S SYNDROME

Symptoms and Signs

- Presenile familial nerve deafness (Bilateral)
- Congenital hemorrhagic nephritis
- Keratoconus and cataracts.

Etiology

- Hereditary familial disorder, more frequently occurring in males.

Management

- Pure tone audiometry and urine examination
- Hearing aid.

ARNOLD-CHIARI SYNDROME OF MALFORMATION

Symptoms

- Stridor, cough due to aspiration, difficulty in feeding.

Signs

- Bilateral vocal cord paralysis, hydrocephalus, meningo-myelocele.

Etiology

- Traction upon the vagus nerve by protrusion of medulla and cerebellum through the foramen magnum.

Diagnostic Procedure

- Computed axial tomography (CAT) scanning, showing protrusion of medulla and cerebellum through foramen magnum.

Therapy

- Treatment of the cause
- Tracheostomy in emergency cases.

ASCHER'S SYNDROME

Symptoms and Signs

- Blepharochalasis, (acquired atrophy of skin of the upper eyelid)
- Adenoma of thyroid gland
- Redundancy of the mucous membrane and submucous tissue of upper lip.

AVELLIS' SYNDROME

- This syndrome is the result of a lesion involving the nucleus ambiguous or the vagus nerve and the cranial portion of accessory nerve. In addition, there is often contralateral loss of pain and temperature sensation due to spinothalamic tract destruction.

Symptoms

- Dysphagia
- Dysphagia due to laryngeal and pharyngeal paralysis, nasal regurgitation and rhinolalia due to paralysis of soft palate. The symptoms may be progressive in that the palatal paralysis may not develop before the laryngeal paralysis
- The cause is usually a vascular or inflammatory lesions in the medulla, but the diseases involving the vagus nerve above the level of nodose ganglion will cause similar paralysis
- Hoarseness of voice
- Nasal twang with regurgitation.

Signs

- Palatolaryngeal hemiplegia.

Etiology

- Effect on the 10th cranial nerve and palatal branch of 11th cranial nerve by an inflammatory or neoplastic lesion near jugular foramen.

Diagnostic Procedures

- CAT scanning showing—tumor mass in the jugular foramen.

Therapy

- Treatment of the cause.

BÁRÁNY'S SYNDROME

Symptoms

- Giddiness
- Deafness
- Tinnitus
- Pain in the back of the head.

Signs

- Vertigo and nystagmus most marked on looking to healthy side
- Falling and past pointing to diseased side.

Etiology

- It is caused by circumscribed serous meningitis in posterior cranial fossa caused after acute suppurative otitis media or after radical mastoidectomy.

Diagnosis

- H/O ASOM or radical mastoidectomy.

Therapy

- Labyrinthine sedatives, antibiotics.

BEHÇET'S SYNDROME

Symptoms

- Massive and indulent ulceration of mucous membranes and sometimes of skin of anogenital region
- Inflammation of eyes
- Pain
- Loss of weight.

Signs

- Ulcerations of mucous membrane and skin
- Iritis, hypopyon, choroiditis, retinitis.

Diagnosis

- Pyrexia
- Leukocytosis
- Increased ESR
- Negative serological test.

Etiology

- Unknown.

Treatment

- Steroids.

BRAIN'S SYNDROME

Symptoms

- Episodic attacks of nausea and vomiting resembling Ménière's disease
- Diplopia
- Vertigo
- Loss of vision
- Drowsiness
- Disturbance of consciousness with incoherent and difficult speech.

Signs

- Nystagmus
- Ataxia
- Hypotonia of limbs
- Bilateral papilloedema.

Etiology

- It is caused by cysticercosis of ventricle with degeneration of vestibular nuclei and also by the tumors of midbrain or cerebellum and of lateral ventricle.

Therapy

- Treatment of cause.

COGAN'S SYNDROME

Symptoms

- Pain in the eye, watering of the eye with diminution of vision
- Deafness
- Vertigo
- Tinnitus
- Nausea and vomiting.

Signs

- Nonsyphilitic interstitial keratitis with vestibuloauditory dysfunction.

Etiology

- Possibly a collagen disorder affecting young adults
- Nonspecific inflammatory disorder
- Degenerative changes found in inner ear, vestibular and spiral ganglia.

Diagnosis

- Characteristic signs and symptoms
- Negative serological tests.

CARDIOAUDITORY SYNDROME OF JERVELL AND LANGE-NIELSEN (1957)

Symptoms

- Deafness
- Fainting attacks.

Signs

- Recessive deafness
- Electrocardiogram (ECG) abnormalities
- Prolonged O-T interval
- Death following syncope due to cardiac arrest or arrhythmia.

Etiology

- Inherited autosomal recessive manner.

Therapy

- Symptomatic treatment.

CHORDA TYMPANI SYNDROME

Symptoms

- Sweating in the submental region.

Etiology

- It is due to misdirection of fibers of chorda tympani nerve after regeneration.

Therapy

- Section of the chorda tympani nerve by endaural route.

COLLET-SICARD SYNDROME

Symptoms

- Hoarseness of voice
- Nasal twang and regurgitation
- Difficulty in speech
- Reduced sense of taste.

Signs

- Homolateral paralysis of tongue, soft palate, larynx, neck muscles, associated with diminished sensation and reduced sense of taste due to simultaneous involvement of last four cranial nerves in the region of jugular foramen.

Etiology

- It is usually caused by neoplastic extension in the jugular foramen, trauma base of skull or basal meningitis.

Therapy

- Treatment of cause.

COSTEN'S SYNDROME

Symptoms

- Pain in the temporomandibular joint with referred otalgia
- Tinnitus and feeling of muffling in the ears.

Signs

- Malocclusion of temporomandibular joint.

Etiology

- Exactly not known. It is supposed to be due to unequal bites on the two sides of the mouth from malocclusion.
- Arthritis or subluxation of joint.

Diagnosis

- X-ray of the temporomandibular joint.

Therapy

- Correction of malocclusion.

CROCODILE TEAR SYNDROME

Symptoms

- Watering of the eye while eating.

Signs

- Gustatory lacrimation.

Etiology

- It is due to misdirection of nerve-fibers going to lacrimal gland after regeneration of facial nerve.

Treatment

- Resection of tympani nerve.

CROUZON'S SYNDROME

Symptoms

- Deafness
- Craniofacial dysostosis with small maxilla.

Signs

- Hypoplasia of maxilla, ectropion and districhiasis
- Additional row of eyelashes at the inner margin
- Hypertelorism
- Oxycephaly
- Bony ankylosis of stapes causing conductive deafness.

Etiology

- Familial hereditary disorder.

Therapy

- For stapes fixation stapedectomy is done.

DOWN'S SYNDROME (TRISOMY-21) (MONGOLISM)

Characteristic features are:

General

- Mental retardation, hypotonia.

Craniofacial Dysostosis

- Flat occiput, oblique palpebral fissure, epicanthic folds, specked iris, protruding tongue, prominent malformed ears, flat nasal bridge.

Thorax

- Congenital heart disease.

Abdomen and Pelvis

- Decreased acetabular and iliac angles, small penis, cryptorchidism.

Hands and Feet

- Simian crease, short broad hands, hypoplasia of middle phalynx of 5th finger, gap between 1st and 2nd toes.

Other Features

- High arched palate, strabismus, broad short neck, small teeth, furrowed tongue, intestinal atresia, imperforate anus.

DUANE'S SYNDROME

Symptoms

- Otic malformation
- Diplopia.

Signs

- Atresia of ear
- Congenital paresis of lateral rectus muscle.

Etiology

- First branchial arch anomaly. Occurs usually due to thalidomide use during pregnancy.

Therapy

- Plastic surgery of ear.

DYSMELIA SYNDROME

Symptoms

- Deafness
- Vestibular disorder
- Facial weakness
- Diplopia.

Signs

- Physical and otic malformations
- Abducent and facial nerve paralysis.

Etiology

- It is caused by the thalidomide, if used by pregnant ladies during first trimester.

EDWARDS' SYNDROME (TRISOMY-18)

Characteristic features are:

General

- Mental retardation, hypertonia, failure to thrive, preponderance in females, low birth weight.

Craniofacies

- Prominent occiput, micrognathia, low set malformed ears.

Thorax

- Congenital heart disease, mainly ventricular septal defect (VSD) and patent ductus arteriosus (PDA).

Abdomen and Pelvis

- Horse-shoe kidney, small pelvis, cryptorchidism, inguinal hernia.

Hands and Feet

- Flexion deformity of fingers, equinovarus.

Other Features

- Cleft lip and palate, ocular anomalies, webbed neck.

FRANCESCHETTI-ZWAHLEN SYNDROME

- Same as Treacher-Collins syndrome.

FREY'S SYNDROME (ALSO CALLED AS BAILLARGER'S SYNDROME AND AURICULOTEMPORAL SYNDROME)

Symptoms

- Flushing and sweating of face during swallowing.

Signs

- Gustatory flushing and sweating of face in the area of auriculotemporal nerve.

Etiology

- It is caused due to disturbance between sympathetic and parasympathetic fibers after parotidectomy or injury to parotid gland.

Therapy

- Resection of tympanic nerve.

GARDNER'S SYNDROME

Symptoms and Signs

- Multiple colonic polyposis which are premalignant
- Generalized multiple soft tissue swellings in the form of fibromas, lipomas, neurofibromas
- Multiple osteomas of facial bones.

Etiology

- It is an autosomal dominent conditions.

GOLDENHAR'S SYNDROME

Symptoms and Signs

- Otic anomalies like atresia of ear
- Facial anomalies like congenital eyelid dermoids notching of upper eyelid
- Vertebral anomalies (cervical).

Etiology

- First, branchial arch anomaly.

Therapy

- Plastic surgery of ear and face.

GRADENIGO'S SYNDROME

Symptoms

- Otorrhea
- Diplopia
- Retro-orbital pain or facial pain.

Signs

- Abducent nerve palsy
- Pain along trigeminal nerve, more retro-orbital.

Etiology

- It is caused by chronic suppurative otitis media (CSOM) with extension of infection to petrous apex.

Therapy

- Radical mastoidectomy with drainage of abscess from petrous apex.

GRISCHE'S SYNDROME

Symptoms

- Neck stiffness
- Palpitations.

Signs

- Stiffness of neck, opisthotonus, tachycardia, painful contracture of cervical muscles.

Treatment

- No pillows to be used, muscle relaxants and sedatives.

HEERFORDT'S SYNDROME

Symptoms

- Swelling of parotid gland
- Fever
- Pain and weakness.

Signs

- Enlarged parotid gland
- Iridocyclitis
- Pyrexia with paralysis of one or more cranial nerves usually facial paralysis. Boeck's sarcoidosis involving mucous membrane of upper respiratory tract.

Etiology

- Sarcoidosis

Therapy

- Treatment of the cause and steroids.

HORNER'S SYNDROME

Symptoms and Signs

- Miosis
- Apparent enophthalmos
- Narrowing of palpebral fissure due to ptosis
- Hyperemia of cheek
- Absence of facial sweating on one side of face due to absence of sympathetic innervation (anhydrosis).

HUGHLINGS JACKSON'S SYNDROME

Symptoms

- Hoarseness of voice
- Difficulty in speech
- Nasal twang and nasal regurgitation.

Signs

- Homolateral paralysis of tongue, soft palate, larynx and neck muscles.

Etiology

- It is due to involvement of 10th, 11th (Spinal part), and 12th cranial nerves by neoplastic extension in the jugular foramen, or intramedullary lesion.

Therapy

- Treatment of cause.

HURLER'S SYNDROME

Symptoms

- Deafness
- Visual disturbance
- Cutaneous lesions.

Signs

- Hereditary conductive deafness
- Skeletal deformities
- Hepatosplenomegaly
- Central nervous system (CNS) and cardiovascular system (CVS) changes (aortic incompetence)
- Inguinal and umbilical hernias
- Cutaneous abnormalities
- Corneal opacities.

Etiology

- It is an autosomal recessive pattern.

JACCOUD'S SYNDROME

Symptoms

- Visual disturbance
- Retro-orbital pain.

Signs

- Blindness
- Ophthalmoplegia
- Pain in the distribution of 5th cranial nerve.

Etiology

- It is caused by extension of nasopharyngeal carcinomas intracranialy.

Therapy

- Radiotherapy.

KALLMANN'S SYNDROME

Symptoms

- Loss of sense of smell.

Signs

- Evidence of anosmia and hypogonadism.

Etiology

- Hypoplasia of olfactory system
- Hypogonadism.

KARTAGENER'S SYNDROME

Symptoms

- Nasal discharge, mild headache.

Signs

- Sinusitis.
- Dextrocardia
- Cong. bronchiectasis
- Situs inversus
- Cystic fibrosis of pancreas.

Etiology

- Developmental abnormality.

Diagnosis

- X-ray chest (PA view)
- X-ray PNS (Water's view).

Klinkert's Syndrome

- It is paralysis of recurrent laryngeal nerve and phrenic nerve.
- Sympathetic paralysis may also be associated.

Etiology

- Neoplastic lesion in the root of neck or in superior mediastinum.
- Occurs mostly on left side.
- May be due to Pancoast's tumor.

KLIPPEL-FEIL SYNDROME

Symptoms

- Deafness
- Atresia of ear.

Signs

- Congenital hereditary deafness
- Congenital short neck due to fusion of cervical and thoracic vertebrae. Low hair line extending to back.

Etiology

- Hereditary disorder.

LAURENCE-MOON-BIEDL SYNDROME

Symptoms

- Visual disturbances
- Gait disturbances
- Voice disorders (remains high pitch).

Signs

- Always familial but never hereditary
- Pigmentary degeneration of retina
- Mental retardation
- Hypogenitalism
- Polydactyly
- Obesity
- Cerebellar ataxia and pituitary dysfunction.

Treatment

- Male hormones.

LERMOYEZ SYNDROME

Symptom

- Deafness and tinnitus precedes an attack of vertigo, after which there is immediate improvement in hearing.

Signs

- Perceptive deafness
- Nystagmus.

Etiology

- Spasm of internal auditory artery.

Therapy

- Antihistamines, e.g. phenargan
- Vasodilators, e.g. nicotinic acid.

MARFAN'S SYNDROME

Symptoms

- Deafness
- Diplopia.

Signs

- High arched palate
- Perceptive deafness
- Convergent squint
- Long tappering fingers
- Some toes are bigger, some are small.

MELKERSSON'S SYNDROME

Symptoms

- Bilateral facial weakness (may be familial)
- Swelling of the upper lip.

Signs

- Peripheral facial nerve palsy often bilateral
- Angioneurotic edema of face especially upper lip
- Lingua-Plicatea (Rosenthal's symptoms), i.e. congenital fissured or furrowed tongue.

Etiology

- Unknown, same as in Bell's palsy.

Treatment

- Same as for Bell's palsy (steroids and electric stimulation of facial nerve on paralysed side).

MÉNIÈRE'S SYNDROME

Symptoms

- Paroxysmal attacks of vertigo
- Deafness and tinnitus
- Heaviness in head
- Nausea and vomiting.

Signs

- Nystagmus present during the attacks of vertigo
- Perceptive deafness.

Etiology

- Various theories
- Thought to be due to spasm of vessels of striavascularis.

Treatment

- Medical
  - Vasodilators like nicotinic acid 100 mg tds
  - Diuretics
  - Tranquilizers
  - Labyrinthine sedatives, e.g. stemetil-5 mg tds or dramamine 50 mg tds.
- Surgical
  - Cervical sympathectomy
  - Myringotomy and grommet insertion
  - Stellate ganglion block
  - Shunt operations
  - Labyrinthectomy, cochlear dialysis.

MIKULICZ'S SYNDROME

Symptoms

- Swelling of salivary glands and lacrimal glands
- Dryness of mouth.

Signs

- Symmetrical enlargement of salivary glands
- Narrowing of palpebral fissure
- Parchment like dryness of mouth
- Usually associated with sarcoidosis.

MOEBIUS SYNDROME

Symptoms

- Deafness perceptive in nature
- Diplopia.

Signs

- Atresia of ear
- Congenital bilateral abducent palsy and aplasia of other brainstem nuclei.

Etiology

- Congenital anomaly.

Treatment

- Plastic surgery of ear.

MONDINI'S DEAFNESS

Symptom

- Deafness.

Sign

- Perceptive deafness (genetic).

Etiology

- Partial aplasia of both the osseous and the membranous labyrinths.

Treatment

- Hearing aid.

MORGAGNI'S SYNDROME

- Frontal intimal hyperostosis.

ORTNER'S SYNDROME (CARDIOVOCAL SYNDROME)

Symptoms

- Hoarseness of voice
- Aphonia.

Signs

- Paralysis of left recurrent laryngeal nerve, aphonia is present when patient turns his head to left. This is due to lack of compensatory movement of right vocal cord in this position, signs of mitral valve disease.

Etiology

- Paralysis of left recurrent laryngeal nerve secondary to mitral valve disease.

Therapy

- Treatment of mitral valve disease.

PANCOAST'S SYNDROME

Symptoms and Signs

- Neuritic pain in the arm
- Atrophy of muscles of arm and hand
- Associated Horner's syndrome
- Osteolysis of ribs and vertebrae
- Coin shadow on X-ray chest at apex of lung.

Etiology

- Usually due to tumor of apex of lung.

PATAU'S SYNDROME (TRISOMY-13)

Characteristic features are:

General

- Mental retardation, failure to thrive, capillary hemangiomas, persistent fetal hemoglobin.

Craniofacies
- Microcephaly, cleft lip and palate, midline scalp dermoids, coloboma, low-set malformed ears, deafness.

Thorax
- Congenital heart disease like PDA and VSD.

Abdomen and Pelvis
- Polycystic kidney, bicornuate uterus, cryptorchidism.

Hand and Feet
- Polydactyly, hyperconvex finger nails, simian crease.

Other Features
- Micrognathia, retroflexible thumb.

PATERSON-BROWN-KELLY SYNDROME (1919)

Symptoms
- Dysphagia.

Signs
- Glossitis with loss of papillae
- Lips and corners of mouth are often cracked
- Koilonychia
- Splenomegaly
- Anemia
- Achlorhydria.

Etiology
- Thought to be due to iron deficiency.

Therapy
- Dilatation of stricture through an esophagoscope
- Blood transfusion—iron preparations orally.

PENDRED'S SYNDROME

Symptoms
- Deafness
- Swelling of thyroid gland.

Signs
- Inherited perceptive deafness (cong. deafness, goiter in nonendemic districts).

Etiology
- Congenital disorder.

Management
- Hearing aid.

PERMANENT PERFORATION SYNDROME

Symptoms
- Deafness
- Discharge from ear.

Signs
- Mechanical defect in the tympanic membrane which exposes the middle ear mucosa to recurrent infections. They are confined to pars tensa and vary in size, shape and position but retain healed edge. Conductive deafness with 20 to 45 dB loss, patient may hear better when ear is discharging due to partial closure of perforation with mucous or loading of the round window.

Therapy
- Keep ear dry
- Myringoplasty.

PEUTZ'S SYNDROME (PEUTZ-JEGHERS SYNDROME)

Symptoms
- Bleeding per rectum
- Severe abdominal pain
- Constipation.

Signs
- Familial intestinal polyposis affecting mainly jejunum, melanosis of the oral mucous membrane.

Therapy
- Snare the polypi by means of a fiberoptic colonoscope.

PICKWICKIAN SYNDROME

Symptoms and Signs
- Exogenous obesity
- Obstructive sleep apnea
- Somnolence
- Hypoventilation of lungs
- Erythrocytosis.

PIERRE ROBIN SYNDROME

Symptoms
- Deaf and dumb, micrognathia.

Signs
- Congenital deaf-mutism
- Deformities of external and middle ear
- Cleft lip and palate
- Hypertelorism
- Mandibular dysostosis
- Glossoptosis.

Etiology
- Abnormal development of first and second branchial arches.

RAMSAY-HUNT SYNDROME (HUNT'S SYNDROME)

Symptoms

- Pain in the ear
- Loss of taste on anterior 2/3rd of tongue
- Facial weakness
- Deafness
- Vertigo.

Signs

- Pain in the ear and palatoglossal arch
- Vesicles along the distribution of nerve of Wrisberg
- Loss of taste on anterior 2/3rd of tongue
- Facial paralysis
- Deafness.

Etiology

- Herpes zoster of geniculate ganglion of facial nerve.

REITER'S SYNDROME

Symptoms

- Pain in the eye with watering of eye
- Pain in joint
- Pain during micturition.

Signs

- Purulent conjunctivitis
- Urethritis
- Arthritis
- Erythrocyte sedimentation rate (ESR) raised
- White blood cell (WBC) count increased.

Etiology

- Veneral in origin.

Treatment

- No specific treatment
- Eye baths and shades
- TAB vaccine.

SCHMIDT'S SYNDROME

Symptoms

- Hoarseness of voice
- Nasal twang with regurgitation.

Signs

- Paralysis of soft palate, pharynx, larynx, sternomastoid and trapezius muscles.

Etiology

- Involvement of 10th and 11th cranial nerves by inflammatory or neoplastic lesion or vascular lesion in caudal portion of medulla.

Therapy

- Treatment of the cause.

SHY-DRAGER SYNDROME

Symptoms

- Hoarseness of voice
- Vocal cord paralysis.

Signs

- Extrapyramidal signs with severe autonomic features.

SJÖGREN'S SYNDROME (KERATOCONJUNCTIVOUVEITIS SICCA)

- Mikulicz syndrome associated with generalized arthritis.

SPRENGEL'S SYNDROME

Symptoms

- Skeletal deformities.

Signs

- Scapula lies at an abnormally high level and is distorted and hypoplastic in shape
- Cervical rib
- Absence or malformation of ribs
- Spina bifida
- Hemivertebrae
- Shortened humerus or clavicle
- Defect in regional muscle (Trapezius).

STEVENS-JOHNSON SYNDROME

Symptoms

- Pain during swallowing
- Fever.

Signs

- Severe stomatitis-ulcerative lesions
- Purulent conjunctivitis
- Acute febrile reaction.

Etiology

Drugs like:

- Sulfonamides
- Thiacetazone

- INH
- Tetracyclines.

STURGE-WEBER SYNDROME

Symptoms and Signs

- Vascular nevi (hemangiomas) along the course of superior and middle branches of trigeminal nerve
- Glaucoma on same side
- Hemangiomas of piamater.

SUBCLAVIAN STEAL SYNDROME

Symptoms and Signs

- Vertigo which is more aggravated by neck twisting.

Etiology

- Deficiency of cerebral circulation as a result of drainage of blood from brain to upper extremity when ipsilateral subclavian artery is obstructed proximal to origin of vertebral artery.
- The compression may occur due to:
  1. Scaleneus anticus muscle
  2. Osteoarthritic spur
  3. Disk herniation
  4. Internal artery sclerotic patch.

Diagnosis

- Arteriography should be done.

TAPIA'S SYNDROME

Symptoms

- Hoarseness of voice
- Difficulty in speaking.

Signs

- Paralysis of larynx and tongue.

Etiology

- Paralysis of 10th and 12th cranial nerves by an inflammatory or neoplastic lesions.

Therapy

- Treatment of the cause.

TAY-SACHS SYNDROME

Symptoms

- Ear discharge
- Visual disturbances
- Jews are usually affected.

Signs

- Amaurotic idiocy
- Cherry red macula
- Otorrhea
- Progressive mental impairment ending in absolute idiocy
- Progressive paralysis of whole body
- Progressive diminution in vision ending in absolute blindness
- Optic atrophy
- Cherry red spots near macula
- Nystagmus
- Hyperacusis.

Etiology

- Due to inborn error in lipid metabolism, usually affecting certain families and certain races like Jews.

Treatment

- No certain treatment, some patients temporarily respond to corticosteroids.

TREACHER-COLLINS SYNDROME

- It is also called a Franceschetti-Zwahlen syndrome.

Symptoms

- Aural abnormalities in the form of anotia or micro-otia
- Deafness.

Signs

- Underdeveloped lower half of face, especially mandible and maxilla
- Notched lower eyelid, called coloboma
- Poorly developed eyelashes (No eyelashes in medial 2/3rd of lower eyelid)
- Microtia or anotia
- Especially the maxilla and mandible
- External auditory canal atresia and middle ear abnormalities
- Abnormal prolongation of hair line on the cheek
- Antimongoloid eyes.

Etiology

- Hereditary malformation of 1st and 2nd branchial arch derivatives.

Treatment

- Plastic surgery of ears and mandible.

TROTTER'S SYNDROME

Symptoms

- Deafness
- Nasal twang of voice
- Facial pain.

Signs

- Soft palate paralysis on ipsilateral side, with curtain movement of palate
- Conductive deafness due to eustachian tube obstruction
- Facial neuralgia due to involvement of maxillary division of trigeminal nerve.

Etiology

- It is caused by local spread of nasopharyngeal tumors.

Diagnostic Aids

- Pure tone audiometry
- X-ray nasopharynx and base of skull.

Treatment

- Radiotherapy.

TURNER'S SYNDROME

- It occurs in females due to chromosomal abnormality.

Symptoms

- Short neck
- Absence of secondary sexual characters.

Signs

- Sexual infantalism
- Cubitus vulgus
- Short webbed neck.

Etiology

- Due to chromosomal abnormality.

USHER'S SYNDROME

Symptoms

- Deafness
- Visual disturbances in the form of night blindness.

Signs

- Perceptive deafness
- Retinitis pigmentosa.

Diagnostic Aids

- Pure tone audiometry
- Funduscopy
- Perimetry.

Treatment

- Hearing aids.

VAN DER HOEVE-DE KLEYN SYNDROME

Symptoms

- Deafness
- Osteogenesis imperfecta
- Blue sclerotics
- Otosclerotic deafness
- Repeated fractures of bones.

Signs

- Otosclerotic deafness
- Brittle bones
- Blue sclerotics
- Osteogenesis imperfecta.

Diagnostic Aids

- Pure tone audiometry
- Skeletal survey by X-rays.

Treatment

- Stapedectomy
- Hearing aids.

VERNET'S SYNDROME

Signs and Symptoms

- Signs and symptoms same as Schmidt's syndrome associated with diminution of taste over posterior third of tongue and loss of pharyngeal sensation.
- Hoarseness of voice.
- Nasal twang with regurgitation.
- Diminution of taste over posterior 2/3rd of tongue.

Etiology

- Paralysis of 9th, 10th and 11th cranial nerves due to inflammatory or neoplastic lesions.
- It is due to 9th, 10th and 11th cranial nerve paralysis due to inflammatory or neoplastic involvements.

Therapy

- Treat the cause
- Radiotherapy in neoplastic lesions and surgical intervention in inflammatory lesions.

Signs

- Laryngeal paralysis (vocal cords)
- Soft palate paralysis
- Loss of pharyngeal sensations.

Diagnostic Aids

- X-ray nasopharynx, jugular bulb and base of skull.

VILLARET'S SYNDROME

It is same as Vernet's syndrome but is also associated with Horner's syndrome and hence its features are:

- 9th, 10th, spinal part of 11th, and hypoglossal paralysis
- Horner's syndrome.

Etiology

- It occurs due to lesions in the space posterior to parotid gland, usually by a tumor.

Treatment

- Excision with radiotherapy.

VOGT-KOYANAGI-HARADA SYNDROME

Symptoms

- Deafness
- Pain along the distribution of nerve
- Patchy loss of hair
- White patches on skins.

Signs

- Perceptive deafness
- Neuralgia
- Alopecia areata
- Vitiligo
- Whitening of eyelashes.

Etiology

- Not known exactly.

Therapy

- Carbamazepine for neuralgic pain and hearing aids for deafness.

VON WILLEBRAND'S SYNDROME

Symptoms

- Epistaxis
- Prolonged bleeding from minor injuries.

Signs

- Purpuric spots
- Prolonged bleeding time.

Etiology

- It is a hereditary disease inherited as autosomal dominant characterised by prolonged bleeding time and factor VIII deficiency.

Diagnostic Aids

- Hemogram.

Treatment

- Replacement of blood with fresh blood or with purified factor VIII.
- Aminocaproic acid may also be helpful.

WAARDENBURG'S SYNDROME (1851)

Symptoms

- Deafness.

Signs

- Hypertelorism (Broad nasal root)
- Congenital perceptive deafness
- Heterochromia iridia
- Frontal bosses
- White fore lock
- Hypertrichosis of medial portion of eyebrows.

Etiology

- Hereditary familial disorder (dominent).

WALLENBERG'S SYNDROME (AUTOSOMAL DOMINANT)

Symptoms

- Dysphagia
- Vertigo
- Diplopia
- Imbalance
- Nystagmus
- Muscular paralysis.

Etiology

- It occurs due to occlusion of posterior inferior cerebellar artery or its branch supplying lower part of brainstem.

Therapy

- Treatment the cause.

WALLENBERG'S SYNDROME (LATERAL MEDULLARY SYNDROME)

Symptom

- Severe paroxysm of vertigo with vomiting.

Signs

- Deafness
- Neurological signs due to medullary infarction.

Etiology

- Thrombosis of posterior inferior cerebellar artery.

Treatment

- Anticoagulants.

WERNICKE'S SYNDROME

Symptoms

- Vertigo
- Pain on moving the eyeball.

Signs

- Nystagmus
- Ophthalmoplegia
- Ataxia.

Etiology

- Acute thiamine deficiency.

Therapy

- Thiamine in large doses.

WHISTLING FACE SYNDROME

Symptoms and Signs

- Microstome, flattended mid face as in whistling, deep seated eyes, coloboma, alterations of nasal wings, kyphoscoliosis, talipes equinovarus, ulnar deviation of fingers.

WILDERVANCK'S SYNDROME

Symptoms

- Short neck
- Diplopia.

Signs

- Cervical dysostosis of Klippel syndrome
- Retraction of eye
- Sixth nerve palsy.

Chapter 77

Otolaryngologic Concerns in the Syndromal Child

More than 3,000 known syndromes have been classified in humans. The evaluation and management of children with these syndromes requires the appropriate knowledge and support of multiple specialists. Otolaryngologists are often consulted in the diagnosis and management of the syndromal child. The focus of this chapter is to identify several common syndromes affecting children, and the otolaryngologic significance of these syndromes.

Airway

Understanding the development of the airway and anatomic variations from normal are critical to the otolaryngologist. Newborns are obligate nasal breathers until about 4 to 6 weeks. Mouth breathing is a learned response. Congenital nasal obstruction or stenosis presents a life-threatening problem. Choanal atresia and midface hypoplasia may present in the neonate as respiratory distress with cyanosis. This is usually effectively initially treated with an oral airway until further surgical management is planned. Micrognathia, retrognathia, glossoptosis, and macroglossia may also significantly obstruct the airway which may be first treated by a nasal airway and prone feeding, and further with adenotonsillectomy when appropriate. A tracheotomy is indicated when other measures have not been successful. In some instance, support and growth of the child is sufficient. Mandibular osteotomies and distraction may be required for malocclusion, when growth is insufficient.

The management of the airway provides a challenge to medical personnel, and it is the responsibility of the otolaryngologist to attain and maintain an appropriate airway for a child with craniofacial anomalies. Communication with the anesthesiologist is critical when operating on a syndromal child. Evaluation of the airway includes examination of the entire airway. This may be achieved by flexible laryngoscopy, direct laryngoscopy, and tracheobronchoscopy. Stertor and the type of stridor provide clues to the level of airway obstruction.

Appropriate management of the pediatric airway requires familiarity with the instruments needed to evaluate and care for the airway. The appropriate size, length, and type of laryngoscope and bronchoscope for each case should be evaluated prior to performing direct laryngoscopy. As a general rule, all instruments should be connected and checked prior to the start of an airway case.

The otolaryngologist may be involved in the management of obstructive sleep apnea in a child with craniofacial anomalies. It is important to understand that functional anomalies contribute to the problem of airway obstruction when developing treatment strategies. Polysomnography is essential in the diagnosis of obstructive sleep apnea. Continuous positive airway pressure may be beneficial in some cases. The management of obstructive sleep apnea (OSA) may require adenotonsillectomy, uvulopalatopharyngoplasty, partial tongue base resection, resection of redundant laryngeal structures, or tracheotomy.

Hearing Loss

Children with craniofacial anomalies are at risk of having or developing hearing loss. Hearing is essential for learning language and verbal communication, as well as education. Therefore, the careful evaluation of the syndromal child includes an appropriate otologic and audiologic examination. Delay in the detection of hearing loss may be very deleterious in the development of the child.

Congenital hearing loss is predominantly conductive in nature, but sensorineural hearing loss may also be involved. Congenital conductive hearing loss may be secondary to microtia, external auditory canal atresia, and ossicular deformity or fixation. In these instances, an appropriate audiologic evaluation with radiography is required prior to surgical correction. If these problems are unilateral, appropriate language development is possible if the hearing in the unaffected ear is optimized. Early detection of otitis media and administration of antibiotics or placement if ventilation tubes, when appropriate, are necessary in the normal ear. Eustachian tube dysfunction (ETD) is common in children with craniofacial anomalies, especially cleft lip/palate, and usually is effectively treated with placement of ventilation tubes. Pressure equalization(PE) tubes may be required into adolescence to prevent hearing loss and complications from ETD.

Speech Disorders

Speech disorders are common in children with craniofacial anomalies, especially in children with nasal obstruction and cleft palate. Hypernasal speech is a common finding in velopharyngeal insufficiency (VPI) following cleft palate repair. Speech therapy is usually sufficient; however, palatopharyngoplasty may be required for children with persistent VPI over the age of 5 years. Hyponasal speech is less common and results from nasal obstruction, which is usually surgically correctable. Hoarseness is another speech abnormality usually due to the development of vocal cord nodules in compensatory laryngeal activity. This may also result from intubation trauma.

Down Syndrome

Down syndrome is the most common syndrome known in humans. It was first described in 1866 by John Landon Down. The prevalence has been estimated as high as 1 in 700 humans. Approximately 95 percent of cases are due to nondisjunction of chromosome 21 in gametogenesis. The remaining cases are from unbalanced translocations. There is a high association with increased maternal age. Maternal age of 33 to 35 carries a 2.8 in 1,000 risk, and maternal age of greater than 44 years carries a 38 in 1,000 risk. There is a 1 percent risk of having a child with Down syndrome if a sibling has this syndrome. Screening methods have been developed and include ultrasonography, alfa-fetoprotein level, human chorionic gonadotropin and unconjugated estriol levels. The average life expectancy of individuals with Down syndrome is 35 years, with highest mortality early in infancy due to congenital heart defects, leukemia, and respiratory distress.

Common signs in a newborn with Down syndrome include hypotonia, poor Moro reflex, hyperextensible joints, loose skin on nape, flattened facial profile, upward slanting palpebral fissures, single palmar crease, flat occiput, and epicanthal folds. Prenatal and postnatal growth deficiency is present in almost all cases. Interestingly, in older patients, Alzheimer disease is common. This is believed to be due to an abnormality of amyloid beta-A4 precursor mapped to chromosome 21.

The craniofacial manifestations of Down syndrome include the absence of the frontal and sphenoid sinuses with maxillary sinus hypoplasia in 90 percent of cases, a flattened nasal bridge with relative mandibular prognathism (midface hypoplasia), small ears with overlapping helix, epicanthal folds and upward slanting palpebral fissures. Atlantoaxial instability is a common finding that must be acknowledged when manipulating the head and neck. Macroglossia with a fissured or geographic tongue is also common. Periodontal disease is found in 90 percent of cases with a relatively low incidence of dental caries.

The otolaryngologic concerns include airway obstruction and hearing loss. Due to midface hypoplasia, the nasopharynx and oropharynx dimensions are smaller and slight adenoid hypertrophy may result in upper airway obstruction. Obstructive sleep apnea is a very common finding ranging from 54 to 100 percent of cases and is due to a combination of anatomic and physiologic abnormalities. Hypotonia with macroglossia and midface hypoplasia contribute to the development of OSA. Polysomnography is diagnostic of OSA, and there are several management options available. Medical management including Continuous positive airway pressure (CPAP) and weight loss when indicated is effective in some cases. However, surgical management is required when medical management in not effective. Adenotonsillectomy alone is a controversial approach due to hypotonia in addition to possible lymphoid hypertrophy. Uvulopalatopharyngoplasty and partial tongue resection are other surgical options. A tracheotomy is the most effective manner to bypass upper airway obstruction when other options have failed. It is also important to note that there is evidence of congenital mild to moderate subglottic narrowing in patients with Down syndrome. Therefore, postextubation stridor is not an uncommon finding.

The otologic issues include a small pinna and stenotic external auditing canal (EAC) which contribute to cerumen impaction in Down syndrome patients. Conductive hearing loss may be secondary to chronic otitis media with effusion and eustachian tube dysfunction. This may be addressed with placement of ventilation tubes. Ossicular fixation is also not uncommon, and may be surgically managed. Sensorineural hearing loss is present in relatively few cases, and is attributed to progressive ossification along outflow pathway of the basal spiral tract.

Cardiovascular anomalies in Down syndrome is present in 40 percent of cases and may range from ventricular septal defects, atrial septal defects, tetralogy of Fallot, and patent ductus arteriosus. Gastrointestinal involvement in 10 to 18 percent includes pyloric stenosis, duodenal atresia, and tracheoesophageal fistula. Of importance is the 20 fold higher incidence of acute lymphocytic leukemia in patients with Down syndrome compared to patients without Down syndrome. It is important to have all systemic issues addressed in the team approach to the management of Down syndrome.

Velocardiofacial Syndrome

Velocardiofacial syndrome (VCFS) is one of the most common syndromes involving the head and neck. The prevalence may be as high as 1 in every 4,000 births. Although patients may appear normal, they have characteristic facial structures. For these reasons, it is essential for otolaryngologists to be familiar with the facial anomalies and physiologic disturbances these patients may display. This syndrome typically has a manifestation of congenital heart disease, hypernasal speech, cleft palate, learning disabilities, and a characteristic facial appearance. An estimated 8 percent of cleft palate clinic patients have VCFS. The inheritance pattern is autosomal dominant with variable expressivity. In 85 percent of cases there is hemizygous microdeletion shared with the DiGeorge sequence at the *22q11.2* locus.

The oropharyngeal findings include structural malformations of the neck in 75 percent of cases, but may vary from readily apparent cleft palate (10–35%), submucous cleft (33%), occult submucous cleft and velar paresis (33%), and a hypernasal speech pattern. Malocclusion is a common finding. The tonsils and adenoids are small or aplastic in 50 percent and 85 percent of cases, respectively. Airway obstruction is not an uncommon finding and up to 50 percent of neonates are diagnosed with obstructive sleep apnea. However, it is very important to avoid tonsillectomy and adenoidectomy in these patients as the obstruction does not improve after this surgery. An oropharyngeal or a nasopharyngeal airway is useful in the urgent setting. Ultimately, repair of the cleft palate or surgical management of velopharyngeal apparatus may be required.

The facial characteristics in VCFS include microcephaly, a long face with vertical maxillary excess, malar flatness, and retrusion of the mandible. The nose is usually prominent with a squared nasal root, hypoplasia of the alae, and narrow nasal passages. The philtrum is usually long with a thin upper lip. Facial asymmetry is not uncommon. In addition, 15 percent of cases exhibit Pierre Robin sequence and 15 percent with Pierre Robin have VCFS. In 35 to 50 percent of cases, the palpebral fissures may appear narrow with allergic shiners. Opthalmologic findings small optic disks, bilateral cataracts, tortuous retinal vessels, and rarely colobomas may be present. Anomalies of the ears are common and include small auricles with thickened helical rims. In 75 percent of cases, CHL is present and likely is due to serous otitis media and cleft palate. SNHL may be present in 8 to 15 percent of cases.

Cardiovascular anomalies are present in 75 to 85 percent cases of VCFS. Ventricular septal defects, right-sided aortic arch, aberrant subclavian artery, and tetralogy of Fallot are common cardiac problems. Approximately 10 percent of infants with VCFS die as a result of congenital cardiac defects. The internal carotid arteries are medially displaced and tortuous in 25 percent of cases, but generally straighten with age. This should always be acknowledged prior to cleft repair.

Mild mental retardation and poor social interaction with a flat affect may be present in some individuals. Renal anomalies may be present in 35 percent of cases. Skeletal growth is also retarded in a large proportion of cases. Hypocalcemia and immunologic findings of T-cell dysfunction, allude to a relationship to the DiGeorge sequence in 15 percent of patients. Both, failure to thrive and frequent infections are present in this population.

The appropriate diagnosis and management of patients with VCFS requires a coordinated team effort of multiple specialties. The most critical factors include appropriate management of cardiac defects early in life and maintenance of good health through early childhood. Hearing and speech impediments must be appropriately managed, as well any disturbances to vision to allow for the greatest academic development. Communication between otolaryngologists, craniofacial surgeons, cardiologists, nephrologists, ophthalmologists, pediatricians, speech pathologists, teachers, and parents is essential in caring for patients with such diverse medical problems.

Branchio-otorenal Syndrome

Branchio-otorenal syndrome (BORS) was first termed by Melnick et al in 1975. It has a prevalence of 1 in every 40,000 newborns and has an autosomal dominant inheritance pattern with high penetrance typically isolated to the gene at the *8q13.3* locus. The characteristics of this syndrome are most commonly branchial cleft cysts or fistulas, preauricular pits, malformed auricles, hearing loss and renal anomalies.

Branchial cleft cysts, sinuses, or fistulas are present in 50 to 60 percent of cases, predominantly found in the lower third of the neck, and are usually bilateral. Fistulas, when present, may open into the tonsillar fossa. Facial nerve paralysis and aplasia/stenosis of the lacrimal duct are not uncommon (10% and 25% of cases, respectively).

The otologic manifestations of BORS range from structural anomalies of the external ear to the inner ear. Auricular malformations are found in 30 to 60 percent of cases and vary from severe microtia to minor anomalies of the pinna. Helical or preauricular pits are present in 70 to 80 percent of cases, and rarely communicate with the tympanic cavity. Hearing loss in present in 75 to 95 percent of affected individuals, composed of conductive (30%), sensorineural (20%), and mixed hearing loss (50%). The onset of hearing loss may vary from early childhood to young adulthood. The middle ear anomalies include malformation and/or fixation of ossicles and abnormal size or structure of the tympanic cavity. In the inner ear, anomalies, although rare, include dilated vestibule and/or endolymphatic duct/sac, bulbous internal auditory canal, small semicircular canals, and hypoplastic cochlea.

The structural anomalies of the urinary system are present in 12 to 20 percent of cases. This is likely under-reported as only 6 percent of those with renal involvement have severe symptoms. The anomalies range from renal agenesis to mild hypoplasia or abnormalities of the renal pelvis or ureters.

Appropriate diagnosis of BORS is dependent upon a thorough history and physical examination. One must keep a high index of suspicion when ear anomalies, hearing loss, neck masses/sinuses, and renal problems are encountered.

Initial management includes antibiotics for infected branchial cleft sinuses/cysts and an audiogram. Profound hearing loss has been found in 1 of 200 individuals with preauricular pits. Further management includes neck CT and possibly temporal bone CT if hearing loss is present. When clinically appropriate a renal ultrasound or intravenous pyelogram may be beneficial. Genetic counseling is beneficial for families.

The treatment for branchial cleft cyst/sinus/fistula is surgical excision to prevent repeated infection and possibility of airway obstruction or dysphagia. The external ear may also be addressed surgically, from microtia repair to simple excision of preauricular pits. Ossicular chain reconstruction may be performed, when indicated, to improve hearing. Hearing aid devices are used frequently when hearing is impaired. Consultation with urologic specialists is appropriate when there is renal involvement.

Treacher Collins Syndrome

Mandibulofacial dysostosis was first described by Thomson and Toynbee in 1846-1847. The essential elements of this syndrome were later described by Treacher Collins in 1960. It is a relatively uncommon syndrome with an incidence of 1 in 50,000 births, and is an autosomal dominant disorder with variable expressivity. The gene called Treacle or *TCOF1*, has been mapped to the *5q32-33.1* locus. Approximately 60 percent of cases are from new mutations, and have an association with increased paternal age. The pathogenesis is likely derived from abnormal migration of neural crest cells into the first and second branchial arch structures. The features of this syndrome are mostly bilateral and symmetric. The characteristics include supraorbital and malar hypoplasia resulting in relatively large appearance of the nose, a narrow face with downward sloping palpebral fissures, malformed pinna, receding chin, and relatively large down-turned mouth.

In addition to malar hypoplasia and nonfused zygomatic arches, the paranasal sinuses are often hypoplastic. The mandibular components are also often hypoplastic, with a concave shape to the undersurface of the mandibular body. The angle of the mandible is also more obtuse than normal. Colobomas of the outer third of the lower eyelid and absence of the lower eyelid cilia may also be present. Cleft palate is found in 35 percent of cases with an additional 30 to 40 percent with palatopharyngeal incompetence.

Abnormalities of the airway include choanal atresia resulting in respiratory distress in the newborn. Obstructive sleep apnea is the most common breathing dysfunction and is frequently caused by mandibular hypoplasia that displaces the tongue posteriorly into the oropharynx. An oral airway may assist ventilation, but a tracheotomy may be performed if needed.

Otologic manifestations include a malformed pinna often misplaced toward the angle of the mandible. One-third of patients with anomalous pinna have EAC atresia or ossicular abnormalities. Conductive hearing loss is common and must be addressed for normal development. It is important to recognize that intelligence is usually normal in patients with Treacher Collins syndrome.

Apert and Crouzon Syndromes

Apert and Crouzon syndromes belong to the family of syndromes with craniosynostoses. Although each is unique, they share some characteristics.

Wheaton first described the features of acrocephalosyndactyly in 1894, but Apert expanded on this syndrome in 1906. Apert syndrome is characterized by craniosynostosis, midfacial malformations, and symmetric syndactyly of the hands and feet. The prevalence of Apert syndrome is 15 to 16 per million newborns and contributes to 4 to 5 percent of all craniosynostoses. It has an autosomal dominant inheritance pattern, but, most cases are sporadic from new mutations associated with increased paternal age.

The coronal sutures are fused in Apert syndrome at birth, with larger than normal heal circumference. The cranial base is malformed and often asymmetric with a short anterior cranial fossa. Shallow orbits result in exophthalmos. The midface is retruded and hypoplastic in some cases, resulting in relative prognathism. The nasal bridge may be depressed and the nose is usually beaked. Hypertelorism, downward slanting palpebral fissures, proptosis, strabismus, and cleft palate are frequently associated.

In 1912, Crouzon first described the characteristics of craniofacial dysostosis. These features were craniosynostosis, maxillary hypoplasia, shallow orbits, and ocular proptosis. It is inherited in an autosomal dominant patter with one-third of cases reported to be sporadic. The prevalence of Crouzon syndrome is also 15 to 16 per million newborns and accounts for 4.5 percent of all craniosynostoses.

In Crouzon syndrome fusion of cranial sutures begins during the first year of life and usually complete by 2 to 3 years of age. Shallow orbits with exophthalmos at birth without involvement of the hands and feet are usually diagnostic for Crouzon syndrome. Midface retrusion, relative prognathism, hypertelorism and a beaked nose are also present as in Apert syndrome.

In both syndromes, the reduced nasopharyngeal dimensions along with choanal stenosis may result in respiratory embarrassment, especially in the newborn. Obstructive sleep apnea and cor pulmonale are associated with airway compromise. In these circumstances, adenoidectomy for hypertrophic lymphoid tissue, endotracheal intubation and tracheotomy may be needed. A polysomnogram is a useful tool for determining airway compromise. Additionally, proptosis results in a high frequency of conjunctivitis and keratitis. The ears may be low set with otitis media and conductive hearing loss resulting from ETD is present in most cases. Congenital fixation of stapes footplate may also be encountered in Apert syndrome. Ventilation tube placement and stapedectomy may be performed when indicated. Fronto-orbital advancement surgery may be required to allow for growth of the brain and expansion of the cranial vault. Orthodontic attention may also be required for abnormalities of the maxillary teeth and crossbite. Cervical spine anomalies are more common in Crouzon syndrome, but may also be present in Apert syndrome.

Pierre-Robin Sequence

The triad of cleft palate, micrognathia, and airway obstruction was first described by St Hilaire in 1822, later by Fairbain in 1846, and by Shukowsky in 1911. Pierre Robin, a French stomatologist, first reported the association of micrognathia with glossoptosis in 1923. He later included cleft palate as part of this sequence. The prevalence of Pierre Robin sequence is reported to be 1 in 8,500 newborns. Children with this disorder are classified into two major categories: nonsyndromic and syndromic. Approximately 80 percent of cases are nonsyndromic and have the potential for normal patterns of growth and development if airway and feeding concerns are addressed early in infancy. Syndromic cases do not have as good a prognosis for growth and development in spite of early intervention. Velocardiofacial syndrome, Treacher Collins syndrome, and fetal alcohol syndrome are three of many conditions that have an association with Pierre Robin sequence.

The initiating factor in Pierre-Robin sequence appears to be mandibular deficiency during fetal development. The hypoplastic and retruded mandible maintains the tongue high in the nasopharynx early in development. The high position of the tongue prevents the medial growth and fusion of the lateral palatal structures which is usually complete at 11 weeks of fetal life. Further into development, the tongue descends into a more normal position; however, at this point the palatal shelves are unable to join. This results in a U-shaped palatal cleft.

Airway obstruction is a major concern in Pierre Robin sequence. The posterior displacement of the tongue and floor of mouth due to retrognathia results in upper airway obstruction. However, airway obstruction in this disorder has anatomic and neuromuscular components. Impairment of the genioglossus and other parapharyngeal musculature are observed and predispose the airway to collapse.

The management of airway obstruction may be achieved by several methods. Prone positioning displaces the tongue anteriorly, and previously was thought to be definitive treatment for glossoptosis. Due to the inability to observe chest retractions, this method has been replaced with the use of mandibular traction devices. The placement of a nasopharyngeal airway may be the most appropriate initial method of managing the airway in infants with Pierre Robin sequence. A tube with an internal diameter of 3.0 mm or 3.5 mm is used and advanced 8 cm or until appropriate ventilation is achieved. This provides some time to prepare for more definitive treatment. Gavage feeds via a nasogastric tube is usually recommended. In addition, tongue-lip adhesion has also been effective in the initial management of some cases. The mucosal surface of the tongue, along the floor of the mouth, over the alveolus, and onto the lower lip is denuded. The tongue is then sutured into a more anterior position. A tongue release is performed at the time of cleft palate repair. Speech is not affected with this method. In some more severe cases, tracheotomy is required when less invasive temporizing methods are unsuccessful. Mandibular distraction osteogenesis provides a definitive means to correct the bony and soft tissue involved in micrognathia. In some cases, patients exhibit catch-up growth and achieve maxillomandibular equilibrium without the need for mandibular corrective surgery.

Otologic concerns in Pierre Robin sequence are primarily due to conductive hearing loss secondary to chronic otitis media with effusion. Approximately 80 percent of patients have bilateral conductive hearing loss. Patients with abnormalities of the palate generally have anomalous anchorage of the muscles associated with the eustachian tube (tensor veli palatine and levator veli palitini). Placement of ventilation tubes is usually sufficient for management of eustachian tube dysfunction and middle ear effusion.

Charge Association

The acronym of CHARGE was first described by Pagon et al in 1981 to identify a nonrandom collection of malformations. The true incidence of this associated is not known. The acronym stands for colobomas, heart abnormalities, atresia choanae, retardation of growth or mental development, genitourinary anomalies, and ear anomalies. In addition to these abnormalities, the head and neck anomalies manifested in this association include facial nerve palsy, pharyngoesophageal dysmotility, laryngomalacia, vocal cord paralysis, obstructive sleep, and gastroesophageal reflux. Anomalies of the temporal bones include hypoplasia of the semicircular canals and Mondini malformation.

The most urgent otolaryngologic concern in a child with this CHARGE is respiratory distress due to bilateral choanal atresia. Chonal atresia should always be included in the differential diagnosis of a newborn child with respiratory distress and cyanosis at rest, with improvement when crying. Diagnosis of chonal atresia may be established by simple auscultation of each nostril with the bell of a stethoscope, use of a mirror to observe fogging under the nostrils, passage of a 6 French nasogastric feeing tube, and direct visualization with flexible laryngoscopy. A CT is a useful radiologic study used preoperatively to determine the abnormal bony structures involved in choanal atresia. Unilateral choanal atresia usually may be managed without any interventions. Management is initially the placement of an oral airway and feeding with a McGovern nipple may be helpful in symptomatic unilateral and bilateral chonal atresia. Surgical treatment of unilateral choanal atresia may be delayed until school-aged. In bilateral cases, surgical intervention is needed earlier in infancy to prevent respiratory decompensation. A tracheotomy is usually performed prior to definitive surgical repair. There are different techiniques including trasnasal and transpalatal approaches, the use of a laser, the use of stents, and use of Mitomycin-C topically (0.3 mg/cc for 2 minutes).

OTOLOGIC ABNORMALITIES

Otologic abnormalities include anomalies of the external, middle, and inner ear. Hearing loss is usually of a mixed type with a characteristic wedge-shaped audiogram. The intervention for chronic otitis media with effusion and eustachian tube dysfunction is usually the placement of ventilation tubes. The use of amplification devices is also useful.

Chapter

78

Head and Neck Cancer Staging

Proper and unified staging of head and neck cancer is important for various reasons, which include:
1. To select an appropriate form of therapy for a patient
2. To provide accurate prognostic information
3. Allow institutional assessment of therapeutic results
4. Allow collation of multi-institutional experiences
5. To provide a foundation for analysis of new forms of treatment.

Rules of the AJCC-UICC System

Components of clinical classification are the tumor, node, and metastasis (TNM). The system is an anatomically based system with weight on prognostic significance of various areas. It is based on physical exam, radiological findings on CT/MRI, endoscopy and biopsy. This system uses the poorer stage when doubt exists and skin, melanoma, sarcoma and lymphoma are considered separately during staging by this system.

T Stage	
Lip and oral cavity	
T1	Tumor <2 cm in greatest dimension
T2	Tumor >2 < 4 cm in greatest dimension
T3	Tumor >4 cm in greatest dimension
T4	*Lip:* Invades adjacent structures (cortical bone, tongue, skin of neck)
T4	*Oral cavity:* Invades adjacent structures (cortical bone, deep (extrinsic) muscle of tongue, maxillary sinus, skin)
Oropharynx	
T1	Tumor <2 cm in greatest dimension
T2	Tumor >2 <4 cm in greatest dimension
T3	Tumor >4 cm in greatest dimension
T4	Invades adjacent structures (cortical bone, soft tissue of neck, deep muscle of tongue)
Nasopharynx	
T1	Tumor limited to one subsite of nasopharynx
T2	Tumor invades more than one subsite
T3	Tumor invades nasal cavity or oropharynx
T4	Tumor invades skull or cranial nerve(s)
Hypopharynx	
T1	Tumor limited to one subsite of hypopharynx
T2	Tumor invades more than one subsite or an adjacent site, without fixation of hemilarynx
T3	Tumor invades more than one subsite or an adjacent site, with fixation of hemilarynx
T4	Invades adjacent structures (cartilage or soft tissues of neck)
Supraglottis	
T1	Tumor limited to one subsite of supraglottis with normal vocal cord mobility
T2	Tumor invades more than one subsite of supraglottis or glottis with normal vocal cord mobility
T3	Tumor limited to larynx with vocal cord fixation or invades postcricoid area, medial wall of piriform sinus, or pre-epiglottic tissues
T4	Tumor invades through thyroid cartilage or extends to other tissues beyond larynx (oropharynx, soft tissues of neck)

- *Subsites:* Suprahyoid epiglottis—lingual and laryngeal surfaces, infrahyoid epiglottis, false cords, arytenoid, aryepiglottic folds (laryngeal aspect).

Glottis	
T1	Tumor limited to vocal cord (T1A) or cords (T1B), may involve anterior and posterior commissures, with normal cord mobility
T2	Tumor extends to supraglottis or subglottis, or with impaired vocal cord mobility
T3	Tumor limited to larynx with vocal cord fixation

Contd...

Contd...

T4	Invades through thyroid cartilage, or extends to tissues beyond the larynx
Subglottis	
T1	Tumor limited to subglottis
T2	Tumor extends to vocal cord(s) with normal or impaired mobility
T3	Tumor limited to larynx with vocal cord fixation
T4	Tumor invades cricoid or thyroid cartilage or tissues beyond the larynx
Maxillary sinus	
T1	Tumor limited to antral mucosa with no erosion/ destruction of bone
T2	Erosion of the infrastructure including hard palate or middle nasal meatus
T3	Invasion of skin of cheek, posterior wall of maxillary sinus, floor of medial wall of orbit, anterior ethmoid sinus
T4	Invades orbital contents or: cribriform plate, posterior ethmoid or sphenoid sinuses, nasopharynx, soft palate, pterygomaxillary or temporal fossae, base of skull
Salivary glands	
T1	Tumor <2 cm
T2	Tumor >2 <4 cm
T3	Tumor >4 <6 cm
T4	Tumor >6
Thyroid	
T1	Tumor <1 cm
T2	Tumor >1 cm <4 cm
T3	Tumor >4 cm but limited to the thyroid
T4	Tumor of any size beyond thyroid capsule

- Measure the largest nodule for classification
- Separate stage groupings
  - Papillary and follicular < 45 years:
    Stage I: M0
    Stage II: M1
  - >45 years:
    Stage I : T1
    Stage II : T2 or T3
    Stage III : T4 or any N1
    Stage IV: M1
- Medullary almost the same as papillary and follicular >45 years grouping:
  - Stage I : T1
  - Stage II : T2 or T3 or T4
  - Stage III: Any N1
  - Stage IV: M1
- Undifferentiated: All are Stage IV (any T, any N, any M)
- For all of the above: TX = primary tumor cannot be assessed, T0 = no evidence of primary tumor, Tis = carcinoma *in situ*.

Lymph node (N)	
NX	Cannot be assessed
N0	No regional lymph node metastasis
N1	Single ipsilateral <3 cm
N2	Divided in a, b, c
N2a	Single ipsilateral >3 < 6 cm
N2b	Multiple ipsilateral < 6 cm
N2c	Bilateral or contralateral nodes <6 cm
N3	Any node >6 cm
Distant metastasis (M)	
Mx	Cannot be assessed
M0	No distant metastasis
M1	Distant metastasis

Basic stage grouping (Stage 0 = Tis)

	N0	N1	N2	N3
T1	I	III	IV	IV
T2	II	III	IV	IV
T3	III	III	IV	IV
T4	IV	IV	IV	IV

COMPONENTS OF PATHOLOGIC STAGING (pTNM)

- *Gx* : Cannot be assessed
- *G1*: Well differentiated
- *G2*: Moderately differentiated
- *G3*: Poorly differentiated
- *G4*: Undifferentiated
- Descriptors may include—Lymphatic invasion, venous invasion.

STAGE GROUPING

Used to indicate prognosis.

REPORTING OF RESULTS ESSENTIAL DATA

Demographic information, description of disease (histology, site and stage), treatment information, start time of 1st mode of therapy, vital status of patient, completeness of follow-up, survival statistics.

OPTIONS FOR CALCULATING SURVIVAL

- *Direct:* Percentage of patients alive at the end of an interval (e.g. 5 years)
- *Actuarial or life table method:* Allows inclusion of patients followed less than a year (establishes survival pattern)
- *Adjusted:* Adjusts for cause of death (one study showed > rate of noncancer deaths in cancer patients)
- *Relative:* Ratio of observed to expected (normal population) adjusted for demographics
- *Kaplan-Meier:* Similar to actuarial.

Future of Staging Strengths of the Current System

- Confidence in the laryngeal staging is the most solid—anatomically precise, uniform surgical procedure, and clear pathology margins
- All sites demonstrate an increase survival in women
- Cervical lymph node metastasis is a poor prognostic indicator (survival decreases by 40%).

WEAKNESSES OF THE CURRENT SYSTEM

Dilemma: Using only one prognostic variable when multiple purposes are sought.

STAGE GROUPINGS

Clustering has resulted in loss of accuracy (inconsistent and biologically inaccurate).

IMPACT OF INADEQUATE STAGING ON MULTI-INSTITUTIONAL STUDIES

- Studies may show a poor outcome
- Need to also include other factors so that specific patient populations can be targeted for their most ideal therapy
- *Problem:* Not large enough numbers.

POTENTIAL MODIFIERS OF STAGING

When developing a new modifier, the researcher must use predetermined end points.

IMAGING

Evaluation of the N0 neck:

	Sensitivity	Specificity	Accuracy
CT	93%	83%	89%
MRI	90%	89%	87%
Clinical	64%	87%	72%

PET scanning may eliminate the Tx category.

ADDITIONAL DESCRIPTORS

- *Term mTNM:* Multiple primary tumors at a single site (use higher stage)
- *Term yTNM:* Classification during or after treatment
- *Term rTNM:* Recurrent tumor after a disease free interval
- *Term aTNM:* 1st classification during autopsy.

Biologic Markers

HOST FACTORS

- *Immunologic*: Anergy to delayed hypersensitivity skin testing = poor prognosis, reduced NK cells, low ratio of CD4: CD8
- *Transfusion:* Immune suppression (monocyte activation and late Ts cell activation up to 12 weeks post-transfusion, decreased T4: T8 ratios and decreased NK cell function)
- *Performance status*: Nutritional (wait loss is poor prognostic indicator), significant additional illness, RTOG—three factors that had independent bearing on treatment outcome—tumor stage, N stage and Karnofsky status
- *Genetic predisposition*: Certain genes (1-myc gene) govern the phenotypic expression
- *Tumor factors*:
  - *Proliferation markers*: For example, loss of MHC is poor prognosis, increased α9 integrin is predictor of tumor aggressiveness
  - *Pathology*: High DNA index demonstrated higher metastatic rate, perineural, angioinvasion, extracapsular spread, all have poor prognosis.

The Future

Medical comorbidity will be an essential component of future staging.

Chapter 79

Histopathology of Common Head and Neck Lesions

This chapter will provide a quick overview of the histopathological picture of common ENT lesions.

Thyroid Lesions

PAPILLARY THYROID CARCINOMA

Histologically, there are papillary fronds of follicular cells with a fibrovascular core. Psammoma bodies may be present. The nuclei have been described as "Orphan Annie" because of their clear or nearly clear appearance; they are often grooved (**Fig. 79.1**).

FOLLICULAR THYROID CARCINOMA

Histologically, the tumor has a microfollicular or trabecular pattern with regular, small, round follicles. The criteria for malignancy are the demonstration of either capsular or vascular invasion. The latter carries a worse prognosis: most cases involve veins at or beyond the capsule (**Fig. 79.2**).

MULTINODULAR GOITER

Histologically, there are benign colloid nodules of widely varying size (**Fig. 79.3**).

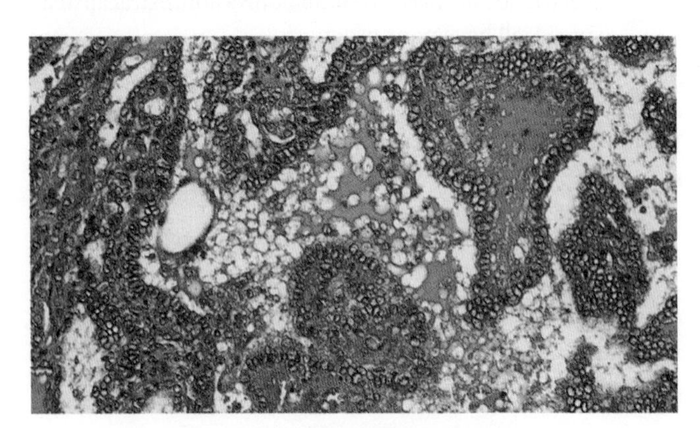

Fig. 79.1: Papillary thyroid carcinoma

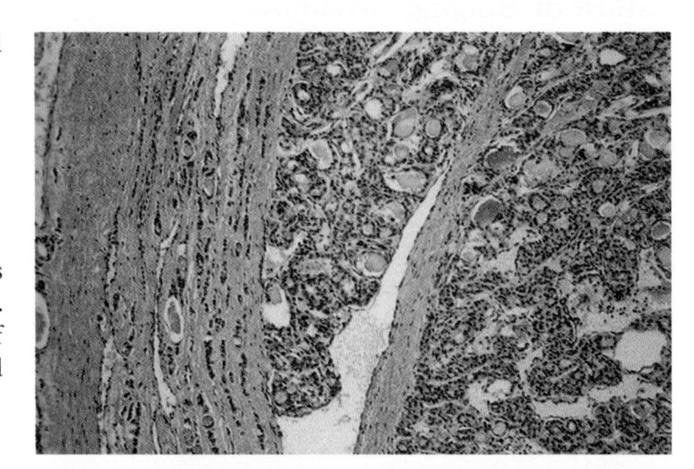

Fig. 79.2: Follicular thyroid carcinoma

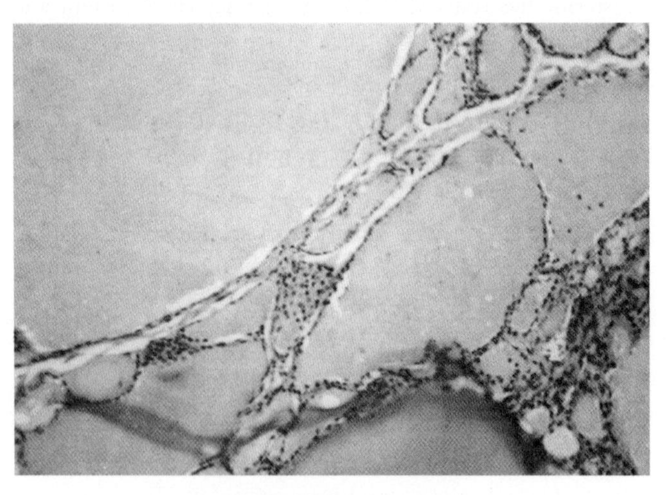

Fig. 79.3: Multinodular goiter

MEDULLARY THYROID CARCINOMA

The tumor is usually infiltrative and grows in nests. Amyloid may be present in the stroma. Special stains like Congo red demonstrates amyloid apple green birefringence on polarized

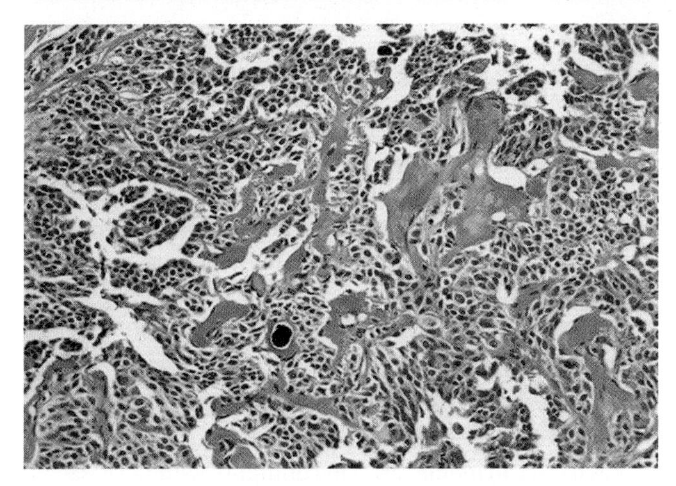

Fig. 79.4: Medullary thyroid carcinoma

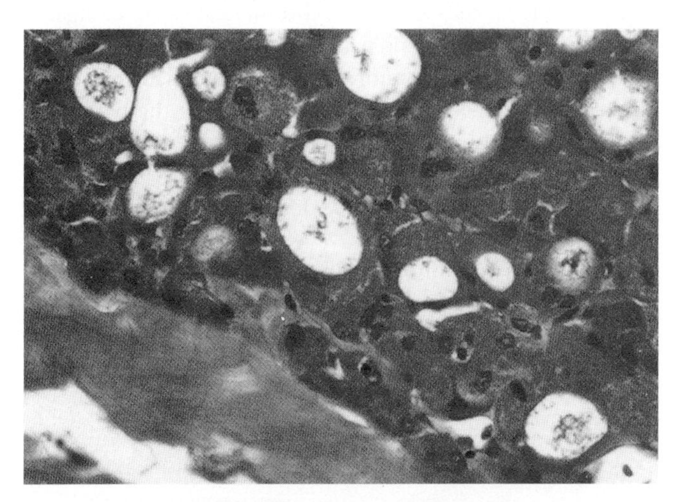

Fig. 79.5: Hurthle cell lesion

light. Calcitonin and chromogranin is identified histologically (Fig. 79.4).

HURTHLE CELL LESION

Hurthle cell neoplasms are most often follicular in pattern, and the criteria for malignancy are the same as for follicular carcinoma or papillary carcinoma, i.e. the presence of vascular or capsular invasion (**Fig. 79.5**).

ANAPLASTIC CARCINOMA

Histologically, the tumor is divided into giant cell, spindle cell, and small cell types. "Bizarre cells" may also be noted (**Fig. 79.6**).

Ear Lesions

ACOUSTIC NEUROMA

Tumors are composed of alternating regions, of compact spindle cells called Antoni 'A' areas, and loose, hypocellular zones called Antoni 'B' areas. In a given tumor, the proportion of these components varies. Nuclei are vesicular to hyperchromatic, elongated and twisted, with indistinct cytoplasmic borders. Cells are arranged in short, interlacing fascicles, and whorling or palisading of nuclei may be seen; nuclear palisading in rows is called Verocay bodies. Antoni 'B' areas display a disorderly cellular arrangement, myxoid stroma, and chronic inflammatory cell infiltrate. Increased vascularity is prominent, composed of large vessels with thickened walls. Changes, including cystic degeneration, necrosis, hyalinization, calcification, and hemorrhage, may be seen (**Fig. 79.7**).

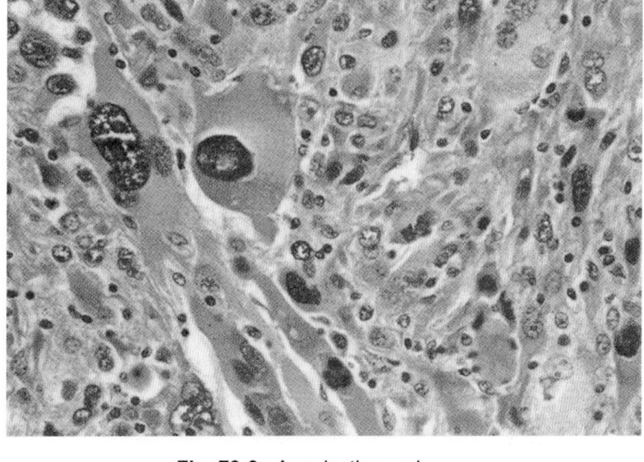

Fig. 79.6: Anaplastic carcinoma

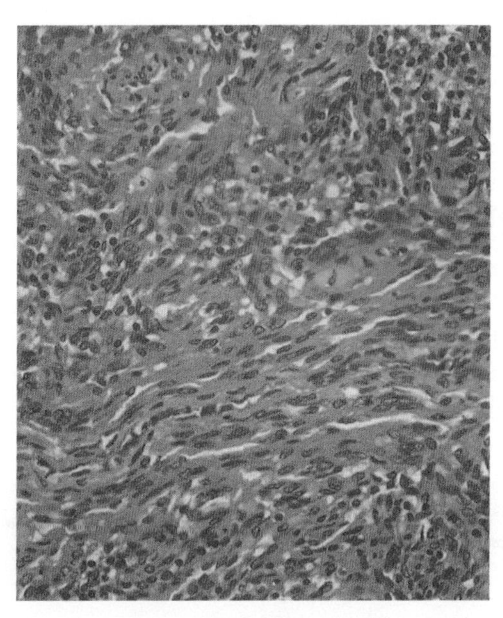

Fig. 79.7: Acoustic neuroma

CHOLESTEATOMA

The diagnosis of cholesteatoma is made in the presence of the following findings (**Fig. 79.8**):

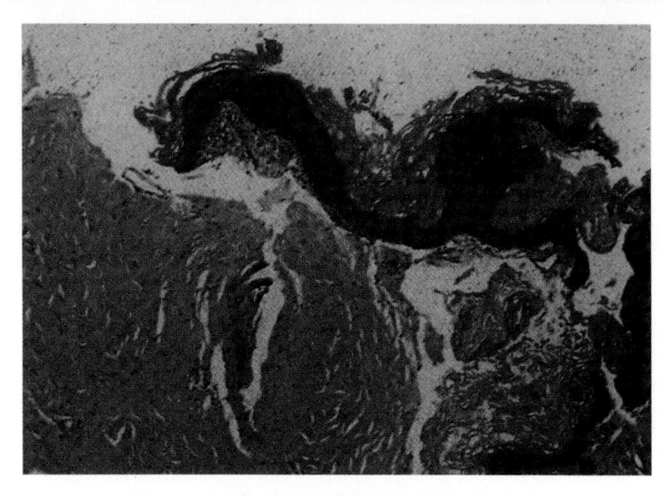

Fig. 79.8: Cholesteatoma

- Stratified keratinizing squamous epithelium
- Subepithelial fibroconnective or granulation tissue
- Keratin debris (the presence of keratin debris alone is not diagnostic).

GLOMUS TUMOR (FIG. 79.9)

Epidemiology

- Ten percent malignant and exhbit invasion, mitoses, necrosis and metastases.
- Ten percent familial, these lesions have increased multifocality.
- Ten percent multifocal
- One percent secretory for vanillylmandelic acid.

Typical histopathological appearance is a cell nest or "zellballen" pattern. These nests are surrounded by a rim of fibrovascular stroma. The neoplasm is composed predominantly of chief cells, which are round or oval with uniform nuclei, dispersed chromatin pattern, and abundant eosinophilic, granular, or vacuolated cytoplasm and sustentacular cells which are modified Schwann cells and lie at the periphery of the cell nests. They are spindle-shaped, basophilic-appearing cells.

BASAL CELL CARCINOMA OF THE EXTERNAL EAR SKIN

All basal cell carcinomas arise in continuity with the basal cell layer of the epithelium or from the adnexae and are composed of fairly uniform cells with hyperchromatic, oval, or elongated nuclei, scant cytoplasm, and palisading appearance of the nuclei at the periphery of the tumor nests; a characteristic retraction (separation) of the surrounding stroma from the peripheral portions of the tumor nests is commonly seen. The various growth patterns include (**Fig. 79.10**):

- Solid type, made up of islands or sheets of tumor cells; most common
- Adenoid type, tumor islands arranged in anastomosing cords, creating a lace-like or adenoid pattern
- Morphea or sclerosing type, in which strands of tumor cells are embedded in a dense, sclerotic stroma.

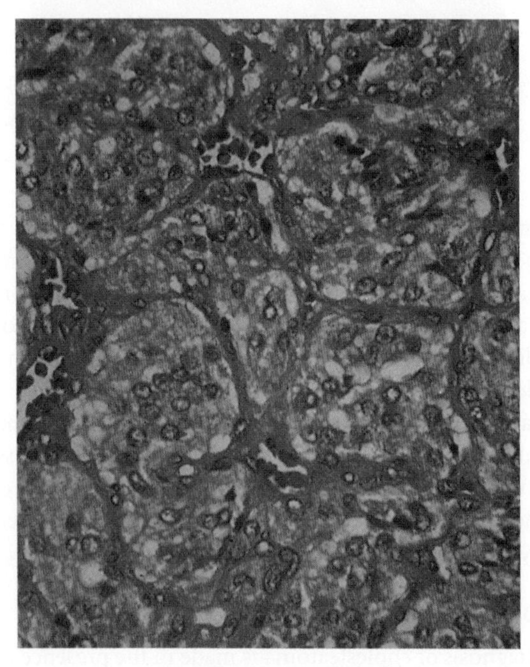

Fig. 79.9: Glomus tumor

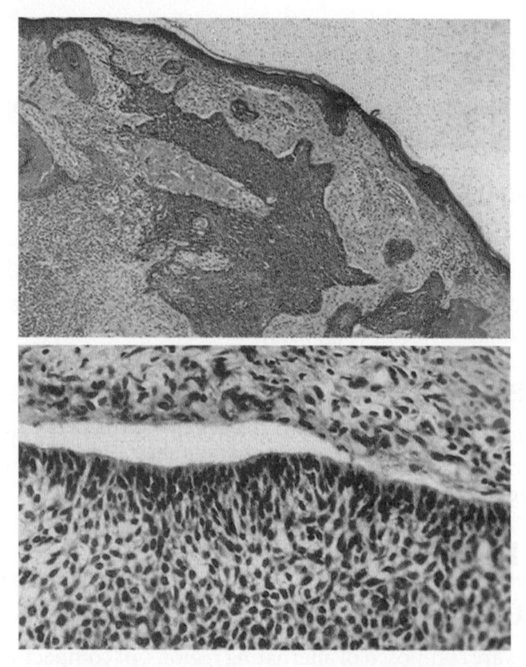

Fig. 79.10: Basal cell carcinoma of the external ear skin

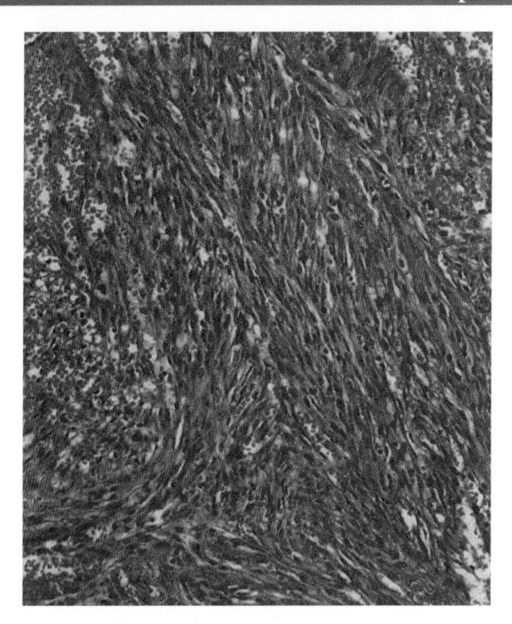

Fig. 79.11: Kaposi's sarcoma

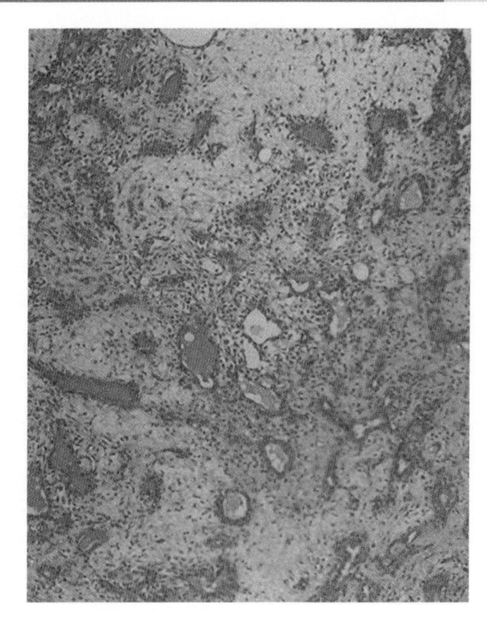

Fig. 79.12: Pleomorphic adenoma

KAPOSI'S SARCOMA

This appears as an unencapsulated and infiltrative lesion composed of spindle cells in a fascicular growth pattern. Pericytes are the cells of origin. Spindle cells are elongated and rather uniform, with scant cytoplasm and indistinct cell borders; scattered mitotic figures can be identified. Erythrocytes commonly extravasate into the spindle cell component (**Fig. 79.11**).

Associated chronic inflammatory cell infiltrates composed of lymphocytes and plasma cells as well as hemosiderin-laden macrophages are seen. Cellular pleomorphism, anaplastic changes, and increased mitoses are indicative of more aggressive tumors.

Salivary Gland Lesions

PLEOMORPHIC ADENOMA

A mixture of epithelial, myoepithelial, and stromal components are the histologic hallmarks of pleomorphic adenoma, with morphologic variability within a single neoplasm.

A fibrous capsule is seen that varies in thickness. Minor salivary gland pleomorphic adenomas are generally not encapsulated, but are well demarcated. Epithelial component may have a variety of growth patterns, including solid, cystic, trabecular, or papillary, consisting of a proliferation of duct lining epithelial cells and myoepithelial cells. Duct-lining epithelial cells that form the inner layer of acini or tubules appear flattened, cuboidal, or columnar, with round to oval nuclei and a variable amount of cytoplasm that appears eosinophilic to amphophilic. Myoepithelial component forms the outer layer and is spindle-shaped in appearance with hyperchromatic nuclei, and may be more than one cell layer. Thick stromal component, the product of myoepithelial cells, varies in appearance from myxoid to chondroid to myxochondroid, and may also appear fibrous and vascular. Any one or all of these components may coexist in the same neoplasm. Any of the components may predominate so that tumors may be diagnosed as epithelial, myoepithelial, or stromal-predominant pleomorphic adenoma. However, all components must be identified in order to diagnose a pleomorphic adenoma (**Fig. 79.12**). Mitoses and necrosis are uncommonly seen.

WARTHIN'S TUMOR

Warthin's tumor is a papillary and cystic lesion composed of epithelial and lymphoid components. The epithelial component that lines the papillary projections is composed of a double layer of granular eosinophilic cells oncocytes. Inner or luminal cells are nonciliated, tall columnar cells with nuclei aligned toward the luminal aspect. Outer or basal cells are round, cuboidal, or polygonal cells with vesicular nuclei. The lymphoid component is mature and has lymphoid follicles with germinal centers (**Fig. 79.13**).

LOW-GRADE MUCOEPIDERMOID CARCINOMA

Characteristic of all grades of mucoepidermoid carcinoma is the presence of mucous cells, epidermoid cells, and intermediate cells; these cellular components vary according to the histologic grade.

Low-grade mucoepidermoid carcinoma is characteristically cystic and has large numbers of mucous cells admixed with less numerous but easily identifiable epidermoid and intermediate cells. Mucous cells are identified lining cystic spaces as large or balloon-shaped with distinct cell borders, and are composed of

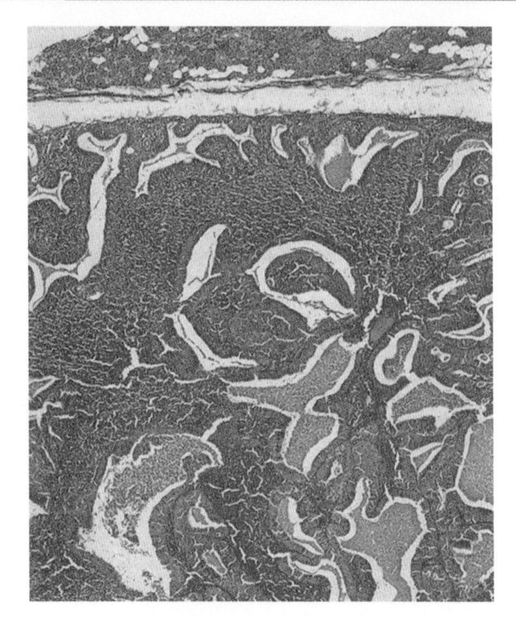

Fig. 79.13: Warthin's tumor

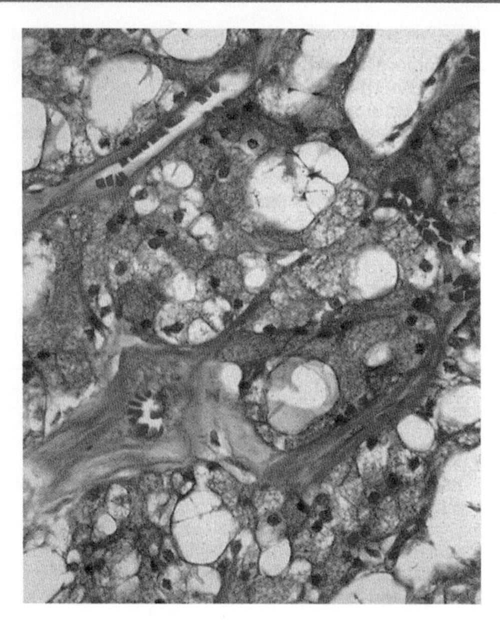

Fig. 79.15: Acinic cell carcinoma

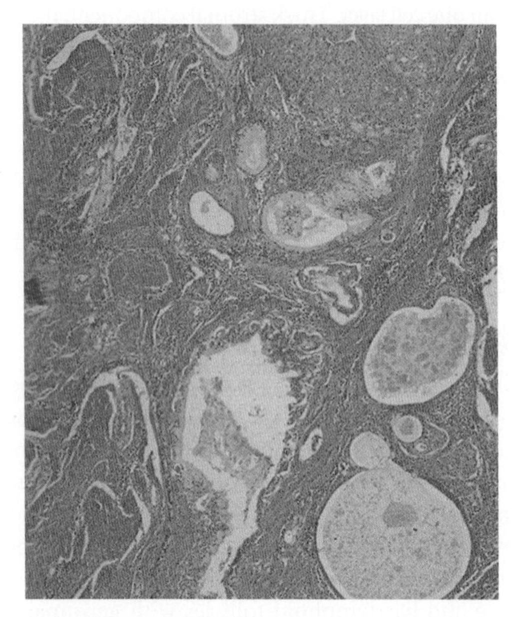

Fig. 79.14: Low-grade mucoepidermoid carcinoma

pale staining or foamy-appearing cytoplasm with peripherally placed, small, dark-staining nuclei. Epidermoid cells form nests or solid areas in conjunction with the mucous cells, have a pavement like arrangement, and are polygonal-shaped with vesicular nuclei and abundant eosinophilic cytoplasm. Intermediate cells are round to oval, contain small, dark-staining nuclei, and have scanty, eosinophilic cytoplasm (**Fig. 79.14**).

Cellular pleomorphism, mitoses, necrosis, and hemorrhage are generally absent. A variable degree of local invasion may be seen; however, neural invasion is not normally a component of the low-grade mucoepidermoid carcinoma. Clear cells, composed of round to oval cells with distinct cell borders, peripherally placed, small, dark nuclei, and their hallmark clear cytoplasm may be seen and, on infrequent occasions, may predominate.

ACINIC CELL CARCINOMA

Acinic cell adenocarcinomas are circumscribed tumors, characterized by a variety of growth patterns including solid, microcystic, papillary-cystic, and follicular. Solid and microcystic are the most common patterns and consist of either sheets of tumor cells in an organoid arrangement or numerous small cystic spaces. Papillary-cystic and follicular are least common patterns and consist of variably sized cystic spaces that are associated with papillary projections supported by a fibrovascular core or follicular spaces which resemble thyroid parenchyma and contain eosinophilic proteinaceous material lined by cuboidal to columnar cells (**Fig. 79.15**).

ADENOID CYSTIC CARCINOMA

Adenoid cystic carcinomas are unencapsulated, infiltrating neoplasms with varied growth patterns, consisting of cribriform, tubular/ductular, trabecular or solid. Individual neoplasms may have a single growth pattern, but characteristically these neoplasms are composed of multiple patterns, any one of which may predominate (**Fig. 79.16**).

Cribriform type: It is considered the classic pattern and has arrangement of cells in a "Swiss cheese" configuration, with

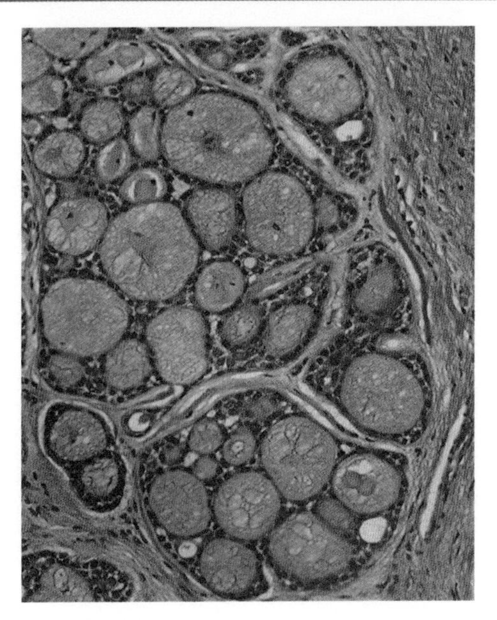

Fig. 79.16: Adenoid cystic carcinoma

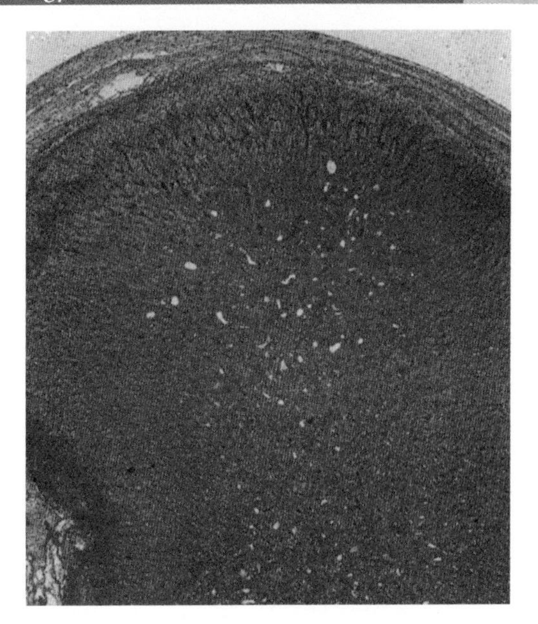

Fig. 79.17: Contact ulcer

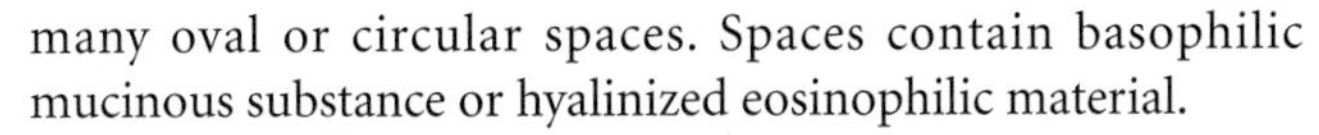

many oval or circular spaces. Spaces contain basophilic mucinous substance or hyalinized eosinophilic material.

Tubular type: It has cells which are arranged in ducts or tubules. Ducts or tubules contain faintly eosinophilic mucinous material. This type carries the best prognosis.

Solid type: Neoplastic cells arranged in sheets or nests of varying size and shape. There is little tendency to form cystic spaces, tubules, or ducts. Carries the worst prognosis.

What is common to all growth patterns is the predilection of these tumors to perineural and intraneural invasion.

Laryngeal Lesions

CONTACT ULCER

Most often appears as an ulcerated lesion with associated fibrinoid necrosis, granulation tissue, showing signs of acute and chronic inflammation.

Chronic lesions may demonstrate a hyperplastic epithelium with no ulcerative component and may include giant cells, with marked vascular proliferation, and spindle cells (fibroblasts). The contact ulcer has histopathological appearance similar to pyogenic granuloma (lobular capillary hemangioma) (**Fig. 79.17**).

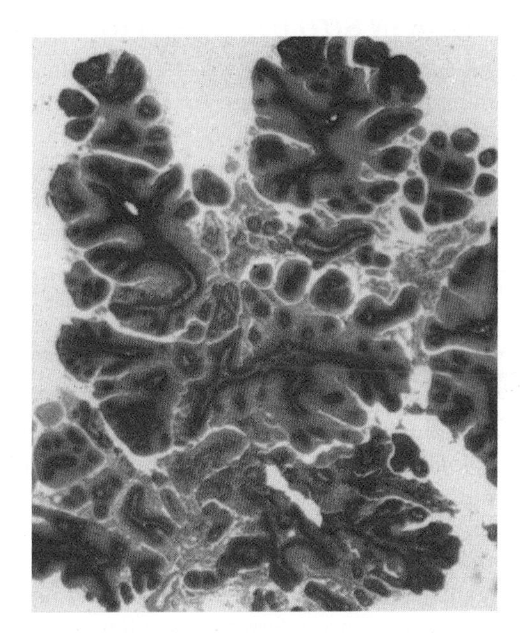

Fig. 79.18: Laryngeal papillomatosis

LARYNGEAL PAPILLOMATOSIS

Typical microscopic findings include papillary fronds of multilayered benign squamous epithelium containing fibrovascular cores. There is little or no keratin production and absence of stromal invasion. A certain degree of cellular atypia may be seen; however, the presence of severe atypia may be indicative of the development of a squamous carcinoma arising in papillomatosis or may in fact represent an exophytic squamous cell carcinoma (**Fig. 79.18**).

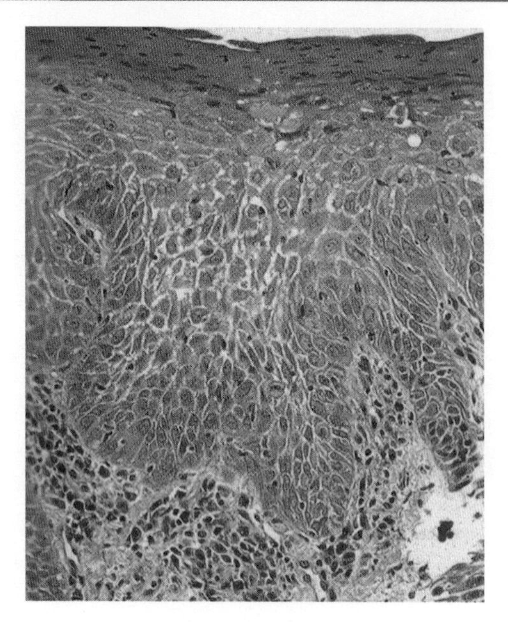

Fig. 79.19: Carcinoma *in situ*

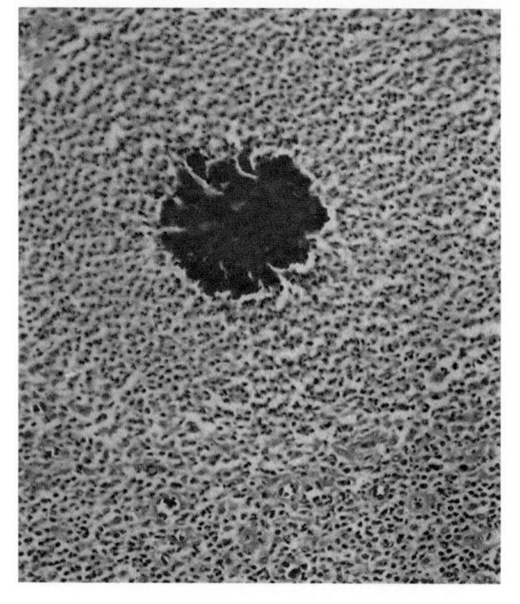

Fig. 79.20: Actinomycosis

CARCINOMA *IN SITU* (LARYNX) (FIG. 79.19)

Typically, the dysplastic process involves the entire thickness of the squamous epithelium which may or may not be thickened. There is loss of cellular maturation and polarity with an increase in the nuclear: cytoplasmic ratio. Presence of mitoses (normal and abnormal) is noted. Keratosis and dyskeratosis may be present and evidence of extension into adjacent seromucous glands may be seen.

Oral Lesions

ACTINOMYCOSIS (FIG. 79.20)

The most common site of these lesions is the tonsils. Microscopically seen as a granulomatous reaction with central accumulation of polymorphonuclear leukocytes (abscess formation) and necrosis.

Within the abscess and enveloped by the neutrophils, microorganism colonies are seen.The organisms form a characteristic appearance, referred to as "sulfur granules". The granules are lobular, deep purple, and composed of a central meshwork of filaments that typically have eosinophilic, club-shaped ends. The organisms stain best with Gram and Gomori methenamine silver (GMS) stains.

SQUAMOUS CARCINOMA (TONGUE) (FIG. 79.21)

The typical microscopic appearance of the squamous carcinoma depends on its degree of differentiation and **Table 79.1** illustrates the differences:

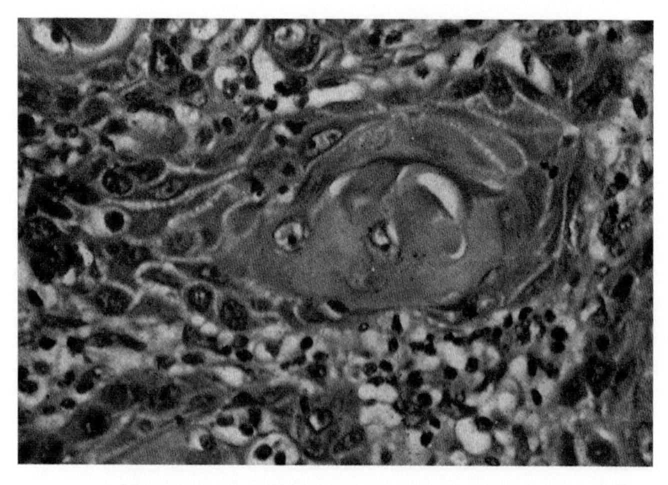

Fig. 79.21: Squamous carcinoma of the tongue

Table 79.1: Histopathological features of squamous cell carcinoma

Feature	Squamous cell carcinoma—degree of differentiation		
	Well	**Moderate**	**Poor**
Keratinization	Present	Focal	Limited
Intercellular bridges	Present	Present	Absent
Pleomorphism	Mild	Moderate	Marked
Mitoses	Few	Prominent	Numerous
Cytoplasm	Distinct	Distinct	Indistinct
Nuclei	Normal	Enlarged	Enlarged

Chapter 80

Common ENT Instruments

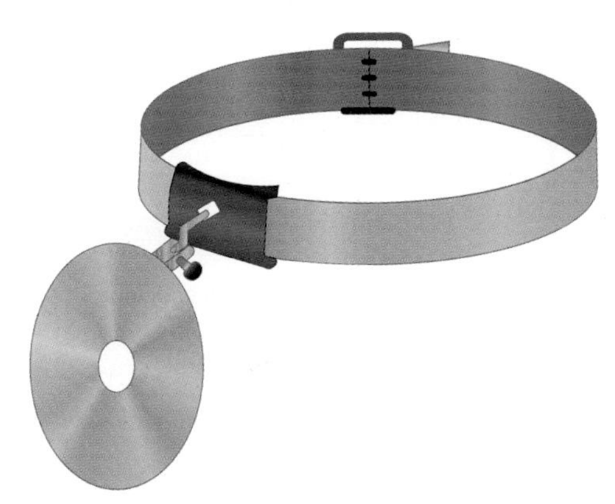

Fig. 80.1: Head mirror

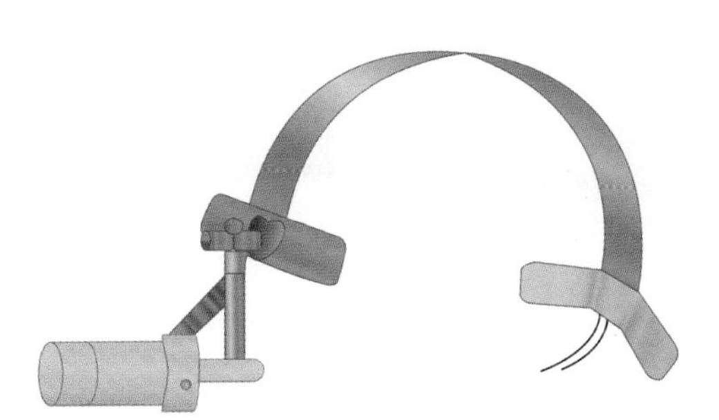

Fig. 80.2: Head light

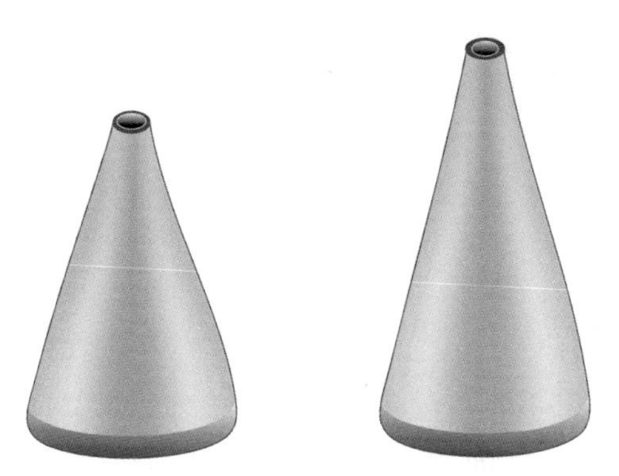

Fig. 80.3: Aural speculum

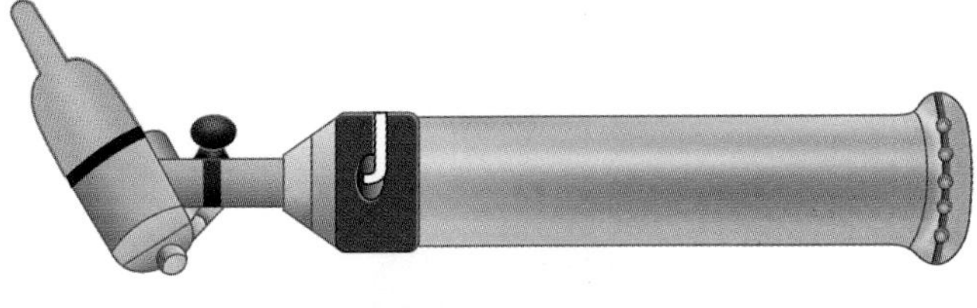

Fig. 80.4: Electrical otoscope

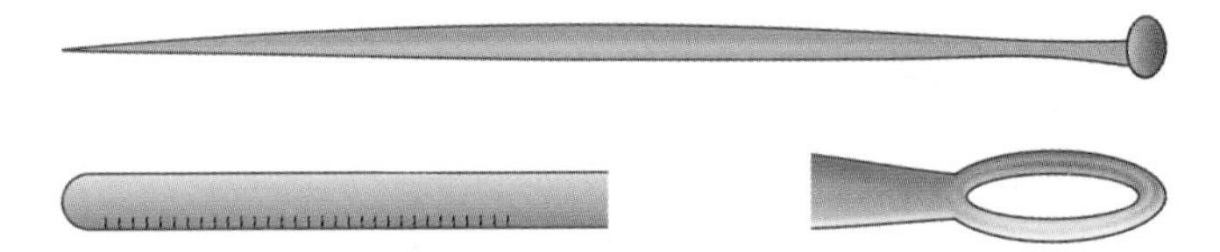

Fig. 80.5: Jobson's aural probe

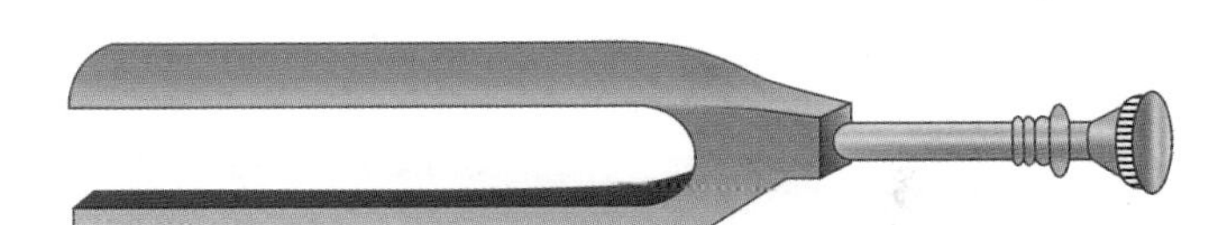

Fig. 80.6: Tuning fork

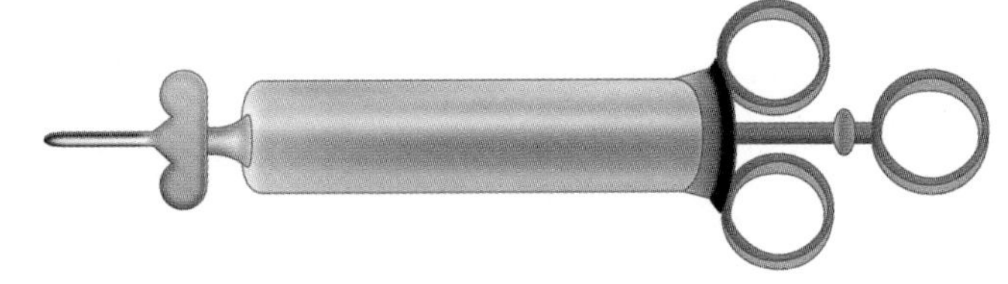

Fig. 80.7: Aural syringe

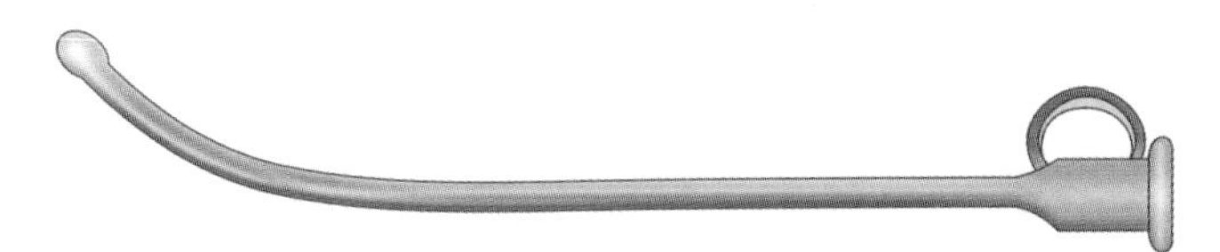

Fig. 80.8: Eustachian catheter

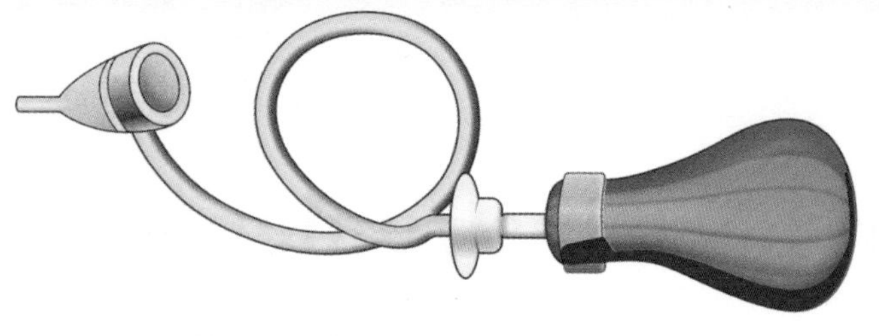

Fig. 80.9: Siegel's pneumatic speculum

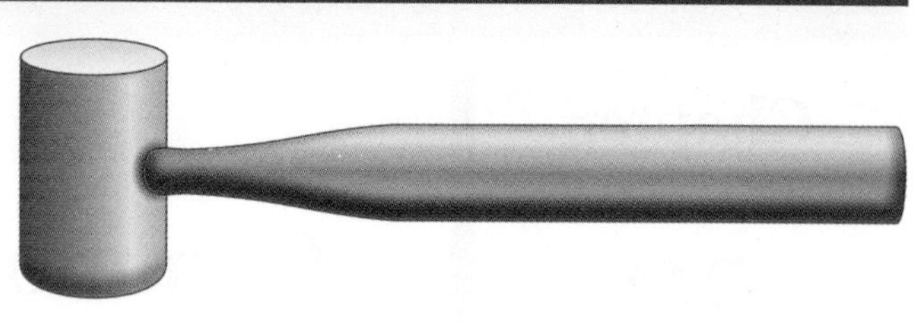

Fig. 80.14: Mallet

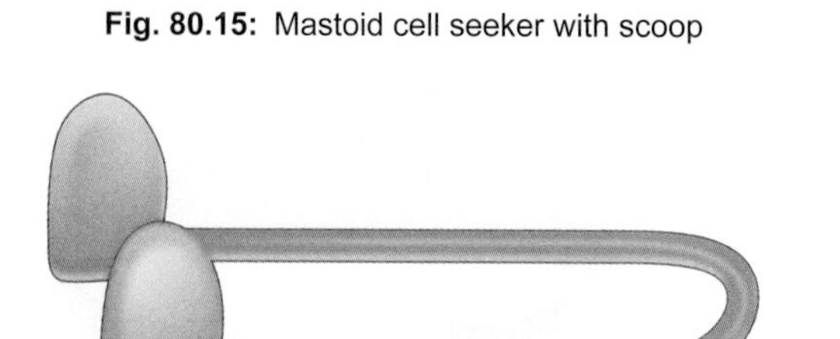

Fig. 80.15: Mastoid cell seeker with scoop

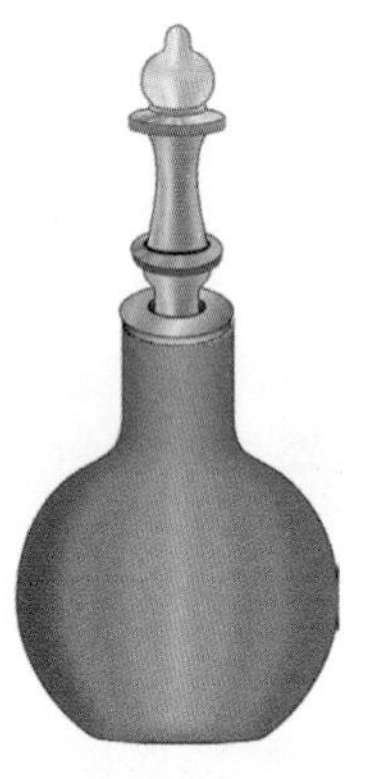

Fig. 80.10: Politzer bag

Fig. 80.16: Thudicum's nasal speculum

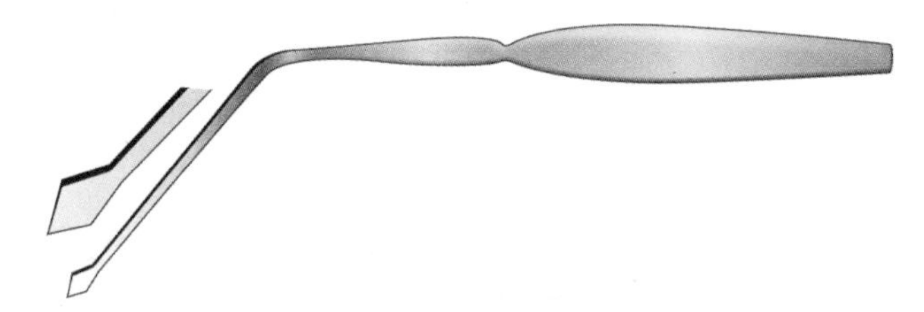

Fig. 80.11: Myringotome

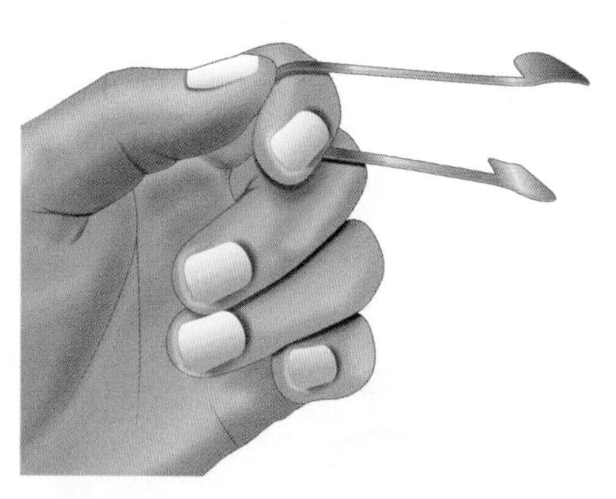

Fig. 80.17: Correct method of holding Thudicum's nasal speculum

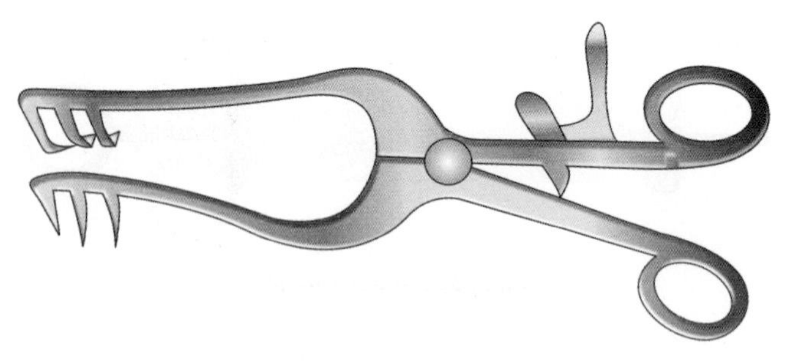

Fig. 80.12: Mastoid retractor

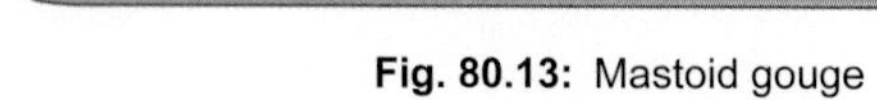

Fig. 80.13: Mastoid gouge

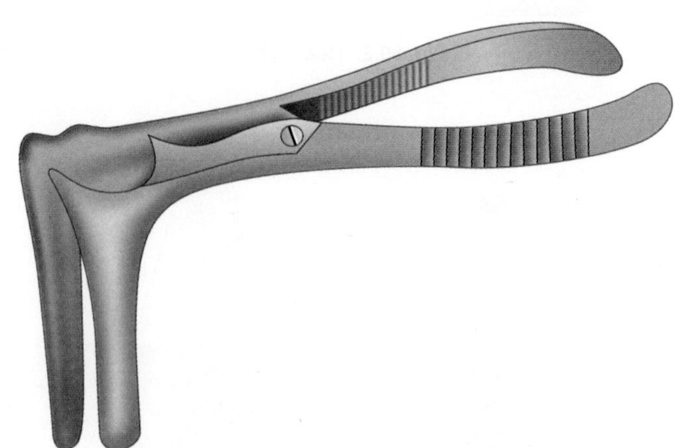

Fig. 80.18: St Clair-Thompson's nasal speculum

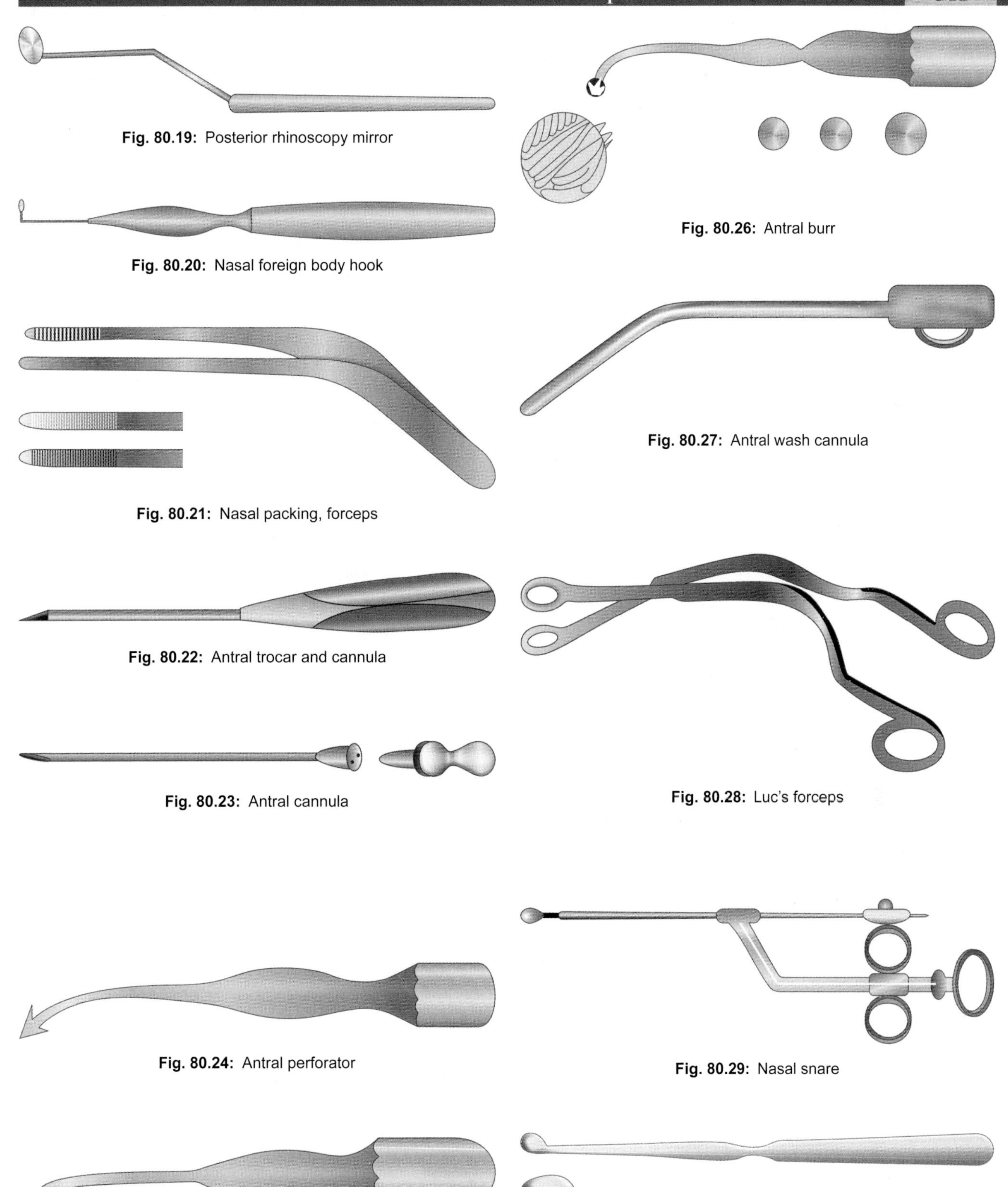

Fig. 80.19: Posterior rhinoscopy mirror

Fig. 80.20: Nasal foreign body hook

Fig. 80.21: Nasal packing, forceps

Fig. 80.22: Antral trocar and cannula

Fig. 80.23: Antral cannula

Fig. 80.24: Antral perforator

Fig. 80.25: Myle's nasoantral perforator

Fig. 80.26: Antral burr

Fig. 80.27: Antral wash cannula

Fig. 80.28: Luc's forceps

Fig. 80.29: Nasal snare

Fig. 80.30: Freer's septal knife

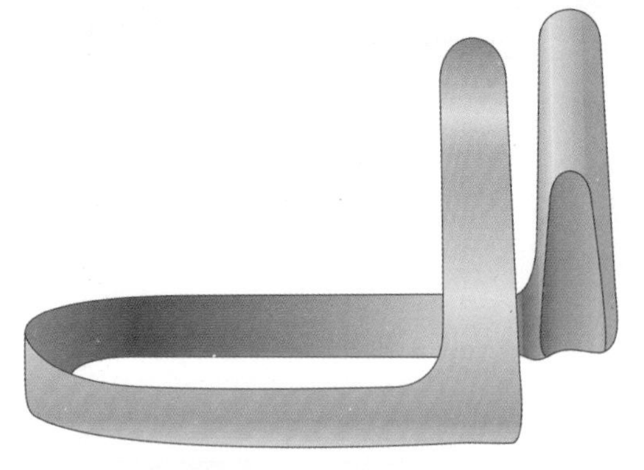

Fig. 80.31: Long-bladed nasal speculum

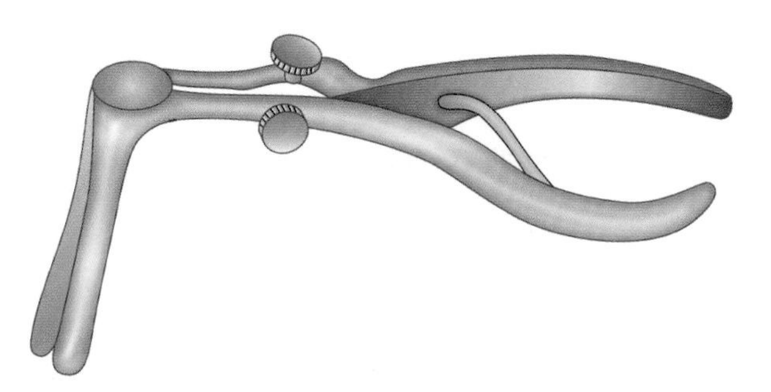

Fig. 80.32: Killian's nasal speculum

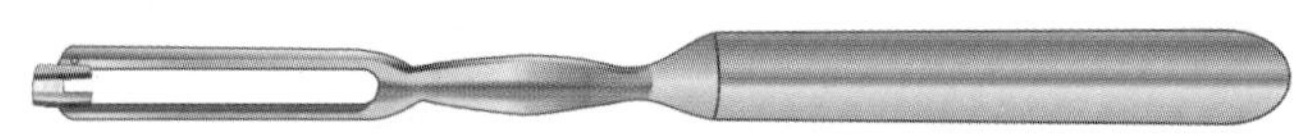

Fig. 80.33: Ballinger's swivel knife

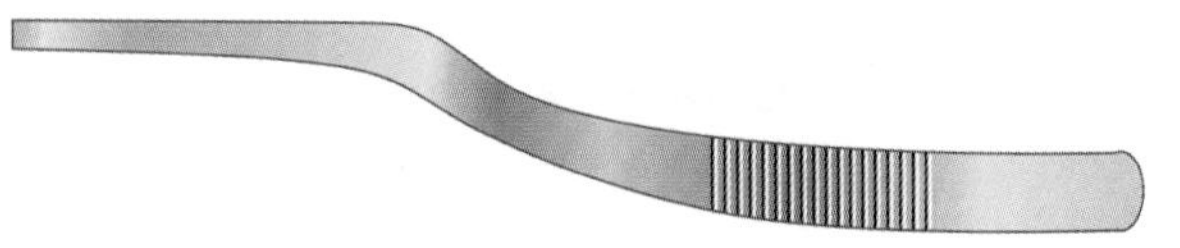

Fig. 80.34: Bayonet-shaped gouge

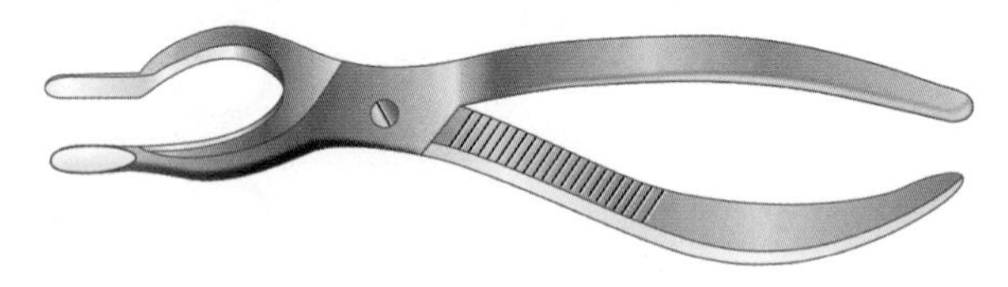

Fig. 80.35: Walsham's forceps

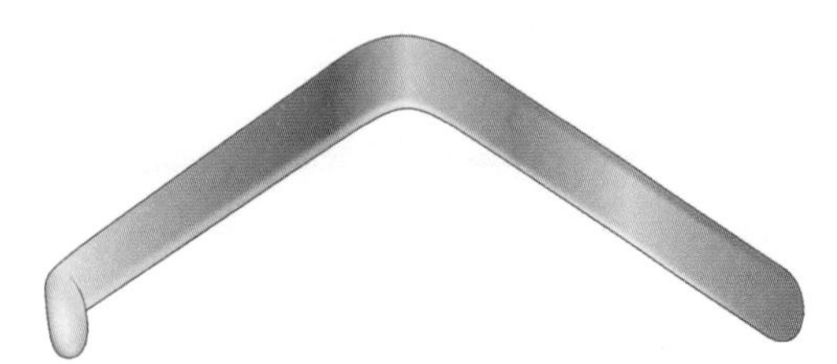

Fig. 80.36: Lack's spatula

Fig. 80.37: Laryngeal mirror

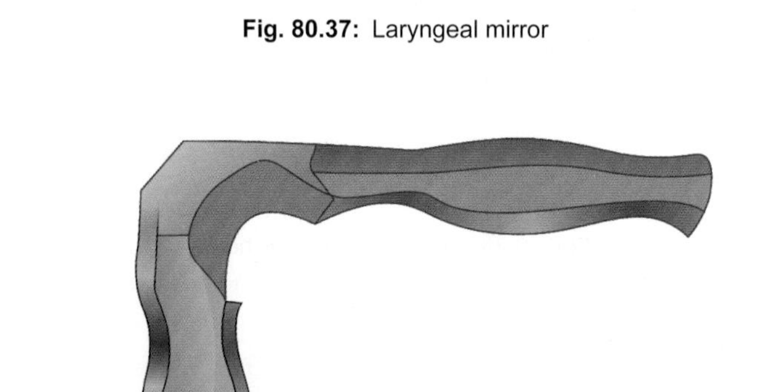

Fig. 80.38: Direct laryngoscope

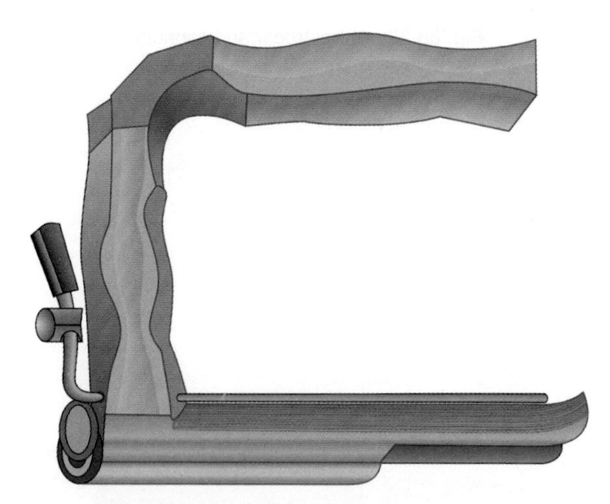

Fig. 80.39: Chevalier-Jackson laryngoscope with removable slide

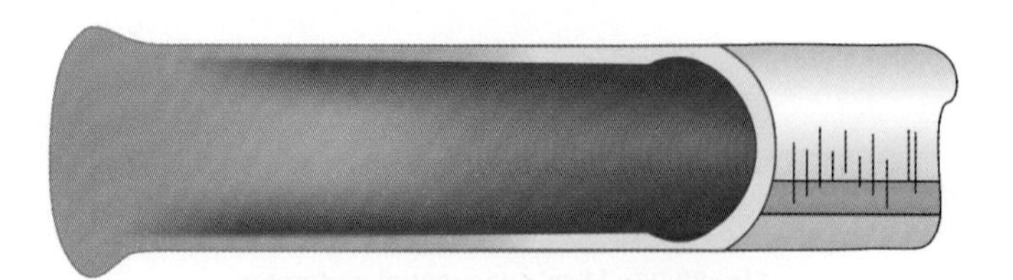

Fig. 80.40: Distal light arrangement

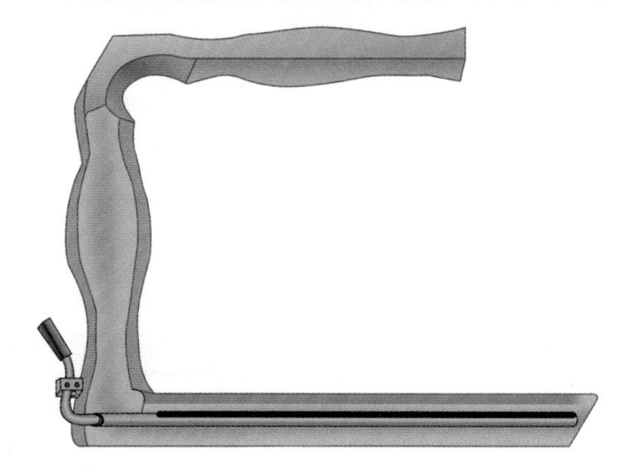

Fig. 80.41: Anterior commissure laryngoscope

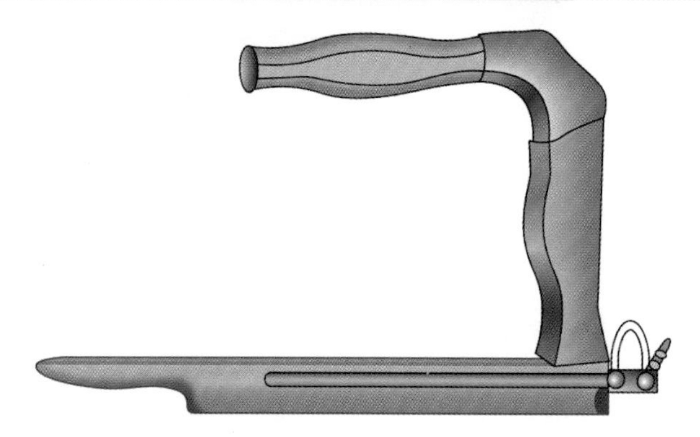

Fig. 80.46: Esophageal speculum

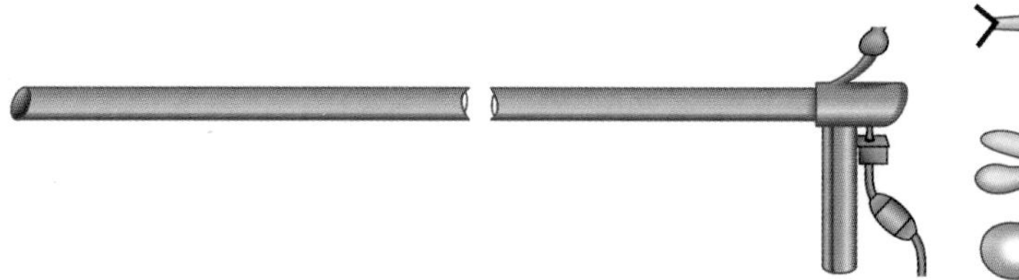

Fig. 80.42: Negus bronchoscope

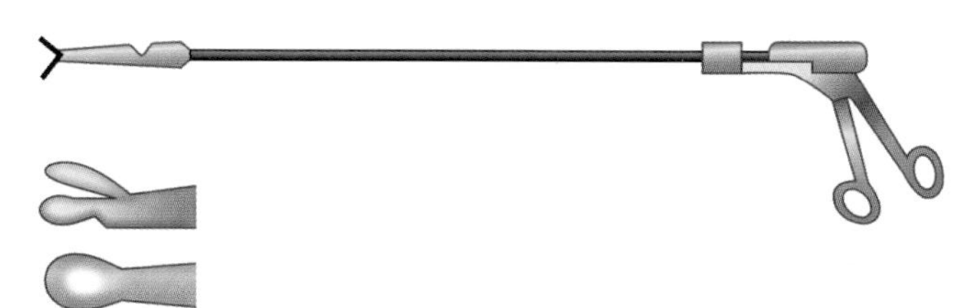

Fig. 80.47: Laryngeal forceps

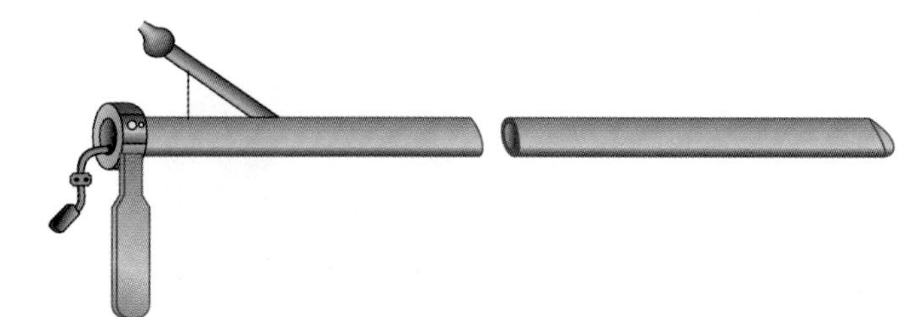

Fig. 80.43: Chevalier-Jackson bronchoscope

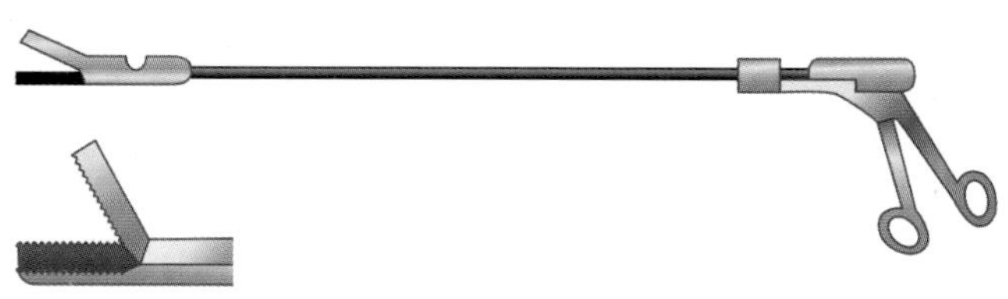

Fig. 80.48: Crocodile punch biopsy forceps

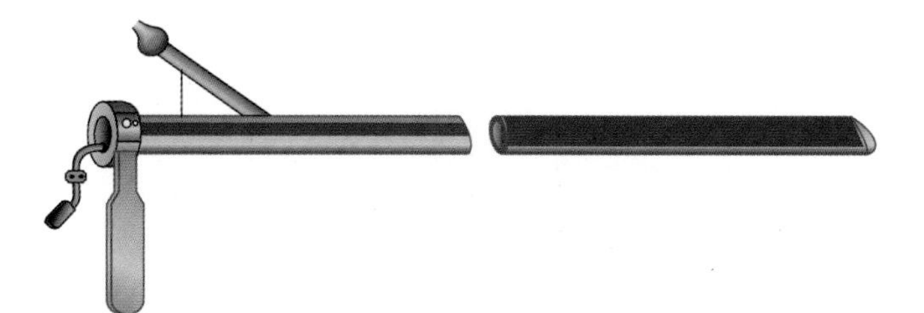

Fig. 80.44: Chevalier-Jackson esophagoscope

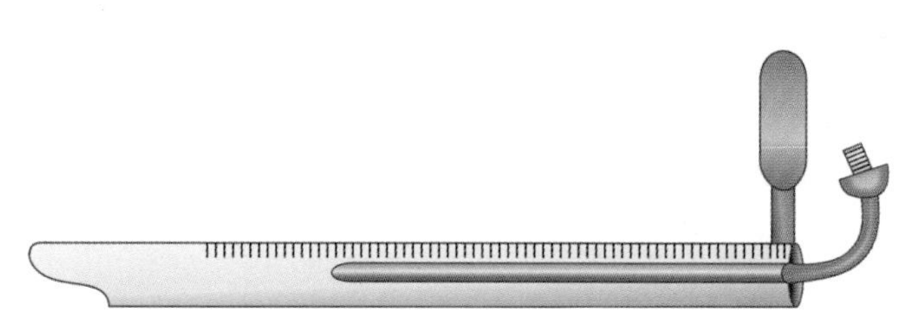

Fig. 80.45: Negus esophagoscope

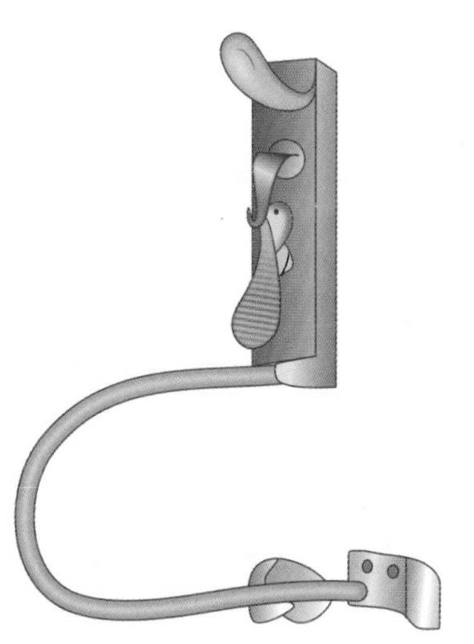

Fig. 80.49: Boyle-Davis mouth gag

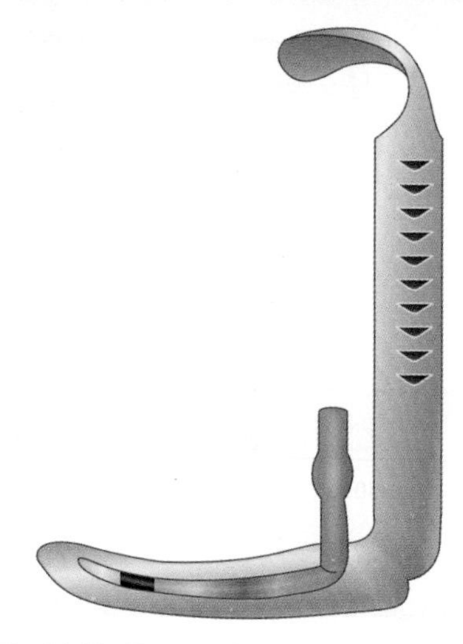

Fig. 80.50: Tongue plate with throat suction

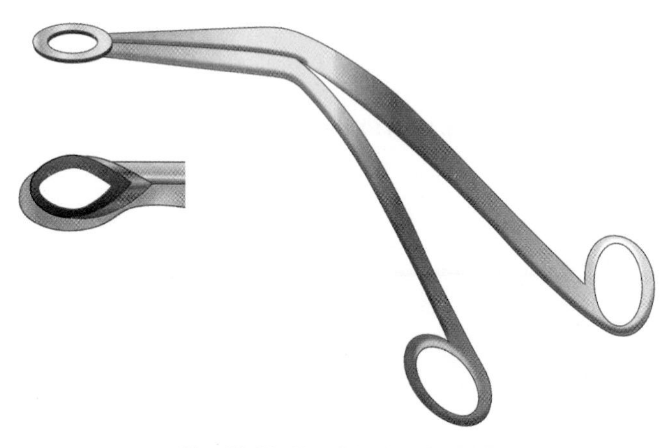

Fig. 80.51: Tonsil holding forceps

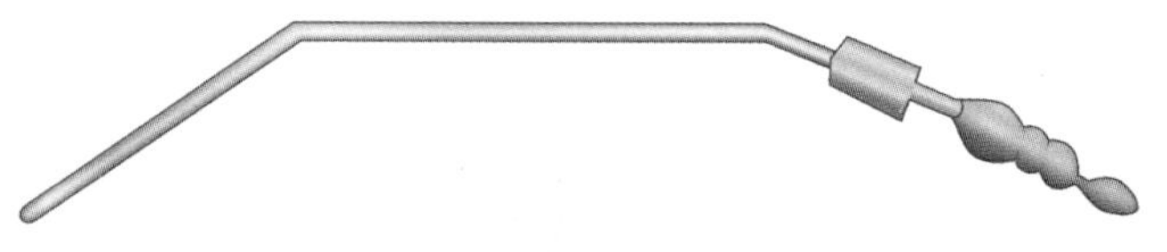

Fig. 80.52: Tonsillar suction

Fig. 80.53: Tonsil pillar retractor and dissector

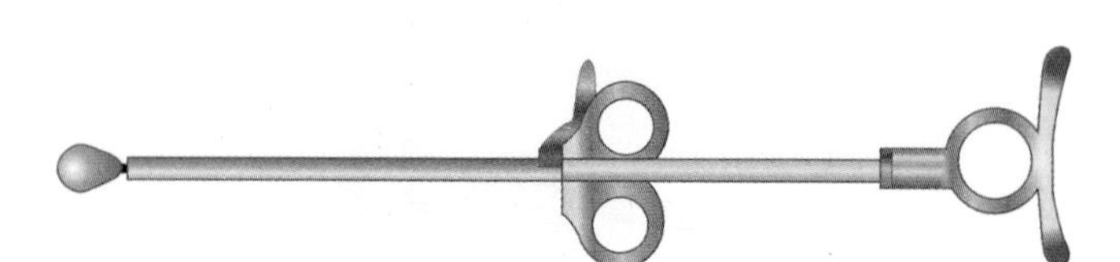

Fig. 80.54: Tonsillar snare

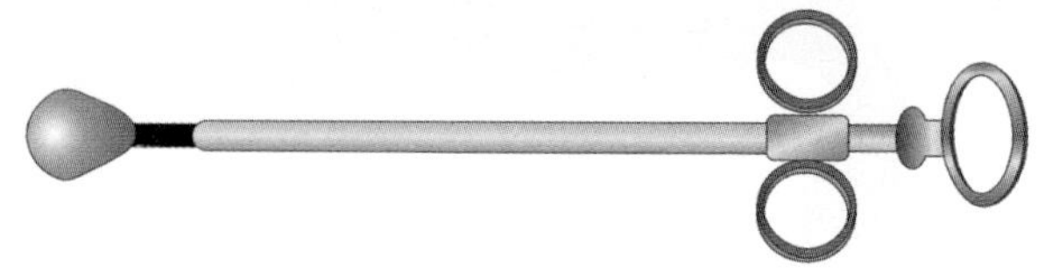

Fig. 80.55: Guillotine

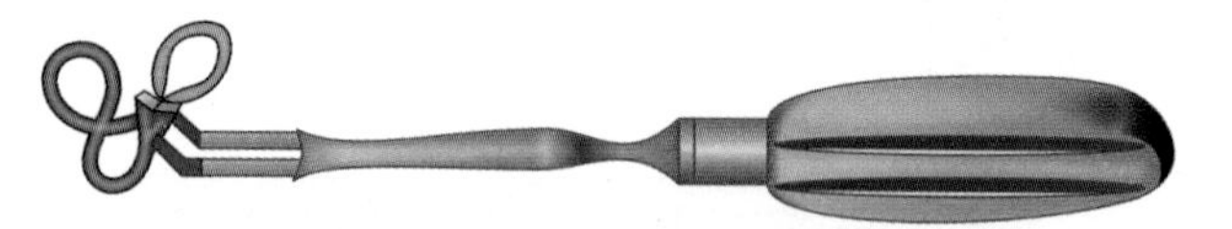

Fig. 80.56: Adenoid curette with cage

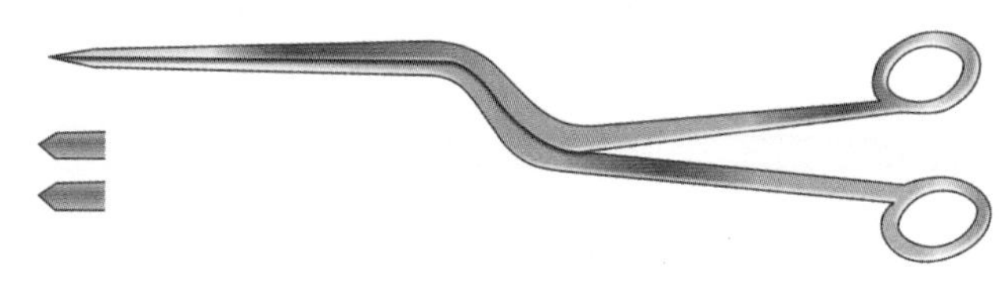

Fig. 80.57: Peritonsillar abscess drainage forceps

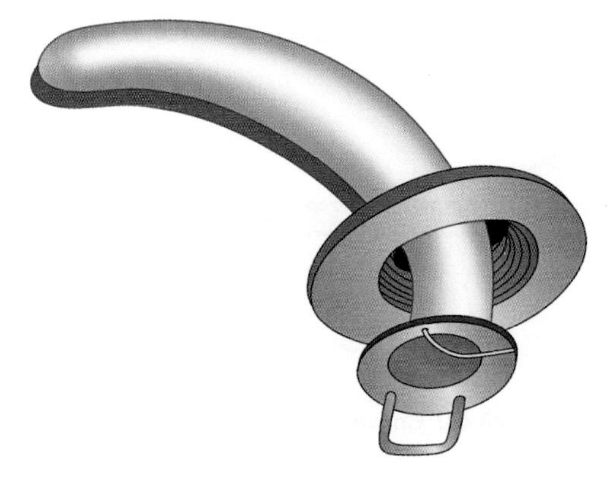

Fig. 80.58: Fuller's tracheostomy tube

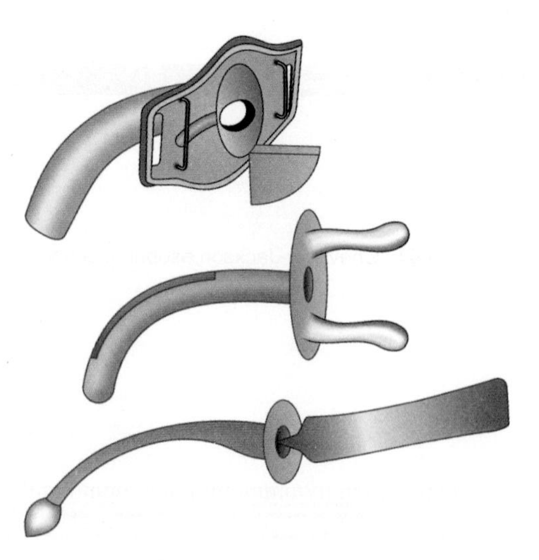

Fig. 80.59: Jackson's tracheostomy tube

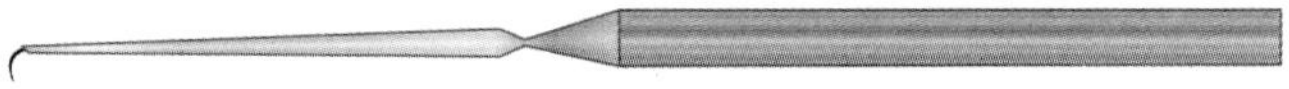

Fig. 80.60: Blunt tracheal hook

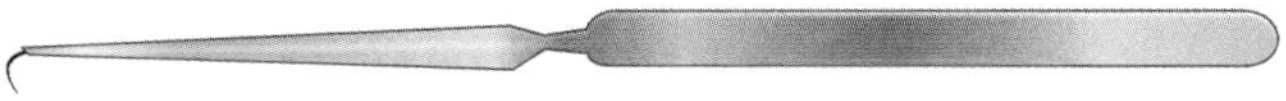

Fig. 80.61: Sharp tracheal hook

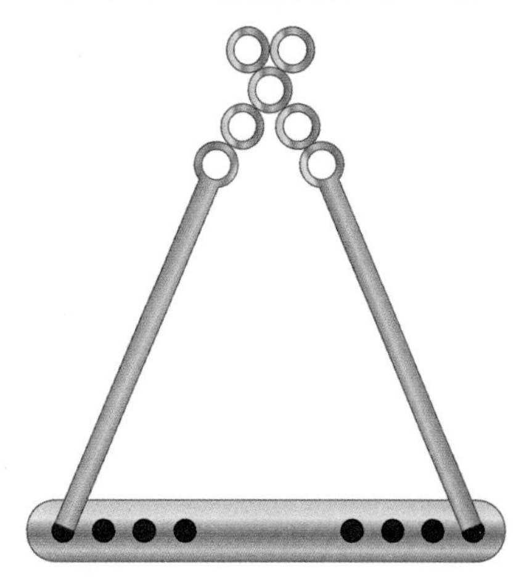

Fig. 80.62: Draffin bipod stand with plate

MCQs on Throat and Larynx

Select one best answer:

1. The arterial blood supply of tonsil includes:
   A. The ascending pharyngeal branch of the external carotid artery
   B. The descending palatine branch of the internal maxillary artery
   C. The ascending palatine branch of the external maxillary artery
   D. All of the above.
2. The thoracic portion of esophagus receives its blood supply from the:
   A. Descending aorta
   B. Bronchial artery
   C. Vertebral arteries
   D. Both A and B.
3. All of the following are true regarding phrenic nerve, except:
   A. Arises from cervical nerves 3, 4, 5
   B. Lies within the carotid sheath
   C. Is located on the anterior surface of the anterior scalene muscle
   D. Supplies the diaphragm.
4. The cervical esophagus receives its blood supply from the:
   A. Superior thyroid artery
   B. Inferior thyroid artery
   C. Facial artery
   D. Lingual artery.
5. In a patient who has undergone submandibular gland resection, asymmetry of the lower lip results from injury to the:
   A. Lingual nerve
   B. Ramus mandibularis nerve
   C. Greater auricular nerve
   D. Hypoglossal nerve.
6. The recurrent laryngeal nerve sends motor branches to all intrinsic laryngeal muscle except the:
   A. Vocalis
   B. Interarytenoid
   C. Cricothyroid
   D. Posterior cricoarytenoid.
7. About 90 percent of tracheoesophageal fistula have:
   A. A blind upper pouch with a lower segment of esophagus from stomach to trachea or left main bronchus
   B. Both upper and lower segment of esophagus enter the trachea
   C. Upper segment of esophagus entering the trachea with blind lowar segment of esophagus
   D. An intact esophagus, aside from the communication.
8. The internal carotid artery:
   A. Is located medial to the external carotid artery in the neck
   B. Has no branches in the neck
   C. Both of the above statements are true
   D. None of the above is true.
9. The most useful preoperative screening test for potential bleeding during adenotonsillectomy is the:
   A. Partial thromboplastin time
   B. Bleeding time
   C. Clotting time
   D. Platelet count.
10. The average amount of saliva produced in 24 hours is:
   A. 50-100 ml
   B. 150-300 ml
   C. 300-500 ml
   D. 1000-1500 ml.
11. Respiratory dead space is about:
   A. 300 ml
   B. 500 ml
   C. 150 ml
   D. 50 ml.
12. Epulis is usually located on the:
   A. Nasal septum
   B. Tonsil
   C. Lip
   D. Gingival or alveolar process.

13. Reinke's space in the larynx is:
    A. Limited above and below by the linea arcuata
    B. Located in the true cord
    C. Associated with vocal polps
    D. Both A and B.
14. The most common type of speech disorder is in the area of:
    A. Phonation-resonation
    B. Aphasia
    C. Stuttering
    D. Articulation
15. The most common cause of oroantral fistula is:
    A. Osteomyelitis of maxilla
    B. Carcinoma of the maxilla
    C. Maxillary sinusitis
    D. Dental extraction.
16. A cardiac condition which may occur secondary to hypertrophied tonsils and adenoids is:
    A. Atrial septal defect
    B. Ventricular septal defect
    C. Bundle branch block
    D. Cor pulmonale.
17. A pulsating swelling on the lateral wall of pharynx suggests:
    A. Pharyngeal hemangioma
    B. Peritonsilar abscess
    C. Aneurysm of the internal carotid artery
    D. Aneurysm of the external carotid artery.
18. The treatment of choice for vincent's angina is:
    A. Mycostatin
    B. Corticosteroids
    C. Penicillin systemically
    D. Streptomycin.
19. A patient with thyroid nodule which revealed Hurthle cell tumor on FNA and the same findings on excision of the nodule, should further undergo:
    A. Completion thyroidectomy
    B. Completion thyroidectomy with radical neck dissection
    C. No further treatment
    D. Contralateral lobectomy.
20. Varicosities on the undersurface of the tongue are often associated with:
    A. Cardiac failure
    B. Cirrhosis of liver
    C. Both
    D. None of these.
21. Aphthous stomatitis is characterized by:
    A. Ulcerations on the oral mucosa
    B. Unknown etiology
    C. Marked pain
    D. All of the above.
22. Contraindications to tonsillectomy includes all of the following, except:
    A. Hemophilia
    B. Attack of tonsillitis in preceding 2 weeks
    C. Poliomyelits epidemic
    D. Sickle cell trait.
23. Gingival hypertrophy may result from:
    A. Dilantin therapy
    B. Monocytic leukemia
    C. Scurvy
    D. All of the above.
24. Ranula:
    A. Usually occurs in children
    B. Originates from the sublingual gland
    C. Is best treated surgically
    D. All of the above.
25. The usual emergency treatment of a person who becomes unable to talk, breathe, or cough while eating a large piece of solid food is:
    A. Slapping the victim on the back
    B. Digital removal
    C. Emergency tracheostomy
    D. Direct laryngoscopic removal.
26. The primary etiologic factor in contact ulcer of the larynx is:
    A. Syphilis
    B. Tuberculosis
    C. Vocal abuse
    D. Smoking.
27. The aphonia of abductor paralysis can be overcome by:
    A. Speech therapy
    B. Teflon injection of the involved vocal cord
    C. Arytenoid mobilization
    D. Arytenoidectomy.
28. Regarding external laryngocele all of the following are true except:
    A. Is congenital
    B. Communicates with the laryngeal ventricle
    C. Herniates through the cricothyroid membrane
    D. Should be removed surgically.
29. Anesthesia of larynx may occur with:
    A. Syphilis
    B. Lead poisoning
    C. Multiple sclerosis
    D. All of the above.
30. Precancerous conditions of the larynx include all except:
    A. Syphilis
    B. Keratosis
    C. Papilloma
    D. Leukoplakia.

31. Dysphagia lusoria:
    A. Results from an abnormal right subclavian artery
    B. Is neurogenic in origin
    C. Is associated with pernicious anemia
    D. Follows ingestion of a caustic
32. Tracheobronchial tuberculosis may be manifested by:
    A. Ulceration
    B. Granulation tissue
    C. Stenosis
    D. Broncholith formation.
33. Attack of stabbing pain in the tonsil area suggests:
    A. Migraine
    B. Glossopharyngeal neuralgia
    C. Temporal arteritis
    D. None of the above.
34. Vernet's syndrome is characterized by:
    A. A lesion at the jugular foramen
    B. Paralysis of the tenth, eleventh and twelfth nerves.
    C. Ipsilateral paralysis of the tenth nerve
    D. Ipsilateral paralysis of the eleventh nerve.
35. The most frequent symptom of the cancer of nasopharynx is:
    A. Blocked nose
    B. Epistaxis
    C. Mass in the neck
    D. Diplopia.
36. The treatment of glossopharyngeal neuralgia is:
    A. Anticonvulsants
    B. Topical anesthetics
    C. NSAID
    D. Ergotamine.
37. Regarding juvenile nasopharyngeal fibroma all are true except:
    A. Begins in prepubescent years
    B. Occurs almost always in males
    C. Is usually treated by surgical excision
    D. Is resistant to radiotherapy.
38. Hypophysectomy may be indicated in all the following conditions, except:
    A. Diabetic retinopathy
    B. Chromophobe adenoma
    C. Nasopharyngeal carcinoma
    D. Metastatic carcinoma of the breast.
39. Tightening of the facial and oral commissure suggests:
    A. Scleroderma
    B. Sarcoidosis
    C. Riboflavin deficiency
    D. Plumbism.
40. Normal flora of the upper respiratory tract includes all of the following, except:
    A. *Streptococcus viridans*
    B. Anaerobic streptococci
    C. *Neisseria caterrhalis*
    D. Pneumococci
41. Oral pemphigus is characterized by:
    A. Painless vasicles or bullae
    B. Profuse salivation
    C. Recurring crops of lesions
    D. All of the above.
42. The differential diagnosis of white oral lesions include:
    A. Leukoplakia
    B. Lichen planus
    C. Syphilis
    D. All of the above.
43. Behcet's syndrome includes:
    A. Recurrent ulcerations of mouth
    B. Ulcerations of genitals
    C. Uveitis
    D. All of the above.
44. Bilateral edematous thickening of vocal cords suggests:
    A. Hypothyroidism
    B. Pachydermia laryngia
    C. Laryngitis sicca
    D. All of the above.
45. The recurrent laryngeal nerve is closely related to the:
    A. Superior thyroid artery
    B. Inferior thyroid artery
    C. Middle thyroid vein
    D. Pyramidal lobe.
46. The external laryngeal nerve is closely related to the:
    A. Superior thyroid artery
    B. Inferior thyroid artery
    C. Middle thyroid vein
    D. Thyrohyoid membrane.
47. Arrhythmia and bradycardia from instrumental stimulation of larynx:
    A. Is mediated via the vagus nerve
    B. Can be controlled by atropine
    C. Both A and B
    D. None of these.
48. The typical case of psychosomatic aphonia presents on laryngeal examination:
    A. Lack of approximation of cords on phonation
    B. Glottic closure on coughing
    C. Both A and B
    D. None of these.
49. Vascular polyps of the vocal cord:
    A. Are usually the results of trauma with sub-epithelial rupture of a small blood vessel
    B. Require no treatment since they absorb with time

C. Both A and B
D. None of these.

50. Congenital angioma of the larynx is:
    A. Usually subglottic in location
    B. Best treated surgically
    C. Both A and B
    D. None of these.
51. Fixation of the vocal cord in carcinoma:
    A. Indicates involvement of the underlying thyroid cartilage
    B. Is a contraindication for hemilaryngectomy
    C. Both A and B
    D. None of these.
52. Following radiation failure for carcinoma of vocal cords, hemilaryngectomy:
    A. Has no place
    B. May be applicable if subglottic extension does not exceed 5 mm
    C. Both A and B
    D. None of these.
53. Regarding carotid body tumor all are true, except:
    A. May be familial
    B. Is a type of chemodectoma
    C. Is supplied by the external carotid artery
    D. Presents as a tender rapidly enlarging mass.
54. Hyperparathyroidism may present as each of the following, except:
    A. Renal calculus
    B. Hypercalcemia
    C. Hypophosphatemia
    D. Hypotension.
55. Treatment of laryngeal diphteria usually includes:
    A. Diphteria antitoxin IM or IV
    B. Airway maintenance often by tracheostomy
    C. Penicillin
    D. All of the above.
56. Mendelson's syndrome refers to:
    A. Aspiration of gastric contents
    B. Transient pneumonitis of allergic origin
    C. Rupture of a tuberculoma into the bronchus
    D. Tracheal compression due to mediastinal growth.
57. The most common site for esophageal perforation during rigid esophagoscopy is:
    A. In areas of esophagitis
    B. At the site of carcinoma
    C. At the site of diverticulum
    D. In the region of cricopharyngeal muscle.
58. Hydrostatic dilatation of esophagus is used in the treatment of:
    A. Plummer-Vinson syndrome
    B. Achalasia
    C. Diffuse spasm
    D. Cricopharyngeal incoordination.
59. Findings suggesting inoperability in bronchogenic carcinoma are:
    A. Pleural effusion with malignant cytology
    B. A lesion located above the level of carina
    C. Vocal cord paralysis
    D. All of the above.
60. Corticosteroids are often necessary after bronchoscopy:
    A. In allergic patients
    B. With bronchograpy
    C. For atelectasis
    D. All of the above.
61. Surgical drainage of Ludwig's angina may require external and/or intraoral drainage because of the:
    A. Buccinator muscle
    B. Digastric muscle
    C. Mylohyoid muscle
    D. Geniohyoid muscle.
62. Regarding parapharyngeal abscess all are true, except:
    A. Is usually accompanied by enlargement or swelling of the tonsil
    B. Is usually accompanied by trismus
    C. Is more likely to occur after tonsillectomy under local anesthesia than under general anesthesia
    D. May result in jugular vein thrombosis.
63. Herpangina:
    A. Is characterized by vesicles on the soft palate and fauces
    B. Is due to Coxsackie virus
    C. Is most often seen below the age 15
    D. All of the above.
64. Mucoepidermoid tumors of salivary glands:
    A. Originate from salivary gland ducts and are not well encapsulated
    B. Tend to recur locally
    C. May metastasize distantly
    D. All of the above.
65. Ludwig's angina is characterized by:
    A. Is most commonly due to intraoral trauma, i.e. dental extraction
    B. Is a severe form of infection of sublingual space
    C. Spreads by continuity
    D. All of the above.
66. Retropharyngeal abscess is characterized by:
    A. Involvement of the prevertebral space
    B. May occur with tuberculosis of cervical vertebrae
    C. Is best seen on CT of neck
    D. All of the above.
67. Carcinoma of the tongue:
    A. Occurs most commonly on the lateral border of the middle third of tongue

B. Metastasizes readily to cervical lymph nodes
C. Is usually radiosensitive
D. All of the above.

68. With regard to epidermoid carcinoma of the tongue, key factors in predicting probable five-year survival rates are:
A. Size of lesion
B. Site of lesion—anterior or posterior
C. Cervical node involvement
D. All of the above.

69. A tracheostomy located between the cricoid cartilage and first tracheal ring is:
A. Called a cricothyrotomy
B. A good procedure in most situations
C. Useful in short necked individuals
D. Often complicated by subglottic stenosis.

70. Pale, smooth, watery edema of supraglottic laryngeal tissue which develops rapidly suggests:
A. Reinke's edema
B. Acute laryngotracheobronchitis
C. Epiglottitis
D. Allergy.

71. The key to surgical removal of a branchial cyst is:
A. Aspiration of cyst prior to surgery
B. Transection of sternocleidomastoid muscle
C. Dissection of the duct to its pharyngeal origin
D. Removal of the medial portion of hyoid bone.

72. Anterior web of larynx is best handled by:
A. Repeated bouginage
B. Excision of scar with skin graft
C. Insertion of silicon keel
D. Steroid.

73. The highest percentage of metastases occur with laryngeal cancer which is:
A. Hypopharyngeal
B. Subglottic
C. Glottic
D. Supraglottic.

74. The usual treatment of congenital laryngeal stridor is:
A. Steroids
B. Tracheostomy
C. Amputation of the epiglottis
D. Reassurance of child's parents.

75. The most common type of thyroid carcinoma is:
A. Papillary
B. Follicular
C. Medullary
D. Hurthie cell.

76. A frequent problem of tracheostomy seen especially in infants is:
A. Granuloma formation
B. Vocal cord paralysis
C. Difficult decannulation
D. Tracheocutaneous fistula.

77. A 21-year-old male presents with unilateral sore throat and earache. Examination shows trismus and displacement of the ipsilateral tonsil medially and inferiorly. The most likely diagnosis is:
A. Acute tonsillitis
B. Peritonsillar abscess
C. Parapharyngeal mass
D. Infectious mononucleosis.

78. A 5-year-old girl presents with a 3-day history of worsening sore throat and earache. She has fever and her tonsils are red, enlarged and have pus on them. The diagnosis is:
A. Acute tonsillitis
B. Glandular fever
C. Peritonsillar abscess
D. Mumps.

79. A 16-year-old-boy complains of severe lethargy and sore throat. His tonsils are large with a white membrane over them. There is also significant cervical lymphadenopathy. The likely diagnosis is:
A. HIV infection
B. Acute leukemia
C. Glandular fever
D. Viral tonsillitis.

ANSWERS

1. D	11. C	21. D	31. A	41. D	51. B	61. C	71. C
2. D	12. D	22. D	32. C	42. D	52. D	62. A	72. C
3. B	13. D	23. D	33. B	43. D	53. D	63. D	73. A
4. B	14. D	24. D	34. B	44. A	54. D	64. D	74. D
5. B	15. D	25. B	35. C	45. B	55. D	65. D	75. B
6. C	16. D	26. C	36. A	46. A	56. A	66. D	76. C
7. A	17. C	27. B	37. D	47. C	57. D	67. D	77. B
8. B	18. C	28. C	38. C	48. C	58. B	68. D	78. A
9. A	19. C	29. D	39. A	49. A	59. D	69. D	79. C
10. D	20. D	30. A	40. D	50. C	60. D	70. D	

Index

Page numbers followed by *f* for figure

B

C

D

T